A TEXTBOOK OF PREVENTIVE DENTISTRY

Robert C. Caldwell, D.M.D., Ph.D.

Late Dean, University of California, Los Angeles, School of Dentistry, Los Angeles, California

Richard E. Stallard, D.D.S., Ph.D.

Dental Director, Group Health Medical Center, Bloomington, Minnesota;
Formerly, Assistant Dean and Director, Clinical Research Center, Boston University, School of Graduate Dentistry, Boston, Massachusetts

W. B. SAUNDERS

Philadelphia • London • Toronto

W. B. Saunders Company: West Washington Square
Philadelphia, PA 19105

1 St. Anne's Road
Eastbourne, East Sussex BN21 3UN, England

1 Goldthorne Avenue
Toronto, Ontario M8Z 5T9, Canada

Library of Congress Cataloging in Publication Data

Main entry under title:

A textbook of preventive dentistry.

Includes index.

1. Preventive dentistry. I. Caldwell, Robert Craig, II. Stallard, Richard E. [DNLM: 1. Oral health. 2. Preventive dentistry. WU113 T355]

RK60.7.T49 617.6'01 73–76184

ISBN 0–7216–2239–9

A Textbook of Preventive Dentistry ISBN 0-7216-2239-9

Print No.: 9 8 7 6 5 4 3 2

In Memory

ROBERT C. CALDWELL

Every man has special qualities that in combination form his character. Bob Caldwell possessed six distinctive characteristics that served as guidelines for his life and work: intelligence, imagination and leadership were tempered with courage, love and humor. Throughout his life, these qualities inspired the respect and admiration of his associates.

Bob loved his family, his people and the sea. He genuinely enjoyed being with friends, or even with strangers. He never ate alone in his laboratory or office, preferring to share the noon hour with someone. On these occasions, it was always surprising to see the number of people from every facet of life whom he knew personally. Chance meetings with these acquaintances prompted responsive smiles and an interesting exchange of enquiries concerning the activities of each. Bob's capacity for love made him warm and friendly with people, and understanding as an administrator.

His intellect was quick, clear and full of insight. These qualities made him recognize the importance of advanced education in his profession. He was highly successful in his graduate studies, and his sensitiveness to the suffering of people led him to maintain a balance in his research between satisfying his scientific curiosity and seeking practical applications of his findings for the benefit of mankind.

Two qualities that contributed much to his successful career and his productivity in the dental field were imagination and leadership; these enabled him to plan and launch the Institute of Dental Research in Birmingham and, subsequently, to set on course the troubled School of Dentistry at U.C.L.A. His vision led him to recognize the value of the concept of an institute where people from different disciplines would work both independently and conjointly to achieve advances in dental health. Bob's strong leadership, colored by his enthusiasm and perception, attracted many men to work together in this dream, which continues today as a reality and a challenge to those who carry on the work he began.

Bob was courageous. He displayed this quality throughout life, especially during his last years. His dignity and his sensitivity for others allowed him to share the truth of his illness only with his wife Marge. The quiet strength of this man, who so courageously faced life and death, is our inspiration.

Bob had two special gifts that enhanced his other qualities: his smile and his wit. These things we remember about Bob: the warmth of his handshake when he greeted you, the warm smile and the ready wit, which could disarm you in a discussion or give you a lift at the end of a weary day. We respect the scholar, the leader, the founder, but we deeply love the smiling, compassionate man whom we were privileged to call our friend.

J. Navia
R. Stallard

CONTRIBUTORS

THOMAS KING BARBER, D.D.S., M.S.

Professor and Chairman, Division of Preventive Dental Sciences, School of Dentistry; Professor of Pediatrics, School of Medicine, Center for Health Sciences, University of California, Los Angeles. Consultant, Veterans Administration Hospital, Brentwood, California.

Prevention of Malocclusion and Minor Orthodontics.

THEODORE E. BOLDEN, D.D.S., Ph.D.

Professor of Dentistry and Chairman, Department of Oral Pathology, School of Dentistry, Meharry Medical College. Attending, George W. Hubbard Hospital, Nashville, Tennessee.

Epidemiology of Oral Cancer. Factors Related to Oral Cancer. The Prevention and Detection of Oral Cancer.

ROBERT C. CALDWELL, D.M.D., Ph.D.

Late Dean, School of Dentistry, University of California at Los Angeles.

Preventive Dentistry and Total Patient Care. Water Fluoridation and Systemic Fluoride Therapy (with Daniel C. Nornoo).

SIDNEY B. FINN, D.M.D., M.S.

Professor Emeritus of Dentistry, University of Alabama School of Dentistry, Birmingham, Alabama.

The Epidemiology of Dental Caries.

WALLACE VERNON MANN, D.M.D., M.S.

Dean, School of Dentistry, University of Mississippi Medical Center; Attending Dentist, University Hospital. Consultant, Veterans Administration Hospital, Jackson, Mississippi.

Oral Hygiene Technics and Home Care.

JUAN M. NAVIA, M.S., Ph.D.

Senior Scientist, Institute of Dental Research; Professor of Dentistry and Comparative Medicine; Director of Research Training, University of Alabama School of Dentistry, Birmingham, Alabama.

Nutrition and Oral Disease.

Ernest Newbrun, D.M.D., Ph.D.

Professor of Oral Biology, and Chairman, Section of Biological Sciences, School of Dentistry, University of California at San Francisco.

Etiology of Dental Caries.

Daniel Codjoh Nornoo, B.D.S., M.Sc.D.

Ministry of Health, Accra, Ghana.

Water Fluoridation and Systemic Fluoride Therapy (with Robert C. Caldwell). *Topical Fluoride Therapy* (with Richard E. Stallard).

Cornelius H. Pameijer, D.M.D., M.Sc.D., D.Sc.

Professor of Prosthodontics, Boston University School of Graduate Dentistry, Boston, Massachusetts.

The Composite Resin: A Preventive Operative Procedure.

Leonard Shapiro, D.M.D., M.S.

Associate Research Professor of Oral Biology, Boston University School of Graduate Dentistry. Associate Staff, Goddard Memorial Hospital, Stoughton, Massachusetts. Active Staff, Jordan Hospital, Plymouth, Massachusetts; Notre Dame Hospital, Central Falls, Rhode Island.

Etiology of Periodontal Disease (with Richard E. Stallard). *Periodontal Disease: Prevention and Control.*

Richard J. Simonsen, D.D.S.

Coordinator of Preventive Dentistry, Group Health Medical Center, Bloomington, Minnesota.

Acid Etch as a Preventive Technique in Dentistry.

Richard Elgin Stallard, D.D.S., M.S., Ph.D.

Dental Director, Group Health Plan, Incorporated; Adjunct Professor, School of Public Health, University of Minnesota, Fairview Hospital, Minneapolis, Minnesota.

Epidemiology of Periodontal Disease. Etiology of Periodontal Disease (with Leonard Shapiro). *Prevention and Control of Dental Caries. Patient and Dentist Education and Motivation* (with Hussein A. Zaki).

Anthony R. Volpe, D.D.S., M.S.

Associate Director, Clinical Investigations, Colgate-Palmolive Research Center. Clinical Associate Professor, Department of Pharmacology, Fairleigh-Dickinson University School of Dentistry, New Jersey.

Dentifrices and Mouth Rinses.

Arthur H. Wuehrmann, D.M.D., A.B.

Professor of Dentistry (Retired), University of Alabama School of Dentistry, Birmingham, Alabama.

Preventive Dental Radiology.

Hussein A. Zaki, M.S.D., M.P.H., B.Ch.D.

Associate Professor of Periodontics, University of Minnesota School of Dentistry. Consultant in Periodontics, Military Hospital, Abu Dhabi, United Arab Emirates.

Patient and Dentist Education and Motivation (with Richard E. Stallard).

PREFACE

This text on preventive dentistry is intended to provide a base on which current concepts can be utilized by those members of the dental profession dedicated to the preservation of the natural dentition. Each subject unit is treated in detail and is in turn linked to the other units to provide a total picture of prevention as it can be practiced today. Both clinical and research data are included upon which sound judgment can be made. Additional reading lists accompany each chapter for those who desire to expand their knowledge in a given area.

I am indebted to all of the contributors to this text for their patience and understanding during the protracted period of preparation resulting, ultimately, in publication. Chapters have been updated and additional references added to include the most current materials available in all areas. I am also indebted to the staff at Saunders for their cooperation and utmost care in preparing the material. Special appreciation is extended to Mrs. Pamela Phillips for her secretarial assistance.

My thanks and appreciation are extended to Mrs. Marge Caldwell for her encouragement, initially to her late husband and finally to me, during all phases of preparation of this book. I am especially grateful to my wife, Jaxon, for her continuing support.

RICHARD E. STALLARD
Minneapolis, Minnesota

CONTENTS

chapter 1

PREVENTIVE DENTISTRY AND TOTAL PATIENT CARE

by
ROBERT C. CALDWELL, D.D.S., PH.D.

Preventive dentistry can be defined as the employment of all measures necessary to attain and maintain optimal oral health. In a general sense, there is primary prevention and secondary prevention. Primary implies the prevention of the initiation of disease and is the highest goal of preventive dentistry. Secondary prevention includes the prevention of additional disease or the recurrence of disease. An example of this is the time-honored concept of "extension for prevention" in operative dentistry.

Preventive dentistry encompasses a broad range of dental science and the scope of the subject includes:

1. factors predisposing to disease, e.g., dental plaque and other deposits;
2. factors encouraging the advance of disease, e.g., host resistance and trauma from occlusion;
3. complications of disease and deformity, e.g., loosening, drifting and malpositioning of the teeth;
4. factors interfering with rehabilitation, e.g., defective restorative dentistry; and
5. factors causing the recurrence of disease, e.g., poor oral hygiene and lack of patient motivation.

The approach to preventive dentistry recommended in this book requires an understanding of certain principles and how they relate to the overall sequence of events in total patient care. Therefore, before describing how preventive dentistry relates to a total patient care program, total patient care should be defined. "Total" clearly implies two things: (a) it is concerned with the whole patient, and (b) the care which is total is the sum of several factors. A definition of "care" includes attending to the patient, which is quite adequately done in most dental practices and clinics. However, a broader meaning suggests watching over the patient, thereby implying a responsibility for the maintenance of oral health. Thus, total patient care consists of the establishment and maintenance of health in addition to treatment of disease and deformity. This comprehensive approach to dental practice includes an effective preventive dentistry program.

PRINCIPLES OF PREVENTIVE DENTISTRY

The principles of preventive dentistry are:

1. Control of disease,
2. Patient education and motivation,
3. Development of host resistance,
4. Restoration of function, and
5. Maintenance of oral health.

Each of these principal areas will now be discussed and synthesized into a logical sequence of events for total patient care. This sequence should be adhered to whenever possible, but flexibility is desirable and professional judgment may alter the recommended order of events.

CONTROL OF DISEASE

It is an established fact that bacteria are one of the causative agents of dental caries and periodontal disease. Thus, the dental practitioner should recognize the importance of reducing the number of bacteria and/or the virulence of the oral microflora. It makes little sense to sew up a festering wound without attending to the cause of the infection. Similarly, it is poor dentistry to place permanent restorations in a mouth in which the infection will continue to be rampant. Some dental authorities recommend that a permanent restoration should not be placed in a mouth with active caries until every carious tooth has been excavated, indirect pulp capping carried out where indicated, and temporary restorations inserted.

Control of infection is equally important in the management of periodontal disease (Fig. 1–1). Periodontists do not undertake extensive treatments where oral hygiene is unsatisfactory. The patient is first brought to the state where the infectious causative factors are controlled and the chance of recurrence of disease has been reduced. The first step in the management of most periodontal disease and caries is to control the infection.

The recommended procedures in this first stage of total patient care are as follows:

1. Emergency treatments for the relief of pain are first on the program. Also, acute problems must receive immediate attention; for example, a chipped tooth which is causing soft tissue ulceration should be smoothed with a disc or covered with a temporary restoration. Similarly, a tooth requiring drainage and therapy to obviate an abscess must receive prompt attention.

2. For children and adults with active carious lesions, the removal of all caries, indirect pulp capping where necessary, and the placement of temporary restorations are next in the care program. The rationale is that the carious infection must be reduced in its intensity as soon as possible. The patient is not well served by the dentist proceeding from one restoration to the next without having attempted to control the caries process in the whole dentition. Thus, all large carious lesions should be excavated and temporary restorations inserted. Permanent restorations will come later.

3. The removal of plaque and calculus by prophylaxis and topical fluoride treatment aids in the control of the infectious carious and periodontal process. In older patients with low or no caries activity, periodontal therapy will usually follow the emergency treatment phase. A plaque control program must be initiated along with the patient education and motivation program.

4. The removal of teeth indicated for extraction is now appropriate. Delaying this step has allowed the dentist to improve the oral health of the patient and has created a more favorable environment for post-extraction healing. Also, the patient has had time to gain confidence in the dentist before facing the worry of having a tooth extracted.

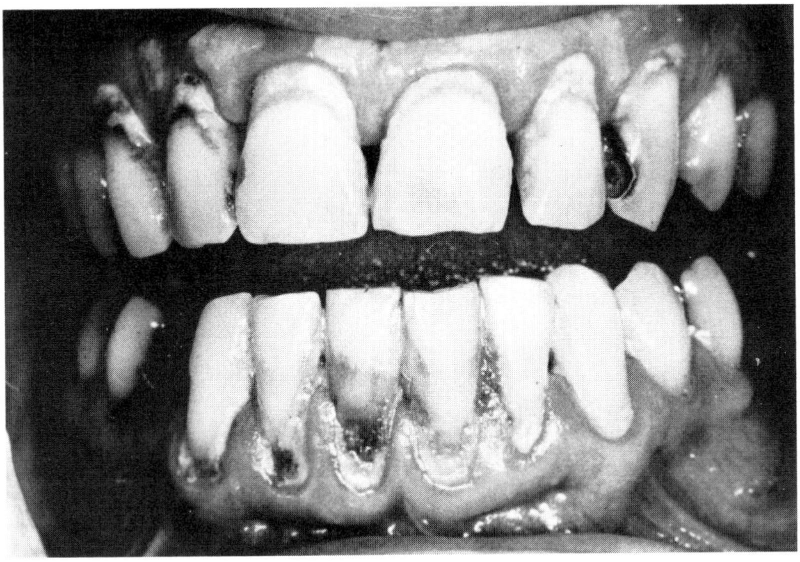

Figure 1–1 Clinical photograph of a 35-year-old patient demonstrating advanced periodontal disease and dental caries. Plaque is acting as a common etiologic factor in both disease processes in this patient.

PATIENT EDUCATION AND MOTIVATION

The intimate relationship of plaque bacterial deposits on the enamel surface and the gingival tissue is a continuing challenge to the integrity of these tissues. The dentist cannot expect to handle this problem successfully alone, and the patient or parent plays a highly significant role in the care of the oral tissues.

Some dentists may not be consciously aware of the deep desire of many patients to achieve optimal dental health. Certainly there are people who place a low priority on dental health, but an encouragingly large percentage of these will change their attitude if dental facts are presented to them in an interesting and positive fashion. Also, dental care is becoming more fashionable and desirable; for example, the sale of electrically powered toothbrushes and water-jet dental appliances has been remarkably increased in the last few years.

The experienced dentist knows that there is no long-range benefit to patient or dentist in technically good restorations in a neglected mouth. To protect the patient's investment and the dentist's reputation, the patient must understand the factors which cause dental problems. It is also important that the patient be motivated to work with the dentist by maintaining a high level of home care and avoiding dietary and mechanical abuses to the dentition.

In the first phase, control of disease, the dentist has laid the biological groundwork for the long-term treatment plan. The temptation at this stage is to press ahead with permanent restorations. This should not be done until a program of patient education and motivation is firmly established.

Evaluation and Education. The condition of the patient's oral health is now evaluated and pertinent information is passed on to the patient. What was the extent of infection? Was the patient in a "caries-rampant" condition? If so, why? Was the extent of gingivitis unusual? Are there periodontal problems which can be attributed to neglect or abusive oral habits? To ask these types of questions, the dentist has to have a mental image of what is normal for the patient at his stage of development and age. A numerical scale relating the average amount of caries and periodontal disease to patient age can be helpful in categorizing the severity of dental disease.

Home Care Instruction. Home care instruction is now begun. The details of oral hygiene techniques and home care are included in Chapter 13. The dentist or his assistant should show the patient that dental plaque is composed mainly of bacteria. This can be done by phase contrast microscopy or by using a patient education film. The patient should be told that brushing does not necessarily mean effective cleaning. In fact, one can over-brush and under-clean. This can be demonstrated by the use of red discoloring wafers which reveal the plaque left *in situ* after the patient has brushed (Fig. 1–2). The proper cleaning technique is then taught, the proper technique being the one which gently removes all the plaque from all surfaces. Flossing usually must supplement brushing for a thorough job.

DEVELOPMENT OF HOST RESISTANCE

Oral health seems to depend on a delicate balance between factors which cause increased susceptibility and those causing increased resistance to disease. The successful treatment and subsequent maintenance of the periodontal structures may depend on increased host resistance. Similarly, dental caries can be controlled to some extent by increasing host resistance even though cariogenic factors may remain active. In both periodontal disease and caries the control of infection is usually of primary importance, but considerable benefits are obtained by the development of host resistance.

Nutrition and Host Resistance. An analysis of the patient's diet should now be made. For the young child and the geriatric patient proper nutrition is especially important. In addition to an adequate caloric intake, the diet should be balanced with respect to protein, fat and carbohydrate. Sufficient variety is important to provide adequate vitamins and trace minerals. Fluoride in water or tablets is also important during the early years.

The importance of avoiding sticky, fermentable sweet foods and between-meal snacks should be emphasized. The Vipeholm study showed that there could be a sevenfold increase in dental caries in subjects eating candies frequently between meals. The diet history should be reviewed with the patient or parent. Patient education films can be used to good advantage in laying the groundwork for necessary changes in the dietary habits.

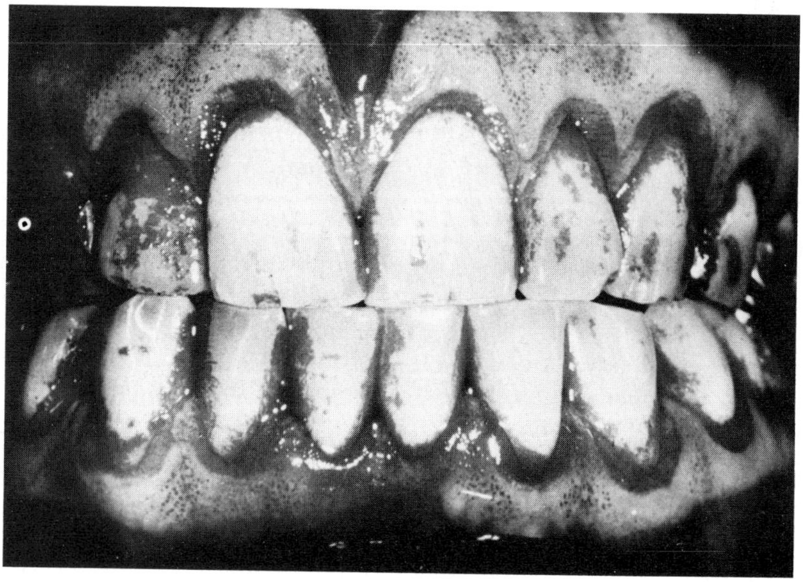

Figure 1–2 The plaque remaining in this patient's mouth has been stained with disclosing tablets. Note that even in a state of reasonably good oral hygiene plaque is present in the non–self-cleansing areas of the teeth.

Fluorides. During the period of tooth formation, the diet is of importance to the future caries resistance of the teeth. The best known and recognized public health method of increasing caries resistance is water fluoridation. However, where the water does not contain fluoride, the dentist or pediatrician should prescribe fluoride tablets for daily use by his child patients. Also, the dentist can increase host resistance by the use of topical fluoride therapy. Fluoride-containing prophylaxis pastes, used regularly in combination with topically applied fluoride solutions such as acid fluoride phosphate, have been reported to reduce caries substantially.

Certain dentifrices and mouthwashes also have active therapeutic properties in addition to the traditionally recognized properties of making oral hygiene more effective and pleasant. Over-the-counter sales of fluoride dentifrices have greatly increased in recent years and it is reasonable to expect more effective products to be available. However, as yet, this approach to increasing the resistance to dental caries is only marginally effective.

RESTORATION OF FUNCTION

To designate restoration of function as a principle of preventive dentistry is fully justified. Until there is complete freedom from dental caries and periodontal disease, the treatment aspect of dentistry will necessarily occupy most of the dentist's time. Even if these diseases are prevented, the development and guidance of an optimally functional definition will continue to be essential to proper oral health.

C. V. Black established "extension for prevention" as a cardinal aspect of cavity preparation. Today's teachers and practitioners of operative dentistry still adhere to Black's general principles and also recognize that occlusal disharmony, missing teeth and improperly contoured restorations all predispose to the recurrence of disease. The placement of permanent restorations and prostheses now is undertaken. On the completion of this phase, the child who requires orthodontic treatment is now ready for the construction of the necessary appliances.

MAINTENANCE OF ORAL HEALTH

The preservation of a disease-free dentition is a noble challenge but, unfortunately, very few individuals can hope to remain in this pristine state of health. At present, most of the population in countries with a high standard of living and a rich diet can expect to experience some degree of dental disease.

The successful management and control of chronic dental infection is not possible without a maintenance program. To many this implies a recall system whereby patients who have been treated are checked periodically for the recurrence of dental problems. This is only a partial solution to the maintenance problem. It has already been emphasized that the control of dental disease is largely in the hands of patient or parent. Thus, at the recall visit, the patient must not only be checked for new evidence of disease but must also be stimulated to continue an effective home-care program. A demonstration of the patient's oral hygiene technique should periodically be requested and checked by means of a disclosing wafer or solution. A prophylaxis is performed for all patients, and children are given a topical fluoride treatment.

The use of so-called caries susceptibility tests can also be a useful tool during a periodic check-up. Although the actual caries susceptibility may not be revealed by any particular test, several such as the Snyder and lactobacillus tests yield some information on the dietary intake of fermentable carbohydrate.

In summary, the sequence of events as dictated by the principles of preventive dentistry are:

1. Control of disease,
2. Patient education and motivation,
3. Development of host resistance,
4. Restoration of function, and
5. Maintenance of oral health.

ADDITIONAL REFERENCE MATERIAL

1. Arnim, S. S.: An effective program of oral hygiene for the arrestment of dental caries and the control of periodontal disease. J. South. Calif. Dent. Hyg. Assoc. *35*:264–280, 1967.
2. Bailey, B. H., and Bennett, G. G.: Psychology of learning applied to dental education. J. Dent. Educ. *30*:297–310, 1966.
3. Barkley, R. F.: Successful Preventive Dental Practices. Macomb, Illinois, Preventive Dentistry Press, 1972.
4. Brandtzaeg, P.: The significance of oral hygiene in the prevention of dental diseases. Odont. Tidskrift *72*:460–486, 1964.
5. Jenkins, G. N.: Current concepts concerning the development of dental caries. Int. Dent. J. *22*:350–362, 1972.
6. Karlsen, Kjell: Traumatic occlusion as a factor in the propagation of periodontal disease. Int. Dent. J. *22*:387–393, 1972.
7. Linn, E. L.: Oral hygiene and periodontal disease: implications for dental health programs. J. Am. Dent. Assoc. *71*:39–42, 1965.
8. Morch, T., and Waerhaug, J.: Quantitative evaluation of the effect of toothbrushing and toothpicking. J. Periodontol. *27*:183–190, 1958.
9. Paffenbarger, George C.: The role of dental materials in the prevention of dental diseases. Int. Dent. J. *22*:343–349, 1972.
10. Shepard, J. E.: Preventive Dentistry for the Patient. Springfield, Illinois, Charles C Thomas, Publisher, 1971.
11. Young, W. O., and Zwermer, J. D.: Objectives and methods of teaching preventive dentistry and community health. J. Dent. Educ. *31*:162–167, 1967.
12. Zaki, H. A., and Stallard, R. E.: An evaluation of the effectiveness of preventive periodontal education. J. Periodont. Res. (Suppl. 3), 1969.

chapter 2

PATIENT AND DENTIST EDUCATION AND MOTIVATION

by

HUSSEIN A. ZAKI, B.Ch.D., M.P.H., M.S.D.

and

RICHARD E. STALLARD, D.D.S., Ph.D.

The technical and mechanical treatment of teeth by restorative dentistry and oral surgery without the active sharing of the responsibility for protecting the dental health of the community should not be the philosophy of dental education, and it is a particular interest of this text to explore the preventive aspects of all phases of dentistry. One has simply to examine the statistics relevant to the incidence and prevalence of dental disease to visualize the magnitude of the problem that faces the dental profession today. Dental manpower has decreased in relation to the growth of the population, and therefore the dental profession has no other solution for such a problem than to direct major effort and attention toward prevention. Prevention, not therapy, is today's problem and hopefully tomorrow's answer.

Oral hygiene procedures and techniques are in reality the substantiating force in preventive dentistry. Their objective is to attain and maintain the health of the oral tissues. These procedures are the most effective way known for the prevention of oral disease (Lobene 1966, Brandtzaeg 1964, and Morch 1958). In a recent survey (Linn 1965) it was shown that only 5 per cent of the 2000 adult participants believed that brushing protects the gingiva. It is believed that a great deal of periodontal disease can be attributed to this lack of instruction and education in the area of oral hygiene. In previous studies (Lovdal 1961, Stanmeyer 1957, and Arnim 1967), it was obvious that most dental diseases can be controlled and "prevented" through proper preparation of today's dentists and through an effective dental health education program for the public. Education, therefore, should be of prime importance for the dental profession onto which a sound preventive program can be built.

Organized dental education has changed tremendously since the first dental school was organized in the United States in 1840. Unfortunately, the changes have been fostered by an overwhelming desire to produce technically competent individuals who are capable of handling the ravages of dental diseases, with particular emphasis on dental caries. The end result has been the graduation of dentists who enter practice with the concept that the bulk of their work is reparative, and who will probably continue with this concept for years to come.

In dental education throughout the world, training is concentrated on skills and knowledge with little emphasis directed toward attitudes and concepts. Prevention first and foremost requires the right attitude and philosophy of practice. Conviction, ideals and enthusiasm are essential to the support of an effective preventive program. It is the obligation of dental educators to see that dental students are constantly stimulated and motivated to develop a strict preventive philosophy which hopefully will grow with them as they practice. The dental students of today, as they assume their positions as practicing dentists, must be responsible for increasing dental public health awareness and for promoting a sound preventive program.

Several research studies have indicated that one of the central problems in preventive dentistry is in motivating the public to take the necessary action for continuous care of their own mouths. An important point often forgotten, however, and not seriously investigated is the motivation of the dentist. To motivate and communicate with others regarding preventive dentistry, it is essential that the dental student, the future dentist, be able to understand his own behavior and be motivated himself.

Since the problem we are facing in preventing oral diseases is one of education, and more specifically one of motivation, it is important to analyze the effectiveness of our present teaching methods as they relate to the dental student. Although the technical aspects of oral hygiene may be recognized, the important question remaining is How well do our instructions affect the student's attitude and behavior toward his own oral health?

In an attempt to evaluate the present status of the effectiveness of preventive periodontal education, a study was carried out at the University of Minnesota (Zaki and Stallard 1969). The study population consisted of approximately 400 dental students distributed equally among freshmen, sophomores, juniors and seniors. The students were evaluated in three areas. First, a clinical examination was conducted to evaluate the degree of oral cleanliness utilizing Greene-Vermillion's Oral Hygiene Index Simplified. Second, after the initial clinical examination each student was given a 20 item questionnaire, which was developed to record existing "attitudes" and behavior patterns regarding different aspects of oral hygiene. This questionnaire provided a general assessment and an overall picture of the commonly used practices in dental care.

A scoring method was devised to give a numerical value to the responses obtained. Only those questions that reflected the student's oral hygiene procedures were considered. A score of 100 was the highest obtainable. Third, in order to assess the student's knowledge regarding preventive periodontal care, a final examination was given. Again, 100 points was the maximum.

The means and standard deviations of scores for the Debris Index Simplified, Calculus Index Simplified, Oral Hygiene Index Simplified test and questionnaire are shown in Table 2–1. They are arranged according to class.

The DI-S, CI-S and OHI-S scores remained stable for all classes. However, the scores were slightly lower for the sophomore class and slightly higher for the seniors. The lowest mean test score was 67.3, calculated for the freshman class, while the highest was 86.4, assigned to the sophomores. The mean test score for the junior class decreased slightly to 83.8 and was followed by a considerable drop to 74.5 for the seniors.

The mean questionnaire score for the whole student body was 73. The scores fluctuated slightly but were essentially the same for the four classes. The senior class, however, had the highest mean score, 74.6.

In order to obtain a better understanding of the relationship of these means,

TABLE 2–1 MEANS AND STANDARD DEVIATIONS OF DI-S, CI-S, OHI-S, TEST AND QUESTIONNAIRE SCORES, ACCORDING TO THE DIFFERENT CLASSES OF DENTAL STUDENTS AND FOR THE GROUP AS A WHOLE

		TYPE OF SCORES									
		DI-S		CI-S		OHI-S		TEST		QUESTIONNAIRE	
DENTAL CLASSES	NUMBERS	*Mean*	*S.D.*	*Mean*	*S.D.*	*Mean*	*S.D.*	*Mean*	*S.D.*	*Mean*	*S.D.*
Freshmen	104	.77	.44	.32	.25	1.09	.60	67.3	10.1	73.0	9.2
Sophomores	106	.69	.31	.29	.27	.98	.46	86.4	7.2	72.6	7.4
Juniors	93	.77	.34	.32	.24	1.09	.49	83.8	7.9	72.0	8.2
Seniors	88	.80	.45	.38	.26	1.18	.61	74.5	10.6	74.6	11.3
Total	391	.75	.38	.33	.26	1.08	.54	78.0	11.9	73.0	9.1

analysis of variance technique was applied. Differences between DI-S, CI-S, OHI-S and questionnaire scores were not statistically significant. The differences between the class means of the test scores, however, were highly significant (P = 0.01).

Additional insight into the oral hygiene levels of the different classes was gained by classifying the students into five groups according to their degree of oral cleanliness: excellent, good, fair, poor and very poor. The criteria for this classification were based upon the number of teeth covered by plaque. Students with no plaque present were categorized as excellent. Such students would have a DI-S score of zero. A student with plaque present on one or two teeth was assigned to a "good" category. Fair oral cleanliness meant three or four surfaces covered by plaque. Poor oral cleanliness meant five or six teeth covered by plaque, and a DI-S score of more than 1 was indicative of very poor oral hygiene. Since the number of students with "excellent" oral hygiene was small (three freshmen, two sophomores, two juniors and two seniors), the good and excellent categories were combined.

A chi-square test was applied to this data to determine whether a significant difference in oral cleanliness existed between the four dental school classes. The chi-square test is highly significant at the P = .005 level. The sophomores contributed fewer students to the "very poor oral cleanliness" category than expected, whereas the seniors contributed more than expected.

Information on frequency of toothbrushing was taken from the questionnaire. In order to verify the students' claims about toothbrushing, the means of DI-S, CI-S and OHI-S were grouped and examined according to the frequency of brushing, and irrespective of class. As the frequency of toothbrushing increased, the scores of DI-S and OHI-S decreased. This negative relation is what one would expect. A similar relation can be seen between CI-S and frequency of brushing. A slight difference exists, however, between those who brush three times and those who brush two times per day. The analysis of variance technique applied disclosed a significant difference at the .01 level for the DI-S, CI-S and OHI-S.

In reviewing the dental literature regarding dental health education and patient motivation many surveys have indicated a remarkable improvement in oral cleanliness associated with oral hygiene instruction even when comparatively little time was spent in instruction. In the case of dental students with an educational program of 4 years, however, the results do not appear consistent and are not proportional. The data, for example, suggest essentially no change in the level of oral hygiene maintained by students as they progressed through the four year dental curriculum. In addition, the fact that toothbrushing alone does not remove the plaque sheltered in the interproximal space does not seem to impress the students. Fifty-six per cent of the students in the study used the toothbrush as the only method to clean their mouths. Only 77 students, or 19 per cent, stated that they floss daily. This lack of behavioral change existed even though the students were giving their patients toothbrushing and flossing instruction.

This study dramatically demonstrates the need for specific oral hygiene instructions to dental students. An effective program must help a student improve his attitudes, as well as contribute to his acquisition and development of oral hygiene skills. It is important from the viewpoint of increasing the effectiveness of oral hygiene practices in the student's own mouth and it is equally, if not more, important from the viewpoint of preparing the student to assume the responsibility for teaching and motivating patients in the oral hygiene procedures.

The dentist's failure to stress effective preventive dental health services and to teach his patients effective oral hygiene has been demonstrated. A recent survey indicated that less than 20 per cent of patients receiving care in dental offices were given oral hygiene instructions. Another study shows that only 18 per cent of patients who see a dentist regularly receive thorough routine dental prophylaxis.

Although the dentist should assume prime responsibility for patient education, it is evident that the enormity of the task requires that implementation be delegated to others on the dental health team, Considering the present status of auxiliaries in dentistry, and the Dental Practice Acts, it appears that the oral hygiene and preventive periodontal responsibilities will be assigned to the dental hygienist. Changes to permit expanded duties for the dental assistant will bring a tremendous influx of qualified personnel to the preventive dentistry program.

Dental hygiene education is already directed toward promoting oral health. There exist many programs that place special emphasis on patient education. When dental hygiene was recommended as a formal educational program by Dr. Fones in 1913, he suggested that dental hygienists be trained and employed mainly in schools to provide preventive treatment for children. In addition, research studies have reported that students in the social sciences tend to care more for people than do students in the physical or biological sciences. In this regard, dental hygienists indeed appear to enjoy a favorable position. Inclusion of social science courses in the dental hygiene curriculum may serve to strengthen their role in providing preventive dental health service.

In light of this feeling for the importance of dental auxiliaries in providing oral hygiene and preventive periodontal instruction, an evaluation similar to the one done with dental students was undertaken to analyze the effectiveness of preventive periodontal education in the dental hygiene curriculum (Zaki and Stallard). The study was expanded to include evaluation one year after graduation for possible changes in attitudes. The final modification was a questionnaire developed to record information regarding different aspects of clinical practice. The questionnaire was administered to the students before graduation and again after one year of practice.

The study population included 42 first year and 38 second year dental hygiene students. The means and standard deviations of scores of DI-S, CI-S, OHI-S, test and questionnaire are listed in Table 2–2. The results are arranged according to the different classes and for the entire group.

TABLE 2–2 MEANS AND STANDARD DEVIATIONS OF DI-S, CI-S, OHI-S, TEST AND QUESTIONNAIRE SCORES, ACCORDING TO THE DIFFERENT CLASSES OF DENTAL HYGIENE STUDENTS AND FOR THE GROUP AS A WHOLE

DENTAL HYGIENE CLASS	NUMBERS	TYPES OF SCORES: DI-S Mean	DI-S S.D.	CI-S Mean	CI-S S.D.	OHI-S Mean	OHI-S S.D.	TEST Mean	TEST S.D.	QUESTIONNAIRE Mean	QUESTIONNAIRE S.D.
Freshmen	42	.73	.40	.28	.20	1.01	.51	76.60	9.0	81.60	5.7
Seniors	38	.49	.30	.18	.15	.67	.39	85.20	6.5	84.2	6.3
Total	80	.61	.37	.23	.18	.84	.48	80.9	7.8	82.9	6.0

The mean OHI-S for the freshmen was 1.01, markedly higher than that for the seniors. The mean test score for the freshman class was 76.60 and increased to 85.20 for the seniors. The mean questionnaire score for the total student body was 82.9. The scores fluctuated slightly but were essentially the same for both classes, with the seniors scoring somewhat higher.

In order to clarify the differences between the means of these variables, the data were statistically analyzed. The differences between DI-S, OHI-S and test scores were statistically significant at the 0.01 level. The differences, however, between questionnaire scores were not statistically significant.

Table 2–3 demonstrates a trend for dental hygiene graduates to move to larger cities. It is evident that the percentage of dental hygienists intending to practice in a city population ranging from 100,000 to 250,000 decreased markedly from 26 per cent to 7 per cent, while the percentage who intended to practice in a city with a population of over 500,000 increased from 27 per cent to 43 per cent. It is interesting to note that the percentage in the smallest communities remained the same.

The number of years senior students predicted, before graduation, that they would practice full-time is illustrated in Table 2–4. The table also demonstrates how these predictions changed after only one year of practice. Thirteen per cent of the senior class stated that they would practice only two years. However, during the first year 42 per cent had already left full-time practice. It is interesting to speculate whether the reason for such large-scale abandonment of full-time practice resulted from disillusionment with the dental hygienists' role or from largely personal reasons, such as marriage.

TABLE 2–4 PREDICTION AS TO LENGTH OF TIME IN FULL-TIME DENTAL HYGIENE PRACTICE

YEARS	PERCENTAGE *Before Graduation*	*After One Year of Practice*
		42% have already left full-time practice
One	0	5
Two	13	25
Three	20	5
Four	7	3
Five	42	6
More than five	18	14
Total	100	100

The dental hygienists' visualization of the nature of their profession before graduation and then after one year of practice can be shown in Table 2–5. Before graduation 90 per cent of the students indicated that they wanted to practice prevention. After one year of practice, however, only 61 per cent indicated that their practice was oriented toward prevention. This group stated that they treated 10 patients a day. In contrast, 39 per cent indicated that their practice was now therapeutic; this group treated an average of 12 patients a day. The number of patients in either category is a heavy work load for even the most efficient dental hygienist. It was also noted on the question-

TABLE 2–3 TENDENCY OF DENTAL HYGIENE GRADUATES TO MOVE TOWARD LARGER CITIES

CITY SIZE	PERCENTAGE *Before Graduation*	*After One Year of Practice*
Under 100,000	27	27
100,000–250,000	26	7
250,000–500,000	20	23
Over 500,000	27	43
Total	100	100

TABLE 2–5 VISUALIZATION OF THE NATURE OF DENTAL HYGIENE PRACTICE

TYPE OF PRACTICE	PERCENTAGE *Before Graduation*	*After One Year of Practice*	*Mean Number of Patients Seen Daily*
Preventive	90	61	10.3
Therapeutic	10	39	12.3
Total	100	100	

naire that many of those who still visualized dental hygiene as preventive in nature admitted that they were unable to practice in that manner because of the office environment.

It is apparent, on the basis of substantial differences in both test scores and oral cleanliness, that the dental hygiene education program is effective in teaching preventive care. The hygienists, however, do not or cannot fully utilize this educational knowledge and skill in preventive dental programs for the public. Before graduation the majority of dental hygiene students strongly believed in stressing preventive dental care and oral hygiene in their practices. In practice they were unable to do so. This is most likely a reflection of the attitudes prevalent in the dental practices in which they are located.

It is surprising to note that many reports have indicated that only 20 per cent of the nation's dentists employ hygienists, and that once hired, 90 per cent of their time is spent on prophylaxis. Obviously, the hygienist is not given sufficient time to adequately educate the patient in home-care techniques.

Millions of people who suffer from dental caries and periodontal disease cannot be treated because of a dental manpower shortage. Taking into consideration the gravity of the disease problem, it becomes evident that prevention is the logical solution. It is important, therefore, to develop a comprehensive and efficient program for patient education. An initial step is to fully realize the importance of the role the hygienist can perform. She can make a major contribution to the prevention and control of dental disease in the general practice of dentistry. Until there are basic changes in the dentists' attitudes about oral hygiene and prevention, and until these changes are reflected in their concept of practice, dental hygienists or any other auxiliaries will not be effectively utilized as teachers in preventive programs.

A fundamental question in the evaluation of preventive dental education concerns the outcome of the learning process. The student evaluation raised serious questions about the methods of education. Obviously, participation in a complete dental curriculum, in and of itself, is not the answer. It is encouraging, however, to note the favorable results of a similar evaluation in the dental hygiene program. Although it too can be improved upon, it is apparent that effective methods for teaching the philosophy and practice of prevention are available.

In addition, there is evidence that new, effective, methods of teaching preventive dentistry can be incorporated into our undergraduate curriculum. Educators, administrators and others are speaking out for prevention. In light of this it is difficult to explain why dental students still spend over 75 per cent of their years in dental school learning to repair and replace teeth. We are desperately asking for prevention, yet we remain actively engaged and oriented toward technical dentistry.

It is obvious that a problem of major proportion exists in the delivery of preventive dental care. Identification of the problem is only the first step. It must be followed by correction with available resources. The next step is application of the preventive procedures as an effective modality in the dental practice.

Model presentation and reinforcement, as the term implies, is a combination of two instructional procedures. Model presentation, a form of imitative learning, consists of demonstrating a problem, and then presenting a solution through the use of motor skills. The problem demonstrated must be made meaningful to the learner. In addition, the learner must have a clear idea of what must be accomplished to solve the problem. By imitating the demonstration, under guidance, the learner acquires the necessary understanding of the movement required. With additional practice, his motor skills develop.

Model presentation approaches the learning process primarily as the motor response to a problem situation. For the attainment of the highest proficiency, it is important to strengthen this response by reinforcement. Reinforcement increases the probability that desired responses will occur in the future. It results, therefore, in improving not only the initial learning

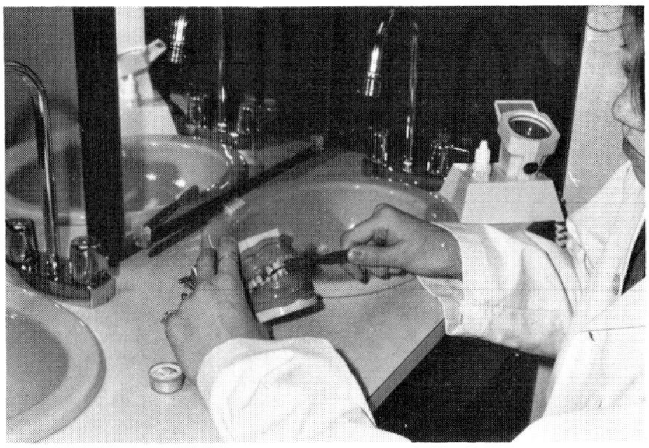

Figure 2–1 During the first session of a preventive program, brushing and flossing techniques are demonstrated to the patient on models. In this illustration the Bass technique of sulcular brushing can be seen.

process but also the retention of what has been learned.

Knowledge of results, frequently referred to as feedback, is a major source of reinforcement. Knowledge of a correct response is reinforcing and strengthens the preceding behavior; it minimizes the chances of producing incorrect responses. The more precise and specific is the feedback, the more readily will the learner determine the correct response. Intelligent practice follows this determination, and a refinement of movement and the development and acquisition of skill results.

The effect of reinforcement is magnified if it immediately follows the response. It has been demonstrated, for example, that students given correct answers immediately following regular hourly quizzes perform better on final examinations than control students who receive the correct answers the next time the class meets.

A student may be highly motivated but learn very little if he is unable to determine whether or not his efforts are adequate. Reinforcement, at the optimum time, is an effective method of preventing this problem.

The effectiveness of model presentation and reinforcement as an instructional procedure can be applied to the development of oral hygiene skills in patients.

SESSION ONE

The first session should be devoted primarily to model presentation. Initially, the learning objectives, methods of operation and importance of the subject are explained. This procedure is intended to make the situation meaningful to the learner.

Toothbrushing techniques and dental flossing are demonstrated on models (Fig. 2–1). The individual components of these techniques are also explained. The patients are given disclosing tablets or the Plak-lite and scored, utilizing the Greene-Vermillion

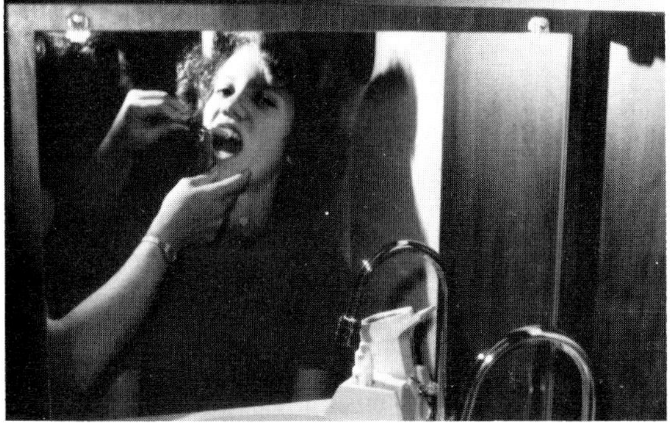

Figure 2–2 The second step in session one is the demonstration and participation by the patient in supervised brushing within her or his own mouth. Here again we can see the use of the Bass technique of sulcular brushing.

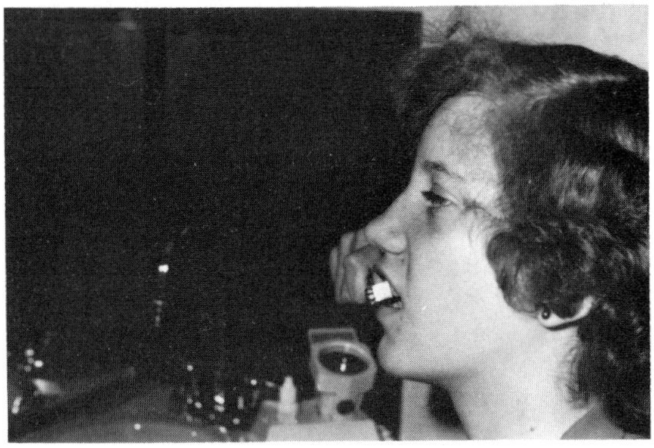

Figure 2–3 Session two is primarily one of reinforcement. During this session the patient is asked to perform the preventive procedures taught in a preceding session. Additional instructions and corrections can be provided at this time to correct any inadequacies in technique.

Debris Index Simplified. In addition, they are instructed to execute the toothbrushing and flossing movements, under supervision, in their own mouths (Fig. 2–2). If shown to be inadequate, the movements are corrected. In this way patients are given a clear idea of what is to be accomplished in order to solve the problem.

DENTAL HEALTH MAINTENANCE RECORD
GROUP HEALTH MEDICAL CENTER

Dental Health Education	Date Conveyed	By Whom	Receptivity*	Literature Dispensed	Comment
tooth brushing	5/21/75	CJS	2	none	patient too young
brushing + floss	11/12/75	CW	4	home care kit	tremendous improvement in oral hygiene
complete preventive	5/3/76	JS	3	home care kit & instructions for flossing	problem c̄ flossing

*5 Point Scale of Receptivity:
1. Hostile
2. Non-receptive
3. Willing to listen
4. Listens carefully
5. Interested in applying instruction to life's pattern

DEN-01 (6/75)

Figure 2–4 Utilizing a single page within the patient's dental record, the dental health maintenance can be recorded and compared. The type of dental health education is recorded, its date, by whom, and the individual patient's receptivity. In addition, literature and materials are dispensed, and any other comments are recorded.

SESSION TWO

The second session is primarily one of reinforcement. It should be conducted approximately three weeks after the first session. Each patient is given a disclosant to observe his level of performance. He is then asked to perform the toothbrushing method of his choice, and to floss his teeth (Fig. 2–3). Additional instruction is provided, when needed, to eliminate undesirable responses, and to focus the patient's attention on the relevant aspects of his task. Further attempts are made to correct the toothbrushing technique. Whenever possible, reinforcement is given by informing the patient how well he is doing.

SESSION THREE

The third session is one of evaluation, although additional instruction is provided when necessary. This session is conducted two months after the start of the program. The Debris Index Simplified is again used to evaluate the degree of oral cleanliness.

Although it has been shown in many studies that the three-session model system is most ideal for reinforcement in establishing changes in patient behavior, this is not always practical in the routine dental practice. For the patient who requires additional dental therapy beyond the routine dental health maintenance, the reinforcement sessions can be built into their appointments, with the result of marked alterations in behavior patterns. To overcome the problem of the single visit, if the patient does not require additional dental care, preventive dental education for the family unit is ideal. Reinforcement is then brought about at home by parents and siblings.

As part of the patient's permanent dental record, progress in dental health maintenance must be recorded. A sample health maintenance chart can be seen in Figure 2–4. Not only is the type of preventive education given recorded but also the patient's receptivity. In addition, space is provided to record the dental health maintenance products and literature dispensed.

Only through a total commitment and effort on the part of the dentist, dental hygienist, dental assistant, patient and family unit can a preventive dental program achieve the maximum effectiveness reported in the literature.

REFERENCES

Arnim, S. S.: An effective program of oral hygiene for the arrestment of dental caries and the control of periodontal disease. J. South. Calif. Dent. Hyg. Assoc. 35:264–280, 1967.

Bailey, B. H., and Bennett, G. G.: Psychology of learning applied to dental education. J. Dent. Educ. *30*: 297–310, 1966.

Brandtzaeg, P.: The significance of oral hygiene in the prevention of dental diseases. Odont. Tidskroft *72*:460–486, 1964.

Bruner, Jerome S.: The Process of Education. New York, Random House, Inc., 1969, p. 17.

Gage, N. L.: Theories of learning. *In* Hilgard, E. R. (Ed.): *Theories of Learning and Instruction.* NSSE Yearbook, Chicago, University of Chicago Press, 1964.

Gardner, A. F.: Education of dental students. J. Dent. Educ. *29*:364–368, 1965.

Greene, J. C., and Vermillion, J. R.: The simplified oral hygiene index. J. Am. Dent. Assoc. *68*:7–13, 1964.

Linn, E. L.: Oral hygiene and periodontal disease: Implication for dental health programs. J. Am. Dent. Assoc. *71*:39–42, 1965.

Lobene, R. R.: The evaluation of oral hygiene in preventive dentistry. J. Mass. Dent. Soc. 1–7, 1966.

Morch, T., and Werhaug, J.: Quantitative evaluation of the effect of toothbrushing and toothpicking. J. Periodont. *27*:183–190, 1958.

Stanmeyer, W. R.: A measure of tissue response to frequency of toothbrushing. J. Periodont. *28*:17–22, 1957.

Trott, J. R.: Evaluation of clinical teaching and teachers. J. Dent. Educ. *31*:229–234, 1967.

Young, W. O., and Zwemer, J. D.: Objectives and methods of teaching preventive dentistry and community health. J. Dent. Educ. *31*:162–167, 1967.

Zaki, H. A., and Bandt, L.: Model presentation and reinforcement—an effective method for teaching oral hygiene skills. J. Perio. *41*:394–397, 1970.

Zaki, H. A., and Stallard, R. E.: An evaluation of the effectiveness of preventive periodontal education. J. Periodont. Res. (Suppl. 3), 1969.

ADDITIONAL REFERENCE MATERIAL

Angell, G. W.: The effect of immediate knowledge of quiz results on final examination scores in freshman chemistry. J. Educ. Res. *42*:391, 1949.

Bass, B. M., and Vaughan, J. A.: Training in industry. The Management of Learning. Belmont, CA, Wadsworth Publishing Company, Inc., 1968, pp. 8, 23.

Berland, T.: What's the truth about "mouthwash magic"? Today's Health *40*:22–23, 72–74, 1962.

Boleo, J. de P.: Prevention of dental caries and treatment of periodontal diseases by means of thermal waters. Rev. Port. Estomatol. Cir. Maxilofac. *12*(1–2):117–128, Jan-June, 1971.

Brandtzaeg, P., and Jamison, H. C.: A study of periodontal health and oral hygiene in Norwegian army recruits. J. Periodont. *35*:302–307, 1964.

Brown, W. E.: Prevention – its role in the curriculum of a new dental school. J. Amer. Coll. Dent. *40*(1): 29–33, Jan, 1973.

Collier, D. R., and Bryan, E. T.: Survey of preventive dental services now being provided to the school-age population of Tennessee. J. Tenn. Dent. Assoc. *53*(3):248–252, July, 1973.

Curson, I., and Manson, J. D.: A study of a group of dental students, including their diet and dental health. Brit. Dent. J. *119*:197–205, 1965.

Greene, J. C., and Vermillion, J. R.: The Simplified Oral Hygiene Index J. Am. Dent. Assoc. *68*:7, 1964.

Horowitz, M. J.: Educating tomorrow's doctors. New York, Appleton-Century-Crofts, 1964.

Lovdal, A., Arno, A., Schei, O., and Waergaug, J.: Combined effect of subgingival scaling and controlled oral hygiene on the incidence of gingivitis. Acta Odont. Scand. *19*:537–555, 1961.

Mork, G. M. A.: Psychology of learning applied in graduate education. Proceedings of a workshop for teachers in periodontology at the University of Minnesota, Ed., Perry A. Ratcliff, Minneapolis, 1960.

Nedelsky, L.: The dental curriculum of tomorrow. J. Dent. Educ. *31*:335–341, 1967.

Orzechowska, K.: Program and methods of field training in the prevention of periodontal diseases for dentists treating adults. Czas Stomat. *26*(9):971–974, Sept., 1973.

Peters, R. S.: The Concepts of Education. London, Routledge and Kegan Paul, 1967.

Schmuth, G. P. F.: Orthodontic prevention and treatment of periodontal diseases. Deutsch Zahnaerztl. Z. *28*(2):138–141, Feb., 1973.

Singer, B.: Preventive dentistry. Oesterr. Z. Stomatol. *70*(9):325–327, Sept., 1973.

Vande Voorde, H. E., and Davis, J. M.: Dental disease control, home treatment program: Case report of patient with severe gingivitis and rampant caries. Illinois Dent. J. *42*(4):231–237, April, 1973.

Witt, E.: Orthodontic measures for the prevention and treatment of periodontal diseases. Deutsch Zahnaerztl. Z. *28*(2):142, Feb., 1973.

chapter 3

THE EPIDEMIOLOGY OF DENTAL CARIES

by

SIDNEY B. FINN, D.M.D., M.S.

Throughout his evolutionary advancement, man has been subjected to a constantly changing environment. Some of these alterations have proved beneficial, others detrimental to his well-being. Among those environmental problems with which man has been unable to cope completely is an increased susceptibility to dental caries. In the United States of America, there are today approximately one billion carious teeth in need of being filled that cannot be cared for professionally for various reasons, such as economy, prevalence of the disease and a lack of complete preventive and corrective measures. In view of this situation, dental caries assumes the enormity of a major national disaster. Man, because of present living habits, is the only species susceptible to this disease in his normal environment, and present attempts at preventing its ravages fall short of approximating the caries freedom enjoyed by other animal species that are subsisting on their natural diet in a wild habitat.

The skulls of prehistoric human beings evidenced a slight susceptibility to dental caries and its sequelae. When man first learned to eat various tubers, grains and berries and to enjoy the sweet taste of honey and other natural sugars, dental caries increased. Skulls found in France dating back 2500 years indicate that even at this early period, one per cent of the teeth were carious.

Primitive man probably ate his food unwashed. The dust on the food combined with the grit from the soft sandstone mortars used in grinding his grain abraded the occlusal surfaces of the teeth and obliterated the pits and fissures. By this means the surfaces were rendered free of dental caries, but the destruction of the normal spillways allowed for the interproximal impaction of food and the development of proximal lesions. Present civilization is characterized by a relatively high caries susceptibility on all tooth surfaces.

In contemporary man the occurrence of dental caries has become universal, affecting all ages and all races from all geographic areas of the world. Figure 3–1 depicts the broad distribution of this disease.

Because of the marked variation in methods of examination and reporting, considerable caution must be exercised in interpreting the data. An increase in dental

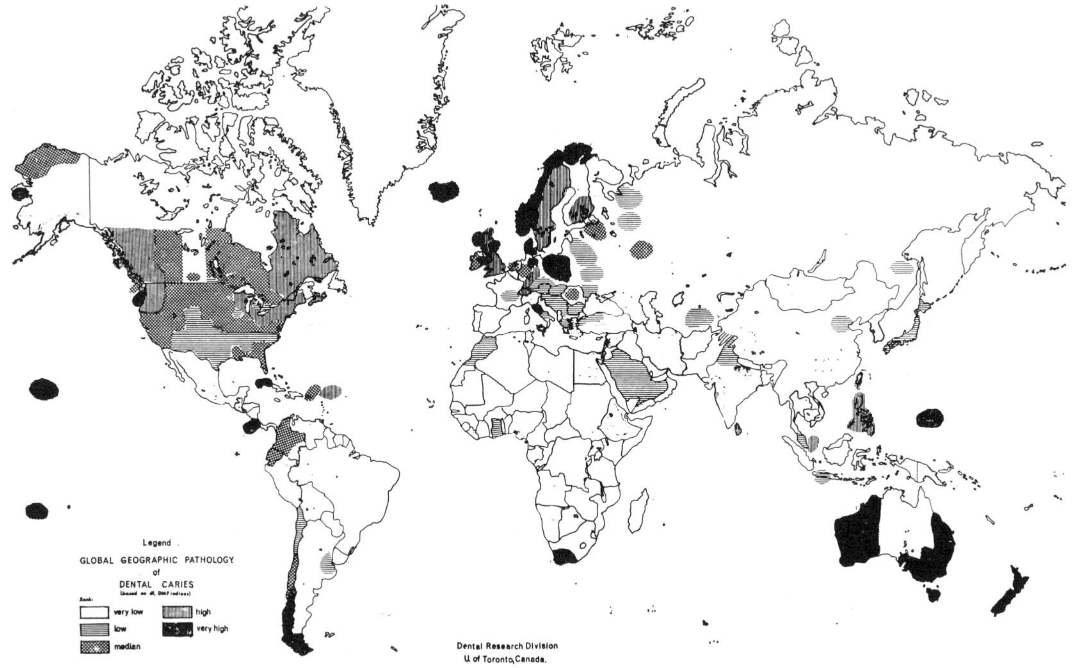

Figure 3–1 Caries distribution throughout the world. (From McPhail and Grainger: A mapping procedure for the geographic pathology of dental caries. Int. Dent. J. *19*:380, 1969.)

caries directly correlates with the densely populated and highly industrialized areas of the world. Easy access to commercially prepared foods with a concomitant change in dietary habits might account for this difference. However, the prevalence rates may vary in limited areas because of other geographic, genetic and environmental factors that will be discussed in subsequent chapters.

Dental caries is progressive. A continuation of the same environmental conditions that induced the lesion will inevitably complete the destruction of the tooth unless the affected area becomes self-cleansing or unless preventive or corrective treatments are employed.

PERMANENT TOOTH INDICES

A comprehensible index to express dental caries experience either of an individual or a population needs to be developed so that all surveys and clinical trials can be universally understood and evaluated on a common basis. Progress is being made toward establishing comparable examination techniques and data compilations.

The index most widely accepted for compiling data for the permanent teeth is based on the number of decayed, missing and filled teeth (DMFT) or surfaces (DMFS) either per individual, per hundred erupted teeth or per thousand erupted surfaces. The missing teeth and surfaces are sometimes excluded from the index (DFT) and (DFS) when the reason for extraction of the teeth is difficult to establish, as with older individuals in whom periodontal disease is a common cause of tooth loss. Another index is based on the number of (DMF) teeth or surfaces as calculated on the basis of a full complement of teeth and surfaces. An index of this type would compensate for age and sex differences. Determining the number of surfaces that were originally carious in a missing tooth presents a problem and affects the reliability of the DMFS index. There are other types of indices, which, because of their infrequent use, are not included in this chapter.

PRIMARY TOOTH INDICES

During the period of changing dentition, it is not possible to make a reliable determination as to whether teeth have been lost because of exfoliation or through extraction. This makes it unsatisfactory to use the same indices that are used for the permanent teeth. Indices for the primary dentition generally employ the terms decayed, indicated for extraction, and filled (def) teeth and surfaces, or decayed and filled (df) teeth and surfaces. Because of the exfoliation factor, the def index is not completely reliable for children over five years of age. An index that counts only the primary cuspid and molar teeth would be reliable until approximately nine years of age, since these teeth are generally lost physiologically, beginning at this age. An index of only df teeth and surfaces ignores missing teeth and would be accurate only if the teeth were lost because of exfoliation and were known to have been caries-free.

The RID index, based on the caries experience of the individual, is calculated from the number of teeth and surfaces present in the mouth. Although not as widely used as the def index, it has several advantages in that the index can be used for the primary, mixed and permanent dentitions and considers only the teeth that are present in the oral cavity. As one gathers from the discussion, there is no perfect index but a few are adequate within expressed limits.

EXAMINATION TECHNIQUES

Examination techniques vary depending upon the goals of the individual study. Competent epidemiological surveys reporting dental caries prevalence should include the use of sharp explorers and mirrors under good light. For limited short-term studies, where testing the efficacy of a preventive agent is the objective, the importance of detecting all lesions as early as possible is critical. In this type of study, radiographs are desirable and perhaps essential, especially if the major inhibition occurs on the proximal surfaces. However, because of the harmful effects of X-ray, caution must be employed to limit the amount of radiation received by the subjects, and the advantages to be gained must be weighed against the essentiality of the additional information.

Surveys concerned only with the

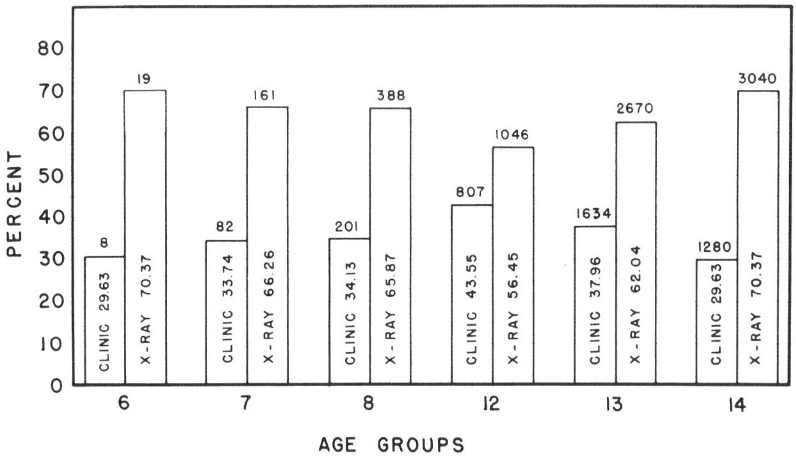

Figure 3–2 Comparison of the number of carious lesions found on proximal surfaces of permanent teeth by direct observation and by radiographic examination. (From Blayney and Hill: Fluorine and dental caries. J. Am. Dent. Assoc. *74*:223, 1967.)

number of missing teeth require less critical precision than those used in detecting caries, since there is only a need for tooth identification.

Figure 3–2 illustrates the number of proximal lesions detected in the Evanston Water Fluoridation Study by direct observation and by radiography. These figures indicate that over 64 per cent of the lesions were found by X-ray.

OTHER CONSIDERATIONS

Such factors as the type of population from which the sample is drawn, the sample size, the elimination of bias and the statistical treatment of data are important to the relevance and reliability of any data presented. Since the dental caries prevalence from community to community or from area to area may vary, it should be clearly understood that the information provided by a study applies specifically to that area studied and only relatively to all communities or areas either in the United States or throughout the world.

DENTAL CARIES IN THE PRIMARY DENTITION

Primary teeth, subject to attack at a very early age, may become carious prior to the eruption of the completed deciduous dentition. Dental caries attack in these teeth is progressive and, until all teeth are exfoliated by 11 to 12 years of age, can create a serious problem in the proper functioning of the masticatory apparatus.

A number of studies have reported positive correlations between the caries experience in the primary teeth and those of the permanent dentition. However, this is not always substantiated and must be qualified. Though the primary dentitions of the children in India and Ceylon develop rampant caries, the permanent teeth are relatively caries-free. Governed to some extent by prenatal and early postnatal environmental factors, this host resistance may account for the susceptibility of the primary teeth and yet have little influence over the permanent dentition.

Since exfoliation of the primary teeth commences at five years of age, surveys of the complete primary dentition must be done on infants and preschool children. There is difficulty in assembling large population groups of preschool children. Therefore, the number of surveys made with this age group has been limited and the number of individuals in each study relatively small. This may account for some of the wide variation in reported findings.

In the midwest, a clinical and radiographic study conducted in a fluoride-free area

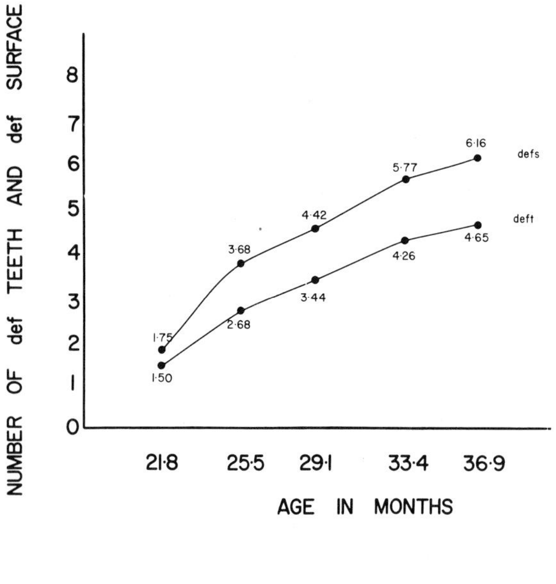

Figure 3–3 Caries experience in the primary teeth in infants and preschool children. (From Hennon, Stookey and Muhler: Prevalence and distribution of dental caries in preschool children. J. Am. Dent. Assoc. 79:1045, 1972.)

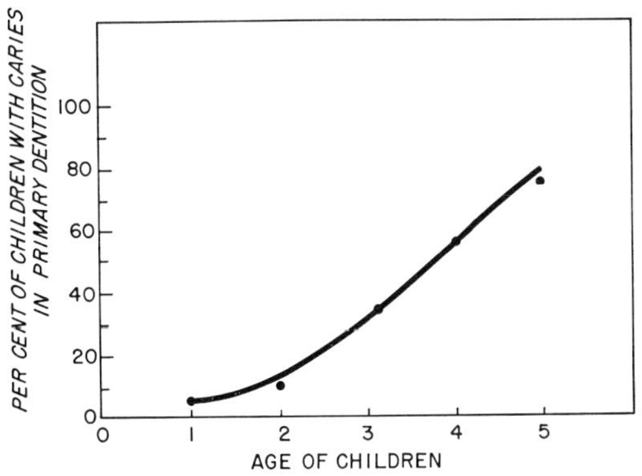

Figure 3–4 Per cent of infants and preschool children with caries experience in the primary dentition. (From Finn, in Toverud et al.: Survey of the Literature of Dental Caries. National Academy of Sciences-National Research Council.)

disclosed that in a group of children under two years of age, there were already 1.5 def teeth per child. The prevalence rate rose rapidly, and by three years of age there were over four def teeth per child, as shown in Figure 3–3.

The number of def surfaces rose more precipitously than the number of involved teeth, from 1.7 at 21 months of age to 6.1 at 37 months, because of the enlargement of existing cavities and the development of new lesions on teeth already cariously involved.

It is of striking importance that the number affected with def teeth rose from 10.3 per cent in children less than two years of age to 75 per cent in children five years of age (Fig. 3–4).

There appears to be no significant difference between sexes concerning caries in the primary dentition, although there is a definite variation between sexes at any specific age in caries experience in the permanent dentition.

Each tooth in both dentitions has a caries susceptibility that is related to the other teeth of the complete dentition. On any individual tooth, there may be different reasons why a carious attack might favor one surface over another. Developmental pits and fissures may foretell the early development of occlusal caries, but other morphologic differences such as the size of the contact area between adjacent teeth or the amount of space between teeth might govern the rate of development of proximal caries. Because of the variation of interprox-

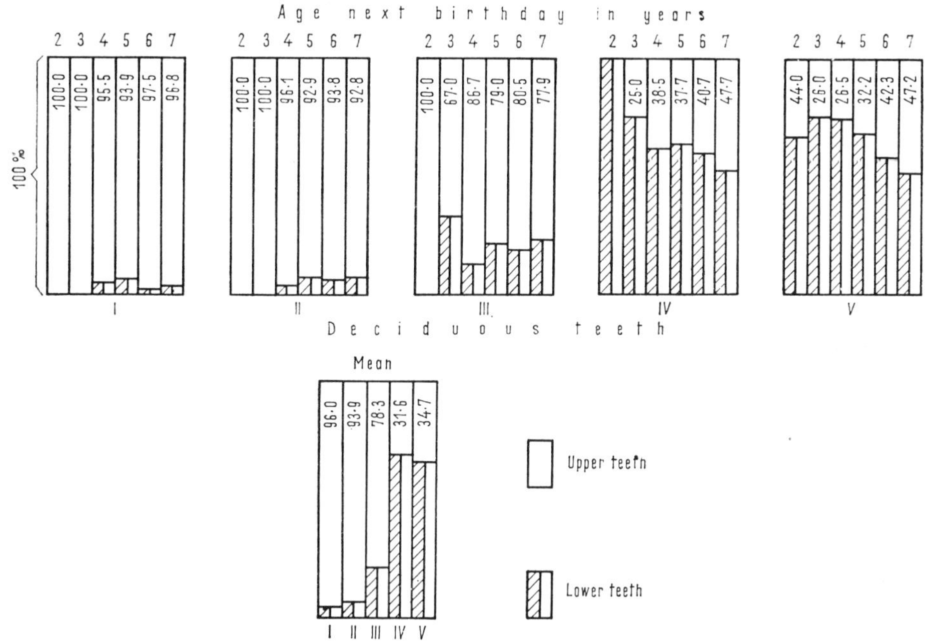

Figure 3–5 Comparison of caries prevalence in the maxillary and mandibular primary teeth. (From Toth: The Epidemiology of Dental Caries in Hungary. Budapest; Akademiai Kiado, 1970.)

imal contact, the surfaces of approximal teeth have a more similar caries experience than the mesial and distal surfaces of either tooth. Proximal surfaces, before there is a tooth in juxtaposition, usually have remained caries-free until the tooth approximating this surface erupts. The presence of an apposing tooth appears to have little effect on the development of occlusal caries.

The lower second molars are the most susceptible teeth in the primary dentition because of the length of the fissures and the broad extent of both proximal contacts. In general the lower incisors are the most resistant, accounting for only about 10 per cent of the total caries experience. The lower molars, being about twice as susceptible as the upper molars, account for about 52 per cent of the total caries experience. If an infant has a caries-free lower dentition, there is a strong implication that the upper dentition will also be decay-free. There are certain exceptions to this observation as exemplified by the early and rampant carious breakdown of the upper anterior teeth seen in nocturnal bottle-feeders given milk sweetened with sugar. Figure 3–5 compares the relative susceptibility of the maxillary and mandibular primary teeth from two through seven years of age. The lower anterior primary teeth at all ages have lower caries scores in contrast to the molar teeth.

DENTAL CARIES IN THE PERMANENT DENTITION

Dental caries experience involving the mixed and permanent dentitions has been surveyed in numerous studies that have included individuals of all ages. The onset, progression and eventual fate of these teeth has been recognized as one of the major public health problems involving present-day man. As early as 14 years of age, 97 per cent of the children have evidenced caries in the permanent teeth, as indicated in Figure 3–6.

Since the first permanent molars erupt between five and six years of age, at which time 20 per cent of the children have experi-

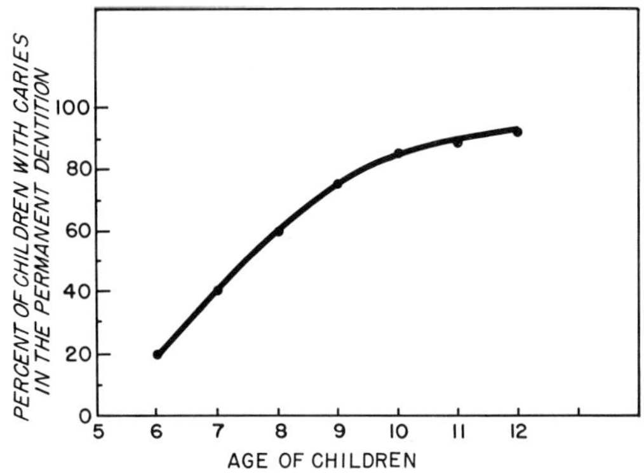

Figure 3–6 The per cent of children with caries experience in the permanent teeth according to age. (From Finn, in Toverud et al.: Survey of the Literature of Dental Caries. National Academy of Sciences-National Research Council.)

enced dental decay, this clearly demonstrates the vulnerability of these teeth to attack.

The number of DMF teeth rises sharply from 0.4 at six years of age to 8.33 at 14 years of age. The yearly increment, approximating .75 of a new tooth per year, involves approximately two surfaces per year. Despite the parallelism between the number of carious surfaces and that on DMF teeth for the chronological period indicated in Figure 3–7, there is an abrupt rise in the number of surfaces attacked. This situation is attributable to the development of new carious surfaces on previously decayed teeth and to increase in the size of some existing lesions, so that these lesions extend to other surfaces.

Although at six years of age there is an average of less than one DMF tooth per child, the rate rises to over five DMF teeth with nearly eight DMF surfaces at about 12 years of age.

Dental caries appears to develop bilaterally; more cavities occur on homologous teeth and surfaces than occur unilaterally. As in the primary dentition, each tooth or each pair of homologous teeth has its specific susceptibility to dental caries. When dental caries is reduced by preventive measures, teeth remain caries-free according to a decreasing order based on original susceptibility, i.e., the teeth that are more resistant to the caries attack are the first to

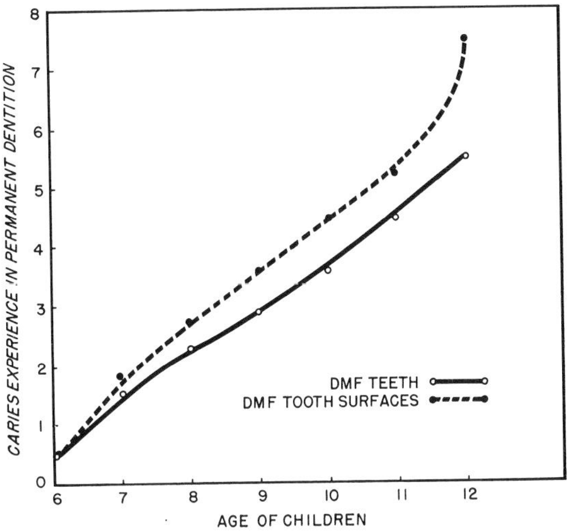

Figure 3–7 DMF teeth and DMF tooth surfaces in the permanent dentition of 6- to 12-year-old children. (From Finn, in Toverud et al.: Survey of the Literature of Dental Caries. National Academy of Sciences-National Research Council.)

remain caries-free. This may possibly explain the observation that currently used caries-preventive agents appear to be more effective on the proximal surfaces than on the occlusal surfaces.

Figure 3–8 shows the percentage of caries experience contributed by each tooth to the total for each child at seven, nine, 11 and 13 years of age.

At seven, nine and 11 years of age the mandibular first molars contribute more than half of the total caries experience, with the maxillary molars contributing approximately 40 per cent. At 11 years of age all other teeth contribute approximately 10 per cent of the total caries experience.

Dental caries increases in a straight-line progression through the teen ages and then levels off as the teeth mature and are consequently less susceptible to attack, and as the number of available susceptible surfaces is reduced by previous carious involvement.

On the molars, pit and fissure areas of the occlusal surfaces usually become carious earlier than the proximal and other smooth-surface areas. Cervical caries is generally the last to develop on the enamel. Root caries develops after gingival recession and is principally a disease of adulthood or old age. Occlusal caries is dependent upon the existence of pits and fissures (original faults of development) and to the steepness of the cusps. Where such faults are nonexistent, especially in the bicuspids, proximal lesions quite commonly occur earlier than those in the occlusal surfaces.

The most susceptible tooth surface in the permanent dentition is the occlusal surface of the mandibular first permanent molar, which may possess a fissure traversing practically the entire mesiodistal diameter of the tooth and by gravity invite impaction of food and debris. The maxillary molars possess a well-defined transverse ridge that divides this surface into two smaller pits. Pits are also present on the buccal surfaces of the lower molars and the lingual surfaces of the upper molars. Cavities appear earlier in these faults than in cervical areas on these same surfaces.

CARIES PROGRESSION

The length of time required for the development of a carious lesion bears an important relation to preventive treatment. Investigators recognize that some lesions never progress beyond the incipient stage and that other identifiable lesions may become benign and progress very slowly. The time required for caries development is highly dependent upon the environment which exists at any particular period. Should this environment change to a less conducive one, because the surface becomes self-cleansing or for some other reason, the caries process may be completely arrested or there is a possibility that incipient lesions may remineralize.

In the United States, children in nonfluoride areas average about 0.75 new lesions a year. Occlusal caries may take from less than three to 48 months for development into recognizable cavitation. In one reported study, 28 per cent of this type of caries progressed beyond the incipient stage in less than six months, but 53 per cent remained in a quiescent state for more than two years. With approximately a quarter of the lesions developing in less than six

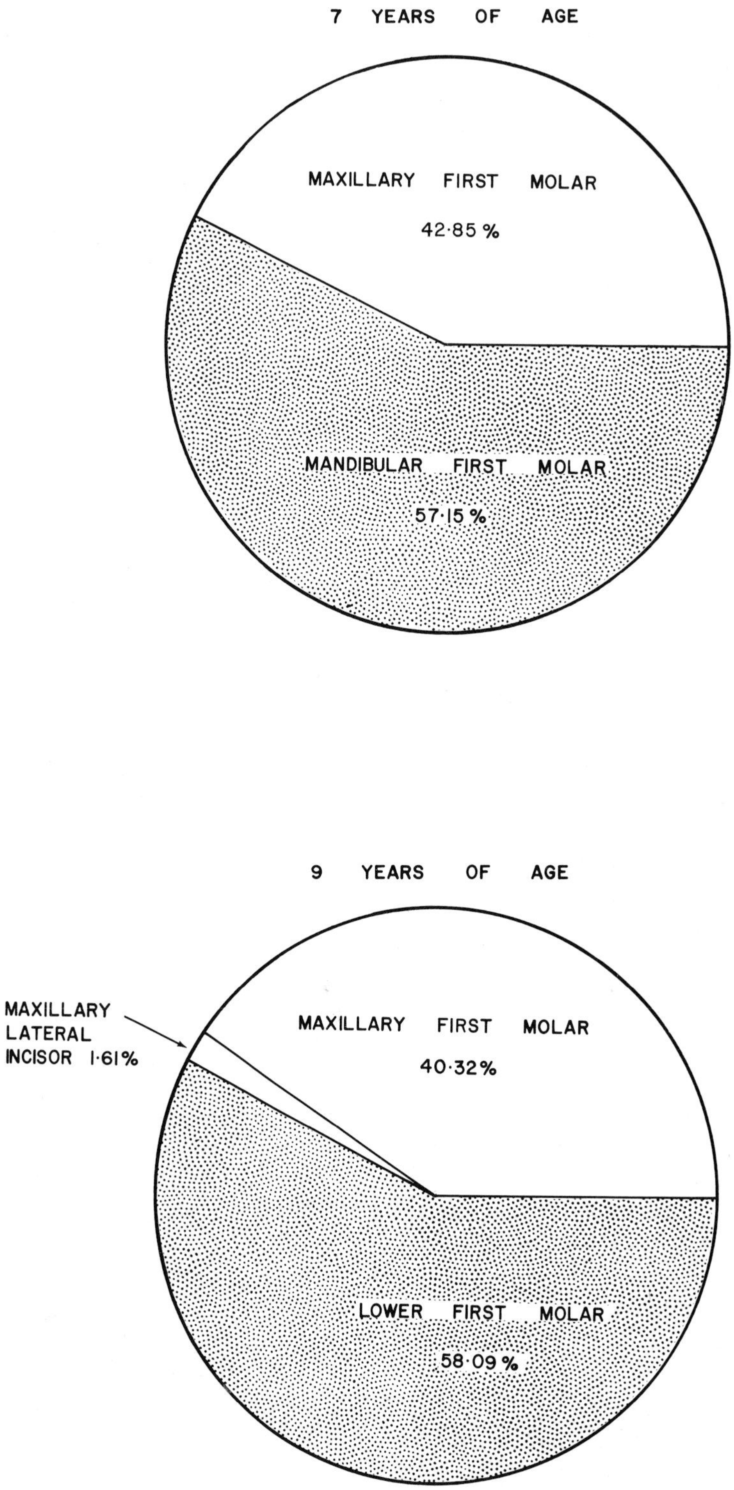

Figure 3–8 Contributions of homologous permanent tooth pairs to the total caries experience in the permanent dentition (155 children).

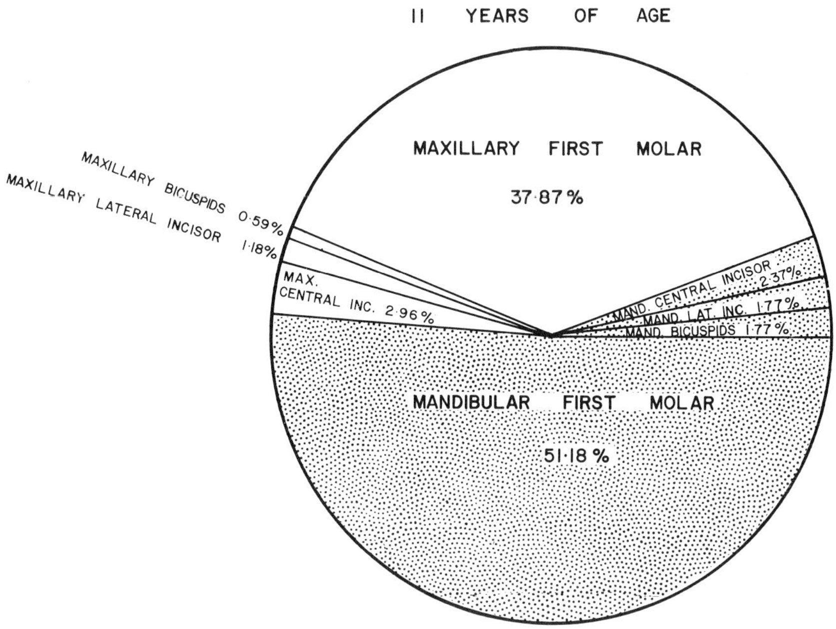

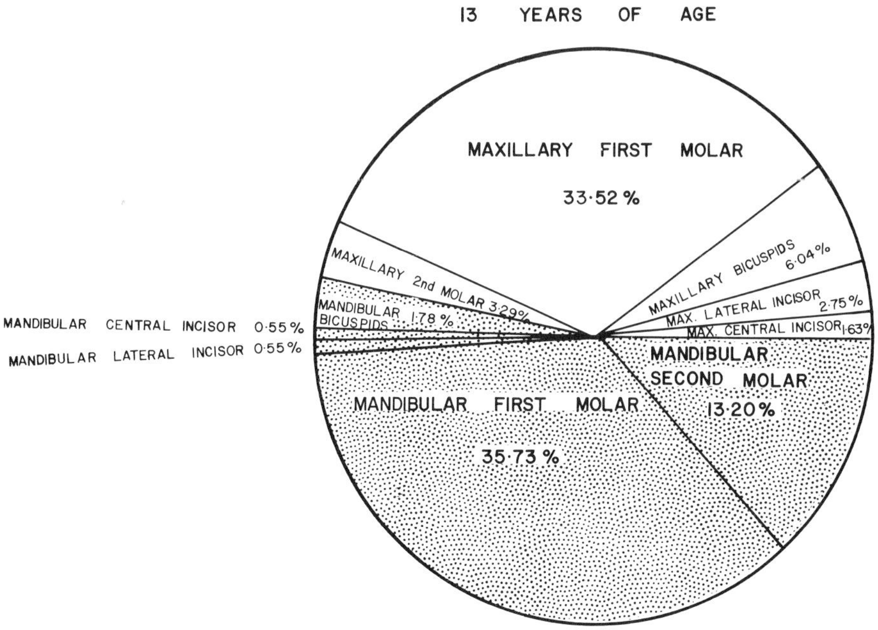

Figure 3–8 *Continued*

months, it would seem prudent to repeat office preventive treatments at intervals of not longer than six months in order to achieve maximum benefit.

SEX DIFFERENCES

Between males and females of the same chronologic age, there is a statistically significant difference in caries prevalence. Girls, especially in adulthood, show a slightly higher prevalence than boys. This difference can be partially explained through the earlier eruption of the teeth in girls, which provides a longer period of exposure for the teeth to the oral environment. Perhaps morphologic differences existing between the teeth of males and females might also account for some of this difference.

HEREDITY AND DENTAL CARIES

Investigators have recognized genetic variations in dental caries prevalence based on two sources of evidence in humans: (1) family studies and (2) twin studies.

The data pertaining to family studies have been derived from information supplied by several investigators. In one study, parents with either low or high caries scores were compared with their siblings. The offspring had caries scores similar to their parents. If both parents had low caries scores, the offspring had low caries scores and the reverse was equally true. If scores of the parents differed, the offspring had intermediate scores. Likewise, the caries-free children in another study had a close resemblance, in this respect, to their siblings.

In another study, caries-free inductees into military service had siblings and parents with significantly lower caries scores than the families of a control group of similar age inductees. It must be recognized, however, that a likeness in dietary and food preferences of members of the same family may account for some of the caries similarities between the inductee and his family.

In a number of twin studies, monozygotic and dizygotic twin pairs of like sex have been compared relative to caries experience. There was a greater concord between the monozygotic than between the dizygotic pairs and an even greater similarity between either type of twin pairs than between pairs of unrelated children of the same sex and age. The unrelated pairs of children, living in different households, may have received unlike diets. This may have accounted for the greater discrepancies that were noted between their caries experience and those of the pairs of twins who lived in the same home. At any given age there was a greater similarity between the number of teeth that were erupted in the monozygotic than in the dizygotic twin pairs, which may explain to some extent why there were greater differences between the dental caries experience in the dizygotic than in the monozygotic twin pairs.

No correlation has been established between the caries experience of an individual and the ages of his parents, the number of children in his family or the relative position of the individual in his family.

RACIAL DIFFERENCES

A number of studies indicate that Negroes of comparable sex and age have a lower caries score than Caucasians. It has not yet been determined whether this difference is a reflection of other dietary modifications, though a recent report suggests that this score does not arise from a difference in sugar consumption. In a Baltimore study, it was found that whites and blacks living under similar environmental conditions had comparable caries scores.

SOCIOECONOMIC STATUS AND DENTAL CARIES

There is ample evidence that an inverse relationship exists between socioeconomic level and dental caries experience in the primary dentition. Such a relationship in the permanent dentition has not been clearly established. The difference, if any, is small.

GEOGRAPHIC VARIATION

There are recognizable geographic variations in dental caries experience in different areas of the United States and throughout the world. In the United States the northeastern region has the highest and the south central region the lowest prevalence caries scores. Intermediate prevalence rates prevail over most of the midwest, the far west and southeastern coastal areas.

Investigators have pointed out the relationship between depleted soil areas and caries prevalence. Similar comparisons have been made in respect to abundance of sunshine, higher temperatures, hardness of water and greater distance from the sea coast. These factors are correlated with lower caries scores. The trace elements selenium, molybdenum, vanadium and fluorine have been studied for their effect on caries. Selenium shows some direct correlation with caries resistance, but fluorine is the only element associated with an unequivocal caries reduction.

Further study will perhaps reveal other essential elements that can be associated with reduced dental caries experience.

DENTAL CARIES IN THE MILITARY

The dental caries status of young adult males has been derived mainly from examination of inductees into the armed services.

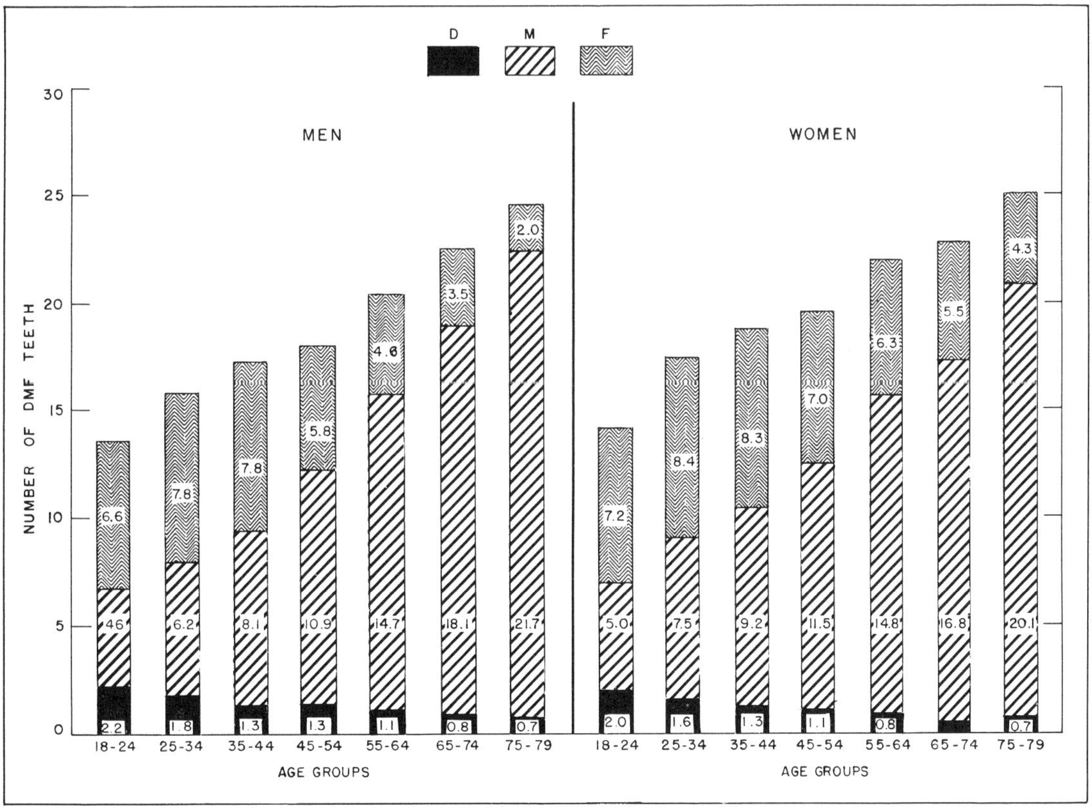

Figure 3–9 Mean number of decayed, missing and filled teeth among dentulous men and women by age group. (From U.S. Department of Health, Education and Welfare Public Health Service: *Decayed, Missing, and Filled Teeth in Adults—United States—1960–1962.* Public Health Service Publication No. 1000, Series 11, No. 23, Washington, D.C.: Superintendent of Documents, February 1967.)

Naval recruits numbering over 2000 were found to have an average of 13.6 DF teeth and 22.5 DF surfaces. Of the 25.6 remaining teeth per individual (excluding third molars), approximately seven were carious and six restored. Of the total DF surfaces, 12.5 were carious and 10 restored.

It is a sad commentary on the dental treatment received by young adults to realize that there were more unfilled than restored teeth in this group.

In 1962, a National Health Survey conducted among the adult population of the United States revealed pertinent facts about the unsatisfactory condition of the teeth or lack of teeth. With advancing age, the adult group exhibited a consistent increase to a total of approximately 25 DMF teeth.

There was a gradual decline in the number of DF teeth since many of the teeth lost through periodontal disease were either carious or restored previous to their loss (Figure 3–9).

Considering all age, sex and racial groups, there were 17.9 DMF teeth per person: 1.4 decayed, 9.4 missing and 7.0 filled. Of the total filled teeth, 90 per cent occurred in only half of the population. Half of the number of carious teeth occurred in one-tenth of the population. Females had higher DMF scores than males and whites higher than blacks. Although the number of edentulous individuals at 75 years of age increased to just under 40 per cent, the number of edentulous persons did not alter the differential between race, sex and age.

CONCLUSION

The magnitude of the dental caries problem is well expressed by the statistics presented in this chapter. With the realization that the number of unfilled teeth in the United States approximates one billion, the enormity of the task of reducing this chronic situation becomes exceedingly important. It is only through an understanding of the problem that there is hope of arriving at a satisfactory solution.

REFERENCES

1. Adler, P.: Correlation between dental caries prevalences at different ages. Caries Res. *2*:79, 1968.
2. American Dental Association: Proceedings of the conference on the clinical testing of cariostatic agents, October 14–16, 1968.
3. Backer-Dirks, O. B.: The distribution of caries resistance in relation to tooth surfaces. *In* Wolstenholme, G. E. W., and O'Connor, M. (eds.): Caries Resistant Teeth. Boston, Little, Brown and Company, 1965, pp.66–85.
4. Baume, L. J., Caries prevalence and caries intensity among 12,344 schoolchildren of French Polynesia. Arch. Oral Biol. *14*(2), February 1969.
5. Blayney, J. R., and Hill, I. N.: Fluorine and dental caries. J. Am. Dent. Assoc. *74*:223, 1967.
6. Dunning, J. M.: Incidence and distribution of dental caries in the United States. Dent. Clin. N. Amer. *6*:291, July, 1962.
7. Finn, S. B.: Prevalence of dental caries. *In* A Survey of the Literature of Dental Caries. Washington, D.C.: National Academy of Sciences–National Research Council, 1952, pp. 117–173.
8. Gisclard, L. F., and Lavergne, J.: Étude Odontologique de Quelques Sites de Prehistoire Recente. Actualites Odonto-Stomat *24*:391–406, 1970.
9. Glass, R. L., Becker, H. M., and Shiere, F. R.: Caries incidence in human primary teeth during the period of the mixed dentition. Arch. Oral Biol. *15*:1007, 1970.
10. Hennon, D. K., Stookey, G. K., and Muhler, J. C.: Prevalence and distribution of dental caries in preschool children. J. Am. Dent. Assoc. *79*:1405–1414, 1969.
11. Hill, I. N., Blayney, J. R., Zimmerman, S. O., and Johnson, D. E.: Deciduous teeth and future caries experience. J. Am. Dent. Assoc. *74*:430, 1967.
12. Jackson, D., and Burch, P. R. J.: Dental caries: Distribution, by age-group between homologous (right-left) mesial and distal surfaces of human permanent maxillary incisors. Arch. Oral Biol. *15*:1059, 1970.
13. Katz, S.: Socio-economic factors and dental caries frequency. J. Indiana State Dent. Assoc. *60*:57, 1967.
14. Knutson, J. W.: Epidemiological trend pattern of dental caries prevalence data. J. Am. Dent. Assoc. *57*:821, 1958.
15. Knutson, J. W., and Klein, H.: Studies of dental caries, Part IV: Tooth mortality in elementary school children, Public Health Rep. (Wash.) *58*: 1701, 1938.
16. Littleton, N. W., Kakehashi, S., and Fitzgerald, R. J.: Study of differences in the occurrence of dental caries in Caucasian and Negro Children. J. Dent. Res. *49*:742, 1970.
17. Ludwig, T. G., and Bibby, B. G.: Geographic variations in the prevalence of dental caries in the United States of America. Caries Res. *3*:32, 1969.
18. McCauley, H. B., and Frazier, T. M.: Dental caries and dental care needs in Baltimore school children (1955). J. Dent. Res. *36*:546, August 1957.

19. McPhail, C. W. B., and Grainger, R. M.: A mapping procedure for the geographic pathology of dental caries. Int. Dent. J. *19*:380, 1969.
20. Miller, J., Hobson, P., and Gaskell, T. J.: The effect on the onset of human fissure caries of the early or late eruption of teeth and the presence of an opponent tooth. Arch. Oral Biol. *13*:661, 1968.
21. National Health Statistic Centre, Department of Health: Dental health status of the New Zealand population in late adolescence and young adulthood. Wellington, New Zealand, 1968.
22. Parfitt, G. J.: The speed of development of the carious cavity. Brit. Dent. J. *100*:204, 1956.
23. Porter, D. R., and Dudman, J. A.: Assessment of dental caries increments— I. Construction of the R.I.D. index. J. Dent. Res. *39*:1056, 1960.
24. Rosenzweig, K. A.: Tooth form as a distinguishing trait between sexes and human population. J. Dent. Res. *49*:1423, 1970.
25. Rovelstad, G. H., Irons, R. P., McGonnell, J. P., Hackman, R. C., and Collevecchio, E. J.: Survey of dental health of the naval recruit. I. Status of dental health. J. Am. Dent. Assoc. *58*:60, 1969.
26. Toth, K.: The Epidemiology of Dental Caries in Hungary, Budapest, Akademiai Kiado, 1970.
27. U. S. Department of Health, Education and Welfare Public Health Service: Decayed, Missing, and Filled Teeth in Adults—United States—1960–1962. Public Health Service Publication No. 1000, Series 11, No. 23, Washington, D.C.: Superintendent of Documents, February 1967.
28. Volker, J. F., and Caldwell, R. C.: The epidemiology of dental caries. *In* Finn, S. B. (ed.): Clinical Pedodontics. 3rd Ed. Philadelphia, W. B. Saunders Co. 1967, pp. 610–653.
29. Williams, E. J., Donnelly C. J., and Fulton, J. T.: An appraisal of the necessity for radiographs in clinical trials of caries-inhibitory agents. J. Public Health *27*:54, 1967.

chapter 4

ETIOLOGY OF DENTAL CARIES*

by

ERNEST NEWBRUN, D.M.D., PH.D.**

INTRODUCTION

Dental caries or tooth decay is a pathological process of localized destruction of tooth tissues by microorganisms (Latin *caries:* rottenness). It is something of a paradox that teeth can be destroyed relatively rapidly *in vivo* and yet are relatively indestructible *post mortem.* A few cases of caries have been found in prehistoric fossils of teeth of dinosaurs, reptiles and early mammals. Caries appears to have accompanied true man (*Homo sapiens*) from the outset of his advent in Palaeolithic times, the incidence increasing during the Neolithic period. Records have been found concerning dental problems of ancient Asia, Africa and America, the earliest being the wall paintings of the Cro-Magnon period (22,000 years ago). In order better to understand the current concepts of the etiology of caries, earlier theories will be considered briefly.

EARLY THEORIES OF CARIES ETIOLOGY

WORMS

An Assyrian legend of the seventh century B.C. ascribed toothache to the worm which drank the blood of the teeth and fed on the roots of the jaws. The idea that caries is caused by a worm was almost universal at one time, being found in the writings of Homer, and is evident also in the popular lore of China, India, Finland and Scotland, to mention only a few instances. Shakespeare alludes to it in *Much Ado About Nothing* (Act III, Scene 2, Line 20). Benedick, complaining of a toothache, is rebuked by his friends:

> What! Sigh for the tooth-ache?
> Where is but a humour or a worm?

*The survey of literature pertaining to this chapter was completed in September, 1971 and revised in April, 1973.

**The author is indebted to many colleagues who have given permission to use figures from original publications and have commented on portions of the manuscript. In particular, the valuable suggestions and constructive criticism of Professor Dr. K. G. König and Professor Dr. B. Guggenheim are deeply appreciated.

At least at the subconscious level this theory survives to our own day when we refer to a toothache as a "gnawing pain."

HUMORS

The ancient Greeks considered that a person's physical and mental constitution was determined by the relative proportions of the four elemental fluids of the body—blood, phlegm, black bile and yellow bile. All diseases, including caries, could be explained by an imbalance of these humors. Hippocrates, while accepting the prevailing Greek philosophy, drew attention to the stagnation of food, suggesting that both local and systemic factors were related to the cause of caries. Aristotle, an astute observer, noticed that soft, sweet figs adhered to the teeth, putrified and produced damage.

VITAL THEORY

The vital theory regarded dental caries as originating within the tooth itself, analogous to bone gangrene. This theory, proposed at the end of the eighteenth century, remained dominant until the middle of the nineteenth century. Clinically, a type of caries with extensive penetration involving the dentine and even the pulp, yet with a barely detectable catch in the fissure, is well known. It is not so surprising, therefore, that the vital theory attracted many supporters.

CHEMICAL THEORY

Parmly (1819) revolted against the then current vital theory and proposed an unidentified "chymical agent" was responsible for caries. He stated that caries began on the enamel surface in locations where food putrified and acquired sufficient dissolving power to produce the disease chemically. Support for the chemical theory came from Robertson (1835) and Regnart (1838), who actually carried out experiments with different dilutions of inorganic acids—sulfuric and nitric—which were found to corrode enamel and dentine.

PARASITIC OR SEPTIC THEORY

In 1843 Erdl described filamentous parasites in the "surface membrane" (plaque?) of teeth. Shortly thereafter, Ficinus, a Dresden physician, observed filamentous microorganisms, which he called *denticolae,* in material taken from carious cavities. He implied that these bacteria were the cause of caries decomposing first the enamel, then the dentine. Neither Erdl nor Ficinus explained exactly how organisms destroyed tooth structure.

CHEMO-PARASITIC THEORY

The chemo-parasitic theory is a blending of the above two theories because it states that caries is caused by the production of acids by microorganisms of the mouth. It has been customary to credit this theory to W. D. Miller (1890), who by his writings and experiments did much to establish this concept on a firm basis. However, Miller owes much to the observations of his predecessors and contemporaries. Pasteur had discovered that microorganisms transform sugars to lactic acid in the process of fermentation. Another Frenchman, Emil Magitot (1867), demonstrated *in vitro* that fermentation of sugars caused dissolution of tooth mineral. Artificial lesions similar to caries were produced in sound adult teeth covered by wax leaving only a small opening and exposing the teeth for an extended period to dilute acids or fermenting mixtures. Magitot also opposed the vital theory on the basis that caries occurred in natural teeth when used in artificial dentures.

Leber and Rottenstein (1867), working in Berlin, presented additional experimental evidence implicating acids (which made enamel porous) and bacteria as the causative agents of caries. They described a specific microorganism, *Leptothrix buccalis,* in tubules of carious dentine and thought it responsible for enlarging the tubules and facilitating the rapid penetration of acids. Micrococci, oval and round-shaped bacteria were found in histological sections of carious dentin by Underwood and Milles (1881). They considered caries absolutely dependent on the presence of organisms which "create an acid which removes the lime salt."

The most profound effect on the thinking about caries etiology and subsequent caries research came from the work of an American, Willoughby D. Miller (1883–1904), at the University of Berlin. Miller learned the methods of isolating, staining and identifying bacteria in the laboratories of Koch. In a series of experiments Miller demonstrated the following:

1. Different kinds of foods (bread, sugar, but not meat) mixed with saliva and incubated at 37° C could decalcify the entire crown of a tooth.

2. Several types of mouth bacteria (at least 30 species were isolated) could produce enough acid to be of significance in dental caries.

3. Lactic acid was an identifiable product in carbohydrate-saliva incubation mixtures.

4. Different microorganisms (filamentous, long and short bacilli and micrococci) invade carious dentine.

Miller wrote: "Dental decay is a chemo-parasitic process consisting of two stages—*decalcification* or softening of the tissues and dissolution of the softened residue. In the case of enamel, however, the second stage is practically wanting, the decalcification of enamel signifying its total destruction." Miller concluded that no single species of microorganism caused caries but rather that the process was mediated by any oral microorganism capable of acid production and protein digestion.

Further weight was added to the chemo-parasitic theory by Williams (1897), who demonstrated dental plaque on the enamel surface. Plaque was considered to be a means of localizing organic acids, formed by microorganisms, in contact with the tooth surface and preventing dilution and neutralization by the saliva.

PROTEOLYTIC THEORY

The classical chemo-parasitic theory has not been accepted universally. Instead it has been proposed that the organic or protein elements are the initial pathway of invasion by microorganisms. Mature enamel is more highly mineralized than any other vertebrate tissue and in the human tooth contains only about 0.5 to two per cent organic material of which 0.3 to 0.4 per cent is protein. According to the proteolytic theory, it is the organic component which is most vulnerable, being attacked by hydrolytic enzymes of microorganisms. This precedes loss of the inorganic phase.

Gottlieb (1944) maintained that the initial action was due to proteolytic enzymes attacking the lamellae, rod sheaths, tufts and walls of the dentinal tubules. He suggested that a coccus, probably *Staphylococcus pyogenes*, was involved because of the yellow pigmentation which he considered pathognomonic of dental caries. According to Gottlieb, acid action alone produces chalky enamel but not true caries. Gottlieb's ideas were based on the observations of histological specimens and on the similarity between carious enamel and enamel whose organic components were stained with silver nitrate. There has been no bacteriological confirmation of his proposal linking caries with *Staph. pyogenes*.

Frisbie (1944) also described caries as a proteolytic process involving depolymerization and liquefaction of the organic matrix of enamel. The less soluble inorganic salts could then be freed from their "organic bond," favoring their solution by acidogenic bacteria which secondarily penetrate along widening paths of ingress.

Pincus (1949) contended that proteolytic organisms first attacked the protein elements such as the dental cuticle and then destroyed the prism sheaths. The loosened prisms would then fall out mechanically. He also suggested that sulfatases of gram-negative bacilli hydrolysed "mucoitin sulfate" of enamel or chondroitin sulfate of dentine, producing sulfuric acid. The released sulfuric acid could combine with the calcium of the mineral phase. It should be noted that the composition of the organic components of enamel do not resemble those of connective tissue and an abundance of sulfated polysaccharides has not been demonstrated. Pincus' theory remains, therefore, without experimental support.

PROTEOLYSIS CHELATION THEORY

A chelate results from a combination of an inorganic metal ion with at least two electron-rich functional groups in a single organic molecule. The chelating agent is a molecule capable of seizing and holding a metal ion in a clawlike grip (Greek *chele:* claw), forming a heterocyclic ring. The atoms holding the metal ion are called *ligands* and are usually oxygen, nitrogen or sulfur. In biology there are many well-known chelates, including hemoglobin (containing iron), chlorophyll (containing magnesium), vitamin B-12 (containing cobalt) and the enzyme cytochrome oxidase (containing both iron and copper) and carboxypeptidase A (containing zinc).

Examples of chelate structures involving lactate or citrate and calcium are shown in Figure 4–1. The calcium is held covalently by two oxygens of the carboxyl groups and in a coordinate covalent bond involving the unshared electrons of the alcohol group. Citrate can effectively form

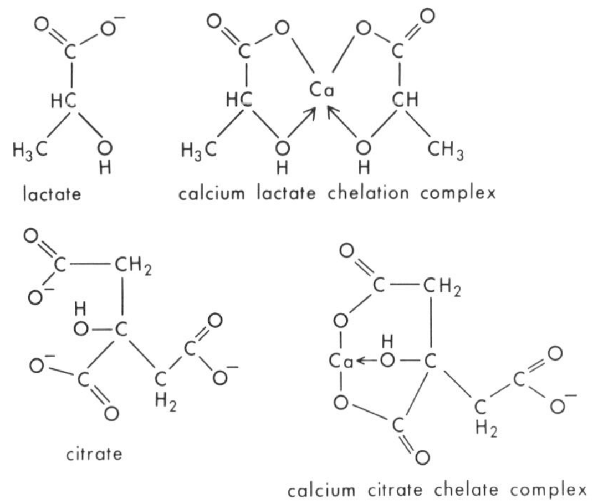

Figure 4–1 The formulae of lactate and citrate and of the calcium chelate compounds which they form. Note the difference between the covalent bonds from the carboxyl groups and the coordinate covalent bonds involving the unshared electrons of the alcohol groups (indicated by arrows).

chelates of calcium and may be important for the physiological mobilization of calcium from the skeleton and transport of complexed calcium to the serum. By comparison, lactate is of negligible importance as an organic chelator of calcium.[117] Of course this does not rule out the role of lactate in acid decalcification.

Chelation has been proposed as an explanation for tooth decay whereby the inorganic components of enamel can be removed at neutral or alkaline pH.[113] The proteolysis-chelation theory considers dental caries to be a bacterial destruction of teeth where the initial attack is essentially on organic components of enamel. The breakdown products of this organic matter have chelating properties and thereby dissolve the enamel minerals. There is thus a simultaneous demolition of both the organic and inorganic constituents.

According to this theory, decalcification is mediated by a variety of complexing agents such as acid anions, amines, amino acids, peptides, polyphosphates or carbohydrate derivatives. These substances arise as microbial breakdown products of either the organic components of enamel and dentine or of food which is ingested and diffuses through the plaque. Oral keratinolytic bacteria are thought to be involved in the process, and possible differences in keratin of children with high caries and low caries experience are considered important. It should be noted that only a small fraction of the protein of enamel bears any resemblance to the keratin of hair.

Schatz and Martin,[135] in challenging the chemo-parasitic theory and advocating proteolysis-chelation, even go so far as to say that acid may prevent tooth decay by interfering with growth and activity of proteolytic bacteria. They suggest that acid protects the enamel organic matter.

The validity of the proteolytic-chelation theory has been seriously questioned[5, 79] primarily because of the lack of experimental supporting data.

Solutions of the sodium salts of various amino acids (alanine, aspartate, glutamate) and lactate at or near neutral pH can increase the uptake of radioactive phosphorus by enamel[114] or loss of calcium from enamel.[126] This has been interpreted as evidence of demineralization occurring at neutral pH. Mörch *et al.*[114] have proposed a caries hypothesis whereby demineralization is initiated by acid dissolution during a low pH phase and continued by complex forming agents while the plaque is neutral.

OTHER THEORIES OF CARIES

Numerous experiments on rodents have demonstrated the potential of phosphate salts to retard dental caries. It is not surprising, therefore, that several theories have been proposed dealing with the role of phosphate in the caries process. Luoma[107] showed that inorganic phosphate, using radioactive phosphorus, is taken up by plaque bacteria during the metabolism of carbohydrates, the phosphate being required for phosphorylation of sugars and for polyphosphates for storing energy. It has been postulated that a steady state equilibrium prevails between the inorganic phosphate of saliva and the mineral phase of enamel. According to the phosphate sequestration theory,[45] as bacteria take up phosphate inorganic phosphate must be removed from enamel. However, *in vivo* there is a continual flow of saliva containing soluble inorganic phosphates which are more readily available to bacteria than the insoluble mineral phase of enamel, provided the saliva can diffuse into the bacteria.

Alternative explanations consider caries as a nutritional deficiency caused either by insufficient phosphate intake[1] or an improper dietary calcium to phosphate ratio.[141] Neither of these latter explanations has adequate statistical or experimental support and they remain primarily conjectural.

Recently, bacterial alkaline phosphatase was found to release phosphate from enamel *in vitro*. It was speculated that this enzyme could participate in caries destruction[101] by acting on phosphoproteins of enamel. A commercial enzyme preparation obtained by ammonium sulfate precipitation was utilized, but it was subsequently observed that ammonium sulfate itself can release phosphate from teeth.[108] Another difficulty with this theory is that the alkaline phosphatase of the bacteria is an intracellular enzyme, therefore the cells would have to lyse to free the enzyme.

EVALUATION OF THE VARIOUS THEORIES OF CARIES

CHEMO-PARASITIC THEORY

There is no doubt that acids are involved in the carious process. A fall in pH has been demonstrated both within carious lesions and in plaque following a rinse with a suitable substrate for bacterial fermentation. Stephan[142] showed, by inserting fine antimony electrodes into plaque on the smooth surface of anterior teeth, that within two to four minutes of rinsing with glucose or sucrose solution there was a fall in pH of from about 6.5 to about five and only a gradual return (up to 40 minutes) to the original pH. More recently, by using telemetry and a miniature glass electrode pH sensor built into a removable appliance, it has been possible to obtain continuous and direct measurements of the pH of interproximal plaques *in situ* at the tooth-plaque interface.[65] These studies indicate that the presence of acid at the tooth plaque interface may be longer-lasting (up to two hours) than observed by Stephan. The recorded pH drop and its duration is influenced by (1) the amount of interdental plaque, (2) the predominant flora,[32] (3) the rate of salivary flow, and (4) the substrate, both type and concentration.

Using specific chromatographic techniques, a variety of organic acids have been identified in dental plaque, in cultures of bacteria isolated from plaque and in carious lesions. The acids detected include lactic, acetic, propionic, formic and butyric; however, the relative concentrations of these acids may vary. This is to be expected, knowing that plaque harbors a mixed bac-

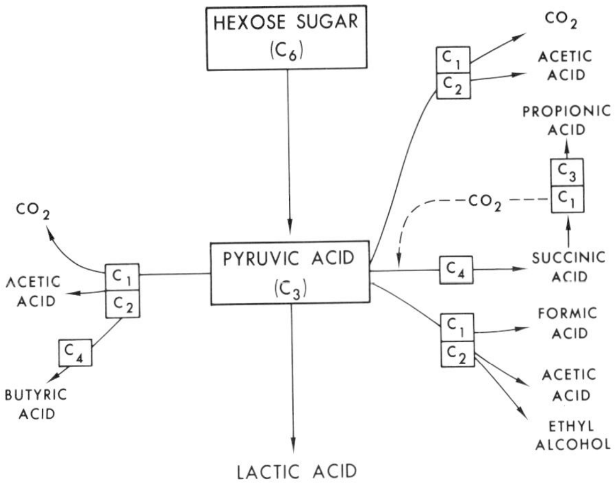

Figure 4–2 Simplified pathway showing how various end-products are derived from hexose sugars in different bacterial fermentations of the glycolytic type.

terial population of homo- and heterolactic fermentative microorganisms, as well as mixed acid fermentative microorganisms, which differ in their fermentative capabilities. Not only are the proportions of these organisms in a dynamic state of flux, but the relative proportions of their end-products are not constant and are influenced by such variables as pH, substrate type and concentration, and oxygen tension.

The pathways whereby the different acid end-products derived from hexose sugars are formed by bacteria are shown in Figure 4–2. Intermediate steps and other end-products have been omitted for simplification. Glycolysis of one six-carbon sugar (C_6) yields two molecules of pyruvate (C_3). In the case of homofermentative lactic acid formers, about 90 per cent of the pyruvic acid is converted to lactic acid with much smaller amounts of the other acids, carbon dioxide and ethyl alcohol. The caries-inducing *Strep. mutans* falls in this category;[153] under aerobic conditions the greater part of glucose is metabolized by way of the Embden-Meyerhoff pathway and a smaller part via the hexose monophosphate shunt. Under anaerobic conditions glucose is mainly metabolized to lactate by the Embden-Meyerhoff pathway.[161] Some of the non-cariogenic oral streptococci do not differ in their fermentation end-products or in the amounts of acids produced[40, 81] (Table 4–1).

Lactobacilli, which numerically are relatively minor components of plaque, are either homofermentative or heterofermentative, the latter forming less than 90 per cent lactic acid and more acetic and other acids. *Neisseria* and *Veillonella*, gram-negative cocci found in plaque, on the other hand, accomplish a propionic acid fermentation.

Most studies have used pure strains of organisms and very little is known about the biochemical capabilities of dental plaque *per se*. According to one report on plaque grown *in vitro*, it was found that the concentration of lactic acid was similar to or less than that of either acetic or propionic acids.[64] Plaques differ inherently in their fermentation, indicating that there are numerical disparities in their content of biochemical types of organisms.

TABLE 4–1 END-PRODUCTS OF GLUCOSE METABOLISM BY RAT STREPTOCOCCI

	mM/100 mM Glucose Used	
	*Strain FAI**	*Strain JR8LG†*
Lactate	181.09	184.54
Acetate	9.18	9.52
CO_2	8.31	10.96
Ethanol	2.77	5.75
Formate	3.42	4.52
Acetoin	.60	.20
Diacetyl	.01	.01
Glycerol	0	0
% glucose utilized	44.17	52.63
% carbon recovered	96.98	100.08

*Caries active
†Caries inactive

Interest in the qualitative and quantitative production of acids is more than merely academic. Table 4–2 shows the dissociation constants of some of these acid end-products, and it can be readily seen that there are significant differences in the amount of available hydrogen ions (i.e., resulting pH). Lactic acid is a much stronger acid than acetic or propionic acid at the same concentration. Accordingly, one would predict that it would be clinically more effective in enamel demineralization.

Formation of propionic acid can occur by a complex pathway involving carbon dioxide fixation, oxaloacetate (C_4) and succinate intermediates by a partial tricarboxylic acid cycle (Fig. 5–2). Lactic acid formed by homofermenters can be dissimilated to the weaker acetic and propionic acids. To what extent this plays a role in altering the plaque pH is not known.

These findings of acid formation by microorganisms using modern sophisticated methods confirm and support the conclusions of the early investigators who first enunciated the Chemo-Parasitic Theory.

PROTEOLYTIC THEORY

The proponents of this idea were primarily histologists and, as such, based their case on the observation of microorganisms within the lamellae or prism sheaths of enamel. However, it is a dangerous trap to interpret biochemical events on the basis of histopathological specimens. There is no doubt that organisms do invade the enamel and can be found in structures of relatively higher organic content, but this neither explains their metabolism nor how they got there. It has been found that gnotobiotic rats inoculated with a single strain of a non-proteolytic streptococcus developed extensive cavitation. The infecting streptococcus could not hydrolyse gelatin, casein, collagen or chondroitin. Although proteolysis of the organic matrix of dentine may indeed occur, probably after decalcification, there is no satisfactory evidence to support the claim that the *initial attack* on enamel is proteolytic. In fact, the gnotobiotic studies show that caries can occur without the presence of highly proteolytic organisms. Furthermore, chemical analysis of early carious enamel lesions shows a rise in nitrogen content and a fall in specific gravity indicative of a persistence or increase in organic matter.

TABLE 4–2 DISSOCIATION CONSTANTS OF ORGANIC ACIDS FOUND IN PLAQUE*

Acid	*Constant for the First Hydrogen*	*pK*[1]
Lactic	74.1×10^{-5}	3.13
Formic	17.6×10^{-5}	3.75
Succinic	6.4×10^{-5}	4.19
Butyric	2.0×10^{-5}	4.70
Acetic	1.8×10^{-5}	4.75
Propionic	1.3×10^{-5}	4.89

*Acids are arranged in decreasing order of available hydrogen ions, at 25°C in aqueous solution.[127]

PROTEOLYSIS-CHELATION THEORY

The weaknesses and strengths of this theory are as follows. Proteolysis is not an important step in the carious process and carious lesions and plaque are acid in the presence of suitable substrate. Chelation, on the other hand, is a widespread biological process and amino acids, citrate and lactate, capable of chelate formation, are present in the saliva and plaque. Whether these chelators are present in sufficient quantities and what proportion of calcium is removed as an ionic salt versus a calcium chelate complex is by no means clear.

CURRENT CONCEPTS OF CARIES ETIOLOGY

Dental caries is a multifactorial disease in which there is an interplay of three principal factors, namely the host (particularly the saliva and teeth), the microflora and their substrate (i.e., the diet). In addition, a fourth dimension, time, must be considered in any discussion of the etiology of caries. These parameters will be examined for the role each plays in the caries

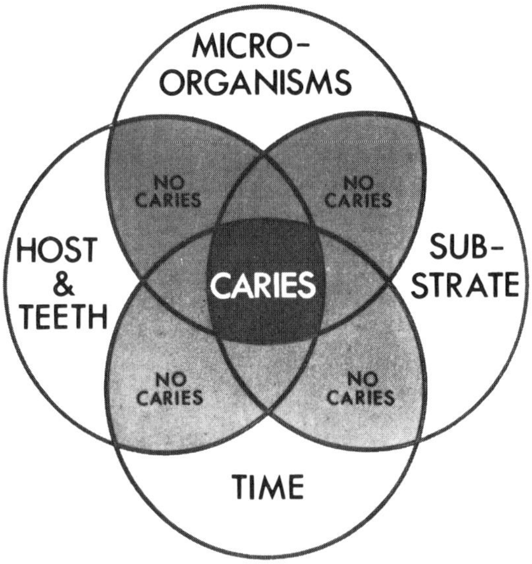

Figure 4–3 The four circles diagrammatically represent the parameters involved in the carious process. All four factors must be acting concurrently (overlapping of the circles) for caries to occur.

process. Diagrammatically, they can be portrayed as four overlapping circles; for caries to occur, conditions in each parameter must be favorable (Fig. 4–3). In other words, caries requires a susceptible host, a cariogenic oral flora, and a suitable substrate which must be present for a sufficient length of time. Conversely, caries prevention is based upon attempts to (1) increase the resistance of the host, (2) lower the numbers of microorganisms in contact with the tooth (plaque control), (3) modify the substrate by selecting noncariogenic foodstuffs, and (4) reduce the time substrate is available in the mouth by limiting the frequency of intake.

Before considering these four factors in some detail, a brief discussion of the clinically observed speed of carious lesion formation is included.

TIME FACTORS IN CARIES DEVELOPMENT

SPEED OF LESION FORMATION

Caries is widely considered to be a chronic disease in man, a lesion developing over a period of months or years. Estimates on the speed at which an incipient lesion (diagnosed by "a catch of the probe") develops into a clinical cavity indicate a wide variation from child to child. The average time of progress through stage of incipient to clinical caries is 18± six months. These conclusions were based on a 5-year longitudinal survey of institutional children presumably using normal oral hygiene.[125] Children residing in institutions generally eat more regular meals and have less opportunity for between-meal eating than other children. Caries progression may be even more rapid.

In the absence of oral hygiene procedures, and by deliberately rinsing nine times a day with a sucrose solution, the caries process can be greatly accelerated. Such frequency of sucrose exposure is not far-fetched; children living at home may actually ingest sucrose-containing foods and beverages this often. By microscopic observations *in vivo*, new lesions ranging from hardly recognizable changes in the optical properties of the enamel to grayish-white spots have been demonstrated in the course of three weeks in humans on such a regimen.[49] Furthermore, these incipient changes can be reversed upon reinstitution of good oral hygiene practice and regular applications of fluoride.

In patients with xerostomia following radiation therapy, total carious destruction of teeth has been observed in as short a time as two months.

Careful epidemiological observation on longitudinal rates and patterns of caries incidence on a large group of children has revealed that all teeth exhibit surprisingly similar patterns of annual attack curves (Fig. 4–4). In general, the annual probability of caries attack reaches a peak two to four years following eruption and declines thereafter, possibly reflecting a post-eruptive "maturation" of the enamel surface.[20] The two-year time interval between eruption and maximum caries incidence is related to the time required for detectable lesions to develop. It also suggests that studies on the effectiveness of any therapeutic procedure in caries pre-

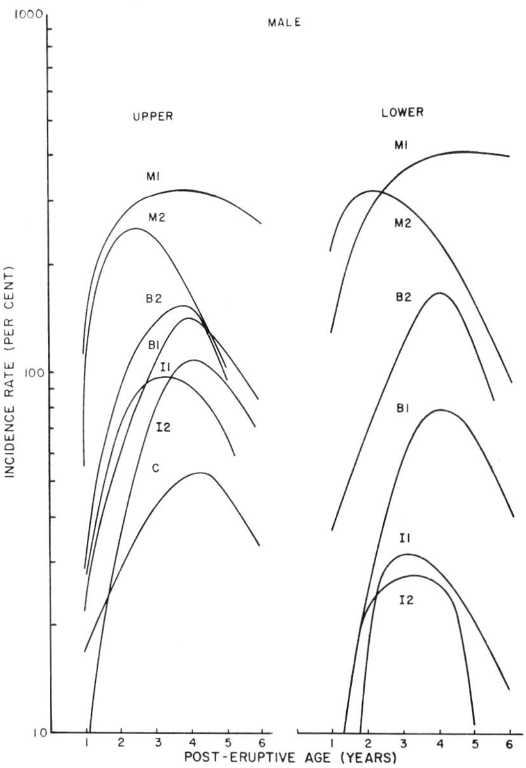

Figure 4–4 Curves showing annual probability of caries attack of the permanent teeth, male children, Kingston, New York. Semilogarithmic scale. M2 = second molars, M1 = first molars, B2 = second premolars, B1 = first premolars, C = canines, I2 = lateral incisors, I1 = central incisors. (Courtesy of Drs. Carlos and Gittelsohn, Arch. Oral Biol., 1965.)

vention must extend over a minimum of a two-year time period.

FREQUENCY OF EATING AND CARIES FORMATION

Undoubtedly the most informative experiment on caries in humans was the classical Vipeholm Dental Caries Study.[73] The main purpose of the investigation was to determine the effect of frequency and quantity of sugar (sucrose) intake on the caries activity. Some of these findings will be discussed in a subsequent section under Diet and Caries. However, the important point to note is that greater caries activity correlated with the longer presence of sugar in the mouth. Of course, the caries activity also depended on the frequency of sugar intake. The Vipeholm study used institutionalized patients so that the composition of the diet and the eating schedule were well controlled. Base line data on a standard diet established the initial caries activity to be low. In those groups which ate sweets in the form of toffee or caramel between meals, a striking increase (up to tenfold) in caries activity occurred.

A survey of the dietary habits of preschool children (average age 5¾) indicates that between-meal items consumed, such as gum, candy, pastries, soft drinks and ice cream, are of high sugar content.[159] A direct and consistent relationship has been disclosed between the between-meal eating frequency and the caries prevalence in the children.

Of course it is much easier to regulate time factors in the diet when using experimental animals. For example, Stephan[143] compared the caries score produced by a high-sugar diet fed to rats twice a day for one hour to the score of animals permitted *ad libitum* feeding (Table 4–3). The differences in caries score are convincing. More elegantly controlled feeding techniques are now available using a programmed feeding machine.[95] The device consists of a circular tray with 18 food cups. A plastic tube leads from each cage to the tray, one cup being accessible at a time. Stepwise movement of the tray is controlled by an endless computer punch card with the 24-hour feeding program kept in motion by a synchronous motor. This machine imposes eating patterns of widely different frequencies on the rats. There is a consistent increase in the average caries incidence with increased frequency of the programmed meals when tested on a particular stock of rats. Moreover, the highly significant positive correlation between frequency of eating and caries incidence is found not only on a sucrose diet but also on a bread (from wheat flour) diet. Of course the caries activity is much lower on the bread diet.[90]

TABLE 4–3 RELATIONSHIP OF CARIES INCIDENCE TO FREQUENCY OF EATING IN RATS FED A CARIOGENIC DIET

FEEDING FREQUENCY	AVAILABILITY OF FOOD (HR)	MEAN CARIES SCORE	STANDARD ERROR	REFERENCE
2	2	11.3	2.03	Stephan[143]
Ad libitum	24	63.0	12.37	
	MEAN DURATION OF EATING (HR)	MEAN FISSURE LESIONS	STANDARD DEVIATION	
12	1	0.7	0.8	König[95]
18	1.5	2.2	0.8	
24	2	4.7	2.4	
30	2.5	4.7	2.3	
Ad libitum	6.25	4.2	4.3	

HOST FACTORS: SALIVA

TERMINOLOGY

In the following discussion, the term "saliva" is used to refer to the mixture of secretions in the oral cavity. This mixture consists of fluids derived not only from the major salivary glands (parotid, submandibular, sublingual) and minor glands of the oral mucosa, but also from the gingival fluid exudate. This latter is not a glandular secretion. Accordingly, it has been proposed that the term "oral fluid," which is more encompassing, be substituted for "saliva." Unless stated otherwise, "saliva" is used synonymously with "oral fluid."

EFFECT OF DESALIVATION ON ANIMAL CARIES

There is no doubt that saliva significantly influences the carious process, as evidenced by animal experiments in which the salivary glands are surgically extirpated.[50] Control hamsters with intact salivary glands developed relatively few carious lesions, whereas desalivated hamsters on an identical diet containing 66 per cent sucrose developed more than five times as many carious teeth and much more extensive lesions (Table 4–4).

These experiments have since been reproduced in several laboratories. It is only fair to point out that such a drastic procedure as salivary gland removal will affect a number of other factors, besides just the saliva, which in themselves influence caries development. These factors include:

1. Differences in food and water consumption.
2. Longer eating time—the animals modify their eating habits to compensate for the lack of saliva.
3. Greater food retention.
4. Possible alterations in the bacterial flora of the mouth.
5. Maturation of the enamel.

It should be noted that in desalivated ani-

TABLE 4–4 EFFECT OF DESALIVATION ON HAMSTER CARIES[50]

GROUP	NUMBER OF HAMSTERS	AVERAGE NUMBER OF CARIOUS TEETH	AVERAGE CARIES SCORE
Intact Salivary glands	20	2.3	4.0
Desalivated*	10	10.5	39.0

*Parotid, submandibular and sublingual glands.

mals a cariogenic substrate is still required for caries to occur. Low carbohydrate or carbohydrate-free diets will not produce caries in these animals, again indicating the multifactorial nature of the carious process.

DECREASED SALIVARY FLOW AND CARIES IN HUMANS

An increase in dental caries and rapid tooth destruction has been reported in humans suffering from decreased, or lack of, salivary secretion. Xerostomia may be the consequence of a variety of different pathological conditions in man such as:

1. Sialolithiasis—a blockage of the salivary duct by calculus.
2. Sarcoidosis which may involve reduced salivary gland function.[4]
3. Sjögren's syndrome—consisting of xerostomia, xerophthalmia and usually a connective tissue disease.
4. Mikulicz's disease—a benign swelling of salivary and lachrymal glands, with histopathology similar to that of Sjögren's syndrome.
5. X-ray irradiation of oral-naso-pharyngeal region—the salivary gland epithelial cells being more sensitive than the surrounding connective tissues.
6. Surgical removal of salivary gland tumors: benign—mixed tumor; malignant—mucoepidermoid carcinoma, adenocystic carcinoma.
7. Iatrogenic—for example, long-term therapy with anticholinergic or atropine-like drugs in the treatment of Parkinson's disease, peptic ulcer and gastrointestinal disorders. Many commonly used "tranquilizers" have atropine-like side effects.
8. Diabetes—a frequent complaint is dryness of the mouth.
9. Post-menopausal women sometimes present with symptoms of xerostomia.

In some of the conditions listed above, the decreased salivary flow has been quantitatively demonstrated; in others it is only a clinical impression. Increased caries associated with xerostomia in cases of Sjögren's syndrome, or following prolonged medication with salivary depressant drugs, has been reported.[144] Rampant caries has been well documented in a number of patients following radiation therapy of the mouth,[57] whether the teeth were inside or outside the field of radiation. The important factor in all patients having such lesions was that the salivary glands had been irradiated and the quantity of saliva greatly reduced. Often the caries is atypical—mostly of cementum and dentin so that the crown is almost amputated.

Under conditions of xerostomia alterations in both the amount and bacteriological composition of plaque are to be expected, and these in turn may be responsible for the increased caries activity.

Not only in pathological states, but also normally during sleep, salivary secretion is virtually absent.[136] This emphasizes the utmost importance of scrupulous oral hygiene and plaque removal before bedtime as part of a comprehensive caries prevention program, for during sleep the protective effect of the saliva is minimal.

SALIVARY COMPOSITION AND CARIES

The above-mentioned findings have led to the conclusion that saliva in some way is necessary for maintaining the integrity of the teeth. Identification of the specific constituents of the saliva which might be involved in protecting against or limiting the caries attack has remained frustratingly elusive. Many physical, chemical and biological characteristics of saliva have, at one time or another, been implicated as playing an important role. The findings to date have been contradictory, with some investigators claiming a relationship between caries prevalence and salivary amylase, urea, ammonia, calcium, phosphate, pH, etc., and others finding no relationship. A major problem in studying the composition of saliva is that it will vary with flow rate, nature of stimulation, duration of stimulation, plasma composition, the time of day at which samples are collected, and the serial dependency of saliva samples, i.e., the effect of previous stimulation on the composition of saliva collected subsequently.[38, 104] Unfortunately, in many salivary studies these variables have not been adequately controlled. In other instances the assay methods were inadequate (e.g., some of the amylase measurements were based on the time required to reach the achromatic point) or the treatment of the data was inadmissible (e.g., the arithmetic averaging of pH which is a logarithmic function). Another difficulty in interpreting results of studies on salivary composition is that saliva is a mixture of the secretions from the three pairs of major salivary glands with contributions from numerous minor mucous glands. The secretion of each type of gland has a unique composition; for example, the secretion of the submandibular salivary glands (6.8 mg calcium/100 ml) contains about 50 per cent more calcium than that of the parotid glands (4.1 mg calcium/100 ml).[118] Such regional differences may in part account for the observed relative immunity of the lower anterior teeth to caries and their higher frequency of calculus.

Reviewing currently available information (Table 4–5), there is no consistent relationship between dental caries prevalence and salivary amylase, ammonia, urea, calcium, phosphate, pH or viscosity.

There is some evidence for an inverse relationship between salivary flow rate and caries; however, the literature is conflicting on this point. The flow rate itself influences the salivary Na^+/HCO_3^- ratio; at higher flow rate there is an increased buffer capacity. The best-established relationship between salivary factors and caries is its buffer capacity (see Ericsson[46, 47]).

TABLE 4–5 RELATIONSHIP BETWEEN SALIVARY CHARACTERISTICS AND CARIES PREVALENCE

PROPERTY	RELATIONSHIP	PROPERTY	RELATIONSHIP
Flow rate	±	pH	–
		Ca	–
Buffer capacity	+	PO_4	–
		NH_3	–
		Amylase	–
		Viscosity	–
		Urea	–

Positive Relation = +
Some Relation = ±
No Relation = –

SALIVARY BUFFERS

A buffer is a solution which tends to maintain a constant pH. A graph of the pH versus equivalent of acid or alkali added to a buffer is the titration curve and the pK marks the point on the curve at which the pH changes the least. This occurs when the concentrations of conjugated base and conjugate acid are equal. In saliva the chief buffer systems are bicarbonate-carbonic acid (HCO_3^-/H_2CO_3, $pK_1 = 6.1$) and phosphate ($HPO_4^=/H_2PO_4^-$, $pK_2 = 6.8$). The bicarbonate is by far the most important salivary buffer because:

1. It can buffer rapidly by losing carbon dioxide (cf. with blood).
2. Its pK is nearer that encountered in plaque, and therefore it is more effective in that range.
3. As the flow rate increases the bicarbonate concentration increases dramatically (as does Na^+), whereas there is a slight fall in phosphate with increased flow rate.
4. After removal of bicarbonate by a current of CO_2-free air at pH 5, the buffering capacity of saliva is markedly reduced.

Dialysis of saliva which removes both bicarbonate and phosphate, but not protein, results in total loss of salivary buffering capacity. This indicates that salivary proteins can be disregarded as buffers in saliva.[80]

Urea is continuously secreted in saliva. Plaque microorganisms can convert urea to non-urea nitrogenous products and ammonia. The ammonia thus formed can also serve as a buffer.

In a longitudinal study of caries increments, a fall in buffer capacity preceded by about 9 months the highest peak in caries increment.[110]

Further evidence of the importance of saliva as a buffer has emerged from studies of the pH of carious lesions and of dental plaque. Within active carious lesions (dentine), a pH gradient exists. The deep-advancing edges of such lesions are more acid than the shallower layers, which are closer to the pH of the saliva. In enlarged and exposed cavities which are emptied of their contents, the carious layer is shallower and more alkaline, probably because of the better access to saliva.[39]

It will be recalled that the plaque pH falls to between pH 4 to 5 following a rinse with a suitable substrate and after a period of time returns to the original "resting" level in the range of pH 6 to 7 (see Evaluation of Various Theories of Caries—Chemo-Parasitic Theory). Recent studies on plaque pH in hamsters infected with *Strep. mutans* have given further insight into the reasons for a return of plaque pH to resting values.[31, 32] When the plaque was exposed to a low concentration of sucrose (2.5 per cent), the pH dropped and after a short while started to rise. However, if the plaque and tooth were isolated with a parafilm cup, the plaque pH decreased further and continued to remain low. In view of the prolonged high levels of acid found when the plaque was isolated, it is presumed that the reversion of pH toward neutrality was due to gradual diffusion of saliva into those areas, coupled with exhaustion of substrate and diffusion out of acid end-products.

ANTIBACTERIAL FACTORS OF GLANDULAR ORIGIN

These include:

1. Lysozyme
2. Peroxidase system
3. Immunoglobulins

Lysozyme

Lysozyme (N-acetylmuramide glycanohydrolase: EC 3.2.1.17) is a hydrolytic enzyme which cleaves the β-1→4 linkage between N-acetylglucosamine and N-acetylmuramic acid which constitute the repeating units of the cell-wall polysaccharides of certain bacteria. Certain organisms such as *Micrococcus lysodeikticus* are rapidly destroyed by the action of this enzyme, others more slowly, and some are resistant to lysozyme action. In 1922 Fleming discovered lysozyme in nasal secretion. This enzyme is also found in saliva, tears, egg white and most tissues and body fluids. There are higher levels of lysozyme in sublingual and submandibular saliva than in parotid saliva.[77] Pure cultures of the predominant cultivable bacteria present in the oral cavity of man are not lysed by lysozyme alone nor prevented from growing by this enzyme.[63] In the presence of a detergent, sodium lauryl sulfate, lysozyme can lyse many cariogenic and noncariogenic streptococci. When lysozyme (from egg white) was added to a cariogenic diet, no cariostatic effect could be found in experimental rats.[94, 116, 150] Although lysozyme may not be effective specifically against cariogenic microorganisms, it probably influences the ecological balance of the oral flora.

Lactoperoxidase

Lactoperoxidase (donor: hydrogen peroxide oxidoreductase EC 1.11.1.7) is a hemoprotein enzyme requiring thiocyanate ions as a cofactor. Thiocyanate has a marked stabilizing effect on lactoperoxidase. It catalyzes the following reaction:

$$\text{peroxidase} + H_2O_2 \rightarrow \text{compound}$$
$$\text{(possibly a ferric peroxide)}$$
$$\text{compound} + AH_2 \text{ (hydrogen donor)} \rightarrow$$
$$\text{peroxidase} + H_2O + A$$

It is active in the absence of an extraneous source of peroxide, against microorganisms which accumulate peroxide—for example, *Lactobacillus acidophilus* and *Streptococcus cremoris.* The system appears to operate by preventing accumulation by the cells of lysine and glutamic acid, both of which are essential for growth.[33] Peroxidase activity has been demonstrated in human saliva by a number of workers. It is present in both submandibular and parotid secretions;[88] in the latter it has been separated into three fractions each of which inhibits the growth of *Lactobacillus casei.*

Pig lactoperoxidase-thiocyanate, when added to pure cultures of strains of *Strep. mutans*, inhibits their growth.[115] Further investigation is necessary to determine whether this enzyme can control cariogenic bacteria *in vivo*. The evidence suggestive of peroxidase involvement in an antibacterial system in saliva is substantial.[140] However, no significant differences in peroxidase levels in parotid or submandibular secretions have been found between caries-resistant and caries-susceptible subjects.[162]

Immunoglobulins and Immunization

Immunoglobulins are specific antibody proteins. The major immunoglobulin in saliva is IgA, which differs from serum IgA by containing an additional glycopeptide, referred to as the "secretory component," SC,[11,13] the origin of SC is the glandular secretory epithelium. The IgA immunoglobulins are synthesized by immunocytes (plasma or mast cells) in the salivary glands, whereas IgG and IgM may be, at least in part, derived from the corresponding serum counterpart; evidence has been presented for both mechanisms. Antibacterial antibodies in unfractionated human saliva have been reported by several investigators.[48,100,156] Salivary IgA adsorbs onto oral bacteria *in vivo*, and the result may be formation of extremely long chains of growing streptococci or enhancement of bacterial phagocytosis.[12] Agglutinating activity against oral isolates of α-hemolytic streptococci, but not *Escherichia coli*, has been found using purified salivary IgA and IgG fractions.[139] IgA antibodies frequently predominate in external secretions. There is increasing evidence that this system may represent a defense mechanism against superficial infections of mucous membranes; antibodies present in serum may play little role in such local infections. IgA isolated from human oral parotid secretion specifically inhibits the adherence of streptococcal strains to human buccal epithelial cells.[159a]

In one study, parotid saliva of 80 per cent of the children examined was reported to have antibodies to the cell wall antigens of cariogenic streptococci. The children with little or no evidence of past or present caries experience had high parotid antibody titers.[76] Another study found no significant differences in parotid salivary IgA levels of caries-resistant and caries-susceptible subjects. Significantly higher IgA levels were found in the submandibular saliva of the caries-resistant persons.[162]

The presence and the titer of serum antibodies to *Strep. mutans* and *Strep. sanguis* increase with age from early infancy to 16 years.[2] This might be expected from the observation[28] that neither *Strep. mutans* nor *Strep. sanguis* become established in the mouth until the teeth have emerged into the oral cavity.

Serum-antibody levels for two strains (HS-6 and FA-1) of *Strep. mutans* were significantly higher in a caries-free group than in a caries-rampant group of young naval recruits.[87] On the other hand, the serum antibody titer to two of seven types of cariogenic streptococci tested and one type of lactobacillus was reported to be higher in subjects with high DMF scores compared to those with a low DMF score.[103] No correlation could be established between caries activity and levels of serum antibody against three strains of *Strep. mutans* and one of *Strep. sanguis*.[2] These anomalous results (inverse, direct and no relationship between caries activity and serum antibody titer) may be due to the techniques employed. *Strep. mutans* strains have several different antigens, one of which forms the specific antigen for identification. The other antigens may also be found in other streptococci (e.g., *Strep. sanguis* and *Strep. salivarius*) which are not caries-inducing. Antibodies against these antigens will react with both *Strep. mutans* and the other bacteria. Such "unwanted" reactions cannot be separated from specific reactions by the agglutination techniques commonly used.

There have been several attempts to prevent caries in experimental animals immunized by repeated injections of cariogenic bacteria. The immunized animals develop high serum levels of antibodies specifically against these bacteria. One study, using gnotobiotic rats infected with a pure culture of *Strep. faecalis*, reported depressed cariogenic activity in immunized rats.[158] It was hypothesized that the caries control of the etiological agent in the oral cavity was via the antibodies secreted in the saliva. A limited study, using three monkeys vaccinated with a dextran-forming streptococcus isolated from human caries, found fewer carious lesions in the vaccinated monkeys than control unvaccinated monkeys.[9] These results were interpreted as encouraging "the belief that vaccination may provide a means of preventing dental caries." Specific pathogen-free rats, when immunized against *Strep. mutans*, developed high levels of antibody in the blood as expected and also developed antibody in the saliva. Such immunized rats were at least partly protected against caries associated with *Strep. mutans*, but the protection was quite variable.[152a]

Other studies using conventional rats, however, found no protection against caries in immunized compared to unimmunized rats.[1a, 70, 152] It should be recognized that immunization raises the serum antibody titers but that plaque bacteria are really outside the body membranes and therefore cannot be attacked by circulating internal antibodies. Furthermore, in these experiments the animals were immunized against only one strain of *Strep. mutans* or glucosyltransferase from one strain. It is now recognized that there are at least five identifiable antigenic groups of *Strep. mutans*,[14] and immunization against only one antigenic group could not be expected to suffice in a situation of mixed oral flora.

The analogy of the pneumococci is relevant. Pneumonococci have been classified into over eighty different types. Using pneumococcal capsular polysaccharide immunization, animals can be protected against pneumococcal infection. However, each polysaccharide antigen has proved effective only against infection with the type of pneumococcus from which it was obtained. Secretory immunoglobulin (IgA) formation against an antigen injected locally has been demonstrated. Rats have been immunized, using vaccine prepared from *Strep. mutans*, by repeated injections in the vicinity of each parotid and submandibular gland. Rats immunized in this fashion produced salivary IgA which agglutinated *Strep. mutans*. These animals had fewer *Strep. mutans* colonies on their teeth and significantly less caries than unimmunized rats.[154a, b]

The question of caries prevention by specific immunization has not been finally answered. We do not yet know how to stimulate formation of local secretory antibodies in human salivary glands. Nor do we know which antibodies are "anticariogenic," those against the cell wall antigens, those against the glucosyltransferase enzymes, or those against some unidentified factors.

Saliva plays an extremely important role in attenuating the caries attack. In part this can be explained simply by the mechanical washing away of some of the food debris, bacteria and their soluble products. Certainly the buffering action of saliva should not be overlooked. Although several different antibacterial factors have been isolated and identified in the individual secretions, there is evidence of a loss of potency of salivary antibacterial activity in whole saliva. To what extent the antibacterial action of saliva contributes to caries prevention is not clear.

HOST FACTORS: TOOTH

TOOTH MORPHOLOGY AND ARCH FORM

A susceptible host, among other factors, is required for caries to occur. Tooth morphology has long been recognized as an important determinant. For example, attempts to induce caries in dogs have been unsuccessful mainly because of the wide spacing and the conical shape of their teeth.

In humans it is known, on the basis of clinical observation, that the pit and fissure areas of the posterior teeth are highly susceptible to caries. Food debris and microorganisms readily impact in the fissures. Investigations of the cusp height and fissure depth have shown a relationship between caries susceptibility and the depth of the fissure.

Irregularities in arch form, crowding and overlapping of the teeth also favor the development of carious lesions. Experimentally this has been verified by the gold plate technique whereby stagnation areas are deliberately created on selected tooth surfaces. These surfaces develop "white spot" lesions within a few weeks, the white appearance being due to optical phenomena associated with increased enamel porosity.

TOOTH COMPOSITION

There is good evidence to indicate that the enamel surface is more caries-resistant than the subsurface. Microradiographs of initial carious lesions frequently reveal marked demineralization of the subsurface enamel beneath an outermost layer which is only slightly affected.[121] Surface enamel is harder than the underlying enamel.[122] These differences are likely to be related to the many differences between the composition of the surface and the rest of the enamel.[15] The enamel surface is more mineralized and has more organic matter but has relatively less water. In addition, certain elements, including fluoride, chloride, zinc, lead and iron, accumulate in the enamel surface, while other constituents, such as carbonate and magnesium, are sparse in surface as compared with subsurface enamel. Changes, including a decrease in density and increase in nitrogen and fluoride content of the enamel, occur with age. These alterations are part of the posteruptive "maturation" process whereby teeth become more resistant to caries with time. The direct relationship between the fluoride content of the enamel surface and its resistance to caries attack is well established and is dealt with in more detail elsewhere.[120a]

MICROFLORA

EVIDENCE OF BACTERIAL ROLE IN CARIES ETIOLOGY

Though there are still some differences in opinion as to the exact mechanism whereby microorganisms produce carious lesions, it is virtually uniformly agreed that without microorganisms no caries can occur. The evidence implicating microorganisms in the etiology of caries is overwhelming. It can be summarized as follows:

1. Germ-free animals do not develop caries.
2. Antibiotics fed to animals are effective in reducing the incidence and severity of caries.
3. Unerupted teeth do not develop caries, yet these same teeth when exposed to the oral environment and microflora can become carious.
4. Oral bacteria can demineralize enamel and dentine *in vitro*, producing caries-like lesions.
5. Microorganisms have been demonstrated histologically invading carious enamel and dentine. They can be isolated and cultivated from carious lesions.

The classic germ-free animal studies of Orland *et al.*[123, 124] firmly established a principle that had been debated for more than a century, namely, that dental caries is a bacterial infection. These studies demonstrated that germ-free rats fed a highly cariogenic sucrose-containing diet do not develop caries. When the gnotobiotic rats on the same diet were infected with combinations of an enterococcus and a proteolytic bacillus or an enterococcus and a pleomorphic bacterium, caries developed. This marked a new epoch in caries research. Independent investigations in various laboratories have since confirmed that germ-free animals will not develop caries, whereas gnotobiotic animals when infected with one or more known pure cultures of microorganisms may develop caries.

The term gnotobiotic animal is used since etymologically it refers to an animal with a known microbiota (Greek *Gnosis:* positive knowledge). Gnotobiote includes both germfree animals and germ-free animals deliberately inoculated with one or more known types of microbes for experimental purposes. Organisms tested and found capable of inducing carious lesions when used as monocontaminants in gnotobiotic rats include *Strep. mutans* (several strains), a *Strep. salivarius* strain, *Strep. sanguis* (several strains), a *Lactobacillus acidophilus* strain, and a *Lactobacillus casei* strain.[54, 132] Using the same animal test system, several types of streptococci and lactobacilli were found incapable of inducing caries. These include *L. fermenti, L. acidophilus, Strep. lactis, Strep. faecalis, Strep. salivarius* and *Strep. sanguis*.[51, 52]

The significance of these findings are:

1. Caries will not occur in the complete absence of microorganisms.
2. Caries can occur in rats that harbor only a single type of organism.
3. Not all types of organisms are cariogenic.
4. Cariogenic organisms need not be proteolytic.

It is not known what determines the cariogenicity of a microorganism. The streptococci with cariogenic potential are a somewhat heterogeneous group of organisms. From the experiments on gnotobiotic rats, it is clear that neither all polysaccharide-forming organisms nor all acid-producing organisms are cariogenic.

There have been attempts to compare the relative cariogenic potency of streptococcal strains within a group known to induce caries. It is very difficult to show definitively innate differences in virulence between any type of pathogen. Large numbers of freshly isolated strains need to be studied before any concrete correlations between virulence and serology can be established.

LOCALIZATION OF THE ORAL FLORA RELATING TO CARIES

Careful evaluation of reports on caries in rodents indicates that different organisms display some selectivity for the tooth surface which they attack and suggests that there are at least three types of processes involved:

1. Organisms which are active in fissures only, with no, or minimal, smooth surface involvement (Table 4–6).
2. The plaque-forming organisms (usually *Streptococcus mutans*) which are essential to the development of lesions on the smooth surfaces and frequently are also active in the sulci.
3. The plaque-forming organisms (e.g., diphtheroids and other gram-positive filamentous bacteria) which usually locate in the gingival crevice area and can initiate cervical type carious lesions in cementum and dentine as well as alveolar bone resorption.

One is obliged to use caution in the extrapolation of findings in the monoinfected gnotobiotic rat model system to naturally occurring caries in humans.

TABLE 4–6 ORAL MICROORGANISMS PRODUCING PRIMARILY FISSURE LESIONS WITH MINIMAL SMOOTH SURFACE INVOLVEMENT IN GNOTOBIOTIC RATS

SPECIES	STRAIN	SOURCE	REFERENCE
Unidentified streptococcus			Fitzgerald[55]
Resembling *Strep. mutans*	PK1 LM7	Fissure lesions from humans with high DMF	Gibbons[59]
Lactobacillus acidophilus	108T	Caries active rats	Fitzgerald[54]
Lactobacillus casei	ATCC 4646	Human carious lesion	Rosen[132]
Strep. salivarius	1A	Human plaque	Kelstrup[86]
Strep. mutans	BHT	Human carious detritus	Duany[41]
Unidentified Streptococcus	D65 D182	Human dento-alveolar abscess	Blackmore[6]

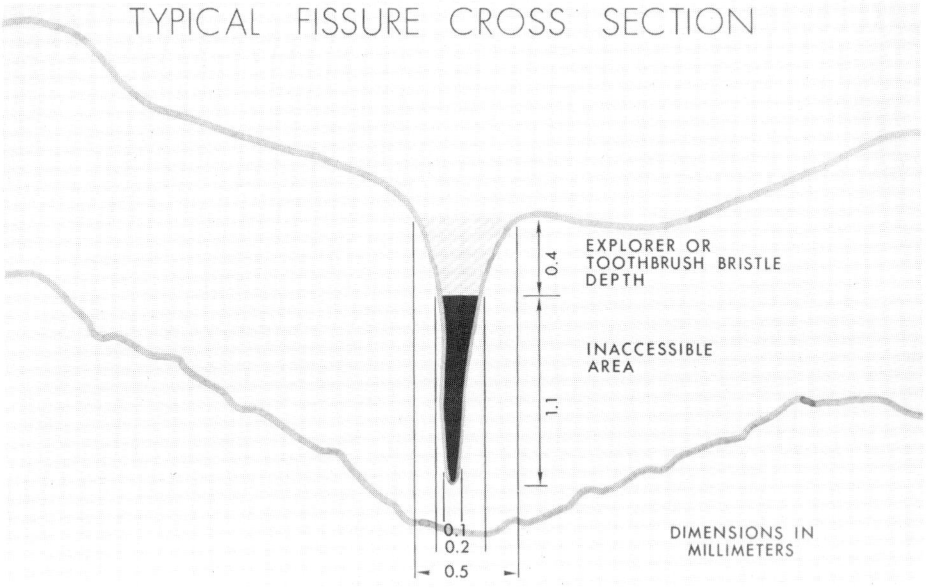

Figure 4–5 Cross-section of an occlusal fissure showing the inability of an explorer or toothbrush bristle to reach the base.

Observations on humans in recent years, however, have generally confirmed the findings in animals. Very little is known about the microbiology of fissure lesions in humans, primarily because of the difficulty of sampling from the base of fissures (Fig. 4–5).

An attempt has been made to follow bacterial colonization using mylar strips acting as "artificial fissures." These strips are inserted into specially designed inlays and may be removed for bacterial sampling or histological preparation.[106] Cultures from such artificial fissures reveal cocci as constituting 75–95 per cent of the microorganisms. *Strep. sanguis* are the predominant viable organism. Lactobacilli are low in early fissure plaque, but increase with time.[155] Mylar strips do not exactly duplicate enamel-pellicle surfaces, and such factors may be of importance in favoring the colonization of specific organisms.

In the case of smooth-surface lesions, *Strep. mutans* has been isolated in high numbers and with high frequency from plaque over human carious lesions. This will be discussed in more detail later. The organisms involved in root caries may be in a different category because the initial lesion involves cementum and dentine, not enamel. Bacteriological sampling of softened human dentine from the depths of such lesions has yielded mainly streptococci and filamentous bacteria. Some of the filamentous bacteria have been identified as *Actinomyces naeslundii* and *Actinomyces viscosus* and another group called *Rothia dentocariosa*.[84, 84a]

TRANSMISSIBILITY OF THE CARIOGENIC FLORA

The specificity of the cariogenic flora has been demonstrated by animal experiments, clearly fulfilling one of Koch's postulates that the infectious agent should be able to produce the disease when transmitted to another animal.[56, 89, 123, 124]

The oral cavity is a highly contaminated field and early attempts at inoculation of organisms thought to be cariogenic gave equivocal results. It is recognized that in an adult animal it may be necessary to depress the existing oral flora with an antibiotic before the establishment of cariogenic microorganisms can take place. Newborn animals do not require antibiotic suppression and, if caged with infected adult animals, transmission of the cariogenic flora will take place. Alternatively, a caries-inducing flora can be transmitted by inoculating young animals with fecal or plaque material from the caries-active animals or with pure cultures of cariogenic organisms.

Evidence of transmission of a specific cariogenic organism is readily apparent in gnotobiotic animals. In conventional animals, however, further proof is necessary to distinguish the infecting or "transmitted" organisms from the existing flora, which may appear to be similar. This has been demonstrated by using "tagged" or "labeled" mutants of microorganisms which have been made resistant to an antibiotic and reisolating these mutants from the infected host animals. Some investigators have also used the technique of fluorescent antibodies prepared against a specific cariogenic strain to show that successful transmission of the cariogenic strain has occurred.

Implantation of *Strep. mutans* in human mouths has been attempted. Recovery of the "labeled" organisms was variable and they were gradually lost over an extended period of time.[82, 98] The failure of the labeled strains to become established in human plaques in high numbers for prolonged periods in these studies is not surprising, as adult subjects were used and their existing oral flora was not suppressed with antibiotics.

BACTERIAL INTERACTIONS

Although innumerable species of organisms have been isolated from the oral cavity, many occur as only transient inhabitants. The ecological balance established in the gingival crevice, the tooth surfaces and other regions in the mouth may depend on several factors, such as local supply of nutrients and adhesion of bacteria to pellicle or epithelial cells. The availability of essential bacterial nutrients is different in the gingival crevice, where there is a flow of gingival fluid exudate, from the situation in the occlusal fissures. There exists a preferential binding of specific microorganisms to the epithelial cells of the oral mucosa.[60, 104a] Once established, such organisms may either favor or hinder the accumulation of other types of organisms at the same site.

The normal oral flora of Osborne-Mendel rats will cause fissure caries. Under similar dietary conditions these rats develop an appreciably higher number of fissure lesions if infected with *Strep. mutans*. This can be considered as evidence of a symbiotic relationship between the indigenous flora and the superimposed cariogenic strain. Often, however, infecting animals with a combination of organisms may actually decrease the amount of caries observed. For example, if the normal flora is depressed and rats are infected with *Strep. mutans* or *Strep. mutans* together with three other organisms, a pronounced interaction between the inoculating organisms can occur (Table 4–7). The rats infected with *Strep. mutans* alone develop a much higher smooth-surface caries score than those infected in combination with the other organisms.[92] Smooth-surface caries is also reduced (Table 4–7) in gnotobiotic rats infected with *Strep. mutans* and Specific Pathogen Free (SPF) flora.

Similarly, a strain of veillonella when introduced with *Strep. mutans* into gnotobiotic rats appears to reduce the cariogenicity of *Strep. mutans* alone (König, personal communication). Veillonella will not ferment glucose or other carbohydrates,[129, 130] but growing cultures can utilize lactate to form the weaker propionic and acetic acids. This may explain the observed altered caries pattern of animals infected with veillonella in combination with *Strep. mutans*.

An interaction between the two dominant streptococcal groups found in plaque has been observed.[26] *Strep. sanguis* grows in a chemically defined medium free of p-aminobenzoic acid, while a strain of

TABLE 4-7 COMPARISON OF CARIES PRODUCED BY *STREP. MUTANS* ALONE OR IN COMBINATION WITH OTHER ORGANISMS

RAT SYSTEM	RELATIVE GNOTOBIOSIS* (ERYTHROMYCIN DEPRESSED)		GNOTOBIOTIC†	
Inoculation	*Strep. mutans*	*Strep. mutans* + Gram-negative rod + Gram-positive rod + Gram-positive coccus	*Strep. mutans*	*Strep. mutans* + SPF feces
Smooth surface caries score	24	8	14.3	5.0

*König[94]
†Van der Hoeven *et al.*[77b]

Strep. mutans does not grow in this medium. In a mixed culture of *Strep. sanguis* and *Strep. mutans* in the p-aminobenzoic acid-free medium both organisms will grow. Presumably, *Strep. sanguis* supplies the necessary growth factor to *Strep. mutans* so that the interaction would be characterized as a parasitism of *Strep. mutans* on *Strep. sanguis.*

Clinically, an apparent inverse relationship has been observed between *Strep. mutans* and *Strep. sanguis* isolated from plaque. When patients followed a strict carbohydrate-free diet, the percentage of *Strep. mutans* found in plaque decreased to a very low or undetectable level, whereas the percentage of *Strep. sanguis* rose significantly. On resuming a normal diet supplemented with sucrose, the percentage of *Strep. mutans* increased markedly and the percentage of *Strep. sanguis* returned to about the original level.[147]

Lactobacilli constitute a minor component of dental plaque. They are usually confined to sites on teeth where there are already clinically detectable carious lesions. Deep in the carious dentine lactobacilli—mostly *casei*—may constitute half of the recoverable flora (Edwardsson, personal communication). Such sites are known to provide an acidic milieu while fermentable carbohydrates are available and therefore selectively favor proliferation of aciduric lactobacilli. This represents another example of symbiotic bacterial interaction.

Bacteriocins are bactericidal substances, synthesized by certain bacterial strains, which are active against some strains of the same or closely related species, but not against unrelated species. Several types of bacteriocins have been detected from streptococci indigenous to the oral cavity.[85] These bacteriocins were all of low molecular weight and sensitive to proteolytic enzymes. Because of their susceptibility to proteolysis, it is not known how significant a role bacteriocins have in maintaining the intra-species stability of the mixed oral microbiota.

It is by no means clear what is involved in such bacterial interactions; such studies are still in their infancy. Careful reconstruction of the normal flora by introducing two or more strains in combination using the gnotobiotic system should further clarify the complex situation existing within the dental plaque.

BACTERIOLOGY OF DENTAL PLAQUE

In direct smears, the early plaque is dominated by cocci and rods, most of which are gram positive. With increasing age, the percentage of cocci in the plaque decreases rapidly and after seven days filaments and fusiforms constitute about 50 per cent of the organisms in plaque. In ecology this change is called *succession.*

On culture a more detailed picture can be obtained, although the same general trend is observed. Both in old and young plaque the streptococci are the predominant organisms. With time, there is a shift in the relative proportions, and in older plaques filamentous organisms, veillonella and corynebacteria form fairly large groups. Lactobacilli comprise less than 1 per cent of the plaque flora and cannot be isolated unless a selective medium is employed.

There is an orderly progression to the growth of dental plaque with shifts in the relative proportions of different microbial populations probably due to (1) redox potential and (2) adhesion between bacteria. One of the problems in identifying and culturing the microorganisms in plaque is that no single culture environment can be used to isolate the multiplicity of microbes that grow in plaque. Some organisms grow only in the absence of oxygen; others require both oxygen and carbon dioxide. Current attempts to increase the viable count recovery of organisms from human plaque samples are based on culturing under a variety of conditions.

Filamentous organisms have long been recognized in plaque and carious dentine. These oral filamentous organisms include *Leptothrix buccalis, Leptothrix dentium (Bacteronema matruchotti),* several Actinomyces species, *Rothia dentocariosus* and *Actinomyces viscosus.* Their role in the etiology of enamel caries has not been established. However, as mentioned previously, certain of these filamentous organisms may initiate root caries.

STREPTOCOCCI OF DENTAL PLAQUE

Irrespective of the age of the plaque and the previous diet, the predominant organisms are gram-positive cocci of the genus *Streptococcus.*[128] These streptococci have been divided into five monothetic groups based on their colonial morphology on mitis salivarius agar and cultural characteristics in sucrose by Carlsson[22] and four categories by Zinner and Jablon.[161]

Streptococcus sanguis

This is one of the predominant groups of streptococci colonizing on the teeth. Formerly it was called *Streptococcus s.b.e.* because of its involvement in subacute bacterial endocarditis. Certain strains within this group have been shown to be cariogenic in animals, but most strains are not. Caries from this strain occurs primarily in sulci and is significantly less than from *Strep. mutans,* which causes smooth-surface caries as well. *Strep. sanguis* grow as small zoogleal colonies, with a firm consistency and form extracellular polysaccharides in sucrose broth. On blood agar *Strep. sanguis* cause α (green) hemolysis. *Strep. sanguis* grown aerobically has relatively complex nutritional requirements for amino acids.[24] It is not clear how these requirements are met on the tooth surface as the dental pellicle is low in cysteine and methionine, both of which are needed by *Strep. sanguis,* but under anaerobic conditions its requirements may be simpler.

Streptococcus mutans

In 1924 Clarke isolated a streptococcus which predominated in many human carious lesions and which he named *Streptococcus mutans* because of the varying morpology. Subsequent studies of dental plaque by different investigators have confirmed the presence of varieties of *Strep. mutans* in plaque. It has further been shown that these specific streptococci almost invariably induce strong to moderate caries activity if implanted in suitable animal model systems (monkey, gerbil, rat or hamster).

Characteristics of this group of streptococci have been described.[42, 67] They are non-motile, catalase-negative, gram-positive cocci in short or medium chains. On mitis salivarius agar they grow as highly convex to pulvinate, the colony is opaque, the surface resembles frosted glass and hemolysis of blood agar may be β (clear) or γ (no change).

Colony morphology is very divergent depending on the culture medium. Although the most common morphology on solid media is that of rough colonies, smooth and mucoid variants are found in about 7 per cent of the samples. These *Strep. mutans* variants also possess caries-inducing properties and on reisolation

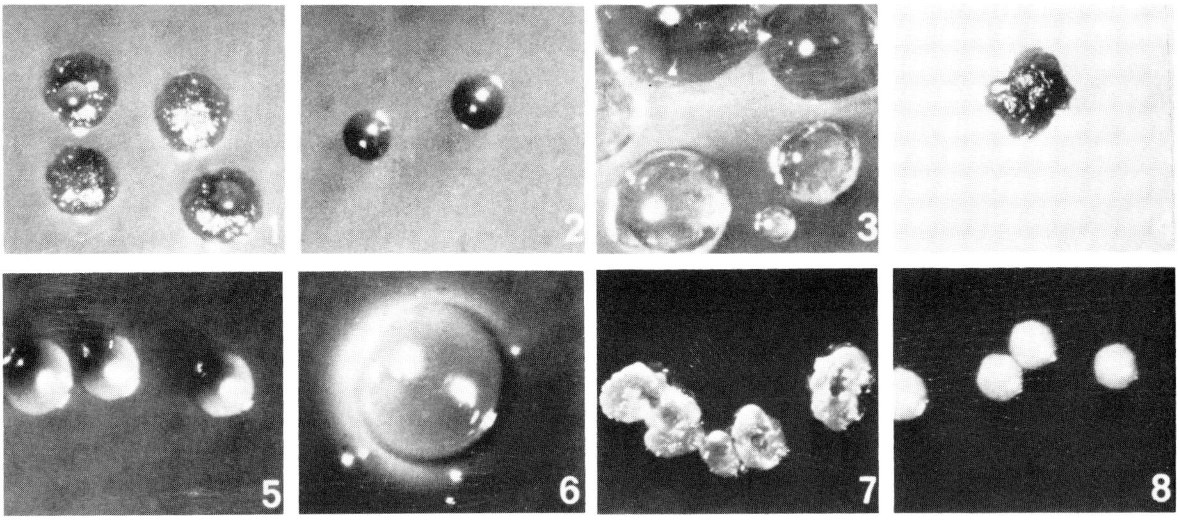

Figure 4–6 Appearance of different colonial variants of *Strep. mutans.* 1. rough; 2. smooth; 3. mucoid variants on Mitis salivarius agar incubated at 37° C for 24 hours in 95 per cent N_2 and 5 per cent CO_2 and 24 hours at room temperature; 4. rough; 5. smooth; 6. mucoid variants on MC-agar incubated 48 hours in 95 per cent N_2 and 5 per cent CO_2; 7. rough; 8. smooth variants on TYC-agar incubated 96 hours in 94 per cent H_2 and 6 per cent CO_2. (Courtesy of Dr. Edwardsson, Odontol. Revy, *21*:153–157, 1970.)

from infected animals may resume the original, rough, colonial form.[43] The appearance of *Strep. mutans* rough, smooth and mucoid variants grown on mitis salivarius agar, mitis salivarius agar with sulfonamide (MC-agar) or trypticase yeast sucrose agar (TYC-agar) is shown in Figure 4–6.

On culture with sucrose they form polysaccharides which are insoluble or can be precipitated with one part ethanol. This property of forming insoluble extracellular polysaccharides from sucrose is widely regarded as an important characteristic contributing to the caries-inducing properties of the *Strep. mutans.* When treated with a mutagenic agent, a strain of *Strep. mutans* lost its property to form sticky deposits on hard surfaces. On testing in gnotobiotic rats this mutant strain had virtually lost its cariogenicity in sharp contrast to the original *Strep. mutans* strain.[148]

Strep. mutans ferment mannitol and sorbitol. They are not as fastidious in their growth requirements as are most streptococci. Except for certain vitamin requirements, the organisms can use ammonia as the sole source of nitrogen. Carlsson[25] speculates that this gives *Strep. mutans* an ecological advantage. It appears to be well adapted for growth in the deepest parts of the microbial aggregations on the teeth, where the anaerobic environment and ammonia may be sufficient to permit survival without exogenous amino acids.

Unlike other oral streptococci, most strains of *Strep. mutans* can be cultured in the presence of noninhibitory (i.e., low) concentrations of sulfonamide. This property has been utilized as a basis for a selective culture medium for isolating *Strep. mutans.*[21] An even better selective medium is Mitis salivarius agar containing 20 per cent sucrose and 0.2 unit/ml. bacitracin. Colonies of *Strep. mutans* could be identified by the typical formazen red color which developed when sprayed with mannitol and tryphenyltetrazolium chloride.[64a]

Strep. mutans exhibit a triad of important properties, namely: (1) synthesis of insoluble polysaccharides from sucrose, (2) acid formation, and (3) implantability on tooth surfaces. However, these are not unique characteristics which can be correlated with cariogenicity. Nor is there any single physiological test that can be used for identification. In other words, mannitol fermentors and polysaccharide formers have been found among noncariogenic strains as well.[97] Furthermore, cariogenic and noncariogenic streptococci grown on glucose reveal no major differences in fermentation end-products or in amounts of acid produced.[40, 81] Compared to *Strep. sanguis*, *Strep. mutans* are more aciduric and can reproduce in a culture medium at a pH as low as 4.3.[145]

Strep. mutans forms a rather homogeneous group based on physiological and morphological characteristics,[22, 42, 67, 163] and has been recognized as a distinct species by the National Communicable Disease Center. However, analyses of the guanosine and cytosine content and hybridization studies on the homologies of the DNA isolated from strains of *Strep. mutans* revealed significant differences.[35, 36] These cariogenic organisms, though phenotypically similar, are genetically heterogeneous and can be further divided into four genetic groups. A detailed study of *Strep. mutans*, isolated by different investigators, separated 69 strains into five serological groups on the basis of specific antigens.[14] Fifty of the strains, including most of those isolated from human plaque or carious lesions, belonged to one serological group. On the basis of common strains, the serological[14] and genetic groups[36] are identical (Table 4–7a).

Dental plaque samples from 14 areas in 10 countries were analyzed with fluorescein-conjugated and absorbed antisera against five serological variants of *Strep. mutans*—groups a, b, c, d and e. The results show that *Strep. mutans* of groups c, d and e have a wide distribution, as they are found in all areas. The other two groups, a and b, were less frequently found. Fluorescein-conjugated antisera against *Strep. mutans* is prepared by repeated I.V. injections of antigens (washed, heated cells). These antisera against *Strep. mutans* react with not only *Strep. mutans* but also *Strep. sanguis*, *Strep. salivarius* and *Strep mitis*. Through absorption it is possible to prepare specific antisera against some of the different antigens of *Strep. mutans* (a, b and d). Plaque

TABLE 4–7A CLASSIFICATION OF STREPTOCOCCUS MUTANS

ORGANISMS *Strains*	CHARACTERISTICS	GROUPING SCHEMES *Coykendall* *DNA Hybridization*	*Bratthall* *Serology*
10449 GS5 JC2 Ingbritt	37–38% GC* Ferment mannitol sorbitol, raffinose. Produce no NH_3 from arginine, low pH in sucrose broth produced	S. *mutans* var. *clarke*	c
BHT FA-1	42–43% GC Ferment mannitol and sorbitol. Produce NH_3 from arginine	S. *mutans* var. *rattus*	b
AHT HS6 E49 OMZ61	43–44% GC Ferment mannitol and sorbitol. Fail to produce low pH in sucrose broth	S. *mutans* var. *cricetus*	a
SL1 KIR OMZ176 6715	44–45% GC Do not ferment raffinose; variable fermentation of mannitol and sorbitol	S. *mutans* var. *sobrinus*	d
LM7 At 10, B14	React with Lancefield group E, (*S. mutans*)	–	E

*GC = Guanidine plus cytosine.

samples are then studied by phase-contrast microscopy and fluorescence of a smear which has been reacted with the specific antisera.[14a]

Strep. mutans b antigen has been isolated and separated into two forms: a polysaccharide and a glycoprotein. Galactose composed about one third and galactosamine about 3 per cent of the total weight of each polymer. Rhamnose was a major component of the polysaccharide (47 per cent). The glycoprotein was about 40 per cent protein. The specificity of the antigen resides in binding sites which contain both D-galactose and D-galactosamine.[106a]

The accumulated evidence on the ecology of *Strep. mutans* and *Strep. sanguis* indicates that these streptococci can only survive in the mouth if solid surfaces such as teeth or dentures are present.[30] Microorganisms with a colonial morphology resembling *Strep. mutans* or *Strep. sanguis* were not detected in the mouths of newborn monkeys until teeth had erupted,[34] and the situation in infants' mouths is similar.[28] On the other hand, *Strep. salivarius,* whose preferable habitat is the tongue, establishes itself early in the mouth of the newborn.[27]

Studies of plaque from humans indicate that *Strep. mutans* is pandemic in many parts of the world.[61, 99, 134, 146] It has been isolated in surveys of populations of diverse ethnic and socio-economic background.[83] *Strep. mutans* is found in large numbers in the plaque isolated from caries-active populations and more frequently in plaque overlying carious lesions than in plaque from sound tooth surfaces.[77a, 105, 138] One report failed to detect *Strep. mutans* in buccal plaque of most subjects, although it was found regularly in deep carious lesions. It must be pointed out that, although several independent studies have found some relationship between dental caries and the occurrence in plaque of *Strep. mutans,* such observations do not prove the cariogenicity of these specific streptococci in human beings.

Streptococcus salivarius

These colonies grow as large, heaped-up, mucoid or gummy colonies on mitis salivarius agar. In sucrose broth they form a water-soluble polymer of fructose, known as levan. They have been found in the plaque, throat, nasopharynx and oral mucosa, but their favorite habitat is the dorsum of the tongue. They can be recovered from the mouths of infants shortly after birth. *Strep. salivarius* can colonize on the teeth of hamsters, resulting in moderate caries activity. In humans they have only a minor degree of cariogenic significance. On blood agar they cause no hemolysis (γ).

Streptococcus miteor

Strep. miteor is a heterogeneous species. On Mitis salivarius agar they form soft, circular, black-brown colonies. They do not form extracellular polysaccharides from sucrose but form intracellular polysaccharides which can be demonstrated by iodine staining. Intracellular polysaccharide synthesis is not unique for this group and is common to almost all carbohydrate-fermenting species found in plaque. On blood agar they cause a green (α) coloration on the plate. The proportion of this group of the total streptococci varies amongst subjects; however, they are found most regularly on the nonkeratinized mucosa, particularly the cheek, lip and ventral tongue surfaces.[104a]

Streptococcus Sp. Miscellaneous

Streptococci with colonial and physiological characteristics other than the previous groups are consistently found in dental plaque. In fact, many streptococci isolated from dental plaque cannot be strictly categorized.

We can summarize that *Strep. mutans* and *Strep. sanguis* preferentially grow on human teeth, i.e., in plaque, and *Strep. salivarius* on the tongue. It has been suggested that plaque-forming strains may evolve from non-plaque-forming strains by natural selection of the more adhesive extracellular polysaccharide-forming microorganisms.[154] Another proposed explanation is that these streptococci have the specific ability to utilize the absorbed glycoproteins on the tooth surface.[96] Gibbons and Spinnell[62] have reported that a high molecular weight fraction in submandibular saliva can cause oral microorganisms to stick together and that saliva-coated enamel particles can bind bacterial cells. Large differences in the degree of sorption and in the susceptibility to agglutination exist among the various oral microorganisms. The selectivity of this process may explain the relative presence or absence of various types of oral bacteria in the initial phase of plaque formation.

LACTOBACILLI AND CARIES

Lactobacilli, or organisms resembling lactobacilli, have been reported in the oral cavity ever since Miller enunciated the Chemo-Parasitic Theory (for a historical review see Burnett and Scherp[16]). In 1925 Bunting and his collaborators claimed that *Bacillus acidophilus* was the specific etiological factor responsible for the initiation of caries. Subsequent investigators have isolated other types of lactobacilli, besides *L. acidophilus,* in the saliva, plaque or carious lesions. The genus *Lactobacillus* includes many species, but the following are the most commonly encountered in the mouth:

Homofermentative	Heterofermentative
L. casei	*L. fermenti*
L. acidophilus	*L. brevis*
L. plantarum	*L. buchneri*
L. salivarius	*L. cellobiosus*

In isolates of lactobacilli from human carious dentine, the homofermentative outnumber the heterofermentative variety.[18, 138a]

The idea that lactobacilli played the major role in the carious process dominated dental literature for about 35 years. It was argued that lactobacilli are both acidogenic and aciduric and could therefore multiply in the low pH of plaque and carious lesions. Using selective culture media, there were indications that a count of lactobacilli present in the saliva could be correlated with the prevalence of dental caries. Furthermore, the growth site of lactobacilli was reported to correspond to sites of clinically diagnosed carious lesions. When such lesions were filled with dental restorations, most of the growth sites of the lactobacilli were removed.

Acceptance of the doctrine that lactobacilli were *the* etiological agents of dental caries was not universal, however. As more information on the microbial composition of dental plaque became available, it became manifest that lactobacilli constituted only a minor fraction (1/10,000) of the plaque flora.[58] The amount of acid which could be formed by the relatively small number of lactobacilli present in plaque is almost insignificant in comparison with that produced by other acidogenic oral organisms.[149] The heavier growth of lactobacilli at active caries lesions does not necessarily establish their causative role, although they could be secondary contributors to the carious process.[106b] An alternative explanation is that plaque conditions which are conducive to caries also favor colonization by lactobacilli. Fitzgerald[53] interprets such data to mean that lactobacilli are more a consequence than a cause of caries initiation.

Evidence implicating certain streptococci as the infectious and transmittable agent in dental caries of experimental animals has undermined the possible role of lactobacilli in the process. Even in gnotobiotic animals very few strains of lactobacilli could induce dental caries. In such cases, the lesions were restricted to the occlusal sulcal regions.

SUBSTRATE: DIET

INFLUENCE OF DIET ON THE CARIES PROCESS

Before discussing the role of diet, it is important that certain terminology be defined. Diet refers to the customary allowance of food and drink taken by any person from day to day. Thus the diet may exert an effect on caries locally in the mouth by reacting with the enamel surface and by serving as a substrate for cariogenic microorganisms. Nutrition concerns the assimilation of foods and their effect on metabolic processes of the body. Nutrition can act only through a systemic route and therefore influence the host during tooth development. It has not been conclusively shown that human teeth are more or less susceptible to caries if affected by various nutritional conditions in early life and before eruption, with the exception of fluoride.

Nutrition and oral disease are dealt with elsewhere, and this section will be restricted to a consideration of diet as it relates to caries.

Diet was suspected of influencing the etiology of caries since the time of the early Greek philosophers. But human volunteers do not subject themselves readily for extended periods (at least two to three years) to strictly controlled diets. Therefore, positive proof of the diet's role in caries in humans has been slow in coming. In an attempt to identify which foods may be particularly cariogenic, many studies have depended on information obtained from the patient's dietary history.[10, 109, 160, 164] A dietary history can be quite useful for purposes of patient education and motivation. However, the reliability and accuracy of such a history for measuring the contribution of diet to the caries prevalence is open to question. Above all, such studies usually lack scientifically acceptable control groups. Nevertheless, a certain pattern has emerged indicating that patients with rampant caries frequently include in their diet sucrose-containing foods so that sucrose has been indicted as "the arch criminal" in the etiology of caries.[119]

EPIDEMIOLOGICAL OBSERVATIONS OF CARIES AND DIET

Circumstantial evidence linking sucrose consumption and human caries prevalence can readily be found in several epidemiological surveys. In England, which depends exclusively on imports for its supply of sucrose, records : over the last hundred years steady increase in per capita sumption, from about 20 lb per year in 1820 to presently over 110 lbs. per capita per year. This represents between 15 to 20 per cent of the individual's caloric requirements. Concomitant with this increased sucrose consumption has been an almost parallel rise in the caries prevalence.[74] Conversely, surveys in Europe and Japan have demonstrated a dramatic reduction in caries accompanying periods of wartime food restrictions.[151, 157]

In Norway during World War II, the consumption of fish, vegetables, potatoes, cod liver oil and flour of high extraction increased, while there was a reduced consumption of fat, meat, flour of low extraction, sugar, syrup and all sugar products. The common feature in each of these countries was the severe rationing of sucrose. It has been proposed that the caries decrease during and after World War II was due to influences (nutritional) exerted during tooth formation rather than simply lack of sucrose substrate (dietary) locally for the oral flora. Marthaler[111] has pointed out that teeth which had already formed showed similar decreased caries as those still forming during 1941 to 1946. On the other hand, matrix formation and mineralization of first molars during periods of maximal sugar restriction did not endow these teeth with any unique caries resistance. In the postwar years, as rationing eased and sugar became more readily available, the caries rate rose again. These findings on the effects of wartime dietary restrictions indicate that the caries process can be influenced by diet.

CONTROLLED HUMAN STUDIES: VIPEHOLM

Vipeholm is a mental institution in southern Sweden. Adult patients were followed for several years on a nutritionally adequate diet and found to develop caries at a slow rate. Subsequently the patients were divided into nine groups to compare the effects of various modifications of carboydrate intake. Sucrose was included in the diet as toffees, chocolate, caramel, in the bread or in liquid form. Significant increase in the caries increment occurred if sucrose-containing foods were ingested between meals. It was further found that not only the frequency but also the form in which sucrose was ingested was important. Sticky or adhesive forms of sucrose-containing foods which can maintain high sugar levels in the mouth were more cariogenic than those forms which were rapidly cleared.[73]

CONTROLLED HUMAN STUDIES: HOPEWOOD HOUSE

Interesting findings on the effect of diet on dental caries have emerged from the study of institutionalized children at Hopewood House in Bowral, N.S.W., Australia. This was a children's home in the country founded in 1942 by a businessman who had recovered his own health by a drastic reorganization of his dietary habits. He had sufficient wealth to attempt to put his dietary theories into practice. Babies were either born at the home or taken into it in the first few weeks of life, gradually building up to a population of 80 children.

From the very beginning, sugar and other refined carbohydrates (e.g., white bread) were excluded from the children's diet. Carbohydrates were given in the form of whole-meal bread, soya beans, wheat germ, oats, rice, potatoes and some treacle and molasses. Dairy products, fruit, raw vegetables and nuts featured prominently in the typical menu. Although this was a vegetarian diet, it nevertheless provided an adequate amount of proteins, fats, minerals and vitamins.

Dental surveys of these children during the ages of five to 13 revealed an average of def and DMFT score of 1.1 or about 10 per cent of the caries prevalence in the general population of that age group. It should be noted that the water supply contained insufficient fluoride (0.1 ppm) and that the children's oral hygiene was poor; about 75 per cent of them suffered from gingivitis. It follows that caries can be reduced to a minimal level by dietary means alone in spite of unfavorable hygiene and fluoride levels. However, it must be recognized that this applies to an institutionalized population and is not valid for other situations. In fact, there is an important postscript to the Hopewood House study. As the children grew older they were relocated and no longer adhered to the original diet which had limited caries almost completely. A steep increase of DMFT experience occurred in the children above 13 years of age[75] corresponding to the deviation in the dietary habits (Fig. 4–7). This indicates that these teeth had not acquired any permanent resistance to caries. The reason that the teeth had not decayed during the prepuberty period was that the local oral environment was favor-

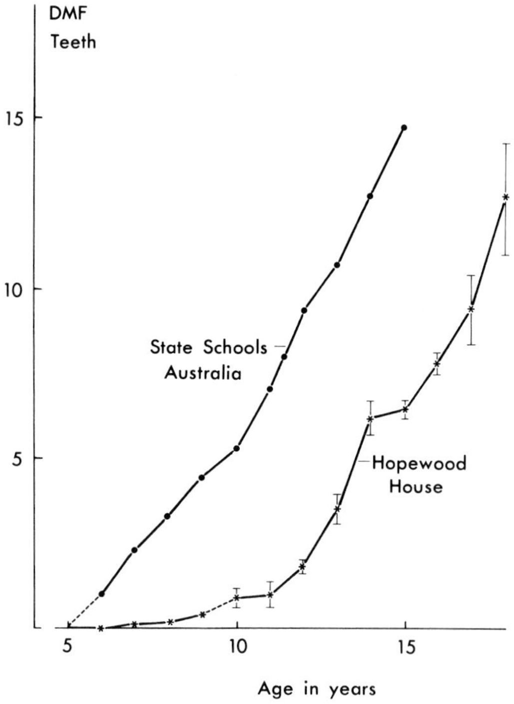

Figure 4–7 Plot of the mean number of DMF teeth per child versus chronological age in State Schools of Australia and in children of Hopewood House (with standard error of means). Note the extremely low caries increment of the institutionalized children while under strict dietary control and the steep increase in caries experience when dietary supervision was no longer in effect—at above 13 years of age. (Courtesy of Prof. Dr. Marthaler, Caries Res., 1967.)

able in that there were few if any cariogenic foods ingested.

HEREDITARY FRUCTOSE INTOLERANCE

With the exception of the Vipeholm and Hopewood House studies, most studies on the relationship of diet to human caries prevalence have relied on information obtained from the patients' dietary history. The limitations of this approach have already been mentioned. Nature, however, has provided a group of subjects who observe a strict dietary pattern because of hereditary fructose intolerance.

Hereditary fructose intolerance (H.F.I.) is an uncommon metabolic disorder believed to be due to an absence of hepatic fructose-1-phosphate aldolase, the enzyme which splits fructose-1-phosphate into two three-carbon fragments which are subsequently metabolized. H.F.I. is characterized by symptoms of nausea, vomiting, malaise, excessive sweating, tremor, coma and convulsions following the ingestion of foods containing fructose. Most of these symptoms can be attributed to a secondary hypoglycemia that occurs after fructose ingestion. Fructosemia and fructosuria are found following a fructose tolerance test.

Fructose occurs in the human diet in certain fruits (e.g., grapes), but by far the commonest source of fructose is sucrose. Patients suffering from this autosomal recessive genetic defect, if they survive early childhood, learn to avoid all forms of sweets, chocolates, candies, cakes, cookies, sweet pastries and other sucrose-containing foods. Of the cases reported in the literature very few provide a sufficiently detailed description of the caries prevalence to express as a DMFT score. One survey, involving patients of both sexes and from six to 41 years of age, revealed eight out of 19 individuals to be caries-free. This is in marked contrast to a random group of naval recruits where there was only one caries-free individual out of 4,887. Furthermore, the DMFT score of those H.F.I. patients which have any decayed, restored, or missing teeth is extremely low compared to the general population in an equivalent age group. Caries, if present at all, is restricted to pits or fissures and is not found on smooth surfaces. Other members of the same families, who are not afflicted by H.F.I., show the usual picture of dental caries including large numbers of fillings and extractions, and full dentures in adults of advanced age.

There is little doubt that the genetic cause of freedom from caries or low caries prevalence can be attributed to a self-imposed dietary regimen involving the elimination of all sucrose-containing foods. These individuals do eat glucose-, galactose-, and lactose- containing items such as milk, dairy products, bread, potatoes, noodles and rice, suggesting that these latter foodstuffs have a minimal cariogenic potential.

FOODS AND CARIES-PRODUCING POTENTIAL

The acid production from various foods has been compared in fermentation tests. Physical tests have measured the adhesiveness of foods and their retention in the mouth. It has been found for example that food is retained not only on the teeth but also on the soft tissues, and that the retention in these locations for the same food item may differ. Of course there are also pronounced differences in oral retention and clearance for different foods. These parameters of retention and acid formation of foods are considered important in caries, but they do not actually measure caries production. Accordingly, it has been difficult to relate the cariogenicity of foods to a single physical property such as adhesion, cohesion or solubility.[17]

EXPERIMENTAL CARIES IN ANIMALS

Serious moral and legal problems arise when caries is deliberately induced in human subjects in order to study factors involved in cariogenicity. Furthermore, it is extremely difficult to secure scientifically adequately controlled and large-enough groups. Accordingly, many investigators have resorted to the use of animals in experimental dental caries, and much useful information has come out of these studies. Rodents (hamsters and rats) have been the favorite species because they are small and therefore economical, and particularly because caries can be produced within a few weeks. In contrast primates, humans and monkeys, usually take somewhere between six to 18 months to develop clinically detectable lesions.

Objections may be raised in applying conclusions reached from animal experiments directly to humans. Certainly there are differences, for example in the composition of the saliva and the morphology of the teeth, between rodents and primates. Even between rodent species there are certain variations as regards eating patterns[93] and genetic differences. Nevertheless, there are also pronounced similarities in the caries process in animals and man as far as cariogenic flora and cariogenic diet are concerned.

TABLE 4–8 COMPARISON OF RAT CARIES SCORES PRODUCED BY DIFFERENT HUMAN FOODS FED *AD LIBITUM*[143]

BASIC DIET 581 S* FOOD MATERIAL ADDED	MEAN CARIES SCORE
Control	0
Corn chips, popcorn, peanuts, milk, sorbitol, lettuce, cabbage, lemons,† oranges†	0
Potato chips	1.6
Carrots	2.1
White bread and peanut butter	5.2
Graham crackers	8.7
White bread and raspberry jam	10.2
Honey graham crackers	19.2
Apples†	19.4
Bananas	21.0
Grapes†	24.1
Candy mints	24.7
Cola†	29.6
Marshmallows	30.1
Raisins	30.9
10% Sucrose water	32.2
Dates	32.7
Milk chocolate	34.1
Sucrose	62.1

*Rats fed 581 S diet 2 × 1 hr./day, test food continuously available.

†Produced dental erosion.

Stephan[143] has compared the cariogenicity of a wide range of human foods and refreshments fed to rats *ad libitum* in addition to their basic diet. This basic diet (581S), consisting of dried skim milk powder and whole dried liver substance, is noncariogenic when fed to the rats twice per day for one hour. Sucrose gave by far the highest caries score. Some of the findings are shown in Table 4–8. Foods producing a caries score of greater than 10.0 were considered significantly cariogenic. It may come as a surprise that certain fruits (apples, bananas, grapes) fall in this category. These fruits contain between 10 to 15 per cent (w/w) available sugars (glucose, fructose and sucrose), whereas citrus fruits (oranges, grapefruits and mandarins) contain seven to eight per cent sugars.[37] This should not be interpreted as condemning the eating of fresh fruits, but it should be recognized that they, too, contain fermentable sugars and therefore one needs to brush thoroughly after partaking of them. Apples do not "clean the teeth" and eating them will not remove plaque.[112] One must observe some caution before relating the findings, of high cariogenicity of some foods offered to rats *ad libitum*, to humans. Rats develop marked food preferences, for example to Coca Cola which they will drink with high frequency. This does not altogether represent the human situation. Nevertheless, one can draw conclusions about the noncariogenic or "safe" food items, which include corn chips, popcorn, peanuts, milk, lettuce and cabbage. These should be kept readily available in the home for children to eat as between-meal snacks.

A comparison of the relative cariogenicity of different between-meal snacks fed to rats *ad libitum*, Table 4–9, reveals a parallelism between the degree of cariogenicity and the amount of sucrose contained in the diet.[78] Other ingredients, and the physical texture in the case of the biscuits, also seemed to be important. The cariogenicity of bread is determined by the garnishing.

TABLE 4–9 COMPARISON OF RAT CARIES SCORES PRODUCED BY HUMAN BETWEEN-MEAL SNACKS FED *AD LIBITUM*[78]

DIET	TOTAL CARIES SCORE PER GROUP		SUCROSE CONTENT
	FISSURE*	SMOOTH SURFACE	(% *w/w*)
Biscuit, Wholemeal Flour, Bran and Nuts	26	0	1.2
Bread 80%, Cheese 20%	27	0	0.4
Bread 80%, Jam 20%	78	3	6.8
Biscuit, Wholemeal Flour, Coarse sugar	80	5	20.2
Biscuit, White Flour, Refined sugar	106	2	13.6
Chocolate Wafers	112	30	10.3
Milk Chocolate with Rice Crispies	129	43	41.6

*Fissure lesions involving dentine (T) for 1st, 2nd and 3rd molars.

CARIOGENICITY OF SUCROSE AND OTHER CARBOHYDRATES

The foregoing findings concerning the role of sucrose in the etiology of caries are based on epidemiological grounds as well as controlled human and animal studies. There have been other animal studies which instead of comparing common human dietary items have compared the cariogenicity of different carbohydrates—starches, sucrose, maltose, lactose, fructose and glucose—usually added to the animal diet in a powdered form. Under such conditions, sucrose invariably proves deleterious by inducing smooth-surface-type lesions more than any other carbohydrate.[66, 72, 133]

This is especially so if the animals are infected with a cariogenic microorganism, such as *Strep. mutans*.[19, 44, 69] However, if comparisons are made on the basis of fissure-type lesions, the distinction between the different carbohydrates is not always as clear-cut,[131, 137] so that some investigators have disputed the importance of sucrose as a caries inducer vis-à-vis the other sugars.[102] But humans do not eat diets consisting of 60–70 per cent powdered carbohydrate, and the relevance of such animal studies can be questioned. The principal carbohydrates available in human diets are starches and sucrose and some lactose, not glucose, fructose or maltose. In both the U.S.A. and Europe wheat, potatoes and sucrose provide about 90 per cent of the total carbohydrate consumed. From a clinical point of view, therefore, the significant comparison is between starches and sucrose, and in this case there can be no doubt that sucrose is the "bad guy."

The key role of sucrose as a dietary substrate in the caries process on smooth surfaces can be explained on biochemical grounds. Smooth-surface caries depends on the growth of a dental plaque. Several independent investigations have clearly demonstrated the presence of extracellular polysaccharides, both glucans and levans, in plaque (Fig. 4–8; see also Guggenheim[68] and Newbrun[119]). The glucans, particularly the water-insoluble fraction, can serve as structural components of the plaque matrix, in effect "gluing" the bacteria to the teeth. The soluble levans and some of the soluble glucans are degradable by the plaque flora and may function as transient reserves of fermentable carbohydrates, thereby prolonging the duration of acid production. Biosynthesis of these polysaccharides occurs by the agency of enzymes which for the most part are extracellular

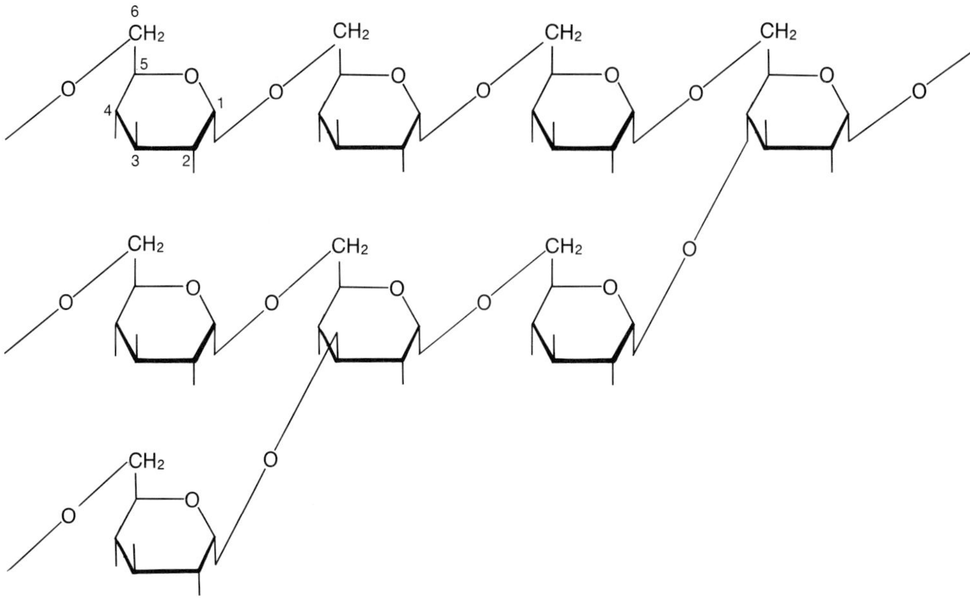

BACTERIAL DEXTRAN

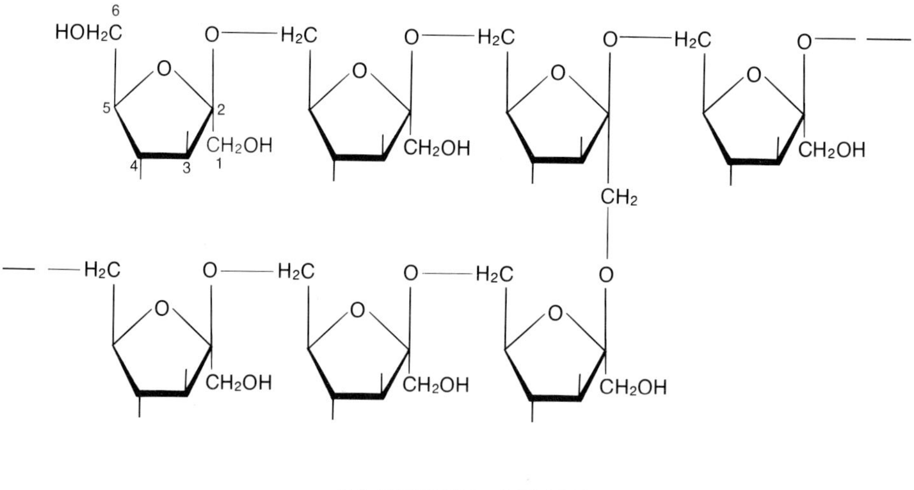

BACTERIAL LEVAN

Figure 4–8 Chemical structure of a portion of bacterial dextran (glucan) and levan (fructan) molecules. Hydroxyl groups are represented by a straight line and hydrogens have been omitted. Dextran is a homologous polymer of D-glucopyranose with predominantly α-(1→6) linkages. Water-insoluble glucans from *Strep. mutans* contain a high proportion of α-(1→3) linkages. Levan is a homologous polymer of D-fructofuranose with predominantly β-(2→6) linkages. The frequency of branching and overall size of these polysaccharides varies with the organism from which it is obtained.

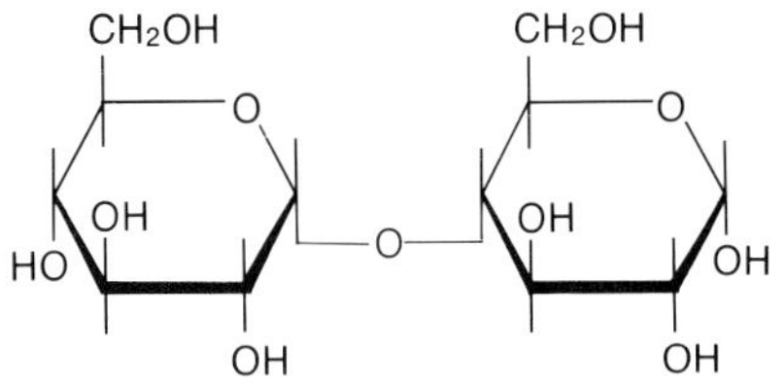

MALTOSE

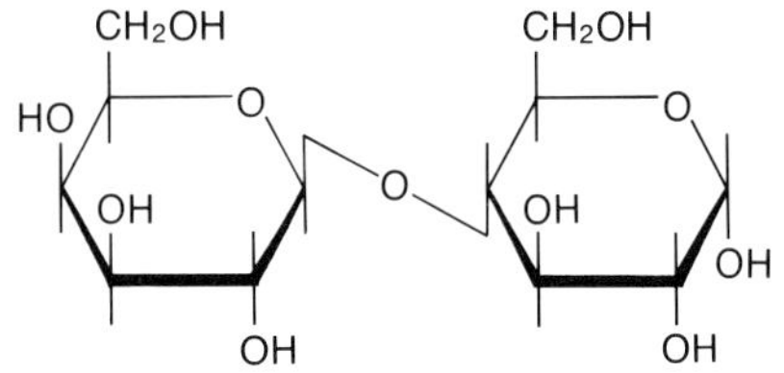

LACTOSE

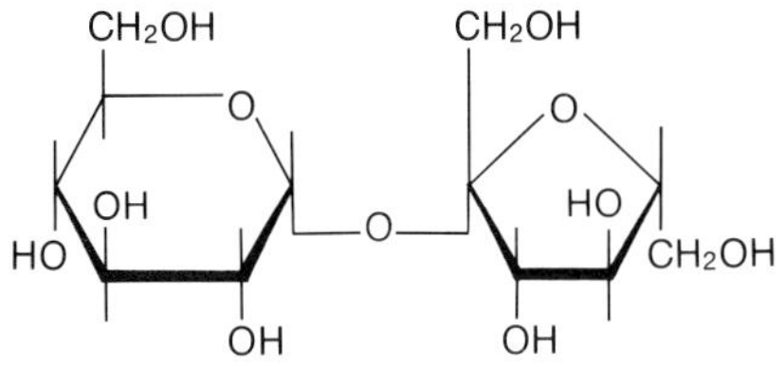

SUCROSE

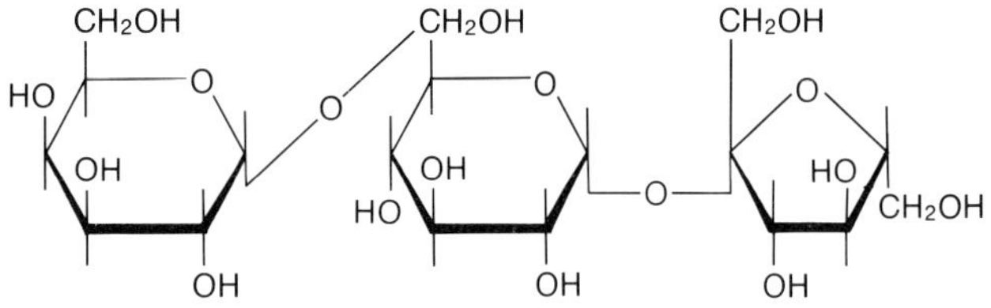

RAFFINOSE

Figure 4–9 Chemical structure of maltose, lactose, sucrose and raffinose. There are potentially high-energy dihemiacetal linkages between the aldehyde and ketone carbons of glucose and fructose respectively in sucrose and raffinose. In maltose, lactose and between glucose and galactose in raffinose the glucosidic link is a hemiacetal between an aldehyde and an alcohol group and is of much lower energy.

or bound to the cell surface and which show a high specificity for sucrose (and sometimes raffinose) as a substrate. Unlike intracellular bacterial, mammalian or plant polysaccharide synthesis which involves sugar-1-phosphate or nucleoside diphosphate-sugar intermediates, this extracellular synthesis transfers glucose or fructose units directly to the growing polymer. The precise mechanism involved is not yet known. Somehow the enzyme conserves the relatively high energy of the link between the two anomeric carbons, C1 of glucose and C2 of fructose, found in sucrose (Fig. 4–9). Disaccharides other than sucrose, such as maltose and lactose, are hemiacetals not dihemiacetals. Therefore, their free energy of hydrolysis is significantly less (Table 4–10), and they cannot serve directly as glycosyl donors in this system. Sucrose, on the other hand, has a free energy of hydrolysis of 6,600 cal/mole which is in the same range as the nucleoside diphosphate sugars, 7,600 cal/mole, and higher than glucose-1-phosphate.[3]

The enzymes involved in the synthesis, glucosyl- and fructosyltransferases, have been isolated and purified from *Strep. sanguis* and *Strep. mutans*.[23, 29, 71, 120] The properties of these enzymes are of con-

TABLE 4–10 FREE ENERGY OF HYDROLYSIS OF GLUCOSYL DONORS AND SOME POLYSACCHARIDES

COMPOUND	STANDARD FREE ENERGY OF HYDROLYSIS ΔG_H *(cal/mole)*
Glucose-1-phosphate	–5000
UDP-glucose	–7600
Sucrose	–6600
Maltose	–3000
Lactose	–3000
Glycogen	–4300
Dextran	–2000
Levan	–4600

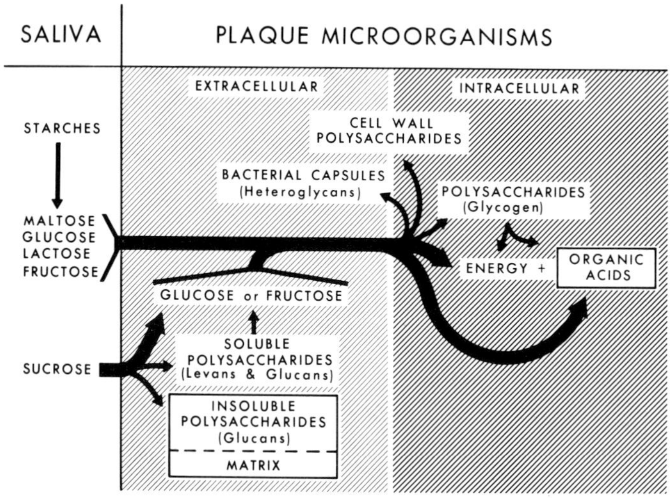

Figure 4–10 Schematic fate of carbohydrates in the plaque.

siderable clinical relevance and can be listed as follows:

1. They are highly specific for sucrose and will not utilize sugars such as fructose, glucose, maltose or lactose.

2. They have a broad pH optimum, 5.2–7.0, coinciding with the pH range prevailing in dental plaque.

3. In the presence of adequate nutrients the enzyme will be made by these organisms and sucrose is not a required inducer. Whenever sucrose is ingested they are ready to synthesize polysaccharides.

4. The equilibrium of the reaction shown below for glucan synthesis is far to the right.

$$\underset{\text{sucrose}}{n\, C_{12}H_{22}O_{11}} \longrightarrow \underset{\text{glucan}}{(C_6H_{10}O_5)_n} + \underset{\text{fructose}}{n\, C_6H_{12}O_6}$$

This means that as long as sucrose is present in the plaque the glucosyltransferase enzymes will continue to utilize it to form plaque matrix material and fructose. The latter can readily be fermented by the plaque flora to form organic acids.

The pathways by which various ingested carbohydrates are used in the plaque are shown schematically in Figure 4–10. Starches are probably prevented from direct entry into the plaque because of limited diffusion of such large molecules. Maltose, lactose, fructose and glucose can be used by the oral flora for the synthesis of bacterial cell wall, capsular and intracellular polysaccharides and for the formation of organic acids. Sucrose is unique in that it can also serve in the formation of insoluble extracellular polysaccharides and thereby enhance plaque formation and microbial aggregation on the tooth surface. Only small amounts of all glucosyl moieties of sucrose are polymerized[151a,b] and insoluble glucans constitute only a small proportion, on a weight basis, of the dental plaque.[77c] The insoluble polysaccharides, though small quantitatively, are important because organisms which have lost this property are no longer caries-inducing.[148] The bulk of the glucosyl and fructosyl moieties of sucrose are fermented to organic acid products as shown by the heavy arrows (Fig. 4–10).

The ability to ferment sucrose is influenced by the previous exposure of the microorganism to sucrose. A strain (PK-1) of *Strep. mutans*, previously grown on sucrose, produced much more lactate when given sucrose as a substrate than the same strain of cells previously grown on glucose.[161] Studies suggest that sucrose phosphorylase and invertase are induced in sucrose-grown streptococci.

REFERENCES

1. Aslander, A. 1961. Lifetime teeth. N.Y.J. Dent., *31*:346–348.

1a. Bahn, A. N., Rosen, S., Dicecco, F. M., and Hayashi, J. A. 1973. Immunization with levan sucrases. 51st Gen. Meeting IADR Abst. 549, p. 196.

2. Berkenbilt, D. A. and Bahn, A. N. 1971. Develop-

ment of antibodies to cariogenic streptococci in children. J. Am. Dent. Assoc., *83*:332–337.
3. Bernfeld, P. 1963. The biogenesis of carbohydrates. *In* Biogenesis of Natural Compounds. P. Bernfeld, Ed., Pergamon Press, Oxford, p. 278.
4. Bhoola, K. D., McNicol, M. W., Oliver, S., and Forna, J. 1969. Changes in salivary enzymes in patients with sarcoidosis. New Eng. J. Med., *28*:877–879.
5. Bibby, B. G., Gustafson, G. and Davies, G. N. 1958. A critique of three theories of caries attack. Int. Dent. J., *8*:685–695.
6. Blackmore, D. K., Drucker, D. B., and Green, R. M. 1970. Caries induction in germ-free rats by streptococci isolated from dental abscesses in man. Arch. Oral Biol., *15*: 1377–1379.
7. De Boever, J., Hirzel, H. C., and Mühlemann, H. R. 1969. The effect of concentrated sucrose solutions on pH of interproximal plaque. Helv. Odontol. Acta, *13*:27–28.
8. De Boever, J., and Mühlemann, H. R. 1969. pH of interproximal plaque with regard to continuous sucrose application. Helv. Odontol. Acta, *13*:97–99.
9. Bowen, W. H. 1969. A vaccine against dental caries. A pilot experiment in monkeys (*Macaca irus*). Br. Dent. J., *126*:159–160.
10. Bradford, E. W., and Crabb, H. S. M. 1961. Carbohydrate restriction and caries incidence. Br. Dent. J., *111*:273–279.
11. Brandtzaeg, P. 1971. Human secretory immunoglobulins. 3.Immunochemical and physiochemical studies of secretory IgA and free secretory piece. Acta Pathol. Microbiol. Scand. [B], *79*:165–188.
12. Brandtzaeg, P., Fjellanger, I., and Gjeruldsen, S. T. 1968. Adsorption of immunoglobulin A onto oral bacteria. J. Bacteriol., *96*:242–249.
13. Brandtzaeg, P., Fjellanger, I., and Gjeruldsen, S. T. 1970. Human secretory immunoglobulins. I. Salivary secretions from individuals with normal or low levels of serum immunoglobulins. Scand. J. Haemat. Suppl. 12, pp. 1–83.
14. Bratthall, D. 1970. Demonstration of five serological groups of streptococcal strains resembling *Streptococcus mutans*. Odontol. Revy, *21*:143–152.
14a. Bratthall, D. 1972. Demonstration of *Streptococcus mutans* strains in some selected areas of the world. Odontol. Revy *23*:401–410.
15. Brudevold, F., and Söremark, R. 1964. Chemistry of the mineral phase of human enamel. *In* Structural and Mineral Organization of Teeth. A.E.W. Miles and R. C. Greulich, Eds., Academic Press, N. Y.
16. Burnett, G. W., and Scherp, H. W. 1968. Oral Microbiology and Infectious Disease. Williams and Wilkins Co., Baltimore, Md., 3rd Ed., p. 352.
17. Caldwell, R. C. 1970. Physical properties of foods and their caries-producing potential. J. Dent. Res., *49*:1293–1298.
18. Camilleri, G. E., and Bowen, W. H. 1963. Classification of lactobacilli isolated from human carious dentin. J. Dent. Res., *42*:1104–1105.
19. Campbell, R. G., and Zinner, D. D. 1970. Effect of certain dietary sugars on hamster caries. J. Nutr., *100*:11–20.
20. Carlos, J. P., and Gittelsohn, A. M. 1965. Longitudinal studies of the natural history of caries II. Arch. Oral Biol., *10*:739–751.
21. Carlsson, J. 1967. A medium for isolation of *Streptococcus mutans*. Arch. Oral Biol., *12*:1657–1658.
22. Carlsson, J. 1968. A numerical taxonomic study of human oral streptococci. Odontol. Revy, *19*:137–160.
23. Carlsson, J. 1970a. A levansucrase isolated from *Streptococcus mutans*. Caries Res., *4*:97–113.
24. Carlsson, J. 1970b. Chemically defined medium for growth of *Streptococcus sanguis*. Caries Res., *4*:297–304.
25. Carlsson, J. 1970c. Nutritional requirements of *Streptococcus mutans*. Caries Res., *4*:305–320.
26. Carlsson, J. 1971. Growth of *Streptococcus mutans* and *Streptococcus sanguis* in mixed culture. Arch. Oral Biol., *16*:963–966.
27. Carlsson, J., Grahnén, H., Jonsson, G., and Wikner, S. 1970a. Early establishment of *Streptococcus salivarius* in the mouths of infants. J. Dent. Res., *49*:415–418.
28. Carlsson, J., Grahnén, H., Jonsson, G. and Wikner, S. 1970b. Establishment of *Streptococcus sanguis* in the mouths of infants. Arch. Oral Biol., *15*:1143–1148.
29. Carlsson, J., Newbrun, E., and Krasse, B. 1969. Purification and properties of dextransucrase from *Streptococcus sanguis*. Arch. Oral Biol., *14*:469–478.
30. Carlsson, J., Söderholm, G., and Almfeldt, I. 1969. Prevalence of *Streptococcus sanguis* and *Streptococcus mutans* in the mouth of persons wearing full-dentures. Arch. Oral Biol., *14*:243–250.
31. Charlton, G., Fitzgerald, R. J., and Keyes, P. H. 1971. Determination of saliva and dental plaque pH in hamsters with glass microelectrodes. Arch. Oral Biol., *16*:649–654.
32. Charlton, G., Fitzgerald, R. J., and Keyes, P. H. 1971. Hydrogen ion activity in dental plaque of hamsters during metabolism of sucrose, glucose and fructose. Arch. Oral Biol., *16*: 655–662.
33. Clem, W. H. and Klebanoff, S. J. 1966. Inhibitory effect of saliva on glutamic acid accumulation by *Lactobacillus acidophilus* and the role of the lactoperoxidase-thiocyanate system. J. Bacteriol., *91*:1848–1853.
34. Cornick, D. E. R., and Bowen, W. H. 1971. Development of the oral flora in newborn monkeys (*Macaca irus*). Br. Dent. J., *130*: 231–234.
35. Coykendall, A. L. 1970. Base composition of deoxyribonucleic acid isolated from cariogenic streptococci. Arch. Oral Biol., *15*: 365–368.
36. Coykendall, A. L. 1971. Genetic heterogenicity in *Streptococcus mutans*. J. Bacteriol., *106*: 192–196.
37. Dako, D. Y., Trautner, K., and Somogyi, J. C. 1970. Der Glukose-, Fruktose- und Saccharosegehalt verschiedener Früchte. Schweiz. Med. Wochenschr., *100*:897–903.
38. Dawes, C. 1970. Effects of diet on salivary secretion and composition. J. Dent. Res., *49*: 1263–1272.
39. Dirksen, T. R., Little, M. F., and Bibby, B. G. 1963. The pH of carious cavities—II. The

pH at different depths in isolated cavities. Arch. Oral Biol., *8*:91–97.
40. Drucker, D. B., and Melville, T. H. 1968. Fermentation end-products of cariogenic and non-cariogenic streptococci. Arch. Oral Biol., *13*:563–570.
41. Duany, L. F., Zinner, D. D., and Landy, J. J. 1971. Bone loss and caries in rats infected with human streptococci. J. Dent. Res., *50*:460–465.
42. Edwardsson, S. 1968. Characteristics of caries-inducing human streptococci resembling *Streptococcus mutans*. Arch. Oral Biol., *13*:637–646.
43. Edwardsson, S. 1970. The caries-inducing property of variants of *Streptococcus mutans*. Odontol. Revy, *21*:153–157.
44. Edwardsson, S., and Krasse, B. 1967. Human streptococci and caries in hamsters fed diets with sucrose or glucose. Arch. Oral Biol., *12*:1015–1016.
45. Eggers Lura, H. 1967. The non-acid complexing and phosphorylating theory of dental caries. Ator Tryk, Holbaek, Denmark.
46. Ericsson, Y. 1959. Clinical investigation of the salivary buffering action. Acta Odontol. *17*:131–165.
47. Ericsson, Y. 1962. Salivary and food factors in dental caries development. Int. Dent. J., *12*:476–495.
48. Evans, R. T., and Mergenhagen, S. E. 1965. Occurrence of natural antibacterial antibody in human parotid fluid. Proc. Soc. Exp. Biol. Med., *119*:815–819.
49. Van Der Fehr, F. R., Löe, H., and Theilade, E. 1970. Experimental caries in man. Caries Res., *4*:131–148.
50. Finn, S. B., Klapper, C. E., and Volker, J. F. 1955. Intra-oral effects upon experimental hamster caries. *In* Advancements in Experimental Caries Research. R. F. Sognnaes, Ed., A.A.A.S., Washington, D.C., pp. 152–168.
51. Fitzgerald, R. J. 1963. Gnotobiotic contribution to oral microbiology. J. Dent. Res., *42*: 549–552.
52. Fitzgerald, R. J. 1968a. Dental caries in gnotobiotic animals. Caries Res., *2*:139–146.
53. Fitzgerald, R. J. 1968b. Plaque microbiology and caries. Ala. J. Med. Sci., *5*:239–246.
54. Fitzgerald, R. J., Jordan, H. V., and Archard, H. O. 1966. Dental caries in gnotobiotic rats infected with a variety of *Lactobacillus acidophilus*. Arch. Oral Biol., *11*:473–476.
55. Fitzgerald, R. J., Jordan, H. V., and Stanley, H. R. 1960. Experimental caries and gingival pathological changes in the gnotobiotic rat. J. Dent. Res., *39*:923–935.
56. Fitzgerald, R. J., and Keyes, P. H. 1960. Demonstration of the etiologic role of streptococci in experimental caries in the hamster. J. Am. Dent. Assoc., *61*:9–19.
57. Frank, R. M., Herdly, J., and Philippe, E. 1965. Acquired dental defects and salivary gland lesions after irradiation for carcinoma. J. Am. Dent. Assoc., *70*:868–883.
57a. Frank, R. M., Guillo, B. and Llory, H. 1972. Caries dentaires chez le rat gnotobiote inocule avec *Actinomyces viscosus* et *Actinomyces naeslundii*. Arch. Oral Biol. *17*: 1249–1253.
58. Gibbons, R. J. 1964. Bacteriology of dental caries. J. Dent. Res., *43*:1021–1028.
59. Gibbons, R. J., Berman, K. S., Knoettner, P. and Kapsimalis, B. 1966. Dental caries and alveolar bone loss in gnotobiotic rats infected with capsule forming streptococci of human origin. Arch. Oral Biol., *11*:549–560.
60. Gibbons, R. J., and Houte, J. van. 1971. Selective bacterial adherence to oral epithelial surfaces and its role as an ecological determinant. Inf. Immun., *3*:567–573.
61. Gibbons, R. J., and Loesche, W. J. 1967. Isolation of cariogenic streptococci from Guatemalan children. Arch. Oral Biol., *12*:1013–1014.
62. Gibbons, R. J., and Spinell, D. M. 1970. Salivary-duced aggregation of plaque bacteria in *"Dental Plaque"*. W. D. McHugh, Ed., E. and S. Livingstone, Edinburgh, pp. 207–215.
63. Gibbons, R. J., Stoppellaar, J. D. de, and Harden, L. 1966. Lysozyme insensitivity of bacteria indigenous to the oral cavity of man. J. Dent. Res., *45*:877–881.
64. Gilmour, M. N., and Poole, A. E. 1967. The fermentative capabilities of dental plaque. Caries Res., *1*:247–260.
64a. Gold, O. G., Jordan, H. V., and van Houte, J. 1973. A medium for selective cultivation of *Streptococcus mutans*. 51st Gen. Meeting IADR Abst. 450, p. 171.
65. Graf, H., and Mühlemann, H. R. 1966. Telemetry of plaque from interdental area. Helv. Odontol. Acta, *10*:94–101.
66. Grenby, T. H. 1963. The effects of some carbohydrates on experimental dental caries in the rat. Arch. Oral Biol., *8*:27–30.
67. Guggenheim, B. 1968. Streptococci of dental plaque. Caries Res., *2*:147–163.
68. Guggenheim, B. 1970. Extracellular polysaccharides and microbial plaque. Int. Dent. J., *20*:657–678.
69. Guggenheim, B., König, K. G., Herzog, E., and Mühlemann, H. R. 1966. The cariogenicity of different carbohydrates tested on rats in relative gnotobiosis with a streptococcus producing extracellular polysaccharides. Helv. Odontol. Acta, *10*:101–113.
70. Guggenheim, B., Mühlemann, H. R., Regolati, B. and Schmid, R. 1970. The effect of immunization against streptococci or glucosyltransferases on plaque formation and dental caries in rats. *In* Dental Plaque. W. D. McHugh, Ed., E. and S. Livingstone, Ltd., Edinburgh, pp. 287–296.
71. Guggenheim, B., and Newbrun, E. 1969. Extracellular glucosyltransferase activity of an HS strain of *Streptococcus mutans*. Helv. Odontol. Acta, *13*:84–97.
71a. Guillo, B., Klein, J. P. and Frank, R. M. 1973. Fissure caries in gnotobiotic rats infected with *Actinomyces naeslundii* and *Actinomyces israelii*.
72. Gustafson, G., Stelling, M., Abramson, Ė., and Brunius, E. 1955. The cariogenic effects of some carbohydrates in dry and moist diets. Experimental dental caries in golden hamsters. V. Odontol. Tidsk., *63*:506–523.
73. Gustafsson, B. E., Quensel, C. E., Lanke, L. S., Ludqvist, C., Grahnén, H., Bonow, B. E., and Krasse, B. 1954. The Vipeholm dental caries study. The effect of different levels

of carbohydrate intake on caries activity in 436 individuals observed for five years. Acta Odontol. Scand., *11*:232–364.

74. Hardwick, J. L. 1960. The incidence and distribution of caries throughout the ages in relation to the Englishman's diet. Br. Dent. J., *108*:9–17.

75. Harris, R. 1963. Biology of the children of Hopewood House, Bowral, Australia. 4. Observations of dental caries experience extending over five years (1957–1961). J. Dent. Res., *42*:1387–1398.

76. Hodgson, H. W., Matsutani, K. K., Shklair, I. L., and Bahn, A. N. 1971. Antibody in parotid saliva of children to cariogenic streptococci. 49th Gen. Session, IADR Abst. 53, p. 66.

77. Hoerman, K. C., Englander, H. R., and Shklair, I. L. 1956. Lysozyme: its characteristics in human parotid and submaxillo-lingual saliva. Proc. Soc. Exp. Biol. Med., *92*:875–878.

77a. Hoerman, K. C., Keene, H. J., Shklair, I. L., and Burmeister, J. A. 1972. The association of *Streptococcus mutans* with early carious lesions in human teeth. J. Am. Dent. Assoc., *85*:1349–1352.

77b. Hoeven, J. S. van der, Mikx, F. H. M., Plasschaert, A. J. M., and König, K. G. 1972. Methodological aspects of gnotobiotic caries experimentation. Caries Res., *6*:203–210.

77c. Hotz, P., Guggenheim, B., and Schmid, R. 1972. Carbohydrates in pooled dental plaque. Caries Res., *6*:103–121.

78. Ishii, T., König, K. G., and Mühlemann, H. R. 1968. The cariogenicity of different between-meal snacks in Osborne-Mendel rats. Helv. Odontol. Acta, *12*:41–47.

79. Jenkins, G. H. 1961. A critique of the proteolysis-chelation theory of caries. Br. Dent. J., *11*:311–330.

80. Jenkins, G. N. 1966. The physiology of the mouth. 3rd Ed., F. A. Davis Co., Philadelphia, p. 318.

81. Jordan, H. V. 1965. Bacteriological aspects of experimental dental caries. Ann. N.Y. Acad. Sci., *131*:905–912.

82. Jordan, H. V., Englander, H. R., Engler, W. O., and Kulczyk, S. 1972. Observations on the implantation and transmission of *Streptococcus mutans* in humans. J. Dent. Res. *51*: 515–518.

83. Jordan, H. V., Englander, H. R., and Lim, S. 1969. Potentially cariogenic streptococci in selected population groups in the western hemisphere. J. Am. Dent. Assoc., *78*:1331–1335.

84. Jordan, H. V., and Hammond, B. F. 1971. Filament-forming bacteria in human cervical caries. 49th Gen. Session, IADR Abst. 193, p. 101.

84a. Jordan, H. V., and Hammond, B. F. 1972. Filamentous bacteria isolated from human root surface caries. Arch. Oral Biol., *17*:1283–1342.

85. Kelstrup, J., and Gibbons, R. J. 1969. Bacteriocins from human and rodent streptococci. Arch. Oral Biol., *14*:251–258.

86. Kelstrup, J., and Gibbons, R. J. 1970. Induction of dental caries and alveolar bone loss by a human isolate resembling *Streptococcus salivarius*. Caries Res., *4*:360–377.

87. Kennedy, A. E., Shklair, I. L., Hayashi, J. A., and Bahn, A. N. 1968. Antibodies to cariogenic streptococci in humans. Arch. Oral Biol., *13*:1275–1278.

88. Kerr, A. C., and Wedderburn, D. L. 1958. Antibacterial factors in the secretions of human parotid and submaxillary glands. Br. Dent. J., *105*:321–326.

89. Keyes, P. H. 1969. The infectious and transmissible nature of experimental dental caries. Arch. Oral Biol., *1*:304–320.

90. König, K. G. 1969. Caries activity induced by frequency-controlled feeding of diets containing sucrose or bread to Osborne-Mendel rats. Arch. Oral Biol., *14*:991–993.

91. König, K. G. 1971. Karies und Kariesprophylaxe. W. Goldmann Verlag, Munich.

92. König, K. G., Guggenheim, B., and Mühlemann, H. R. 1965. Modifications of the oral flora and their influence on dental caries in the rat. II. Inoculation of a cariogenic streptococcus and its effect in relation to varying time of depression of the indigenous flora. Helv. Odontol. Acta, *9*:130–134.

93. König, K. C., Larson, R. H., and Guggenheim, B. 1969. A strain specific eating pattern as a factor limiting the transmissibility of caries activity in rats. Arch. Oral Biol., *14*:91–103.

94. König, K. G., and Mühlemann, H. R. 1964. Further investigations into a possible effect of dietary lysozyme on caries incidence in rats. Helv. Odontol. Acta, *8*:22–24.

95. König, K. G., Schmid, P., and Schmid, R. 1968. An apparatus for frequency-controlled feeding of small rodents and its use in dental caries experiments. Arch. Oral Biol., *13*: 13–26.

96. Krasse, B. 1970. A review of the bacteriology of dental plaque. *In* Dental Plaque. W. D. McHugh Ed., E. and S. Livingstone, Edinburgh, pp. 199–205.

97. Krasse, B., and Carlsson, J. 1970. Various types of streptococci and experimental caries in hamsters. Arch. Oral Biol., *15*:25–32.

98. Krasse, B., Edwardsson, S., Svensson, I., and Trell, L. 1967. Implantation of caries inducing streptococci in the human oral cavity. Arch. Oral Biol., *12*:231–236.

99. Krasse, B., Jordan, H. V., Edwardsson, S., Svensson, I., and Trell, L. 1968. The occurrence of certain "caries-inducing" streptococci in human dental plaque material. Arch. Oral Biol., *13*:911–918.

100. Kraus, F. W., and Konno, J. 1965. The salivary secretion of antibody. Ala. J. Med. Sci., *2*:15–22.

101. Kreitzman, S. N., Irving, S., Navia, J. M., and Harris, R. S. 1969. Enzymatic release of phosphate from rat molar enamel by phosphoprotein phosphatase. Nature, *223*:520–521.

102. Leach, S. A., Green, R. M., Hayes, M. L., and Dada, O. A. 1969. Biochemical studies on the formation and composition of dental plaque in relationship to dental caries: extracellular polysaccharides. J. Dent. Res., *48*:811–817.

103. Lehner, T., Wilton, J. M. A., and Ward, R. G. 1970. Serum antibodies in dental caries in man. Arch. Oral Biol., *15*:481–490.

104. Leung, S. W. 1962. Saliva and dental caries. Dent. Clin. North Am., July, pp. 347–355.

104a. Liljemark, W. F., and Gibbons, R. J. 1972. Pro-

portional distribution and relative adherence of *Streptococcus miteor* (mitis) on various surfaces in the human oral cavity. Inf. Immun., *6*:852–859.
105. Littleton, N. W., Kakehashi, S., and Fitzgerald, R. J. 1970. Recovery of specific "Caries-inducing" streptococci from carious lesions in the teeth of children. Arch. Oral Biol., *15*:461–463.
106. Löe, H., Karring, T., and Theilade, E. 1973. An *in vivo* method for the study of the microbiology of occlusal fissures. Caries Res., *7*: 120–129.
106a. Mukasa, H. and Slade, H. D. 1973. Structure and immunological specificity of the *Streptococcus mutans* group b cell wall antigen. Inf. Imm. *7*:578–585.
106b. Loesche, W. and Syed, S. A. 1973. The predominant cultivable flora of carious plaque and carious dentine. Caries Res. *7*:201–206.
107. Luoma, H. 1964. Lability of inorganic phosphate in dental plaque and saliva. Acta Odontol. Scand., *22*, Suppl. 41.
108. Makinen, K. K., and Paunio, I. K. 1970. The pH-dependent liberation of phosphate from human dental enamel and dentine by ammonium sulphate. Acta Chem. Scand., *24*: 1541–1550.
109. Mansbridge, J. N. 1960. The effect of oral hygiene and sweet consumption on the prevalence of dental caries. Br. Dent. J., *109*: 343–354.
110. Marlay, E. 1970. The relationship between dental caries and salivary properties at adolescence. Aust. Dent. J., *5*:412–422.
111. Marthaler, T. 1967. Epidemiological and clinical dental findings in relation to intake of carbohydrates. Caries Res., *1*:222–238.
112. Marthaler, Y. 1968. Apfel, Gesundheit und Kauorgan. Schweiz. Monatsschr. Zahnheilkd., *78*:823–836.
113. Martin, J. J., Isenberg, H. D., Schatz, V., Trelawny, B. S., and Schatz, A. 1954. Chelation, or metal-binding, as a new approach to the problem of dental caries. Rev. Euclides, *14*:311–317.
114. Mörch, T., Punwani, I., and Greve, E. 1971. The possible role of complex forming substances in the decalcification phase of the caries process. Caries Res., *5*:135–143.
115. Morrison, M., and Steele, W. F. 1968. Lactoperoxidase, the peroxidase in the salivary gland. *In* Biology of the Mouth. P. Person, Ed., A.A.A.S., Washington, D.C., pp. 89–110.
116. Mühlemann, H. R., and König, K. G. 1962. The effect of lysozyme on experimental caries. Helv. Odontol. Acta, *6*:33–37.
117. Neuman, W. F., and Neuman, M. W. 1958. The chemical dynamics of bone mineral. Univ. Chicago Press, pp. 142–143.
118. Newbrun, E. 1961. Application of atomic absorption spectroscopy to the determination of calcium in saliva. Nature, *192*:1182–1183.
119. Newbrun, E. 1967. Sucrose, the arch criminal of dental caries. Odontol. Revy, *18*:373–386.
120. Newbrun, E. 1971. Dextransucrase from *Streptococcus sanguis*. Further characterization. Caries Res., *5*:124–134.
120a. Newbrun, E. 1975. *Fluorides and Dental Caries.* Second Edition. Springfield, Ill., Charles C Thomas, Publisher.
121. Newbrun, E., Brudevold, F., and Mermagen, H. 1959. A microradiographic evaluation of occlusal fissures and grooves. J. Am. Dent. Assoc., *58*:26–31.
122. Newbrun, E., and Pigman, W. 1960. The hardness of enamel and dentine. Aust. Dent. J., *5*: 210–217.
123. Orland, F. J., Blayney, J. R., Harrison, R. W., Reyniers, J. A., Trexler, P. C., Ervin, R. F., Gordon, H. A., and Wagner, M. 1955. Experimental caries in germfree rats inoculated with enterococci. J. Am. Dent. Assoc., *50*: 259–272.
124. Orland, F. J., Blayney, J. R., Harrison, J. W., Reyniers, J. A., Trexler, P. C., Wagner, M., Gordon, H. A., and Luckey, T. D. 1954. The use of germfree animal technics in the study of experimental dental caries. I. Basic observations on rats reared free of all microorganisms. J. Dent. Res., *33*:147–174.
125. Parfitt, G. J. 1956. The speed of development of the carious cavity. Br. Dent. J., *100*:204–207.
126. Plasschaert, A. J. M., Mörch, T., and König, K. G. 1972. Effect of sodium lactate under conditions of neutral pH on the release of calcium from the enamel surface. Caries Res., *6*: 334–345.
127. Rauen, H. M. Biochemisches Taschenbuch, I. Springer Verlag, 1964, pp. 219–239.
128. Ritz, H. L. 1967. Microbial population shifts in developing human dental plaque. Arch. Oral Biol., *12*:1561–1568.
129. Rogosa, M. 1964. The genus *Veillonella*. I. General cultural, ecological and biochemical considerations. J. Bacteriol., *87*:162–170.
130. Rogosa, M., Krichevsky, M. I., and Bishop, F. S. 1965. Truncated glycolytic system in *Veillonella*. J. Bacteriol., *90*:164–171.
131. Rosen, S. 1969. Comparison of sucrose and glucose in the causation of dental caries in gnotobiotic rats. Arch. Oral Biol., *14*:445–450.
132. Rosen, S., Lenney, W. S., and O'Malley, J. E. 1968. Dental caries in gnotobiotic rats inoculated with *Lactobacillus casei*. J. Dent. Res., *47*:358–363.
133. Schafer, W. G. 1949. The caries-producing capacity of starch, glucose and sucrose diets in the Syrian hamster. Science, *110*: 143–144.
134. Schamschula, R. G., and Charlton, G. 1971. A study of caries etiology in New South Wales schoolchildren. I. The streptococcal flora of plaque and caries prevalence. Aust. Dent. J., *16*:77–82.
135. Schatz, A., and Martin, J. J. 1955. Speculation on lactobacilli and acid as possible anticaries factors. N.Y. State Dent. J., *21*:367–379.
136. Schneyer, L. H., Pigman, W., Hanahan, L., and Gilmour, R. W. 1956. Rate of flow of human parotid, sublingual and submaxillary secretions during sleep. J. Dent. Res., *35*:109–114.
137. Shaw, J. H., Krumins, F., and Gibbons, R. J. 1967. Comparison of sucrose, lactose, maltose and glucose in causation of experimental oral diseases. Arch. Oral Biol., *12*:755–768.
138. Shklair, I. L., Keene, H. J., and Simonson, L. G. 1972. Distribution and frequency of *Streptococcus mutans* in caries active individuals. J. Dent. Res., *51*:882.

138a. Shovlin, F. E. and Gillis, R. E. 1969. Biochemical and antigenic studies of lactobacilli isolated from deep dentinal caries: I Biochemical aspects. J. Dent. Res. *48*:356–360.
139. Sirisinha, S. 1970. Reactions of human salivary immunoglobulins with indigenous bacteria. Arch. Oral Biol., *15*:551–554.
140. Slowey, R. R., Eidelman, S., and Klebanoff, S. J. 1968. Antibacterial activity of the purified peroxidase from human parotid saliva. J. Bacteriol., *96*:575–579.
141. Stanton, G. 1969. Diet and dental caries. The phosphate sequestration hypothesis. N.Y. State Dent. J., *35*:399–407.
142. Stephan, R. M. 1940. Changes in the hydrogen ion concentration on tooth surfaces and in carious lesions. J. Am. Dent. Assoc., *27*:718.
143. Stephan, R. M. 1966. Effect of different types of human foods on dental health in experimental animals. J. Dent. Res., *45*:1551–1561.
144. Stephan, R. M. 1971. Clinical study of etiology and control of rampant dental caries. 49th Gen. Session, IADR Abst. 636, p. 211.
145. Stoppelaar, J. D. de. 1971. *Streptococcus mutans, Streptococcus sanguis* and dental caries. Thesis, University of Utrecht, The Netherlands.
146. Stoppelaar, J. D. de., Houte, J. van, and Backer Dirks, O. 1969. The relationship between extracellular polysaccharide-producing streptococci and smooth surface caries in 13-year-old children. Caries Res., *3*:190–199.
147. Stoppelaar, J. D. de., Houte, J. van, and Backer Dirks, O. 1970. The effect of carbohydrate restriction on the presence of *Streptococcus mutans, Streptococcus sanguis* and Iodophilic polysaccharide-producing bacteria in human dental plaque. Caries Res., *4*:114–123.
148. Stoppelaar, J. D. de, König, K. G., Plasschaert, A. J. M., and Hoeven, J. S. van der. 1971. Decreased cariogenicity of a mutant strain of *Streptococcus mutans*. Arch. Oral Biol., *16*:971–975.
149. Strålfors, A. 1950. Investigations into the bacterial chemistry of dental plaques. Odontol. Tidsk., *58*:155–341.
150. Sweeney, E. A., and Shaw, J. H. 1963. The effect of dietary lysozyme supplements on caries incidence in rats. Arch. Oral Biol., *8*:775–776.
151. Takeuchi, M. 1961. Epidemiological study on dental caries in Japanese children before, during, and after World War II. Int. Dent. J., *11*:443–457.
151a. Tanzer, J. M. 1972. Studies on the fate of the glucosyl moiety of sucrose metabolized by *Streptococcus mutans*. J. Dent. Res., *51*: 415–423.
151b. Tanzer, J. M., Chassy, B. M., and Krichevsky, M. I. 1972. Sucrose metabolism by *Streptococcus mutans*, SL-1. Biochim. Biophys. Acta, *261*:379–387.
152. Tanzer, J. M., Hageage, G. J., and Larson, R. H. 1970. Inability to immunologically protect rats against smooth surface caries. 48th Gen. Meeting, IADR Abst. 466, p. 165.
152a. Tanzer, J. M., Hageage, G. J., and Larson, R. H. 1973. Immunization of rats against *Streptococcus mutans*-dependent caries. 51st Gen. Meeting IADR Abst. 546, p. 195.
153. Tanzer, J. M., Krichevsky, M. I., and Keyes, P. H. 1969. The metabolic fate of glucose catabolized by a washed stationary phase caries-conductive streptococcus. Caries Res., *3*:167–177.
154. Tanzer, J. M., and McCabe, R. M. 1968. Selection of plaque-forming streptococci by the serial passage of wires through sucrose-containing broth. Arch. Oral Biol., *13*:139–143.
154a. Taubman, M. A. 1973. Role of immunization in dental disease. Comparative Immunology of the Oral Cavity. S. Mergenhagen and H. W. Scherp, Eds. DHEW Publ. No. 73-438, U.S.G.P.O. Washington, D.C. pp. 138–158.
154b. Taubman, M. A., and Smith, D. J. 1973. Salivary IgA antibody: Possible effects on experimental dental caries. 51st Gen. Meeting IADR Abst. 873, p. 277.
155. Theilade, E., Larson, R. H., and Karring, T. 1973. Microbiological studies of plaque in artificial fissures implanted in human teeth. Caries Res., *7*:130–138.
156. Tourville, D., Bienenstock, J., and Tomasi, T. B., Jr. 1968. Natural antibodies of human serum, saliva and urine reactive with *Escherichia coli*. Proc. Soc. Exp. Biol. Med., *128*:722–727.
157. Toverud, G. 1964. Child dental health. Br. Dent. J., *116*:299–304.
158. Wagner, M. 1968. Specific immunization against dental caries in the gnotobiotic rat. *In* Adv. Germfree Res. and Gnotobiology. M. Miyahawa and T. D. Luckey, Eds. The Chemical Rubber Co., Cleveland, Ohio, p. 264.
159. Weiss, R. L., and Trithart, A. H. 1960. Between-meal eating habits and dental caries experience in preschool children. Am. J. Public Health, *50*:1097–1104.
159a. Williams, R. C., and Gibbons, R. J. 1972. Inhibition of bacterial adherence by secretory immunoglobulin A: a mechanism of antigen disposal. Science, *177*:697–699.
160. Winter, G. B., Hamilton, M. C., and James, P. M. C. 1966. Role of the comforter as an aetiological factor in rampant caries of the deciduous dentition. Arch. Dis. Child., *41*:207–212.
161. Yamada, T., Hojo, S., Kobayashi, K., Asano, Y., and Araya, S. 1970. Studies on the carbohydrate metabolism of cariogenic *Streptococcus mutans* strain PK-1. Arch. Oral Biol. *15*:1205–1217.
162. Zengo, A. N., Mandel, I. D., Goldman, R., and Khurana, H. S. 1971. Salivary studies in human caries resistance. Arch. Oral Biol. *16*: 557–560.
163. Zinner, D., and Jablon, J. M. 1968. Human streptococcal strains in experimental caries. In "*Art and Science of Dental Caries Research*." R. S. Harris, Ed., Academic Press, N.Y., pp. 87–108.
164. Zita, A. C., McDonald, R. E., and Andrews, A. L. 1959. Dietary habits and dental caries. J. Dent. Res., *38*:860–865.

chapter 5

EPIDEMIOLOGY OF PERIODONTAL DISEASE

by

RICHARD E. STALLARD, D.D.S., PH.D.

The significance of epidemiologic investigations into the occurrence of any disease is becoming increasingly important. The data assembled are not only of statistical curiosity, but also of great value in correlating etiologic factors with the disease to bring about successful therapeutic measures.

In the area of periodontal disease it has been stated that the exact prevalence is unknown because of the lack of generally accepted epidemiological tools with which to measure it; however, many reports have indicated a universal distribution of periodontal pathology in the world's population.[1–4] The apparent increase in periodontal disease is not due entirely to an increase in the incidence of disease itself but rather to a better understanding by both the dental profession and the public of periodontal problems.

If maintenance of an efficient natural dentition throughout the life of the individual is a principal objective, then periodontal disease must rank with dental caries as a matter of immediate concern in the practice of dental public health. According to a United States H.E.W. study[5] dental decay accounted for 41.4 per cent of required extractions, and periodontal disease for 38.3 per cent. It was found that the average need for extractions due to decay did not decline greatly with age, but the number of extractions due to periodontal disease increased markedly. The incidence of extraction due to periodontal disease in males over 35 and females over 40 years of age ranked higher than extraction because of caries at a ratio of 3:1.

It can be demonstrated that nearly every adult shows some deviation from the ideal condition of the periodontium. Gross deviation from normal was found to affect half the population over 70 years of age[6] despite the fact that many of the causative factors in periodontal disease are accessible, controllable and correctable (Figures 5–1 and 5–2).

Let us now examine in detail the current epidemiologic tools utilized in assessing the occurrence of periodontal disease. The present indexes are basically measurements of specific factors that in theory express the status of a group or population with respect to the disease. The fact that there are many indexes with a multitude of variations and modifications leads one to the realization that there is apparently no perfect index. Each investigator has selected various etiologic factors or symp-

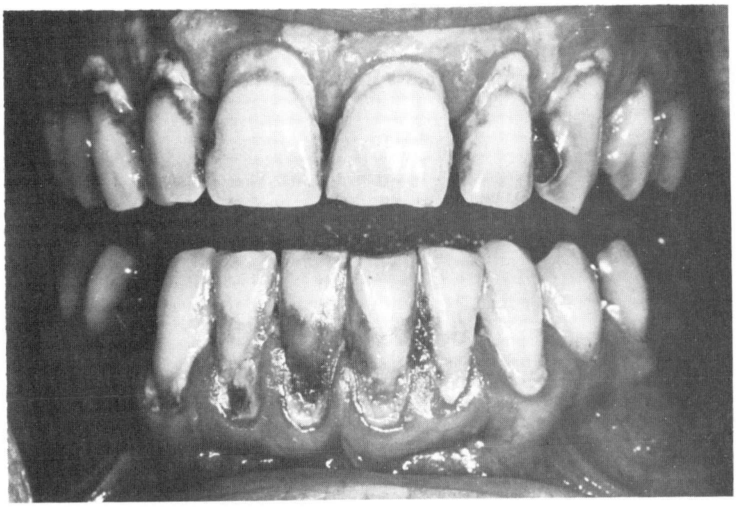

Figure 5–1 Clinical photograph of a 35-year-old male patient from the United States. The gross dental pathology appears to be a direct result of inadequate preventive measures and poor oral hygiene.

toms that in his opinion most accurately reflect, clinically, the periodontal health of an individual. Inherent weaknesses, such as subjectivity, inadequate methods, untrained examiners, or improperly weighted scoring systems, are built into every index. Many of the weaknesses have arisen because the various indexes were originally designed to evaluate specific problems but were subsequently used and modified for other evaluations.

One of the early attempts to assess periodontal disease quantitatively was the PMA Index.[7] Many other indexes designed specifically for large-scale epidemiologic investigations,[8] the evaluation of oral hygiene,[9] and other specific etiologic factors[10] followed. Additional attempts have been made to assess the relationships of etiologic factors to periodontal disease.[11, 12]

Crevicular fluid flow measurements have also become a widely used and accepted method of determining and evaluating inflammatory changes in gingival tissues in response to systemic and local factors,[13, 14] and may be of value in assessing gingival health. In addition, bacterial and cytologic smears have been suggested as possible methods of evaluating gingival health.[15] Ultimately, in studying the health of gingival tissues, it is necessary that a biopsy be taken to assess the state of health; only by this method can one accurately determine the extent and type of inflammation present.

In evaluating dental indexes, it be-

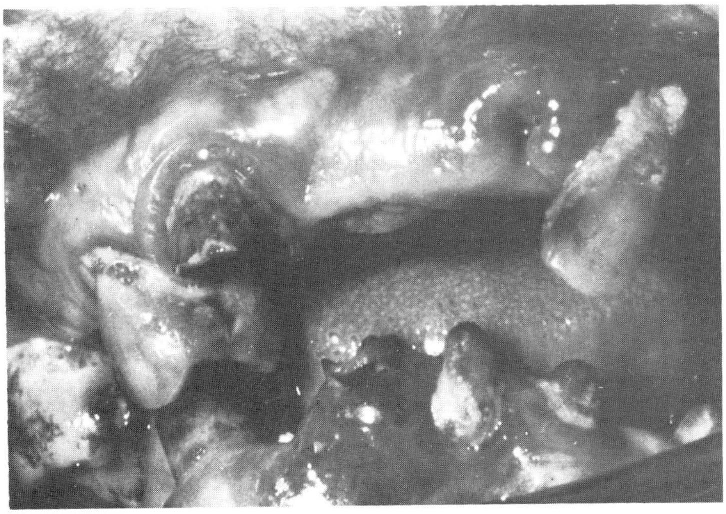

Figure 5–2 Clinical photograph of a 35-year-old male South Vietnamese patient. As in the case of Figure 5–1 a mutilated dentition already manifests itself by the age of 35. Possible genetic and environmental factors may account for the differences observed in the severity of the disease process. Dental plaque, however, has been implicated as the primary etiologic factor in both dental caries and periodontal disease, with the host factors acting only as modifying influences.

comes apparent that the ideal index has probably not yet been developed. Confusion exists because of the disagreement between investigators regarding the clinical signs, symptoms, and etiologic factors related to periodontal disease. Our inability to agree on the primary etiologic factors and their control has resulted in the establishment of many indexes representative of investigators' particular interests and opinions. It would seem important that an index evaluating oral health be as sensitive in the individual evaluation as it is in group evaluations, particularly if it is used in clinical investigations. In this regard, it is essential to know the relation between individual clinical scores and the histologic status of gingival health. From this point of view, it is essential to assess the validity of the commonly used indexes and their components on an individual and population basis.

The various indexes and their respective components were investigated in a recent study[16] and compared to biopsy scores which were considered to be the most accurate evaluation of gingival health. As a method of predicting or evaluating gingival health, the inflammatory condition and calculus scores were unreliable and inaccurate. Crevicular fluid flow measurements also proved to be only as accurate in predicting gingival health as were the calculus scores.

The relationship between oral hygiene, gingivitis, and periodontitis has been accepted for years. It is not surprising, therefore, to find a highly significant relationship between OHI-S scores and biopsy scores ($r = 0.60$ at the .01 level). This is a combination, however, of two possible etiologic factors, oral debris and calculus. From the data obtained, it is suggested that calculus has less influence on the combined scores

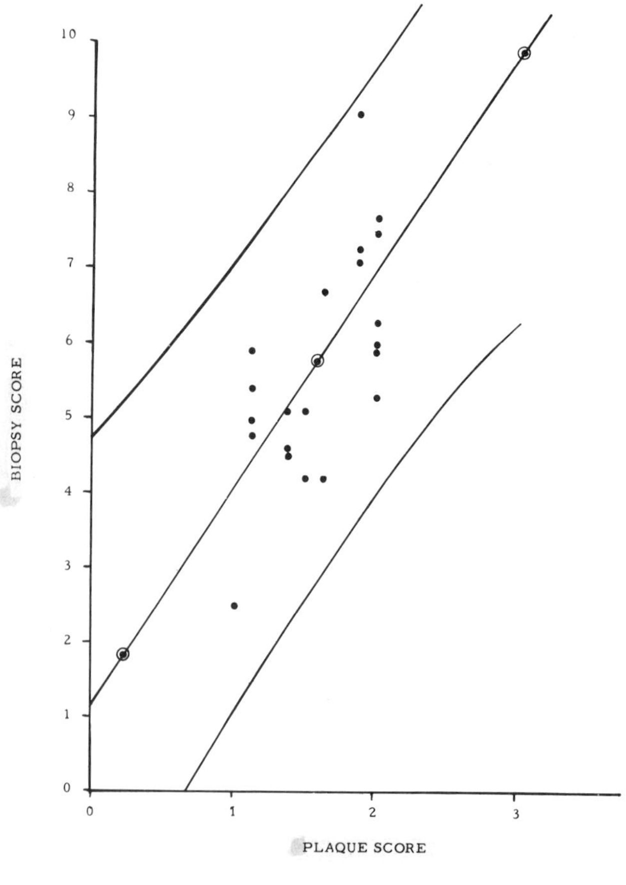

Figure 5–3 This scatter diagram, with its computed regression line, demonstrates clearly the nearly linear relationship between the quality of dental plaque present and the inflammatory status of the tissue as revealed by a biopsy. (Orban, J. E., Stallard, R. E., and Bandt, C. L.: An evaluation of indexes for periodontal health. J. Am. Dent. Assoc. *81*:683–687, 1970.)

than plaque measurements.[16] Gingivitis scores had the second highest correlation; however, the direct correlation with the biopsy scores is lost because etiologic factors and clinical symptoms are again combined.

The fact that plaque exerts a significant effect on tissue health (Fig. 5–3) is of great importance not only to the epidemiologist but to the clinician, as periodontal disease appears to be the result of local factors combined with systemic influences and the host resistance. Thus the control, reduction, or elimination of plaque accumulations appears to be the most effective measure in rendering a preventive dental service, whether on a population or an individual basis.

Epidemiologic studies on the relationship between genetic factors and periodontal disease have been meager. In patients with acatalasia, hypophosphatasia or cyclic neutropenia, which are the result of single mutant genes, periodontal disease is a constant finding.[17] These genes cause their effect on periodontal structures in all environments and thereby illustrate that inborn characteristics can be extremely potent in producing periodontal pathology. However, these conditions are obviously rare and do not represent common periodontal disease, which is clearly caused by a multitude of factors. Nevertheless, it is equally apparent that these causative agents act on tissues that possess inborn potentials of reaction. Therefore, the contribution of hereditary factors in general must be considered in their relationship to other etiological agents which act on the organism to produce the diseased state (Fig. 5–4).

In a detailed review of the literature[18] several major categories of genetic investigations of periodontal disease were enumerated, including family, twin and racial studies. Numerous attempts have been made to detect in families genetic factors related to periodontal disease.[19, 20, 21] Unfortunately the genetic tools that provide the most precise answers are also those that are most fastidious. Simple pedigree analysis can be rewarding but must be used for rare, clearly defined entities caused by single abnormal genes. It is certain that the common form of the disease is not caused by a single gene segregating within families. Family studies may provide confirmation if specific factors are examined, such as calculus formation.

Twin investigations have also been used to ascertain genetic influences in the production of periodontal disease.[21, 22] Identical twins have all of their genes in common, while in sibs, fraternal twins and in parents and children, half the genes are shared. More distant relatives are less valuable since they share a quarter or less genes.

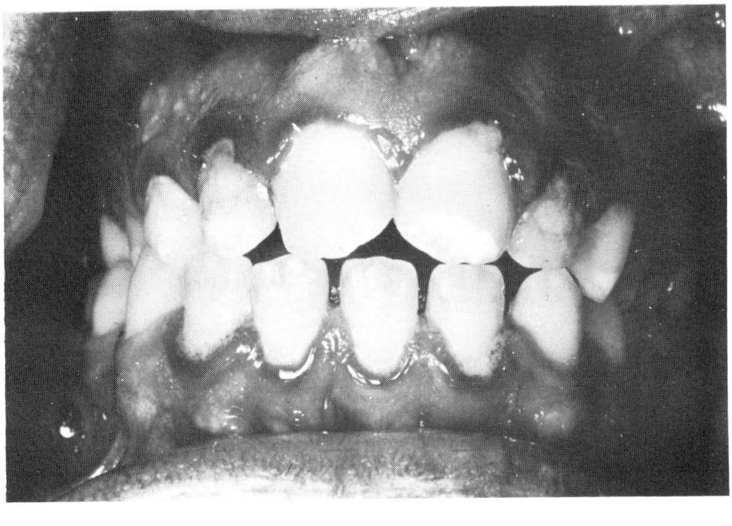

Figure 5–4 Clinical photograph of an adolescent demonstrating crowding and tipping of teeth. The tendency toward malalignment of teeth may be inherited. The neglect, as exemplified in poor oral hygiene, however, represents the most significant variable in production of the disease process.

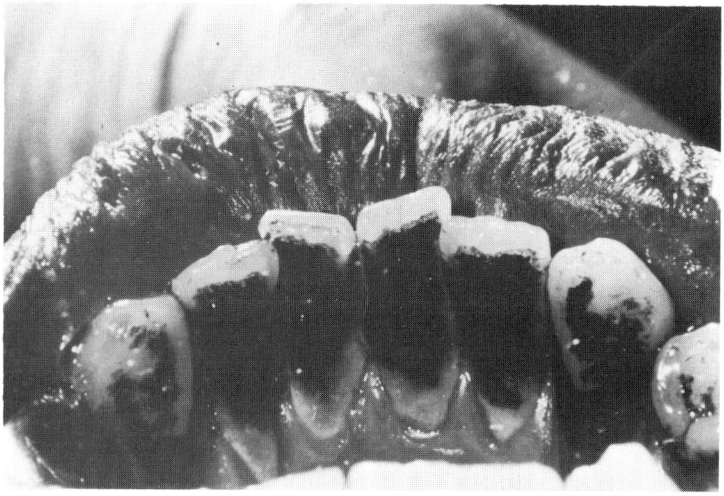

Figure 5–5 Clinical photograph of a patient from India demonstrating additional local environmental factors which may influence the sequence of events in the natural history of periodontal disease. Environmental factors must be weighed carefully before any conclusions are drawn regarding racial tendencies and periodontal disease.

The technique employed in twin studies involves ascertaining whether a trait is present in one twin and then deciding whether the other twin is affected and whether or not the condition is identical.

Of significance was a study carried out in 1958[23] on the occurrence of subgingival calculus. Analysis of 82 identical and 79 non-identical pairs of twins revealed a greater discordance and intra-pair variation among the fraternal twins, suggesting some genetic relationship in subgingival calculus formation.

The importance of race and the tendency of various racial groups to exhibit different incidence of periodontal disease have been discussed by many authors.[24, 25, 26] The differences between races in frequency of a condition such as periodontal disease suggest a genetic basis for the disease, provided it is not due to environmental differences among the races. Nevertheless, detection of differences, whether they be genetic or environmental, suggests the need for further study (Fig. 5–5).

While there is no universally accepted epidemiologic index to evaluate the incidence of periodontal disease, many investigators have established its enormity as a dental health problem. The definitive cause of periodontal disease is also not fully understood; however, it is accepted that there is an interplay of a multiplicity of etiological factors. The human resource of trained personnel necessary for the administration of periodontal therapeutic procedures throughout the world is overwhelmed by the need; therefore, it is necessary to look increasingly to the primary prevention of oral disease as the ultimate answer to this costly area in national health.

REFERENCES

1. Maxcy, K. F., and Rosenau, M. J., eds.: Preventive medicine and public health. 9th Ed., Appleton-Century-Crofts, New York, 1965.
2. W.H.O. Technical Report Series, No. 207: Periodontal disease: Report of an expert committee on dental health. Int. Dent. J. *11*:544, 1961.
3. Marshall-Day, C. D., and Stephens, R. E.: Periodontal disease: prevalence and incidence. J. Periodontol. *26*:185, 1955.
4. Littleton, N. W.: Dental caries and periodontal disease among Ethiopian civilians. Public Health Res. *78*:631, 1963.
5. U.S. Department of Health, Education and Welfare: Selected dental findings in adults by age, race and sex. Publication No. 1000, Series 11, No. 7, 1952.
6. U.S. Department of Health, Education and Welfare: Periodontal disease in adults. Publication No. 1000, Series 11, No. 12.
7. Schour, I., and Massler, M.: Prevalence of gingivitis in young adults. J. Dent. Res. *27*:733, 1948.
8. Ramfjord, S. P., and others: Epidemiological studies of periodontal diseases. Am. J. Public Health 58:1713, 1968.
9. Greene, J. C., and Vermillion, J. R.: Oral hygiene index: a method for classifying oral hygiene status. J. Am. Dent. Assoc. *61*:172, 1960.
10. Volpe, A. R., Kupczak, L. J., and King, W. J.:

In vivo calculus assessment III. Scoring techniques, rate of calculus formation, partial mouth exams vs. full mouth exams and intraexaminer reproducibility. Periodontics *5*: 184, 1967.
11. Lindhe, J., and Koch, G.: The effect of supervised oral hygiene on the gingiva of children. J. Periodont. Res. *1*:260, 1966.
12. Loe, H., and Silness, J.: Periodontal disease in pregnancy. Acta Odont. Scand. *21*:533, 1963.
13. Mann, W. V.: The correlation of gingivitis, pocket depth, and exudate from the gingival crevice. J. Periodontol. *34*:379, 1963.
14. Linhe, J., and Attstrom, R.: Gingival exudation during the menstrual cycle. J. Periodont. Res. *2*:194, 1967.
15. Egelberg, J., and Crowley, G.: The bacterial state of different regions within the clinically healthy gingival crevice. Acta Odontol. Scand. *21*:289, 1963.
16. Orban, J. E., Stallard, R. E., and Bandt, C. L.: An evaluation of indexes for periodontal health. J. Am. Dent. Assoc. *81*:683, 1970.
17. Gorlin, R. J., and Pindborg, J. J.: Syndromes of the head and neck. New York, McGraw-Hill Book Co., 1964.
18. Gorlin, R. J., Stallard, R. E., and Shapiro, B. L.: Genetics and periodontal disease. J. Periodontol. *38*:5, 1967.
19. Denney, R. E.: Heredity and its influence on the teeth. Dent. Cosmos *72*:596, 1930.
20. Roccia, B.: Krankheiten des Stoffwechsels und des endokrinen Systems bei der Ätiologie der Parodontose und der Paradentitiden. (Alveolaryphyorrhoe). Zahnaerztl. Rdsch., *49*:1057, 1940.
21. Korkhaus, G.: Über die erbliche Disposition zur Paradentose. Dtsch. Zahnaerztl. Z., *7*:441, 1952.
22. Noack, B.: Die Parodontoseätiologic im Lichte der Vererbung. Untersuchungen an erbverschiedenen und erbgleichen Zwillingspaaren. Osterr. Z. Stomatol. *38*:267–278, 369–377, 395, 1940.
23. Reiser, H. E., and Vogel, F.: Über die Erblichkeit der Zahnsteinbildung beim Menschen. Dtsch. Zahnaerztl. Z., *13*:1355, 1958.
24. Hruska, A.: Die frühzeitige Zahnlockerung in ihrer geographischen Verbreitung als Rassenfaktor und Pathoheredität trachtet. Żahnaerztl. Welt. *6*:95, 1951.
25. Dabbert, A.: Beobachtungen über Parodontose in Abessinien. Zahnaertzl. Rdsch. *44*:1443, 1935.
26. Leguay, J., and Mantelin, E.: Étude statistique sur les gingivopathies et les parodontolyses de la race berbère. Paradentologie *6*:52, 1952.

ADDITIONAL READING LIST

1. Greene, J. C., and Vermillion, J. R.: The simplified oral hygiene index. J. Am. Dent. Assoc. *68*:7, 1964.
2. Hruska, A.: Zahnanthropologisch-geographische Studien in Lappland. Zahnaerztl. Rdsch., *43*:2163, 1934.
3. Hruska, A.: Die Paradentose als Vererbungsfaktor. Osterr. Z. Stomatol., *37*:1348, 1939.
4. Kapellusch, W.: Anthropogeographische Paradentoseforschung. Paradentologie (Zurich), *7*:90, 1953.
5. Lovdal, A., Arno, A., and Waerhaug, J.: Incidence of clinical manifestations of periodontal disease in light of oral hygiene and calculus formation. J. Am. Dent. Assoc. *56*:21, 1958.
6. O'Leary, T. J., et al.: A screening examination for detection of gingival and periodontal breakdown and local irritants. Periodontics *1*:167, 1963.
7. Ramfjord, S. P.: Indices for prevalence and incidence of periodontal disease. J. Periodontol. *30*:51, 1959.
8. Russell, A. L.: International nutrition surveys: A summary of preliminary dental findings. J. Dent. Res. *42*:233, 1963.
9. Russell, A. L.: A system of classification and scoring for prevalence surveys of periodontal disease. J. Dent. Res. *35*:350, 1956.
10. Volpe, A. R., Manhold, J. H., and Hazen, S. P.: In vivo calculus assessment. I. A method and its examiner reproducibility. J. Periodontol. *36*:292, 1965.
11. Williams, N. B., Parfitt, G. J., and Richards, M. D.: A preliminary study of microbial smears as an aid in diagnosis of gingival health. J. Periodontol. *35*:197, 1964.
12. Zimmerman, E. R., and Baker, W. A.: Effect of geographic location and race on gingival disease in children. J. Am. Dent. Assoc. *61*: 542, 1960.

chapter 6

ETIOLOGY OF PERIODONTAL DISEASE

by

LEONARD SHAPIRO, D.M.D., M.S.,

and

RICHARD E. STALLARD, D.D.S., PH.D.

The etiology of the inflammatory periodontal lesion is complex and, to a certain degree, obscure. It represents the interaction of extrinsic and intrinsic factors which result in the production of a group of symptoms collectively termed periodontal disease. While the lesion is the result of an interaction of various agents and circumstances, the nature and extent of the disease will vary from patient to patient and even from site to site in the same patient.

ANATOMICAL CONSIDERATIONS

The anatomy of the periodontium and the dentition must be considered as significant contributing factors in the development of the inflammatory lesion. While the external surface of the gingiva presents with a relatively keratinized surface which acts as a barrier to extrinsic irritants, the lining of the sulcus (Fig. 6–1) and the col area are relatively unkeratinized and are therefore not afforded the protection of a keratin shield.[16] The col area has been described as the weakest link in the periodontal chain of defense.[11] While a sufficient zone of attached gingiva which can withstand functional forces can be subjected to a plethora of noxious stimuli and still main-

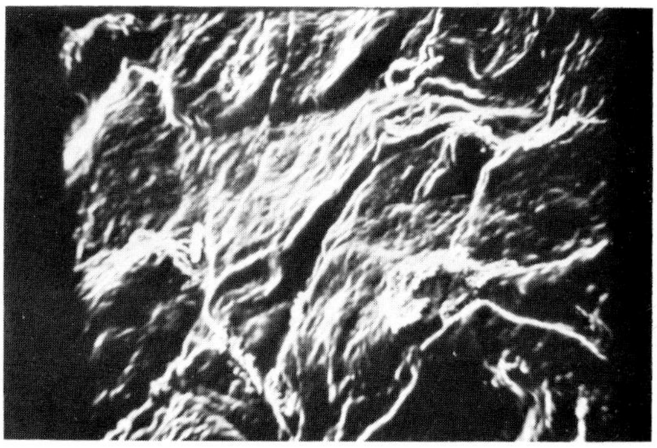

Figure 6–1 Scanning electron micrograph of the epithelium lining the gingival sulcus. Note the integrity of the epithelium and very little intercellular spaces. It is this epithelium that acts as a primary barrier in etiology of periodontal disease.

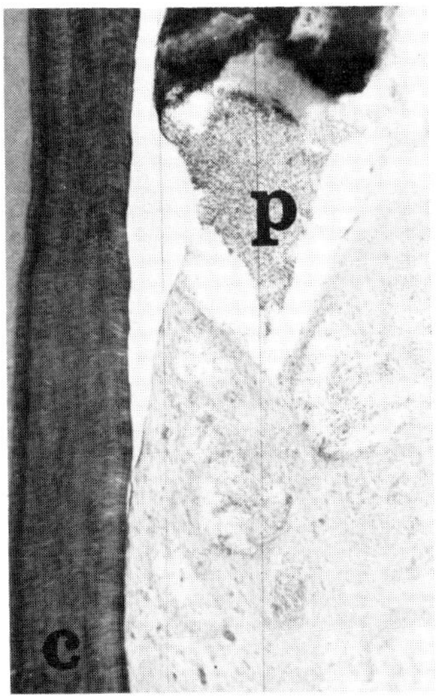

Figure 6–2 With the accumulation of dental plaque and calculus, downgrowth of the epithelium occurs, with destruction of underlying connective tissue. Note the v-shaped defect in the epithelium corresponding to the morphology of dental plaque, indicating the importance of dental plaque as the primary etiologic factor of periodontal disease (C-cementum, P-plaque).

tain its structural integrity, the unkeratinized areas of the attachment apparatus react by undergoing successive inflammatory and degenerative changes, eventually leading to their destruction. An insufficient zone of attached gingiva resulting in detachment of the marginal tissue, on the other hand, reacts in a manner similar to that of the unkeratinized tissues, i.e., marked inflammatory changes and apical migration of the epithelial adherence (Fig. 6–2).

The anatomy and integrity of the dental arch also present an important factor in the defense mechanism of the periodontium and conversely, an absence of this integrity contributes to the breakdown associated with the inflammatory lesion. Constricted arches and malposed teeth (Fig. 6–3) are associated with the relative absence of supporting bone. Rather than the osseous structures being relatively thick with an endosteal and periosteal blood supply, the endosteal supply is compromised, and nourishment is almost completely periosteal. Inflammatory reactions in the periodontium will affect the periosteal blood supply and lead to an early loss of osseous support. Missing and malaligned teeth also play an important role, owing to the lack of contiguous integrity of the dental arch (Fig. 6–4). With the resultant absence or malalignment of proximal contact, these areas become affected by inordinate pressures by such extrinsic factors as food, leading to a breakdown of support.[4]

Dental anatomy also plays a role in the etiology of the inflammatory lesion. While the adherence of the periodontal fibers to cementum is relatively firm, there is an absence of adherence between periodontal fibers and enamel. A groove on the lingual surface of an upper incisor (Fig. 6–5) or an enamel projection into a furcation area pro-

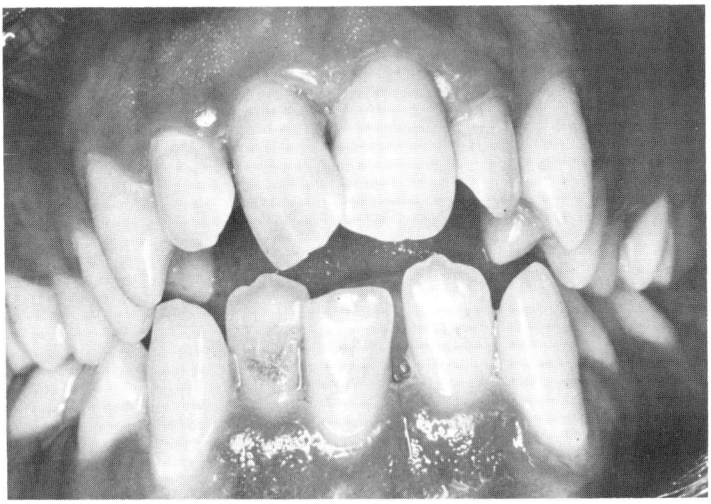

Figure 6–3 Constricted dental arches with accompanying malpositioning of the teeth often results in a deficiency of alveolar bone with the appearance of fenestrations or dehiscences. Any periodontal breakdown in this situation will result in rapid loss of periodontal supporting tissue.

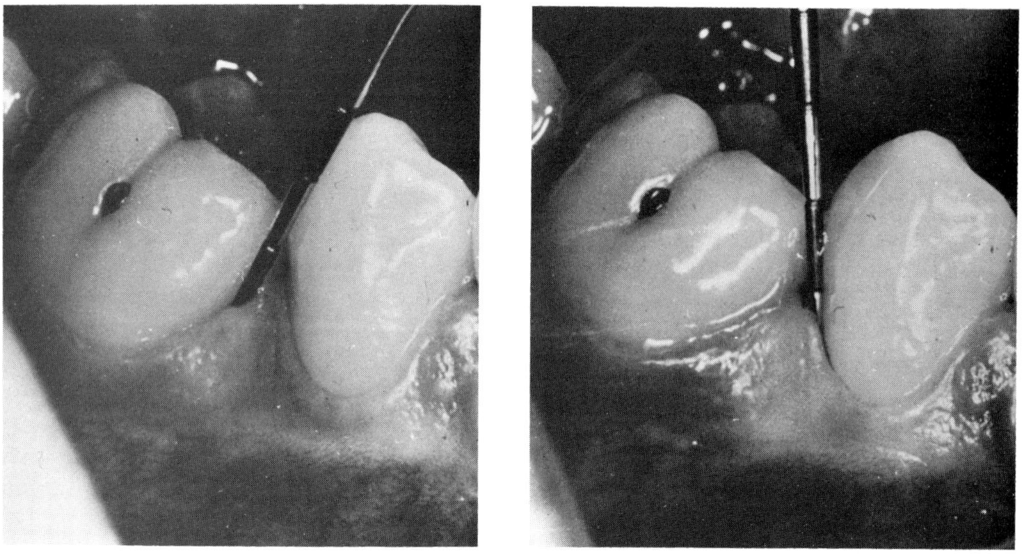

Figure 6–4 Loss of the second premolar and the resultant mesial migration and tipping of the first molar creates initially an apparent increase in sulcular depth on the mesial of the first molar. Difficulty in maintaining oral hygiene in this area subsequently results in true pocket formation.

vides a means of ingress[10] for noxious agents directly into the periodontal structures. These areas are not afforded a fiber barrier system as are the areas of the attachment apparatus which abut cementum.[16]

The fiber system of the periodontium has been well documented and is composed of fibers running between the soft and hard tissues consisting of relatively strong collagen fibers.[3] A thick network of these fibers in both the gingiva and the periodontal ligament affords a mechanism that protects the underlying structures from external irritants. Once the integrity of the fiber barrier system has been compromised, an avenue of ingress is afforded to extrinsic factors and

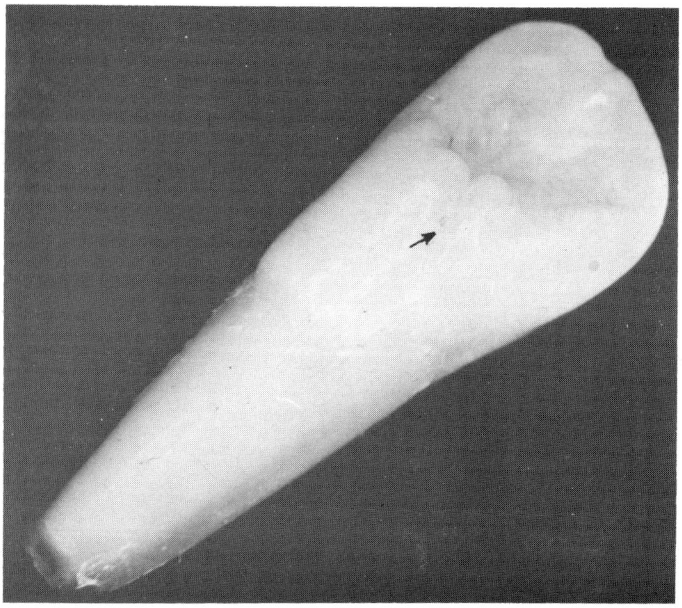

Figure 6–5 The groove on the lingual surface of this tooth provided ingress for toxic materials from dental plaque, contributing to the premature loss of this tooth from periodontal disease.

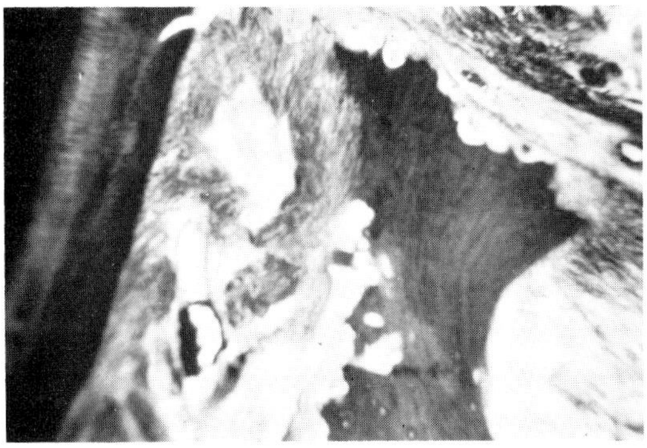

Figure 6–6 In this photomicrograph of human periodontal disease, disruption of the connective tissue elements of the periodontal ligament and gingiva affords ready access of extrinsic factors into the remaining supporting structures, with the resultant rapid continued periodontal breakdown.

also allows for an apical progression of the inflammatory process (Fig. 6–6).

It is apparent, therefore, that the anatomy of the periodontium and the dentition plays a role in the protective mechanism of the host against external stimuli, and conversely, a lack of anatomic integrity will affect the host response to noxious agents and hence play an indirect role in the etiology of the lesion.

BACTERIAL FACTORS

A logical progression from anatomic factors is a consideration of bacterial factors which will affect the integrity of the periodontium. Bacterial plaque appears to be the single most important extrinsic etiologic agent in the development of the inflammatory periodontal lesion.[7] Bacterial plaque has been implicated more by its presence than by a fulfillment of Koch's postulates for infectious diseases. Conversely, the absence of bacterial plaque has led to a reversal of the inflammatory process and, as a logical consequence of this reasoning, it has been argued that the bacterial plaque is the etiologic factor in the disease process.

Bacterial plaque begins as a pellicle deposition on tooth structure.[13] The primary source of the acquired pellicle is saliva, and it forms by a selective absorption of selected glycoproteins on the tooth. The acquired pellicle is covered by a bacteria-free matrix which is then colonized by bacteria. As the plaque develops, it changes from a predominantly gram-positive colonization to a relatively gram-negative population.[15] As the bacterial cells undergo metabolic changes and replicate, selected products are secreted into the surrounding sulcular exudate and thus are in direct contact with the gingival sulcular lining. The metabolic products of the bacteria rather than the bacteria themselves are responsible for the inflammatory changes occurring in the periodontium.[9] Bacterial enzymes such as collagenase and hyaluronidase are present, are capable of degrading natural collagen, and may play a significant role in the initiation of the inflammatory lesion (Fig. 6–7). As a secondary stage, gram-negative bacteria produce endotoxin which may be responsible for the inflammatory reactions in the gingival tissue (Table 6–1).[18] The antigenic potential of these bacterial metabolites has been established, and the resultant immunologic reaction with the subsequent activation of the complement system is ca-

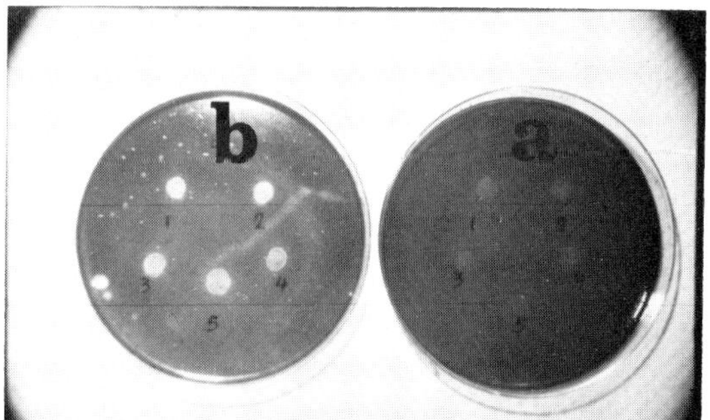

Figure 6–7 The activity of proteolytic enzymes present in dental plaque is demonstrated in this illustration. The media consists of reconstituted collagen onto which a measured quantity of sonicated human dental plaque was placed. All five patients demonstrate the presence of the enzymes by digestion of the material as seen in Petri dish b. At this time a complete dental prophylaxis was performed. One week later similar samples were taken. Note the diminished enzymatic activity of the immature dental plaque (a).

TABLE 6-1 SUMMARY OF MEDIAN VALUES

SEVERITY OF INFLAMMATION	SALIVA *mcg/ml.*	TISSUE *mcg/ml.*	SULCULAR FLUID *mcg/ml.*	PLAQUE *mcg/ml.*
1	.130	.006	.002	1.6
2	.380	.0009	.768	2.4
3	.464	.003	.656	2.4
NUG	.544	.02	1.024	3.0
	$p < .01$	$p < .001$	$p < .001$	$p < .01$

pable of inducing the changes present in the inflamed gingiva.[14]

DENTAL CALCULUS

While bacterial plaque may be the culprit in the initiation of the lesion, other secondary factors are present which contribute significantly to the etiology of the lesion. Calculus formation is the mineralized end product of plaque accumulation on the tooth surface.[22] With plaque acting as a nidus, there is a selective deposition of calcium and phosphate ions, with resultant calculus formation. The calculus which has formed acts as both a mechanical irritant and a porous surface for additional plaque deposition with the consequent continuation of the inflammatory reaction.

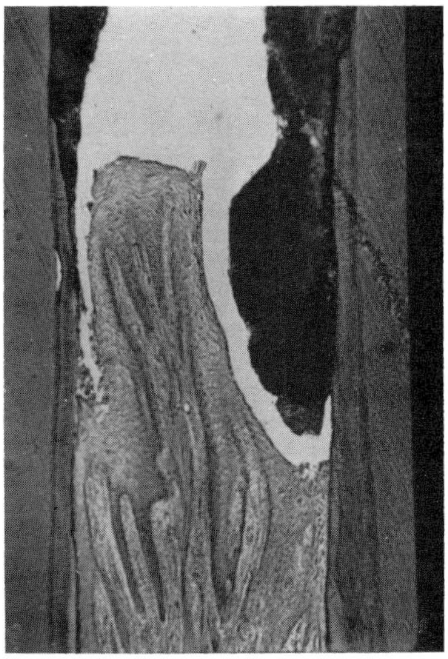

Figure 6–8 In this human biopsy specimen subgingival calculus can be observed. The calculus represents mineralized dental plaque, and in the case of subgingival calculus gingival crevicular fluid represents a major component of the matrix.

Subgingival calculus, on the other hand, differs from supragingival calculus in its formation and composition.[21, 24] Rather than being a direct etiologic agent of the inflammatory reaction, it is a product of the reaction (Fig. 6–8). Selective deposition of mineral ions from the sulcular exudate precipitates the formation of subgingival calculus and then acts as an irritant to further the inflammatory reaction.

OTHER FACTORS

The bacterial plaque and its resultant inflammatory reaction affect the supporting mechanisms of the tooth. If the fiber system of the attachment apparatus remains intact, an adequate barrier to the apical progression of the inflammatory exudate is present. If the bacterial products, however, react with the collagenous substances making up the fiber barrier system, breakdown occurs and the lesion progresses from a self-contained marginal lesion to one which attacks the support of the tooth. As the integrity of the fiber system is compromised, there is a progressive apical migration of the epithelial adherence, with subsequent destruction of the hard structures of the attachment apparatus (Fig. 6–9).[19] Recent investigations have demonstrated that products of the gram-negative population of the dental plaque are capable of inducing osseous destruction[26] or preventing new bone formation.[27] Prostaglandins, also abundant in the inflammatory exudate, may play a significant role in the destructive process when they are combined with bacterial products.[25]

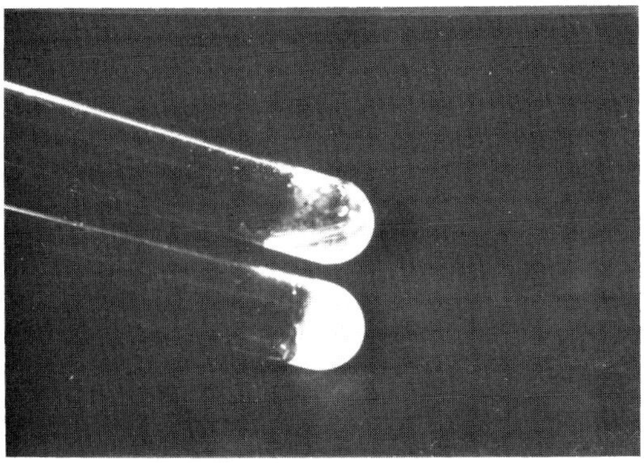

Figure 6–9 The presence of endotoxins produced by gram-negative organisms in human dental plaque can be visualized in these test tubes. Gel formation of the Limulus lysate occurred in the lower tube as a result of the presence of endotoxins. In the upper tube the lysate remains liquid, demonstrating the absence of endotoxins.

Other factors must also be given consideration in the secondary etiology and progression of the lesion. Much stress has been placed on the role of the occlusion in the pathogenesis and progression of the lesion.[8] Traumatic occlusal forces may alter the arrangement of the fiber barrier system and allow the inflammatory exudate to progress directly into the osseous structures with the consequent development of intraosseous lesions (Fig. 6–10).[2] Abnormal occlusal forces alone cannot initiate the lesion, but they are probably capable of altering the progression of the inflammatory exudate into the attachment apparatus.

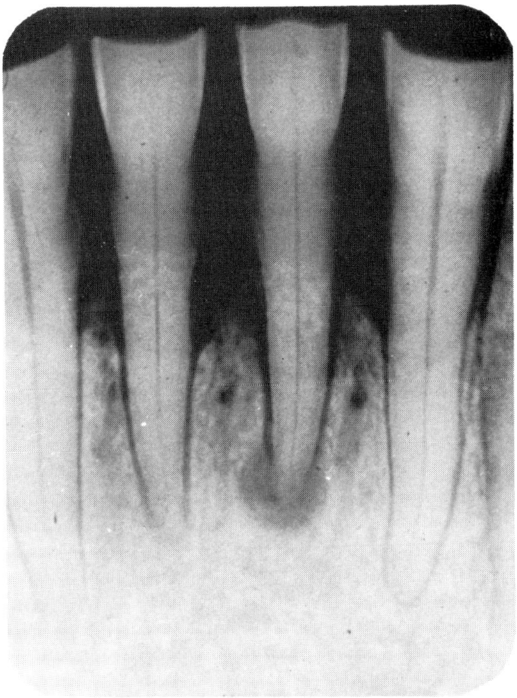

Figure 6–10 This radiograph demonstrates both horizontal and vertical bone loss accompanying trauma from occlusion combined with gingival inflammation resulting from accumulation of dental plaque and calculus. Note the significant incisal wear and periapical lesion that has developed on the right central incisor.

Also concerned with the occlusion is the iatrogenic consequence of faulty restorative dentistry. Like the occlusion, improper restorative dentistry cannot initiate a

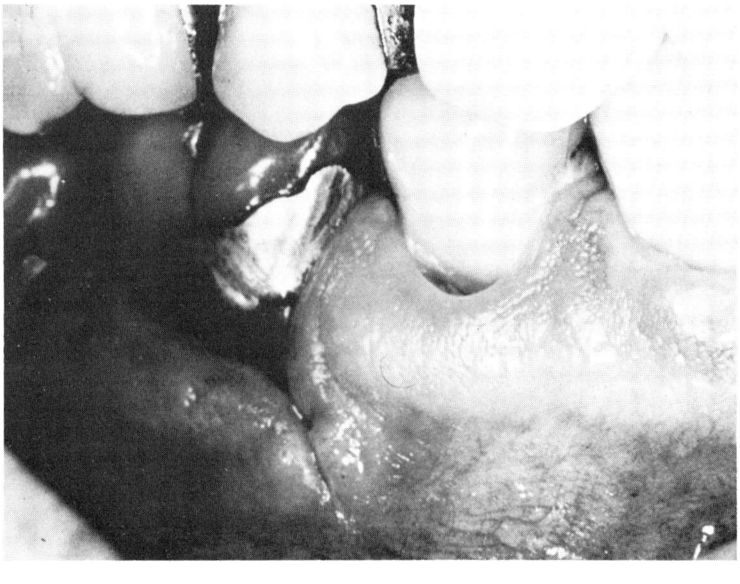

Figure 6–11 Placement of an improperly contoured buccal amalgam restoration has allowed further accumulation of dental plaque with alterations in the gingival morphology and cleft formation, together with bone loss.

lesion. Improperly contoured restorations, however, act as a reservoir for plaque accumulation and are therefore capable of playing a significant role in the development of the lesion (Fig. 6–11).[20] Improper tooth contacts also allow for food impaction which causes pressure degenerative changes in the periodontium. Tooth contacts which are too broad compromise the interdental papilla, making it more susceptible to inflammatory insults.

While the etiology of the inflammatory periodontal lesion is basically extrinsic, certain intrinsic humoral factors may be present which are capable of altering the host response to external factors. Any systemic factors,[12] such as diabetes, pregnancy, and blood dyscrasias,[6] which alter host resistance, are capable of altering host responses to external irritants. The response of periodontal tissues to a generalized disease state can be expressed as being part of the overall tissue response to stress. Generalized disease states must be considered as modifying rather than initiating factors. It is reasonable to assume that patients with generalized disease states will react in an accentuated manner to local factors. This may be due to an altered resistance or an interference with repair in the local tissues. The initiating insult, however, must be extrinsic in origin.

All the available data indicate that the periodontal lesion is extrinsic in nature, most likely of bacterial origin, and can be modified by intrinsic factors which can alter the host resistance.

REFERENCES

1. Cohen, B.: Morphological factors in the pathogenesis of periodontal disease. Br. Dent. J. *107*:31–39, 1959.
2. Glickman, I., and Weiss, L. A.: Role of trauma from occlusion in initiation of periodontal pocket formation in experimental animals. J. Periodontol. *26*:14, 1955.
3. Goldman, H. M.: The behavior of transseptal fibers in periodontal disease. J. Periodontol. *30*:249, 1957.
4. Hirschfield, I.: Food impaction. J. Am. Dent. Assoc. *17*:1504, 1930.
5. Hodge, H. C., and Lueng, S. W.: Calculus formation. J. Periodontol. *31*:211, 1960.
6. Loe, H., and Silness, J.: Periodontal disease in pregnancy. I. Prevalence and severity. Acta Odontol. Scand. *21*:533, 1963.
7. Loe, H., Tgeukade, E., and Jensen, S. B.: Experimental gingivitis in man. J. Periodontol. *36*:177, 1965.
8. MacApanpan, I. C., and Weinmann, J. P.: The influence of injury to the periodontal membrane on the spread of gingival inflammation. J. Dent. Res. *33*:263, 1957.
9. MacDonald, J. B., Gibbons, R. J., and Socransky, S.: Bacterial mechanism in periodontal disease. Ann. N.Y. Acad. Sci. *85*:467, 1960.
10. Masters, D. H., and Hoskins, S. W.: Projection of cervical enamel into molar furca bone. J. Periodontol. *35*:49, 1964.
11. McHugh, W. D.: Some aspects of the development of gingival epithelium. Periodontics *1*:239, 1963.
12. McMullen, J., Gottsegen, R., Legg, M., and Camerini-Davalos, R.: Microangiopathy in the gingival tissues in prediabetes. I.A.D.R. Abstracts. Abst. 56, 1965.
13. Meckel, A. H.: The formation and properties of organic films on teeth. Arch. Oral Biol. *10*:585, 1965.
14. Mergenhagen, S.: Complement as a mediator of inflammation. Formation of a biologically active product after interaction of serum complement with endotoxins and antigen-antibody complexes. J. Periodontol. *41*:202, 1970.
15. Ritz, H. L.: Microbiology population shifts in developing dental plaque. Arch. Oral Biol. *12*:1561, 1967.
16. Schultz-Haudt, S. D., and Aas, E.: Dynamics of the periodontal tissues. II. The connective tissue. Odontol. Tidskr. *70*:397, 1962.
17. Schultz-Haudt, S. D., and From, S.: Dynamics of the periodontal tissues. I. The epithelium. Odontol. Tidskr. *69*:431, 1961.
18. Shapiro, L., Lodato, F. M., Courant, P. R., and Stallard, R. E.: Endotoxin determinations in gingival inflammation. J. Periodontol. *43*:591, 1972.
19. Stallard, R. E., Orban, J. E., and Hove, K. A.: Clinical significance of the inflammatory process. J. Periodontol. *41*:20–24, 1970.
20. Waerhaug, J.: Effect of rough surfaces upon gingival tissues. J. Dent. Res. *35*:323, 1956.
21. Waerhaug, J.: The source of mineral salts in subgingival calculus. J. Dent. Res. *34*:563, 1955.
22. Wasserman, B. H., Mandel, I. D., and Levy, B. M.: *In vitro* calcification of dental calculus. J. Periodontol. *29*:144, 1958.
23. Weinstein, E., and Mandel, I. D.: The fluid of the gingival sulcus. Periodontics *2*:147, 1964.
24. Zander, H. A.: The attachment of calculus to root surfaces. J. Periodontol. *24*:16, 1953.

ADDITIONAL REFERENCES

25. Goodson, J. M.: Prostaglandins: Potential mediators of periodontal disease. I.A.D.R. Abstracts. Abst. 375, 1972.
26. Hausman, E., Raisz, L. G., and Miller, W. A.: Endotoxin: Stimulation of bone resorption in tissue culture. Science *168*:862, 1969.
27. Norton, L. A., Proffit, W. R., and Moore, R. R.: Inhibition of bone growth *in vitro* by endotoxin: Histamine effect. Nature *221*:469, 1969.

chapter 7

EPIDEMIOLOGY OF ORAL CANCER

by

THEODORE E. BOLDEN, D.D.S., PH.D.

INCIDENCE AND PREVALENCE

The incidence of oral cancer varies in different populations. In decreasing order for males between 35–64 years of age, the six highest rates are reported in:

Bombay, India	61.3
Puerto Rico	26.6
Oceania (Caucasian)	16.8
Connecticut	11.5
Durban, South Africa	10.9
Cali, Colombia	9.0

The lowest rate, 1.3, is seen in Finland.[14]

Cancers of the mouth constitute three per cent to five per cent of all human cancers.[29] They are most commonly seen on the tongue, on the lateral margin of the anterior two-thirds. The disease may occur at any age in either sex but is seen more frequently between the fifth and sixth decade and in males nine times more frequently than in females. Presenting symptoms are usually an ulcer or a swelling which is painful. The symptoms of more advanced stages include dysphagia, dysphonia, a lump in the neck and/or a pain in the ear.[29]

Approximately 7000 Americans die each year of oral cancer. Oral cancer is a disease that strikes children as well as adults, but it occurs with increasing frequency with advancing age. Also, it is a disease that occurs more frequently in men than women. Of the estimated 6950 deaths that resulted from oral cancer in 1967, approximately 5200 deaths occurred in men and 1750 in women.[33]

For 1971, it was predicted that 14,200 Americans would present with new cases of oral cancer and that 7000 would die of oral cancer (buccal cavity and pharynx) (Table 7–1 *A*).

Three hundred new cases of oral cancer were estimated for Tennessee as compared to 100 for Mississippi.[28] In 1976, it was estimated that 23,800 Americans will present with new cases of oral cancer and that 8300 will die of oral cancer (buccal cavity and pharynx) (Table 7–1 *B*).[7a] In Britain more than 1850 cases of oral cancer are reported per annum (1963–1964). Approximately 900 deaths per year occur from oral cancer.[8] Death from oral cancer is a worldwide problem. Per 100,000 population, those countries with highest death rates from oral cancer are shown in Table 7–2.

The United States male ranks eighth in death rate from oral cancer, while the United States female ranks twelfth. The highest death rate for both male and female is seen in Hong Kong.

TABLE 7-1A ESTIMATED CANCER DEATHS AND NEW CASES BY SEX AND SITE—(1971)*

SITE	ESTIMATED DEATHS			ESTIMATED NEW CASES		
	Total	*Male*	*Female*	*Total*	*Male*	*Female*
All Sites	335,000	183,000	152,000	635,000	333,800	301,200
Buccal Cavity and Pharynx (Oral)	7,000	5,100	1,900	14,200	9,800	4,400
Lip	125	100	25	1,500	1,300	200
Tongue	1,625	1,200	425	2,700	2,000	700
Salivary Glands	650	400	250			
Floor of Mouth	500	400	100			
Other and Unspecified Oral	1,100	700	400	5,900	3,600	2,300
Pharynx	3,000	2,300	700	4,100	2,900	1,200

*From '71 Cancer Facts and Figures, American Cancer Society.

TABLE 7-1*B* ESTIMATED CANCER DEATHS AND NEW CASES BY SEX AND SITE—1976*

SITE	ESTIMATED DEATHS			ESTIMATED NEW CASES		
	Total	*Male*	*Female*	*Total*	*Male*	*Female*
All Sites	370,000	202,000	168,000	675,000	339,000	336,000
Buccal Cavity and Pharynx (Oral)	8300	5900	2400	23,800	16,900	6,900
Lip	225	200	25	4100	3800	300
Tongue	2000	1400	600	4500	3100	1400
Salivary Gland	650	400	250	}		
Floor of Mouth	525	400	125	8600	5100	3500
Other & Unspecified Mouth	1250	800	450	}		
Pharynx	3650	2700	950	6600	4900	1700

*Adapted from Ca-A Cancer Journal for Clinicians 26(1) 22, 23, 1976. American Cancer Society.

TABLE 7-2 DEATH RATES FROM ORAL CANCER BY COUNTRY HIGHEST INCIDENCE BY SEX

	MALE	FEMALE	FEMALE	
Hong Kong	17.95 (1)	6.29 (1)	6.29 (1)	Hong Kong
France	9.17 (2)	0.78 (28)	3.20 (2)	Taiwan
Puerto Rico	8.73 (3)	2.05 (7)	3.05 (3)	Venezuela
Switzerland	6.95 (4)	0.78 (29)	2.82 (4)	Philippines
Taiwan	6.60 (5)	3.20 (2)	2.36 (5)	Northern Ireland
South Africa	5.92 (6)	1.23 (13)	2.07 (6)	Ireland
Italy	5.44 (7)	0.88 (24)	2.05 (7)	Puerto Rico
United States	4.58 (8)	1.25 (12)	1.77 (8)	Panama
Portugal	4.57 (9)	1.07 (20)	1.47 (9)	England—Wales
Ireland	4.33 (10)	2.07 (6)	1.47 (10)	Sweden

SEX AND SITE DIFFERENCES

The probability of a woman developing a cancer of the lip is between 40 and 70 per cent of that of a man doing so; the incidence of salivary gland tumors is equal in the two sexes; malignant melanoma is more common in women than in men.[3]

The frequency at which oral cancer may occur at any intraoral site has been tabulated by the Cancer Control Branch (CCB) of the United States Public Health Service as follows:

27%	lip
22%	tongue
16%	other oral mucosa
14%	salivary glands
11%	floor of mouth
10%	oral mesopharynx, including tonsil

TABLE 7–3 INCIDENCE OF DIFFERENT TYPES OF CANCER IN DIFFERENT POPULATIONS: ANNUAL RATES PER 100,000 PERSONS AGED 35–64 YEARS, STANDARDIZED FOR AGE

POPULATION	INCIDENCE OF CANCER *Oral* *(141, 143–4)*	*Leukemia* *(204)*
AFRICA		
Mozambique,		
Lourenco Marques	8.5	4.2
Nigeria, Ibadan	2.3	9.1
S. Africa		
*(coloured)	–	3.0
*(white)	–	8.0
Durban		
(African)	10.9	4.8
(Indian)	3.3	7.5
Johannesburg (African)	7.9	2.6
Uganda, Kyadondo	1.9	3.7
AMERICA		
Canada,		
Alberta	4.5	6.7
Manitoba	2.9	12.3
New Brunswick	5.4	4.7
Newfoundland	3.8	4.2
Saskatchewan	3.2	11.0
Chile	2.3	4.4
Colombia, Cali	9.0	4.5
Jamaica, Kingston	7.9	5.7
Puerto Rico	26.6	5.9
*Uruguay	–	9.4
*Venezuela	–	4.1
U.S.A.		
*(non-white)	–	8.3
*(white)	–	10.6
Connecticut	11.5	11.6
New York State	7.7	8.9
ASIA		
*Hong Kong	–	3.1
India, Bombay	61.3	3.7
Israel	3.0	10.6
Japan, Miyagi	1.9	3.2
Singapore (Chinese)	4.6	1.3
*Taiwan	–	–

POPULATION	INCIDENCE OF CANCER *Oral* *(141,143–4)*	*Leukemia* *(204)*
EUROPE		
*Austria	–	9.4
*Belgium	–	9.8
*†Bulgaria	–	8.7
*Czechoslovakia	–	8.8
Denmark	2.2	9.0
England and Wales		
Birmingham region	4.4	6.2
Liverpool region	3.7	6.6
S. Metropolitan region	3.1	6.8
S. Western region	2.5	6.4
Finland	2.4	8.1
*France	–	9.4
*‡Germany F.R.	–	9.2
*Greece	–	9.0
*Hungary	–	11.2
Iceland	1.3	10.7
*Ireland	–	9.7
*Italy	–	9.0
Netherlands (3 provinces)	3.1	5.4
*N. Ireland	–	7.9
Norway	3.1	7.5
*Poland	–	11.4
*Portugal	–	6.7
*Roumania	–	6.5
*Scotland	–	7.2
Sweden	2.6	11.3
*Switzerland	–	8.8
*Yugoslavia	–	6.6
Yugoslavia, Slovenia	5.0	6.5
OCEANIA		
*Australia	–	8.3
New Zealand	3.9	7.8
U.S.A., Hawaii		
(Caucasian)	16.8	5.9
(Hawaiian)	5.9	15.6
(Japanese)	1.9	6.7

*Estimated from mortality data.
†Estimated from data for ages 30–59 years.
‡Figures in parentheses refer to Hamburg only.

The CCB has stated that the risk of oral cancer is highest at ages 45 to 54 for males and 65 to 74 for females. The incidence is 10 in 100,000 or greater.[25] The rate is highest among those who use alcohol and tobacco products. The older the population and the greater the proportion of males, the greater the chances are that a significant number of oral cancers will be found.[38]

When the incidence of mouth cancer is compared to the world population between the ages of 35 and 64 years of age, it can be shown that in the populations of Bombay, Puerto Rico and Hawaii, Caucasians have the highest incidence of mouth cancer, while Caucasian citizens of Hawaii, Manitoba and Connecticut have the highest incidence of leukemia (Table 7–3).

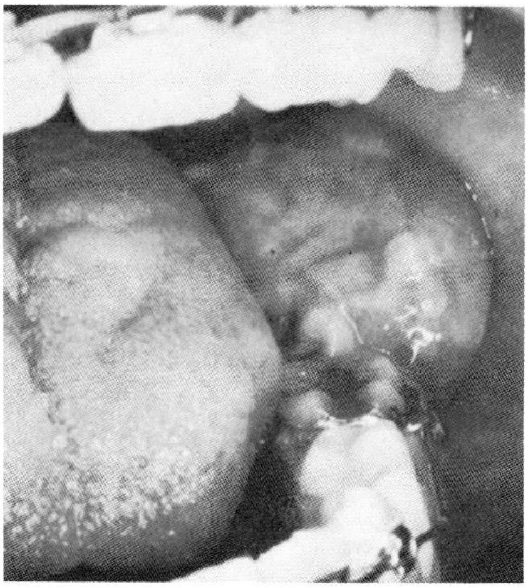

Figure 7–1 This rapidly growing lesion immediately distal to the mandibular left second molar in a 12-year-old girl under orthodontic treatment was clinically diagnosed as pyogenic granuloma, but was later identified by biopsy to be, in reality, a fibrosarcoma. (From Rowe, N. H., and Kwapis, B. W.: Oral and perioral cancer detection. Dent. Clin. N. Amer. *12*:189–201, March 1968.)

ORAL CANCER BEHAVIORIAL CHARACTERISTICS

Oral cancer is essentially of two types – carcinoma and sarcoma. The carcinoma originates in the epithelium; the sarcoma originates in muscle, nerve, blood or connective tissue.

The initial oral carcinoma has specific growth characteristics: (a) remarkable surface differentiation of epithelial growth with ortho- and parakeratosis; (b) neoplastic growth along minor salivary ducts; (c) lateral cancerization (Slaughter); (d) multicentric intraoral origin (Slaughter); and (e) multiple extraoral malignancies.[9] The squamous cell carcinoma may be indurated with a central depression or ulceration late in the disease. Pain is a late sign.[27] Salivary gland tumors present as slow growing, often asymptomatic swellings which seldom ulcerate.[27]

Sarcomas tend to grow fast, appear most often in the mandible, and either destroy bone or produce bone sclerosis (chrondrosarcoma, osteosarcoma).[27] Patients are uniformly young, not aged (Fig. 7–1). When patients first present with tumors more than 2 cm. in diameter, many are advanced and already involve lymph nodes. Oral sepsis, malnutrition and gross loss of weight, anemia, protein deficiency, avitaminosis and bronchopneumonia, emphysema, chronic bronchitis, atherosclerosis and congestive heart failure are current diseases which may accompany oral malignancy,[18] especially cancer of the floor of the mouth in males aged 60 years or more and females aged 70 years or more.

Less than one per cent of oral cancers metastasizes to the oral cavity from a silent, primary site. Swelling and pain and loosening of one or more teeth in the area of the mandible or maxilla are common.[27] The spread is frequently hematogenous.[5]

SURVIVAL PATTERNS

The appearance of regional lymph node metastasis tends to cut the survival rate in half. When lymph node metastasis becomes fixed, survival is again cut in half (Table 7–4). Persons with bilateral lymph node metastasis tend to have the same survival experience as individuals with fixed nodes.[31]

Death from oral cancer is directly related to metastatic disease beyond the neck

TABLE 7–4 SURVIVAL RESULTS OF ORAL CAVITY CANCERS ACCORDING TO STAGE, SIZE OF PRIMARY LESION AND SIZE AND FIXATION OF REGIONAL LYMPH NODE METASTASES*

STAGE	PRIMARY SIZE AND FIXATION	SURVIVAL RESULTS
Stage I	2 cm. or less No metastasis	Best
Stage II	2 and 4 cm. No metastasis	Decreased over Stage I
Stage III	Greater than 4 cm. Regional metastasis Not fixed	One-half that for Stage I Cancers
Stage IV	Metastasis in both sides of neck or metastasis fixed	Decreased over one-half

*Adapted from Smith, R. R.: Stage Classification and End Result Reporting for Oral Cavity Carcinoma. Sixth National Cancer Conference Proceedings. Philadelphia, J. B. Lippincott Co. 1968, pp. 647–653.

or to recurrent or uncontrollable disease above the clavicle.[36] Table 7–5 shows the total number of patients admitted to the University of Texas M. D. Anderson Hospital and Clinic over a period of 25 years with a diagnosis of oral cancer, confirmed by biopsy, and who died in the institution. All tumors were squamous cell carcinomas except one embryonal rhabdomyosarcoma in a three-year-old child and three malignant salivary gland tumors of the palate.

The total number of cases falling into the five divisions of the cause of death is summarized in Table 7–6. The majority (28 per cent) died as a direct consequence of primary oral disease.

TABLE 7–5 ADMISSIONS TO THE M.D. ANDERSON HOSPITAL

SITE	TOTAL ADMISSIONS (1944–1969)	AUTOPSIES	PERCENTAGE
Lip	1298	35	2.7
Buccal Mucosa	287	12	4.2
Gingiva	576	16	2.8
Palate	294	13	4.4
Floor of Mouth	420	24	5.7
RMT–Tonsil	438	25	5.7
Tongue	947	55	5.8
	4260	180	4.47 (Avg.)
Too large to classify		7	
		187	

BREAKDOWN BY SITES†

Gingiva	16	RMT and T	25
Lower	13	Tonsil	5
Upper	3	Pillar	5
Floor of Mouth	24‡	RMT	15
Palate	13	Tongue	55
Soft	9	Base	26
Hard	4‡	Lateral	12
		Tip	2
		Too large to tell	15

*From Thoma, G. W.: Causes of death in patients with oral cancer. Oral Surg. *30*(6):817–823, December 1970.

†Age range: 3–93; all tumors were squamous cell carcinomas except for (‡) one embryonal rhabdomyosarcoma, one mucoepidermoid tumor and two malignant mixed tumors.

TABLE 7–6 CAUSE OF DEATH*

Summary of all Sites		187
Local	20	52
Metastatic	32	
Complication P_x		46
Unrelated: Malignant		46
Non-Malignant		43

*From Thoma, *ibid.*

Prognosis for oral cancer is more influenced by the *stage* of the disease than by any other parameter (Table 7–5).[37]

Survival for cancer of the oral cavity by *stage* ranged from 5 to 90 per cent (Table 7–7). The posterior or base of the tongue (Stages II and IV) offers the poorest prognosis.[37]

Survival for advanced oral cancer would appear to be greater with surgery than from radiotherapy (63/50 Stage II; 43/8 Stage III) (Table 7–7).[37]

Survival by Negroes for five years is one-half that of American whites.[37] Tables 7–9 and 7–10 show data on 58 posterior tongue carcinomas. Of the 16 survivors, seven had glossectomies, seven had primary irradiation and two had glossectomy plus irradiation.

Table 7–11 shows the survival of 56 patients with carcinoma of the floor of the mouth. In the 22 survivors, 18 had surgery and four had radiotherapy. The results of 41 patients with soft-palate carcinoma are illustrated in Table 7–12. The primary therapy for three of the 10 survivors was surgery and for seven, radiotherapy. Three of the latter required subsequent surgery.

Finally, in Table 7–13, the data on 37 patients with carcinoma of the anterior two-thirds of the tongue are recorded. Seventeen survived—16 had glossectomies, one (Stage II) had irradiation.

TABLE 7–7 SURVIVAL RELATED TO STAGE IN 233 PATIENTS WITH CARCINOMA OF THE ORAL CAVITY*

SURVIVAL TIME (MONTHS)	STAGE I *19 Patients* (%)	STAGE II *69 Patients* (%)	STAGE III *100 Patients* (%)	STAGE IV *45 Patients* (%)	TOTAL *233 Patients* (%)
6	100	100	98	73	94
12	100	96	86	33	80
24	100	88	56	8	60
36	100	77	42	5	50
48	94	72	33	5	44
60	94	65	27	5	40

*From Trimble, W. M.: Cancer of the oral cavity: Five-year end results in 237 patients. Ann. Otol. Rhinol. Laryngol. 78:716–723, 1969.

TABLE 7–8 "ESTIMATED" FIVE-YEAR SURVIVAL RELATED TO TREATMENT AND STAGE IN 200 PATIENTS WITH ORAL CAVITY CARCINOMA*

STAGE	SURGERY	RADIOTHERAPY†	COMBINED‡
I	92% of 14	100% of 4	
II	63% of 35	50% of 26	0% of 11
III	43% of 42	8% of 26	18% of 11
IV	6% of 17	6% of 17	0% of 7

*Indeterminate and supportive-therapy-only patients discarded, causing higher "estimated" figures for comparison.

†Usually supervoltage (2 mev).

‡Considered combined therapy if both modalities planned initially and completed within four months. (From Trimble, *ibid.*)

TABLE 7-9 FIVE-YEAR SURVIVAL RATES OF 58 PATIENTS WITH CARCINOMA OF THE BASE OF TONGUE TREATED FROM 1958 THROUGH 1963 (All Stages)[a]

	(1)	(2)	(3)	(4)	(5)	(6)	(7)	(8)
TIME OBSERVED IN MONTHS	TOTAL NUMBER PATIENTS	DIED TONGUE CARCINOMA	DIED OTHER CAUSES[b]	LOST FOLLOW-UP[b]	NUMBER AT RISK[c]	PROPORTION DYING[d]	PROPORTION LIVING[e]	CUMULATIVE PROPORTION SURVIVING (%)[f]
0–6	58	5	2		57.0	.088	.912	91
7–12	51	15	1	1	50.0	.300	.700	64
13–24	34	10		1	33.5	.299	.701	45
25–36	23	6			23.0	.261	.739	33
37–48	17				17.0	.000	1.000	33
49–60	17	1			17.0	.059	.941	31
60+	16				16.0	.000	1.000	31

[a]Similar tables prepared for each stage and site. [b]Without evidence of base of tongue carcinoma. [c]Number in column 1 minus one-half of columns 3 and 4. [d]Column 2 divided by column 5. [e]One minus column 6. [f]Column 7 times preceding column 8, expressed to nearest whole per cent. (From Trimble, *ibid.*)

TABLE 7-10 SURVIVAL RELATED TO STAGE OF DISEASE IN 58 PATIENTS WITH CARCINOMA OF THE BASE OF TONGUE*

SURVIVAL TIME (MONTHS)	STAGE II *10 Patients* (%)	STAGE III *25 Patients* (%)	STAGE IV *21 Patients* (%)
6	100	100	76
12	100	80	23
24	88	51	12
36	63	38	6
48	63	38	6
60	63	34	6

*There were only two Stage I patients, both surviving five years. The "total" column is given in Table 8–7. (From Trimble, *ibid.*)

TABLE 7-11 SURVIVAL RELATED TO STAGE OF DISEASE IN 56 PATIENTS WITH FLOOR OF MOUTH CARCINOMA TREATED FROM 1958 THROUGH 1963*

SURVIVAL TIME (MONTHS)	STAGE I *5 Patients* (%)	STAGE II *16 Patients* (%)	STAGE III *26 Patients* (%)	STAGE IV *9 Patients* (%)	TOTAL *56 Patients* (%)
6	100	100	100	78	96
12	100	93	88	45	84
24	100	93	80	11	74
36	100	87	72	11	68
48	100	80	51	11	56
60	100	65	37	11	46

*From Trimble, *ibid.*

TABLE 7-12 SURVIVAL RELATED TO STAGE OF DISEASE IN 41 PATIENTS WITH SOFT PALATE CARCINOMA*

SURVIVAL TIME (MONTHS)	STAGE II *14 Patients* (%)	STAGE III *16 Patients* (%)	STAGE IV *9 Patients* (%)	TOTAL *41 Patients*† (%)
6	100	100	56	90
12	100	88	45	83
24	79	49	0	51
36	64	21	0	35
48	57	14	0	31
60	43	14	0	26

*From Trimble, *ibid.*
†There were only two patients in Stage I; both survived 5 years (100%).

GEOGRAPHIC CONSIDERATIONS

WESTERN CANADA

Oral cancer susceptibility in western Canada increases with age with 45 years or over being the high risk range. Men seem to be more susceptible, but this is decreasing. For Ontario (males over 45 years), in decreasing order, the most susceptible oral sites are lower lip (in rural residents), lateral margins of the tongue, anterior floor of the mouth, remainder of tongue, buccal mucosa and lower gingiva.

A 1965 cancer incidence survey in Ontario by site and status revealed 26,542 cases of cancer. There were 616 new cases of cancer involving the lip (268), tongue (100) and mouth (248), and 137 new cases of cancer of the pharynx. There were 9282 deaths from cancer. Males had a higher incidence of cancer than females under 25 years and at 65 years and over. There were 16 males to every one female with lip cancer, four to one for cancer of the pharynx and about three to one for tongue and bladder cancer.[22]

Manitoba and Saskatchewan have a much higher incidence of lip cancer than Quebec and Ontario, with the reverse being true for intraoral cancer.

Age and sex are very significant factors in oral cancer incidence with older men having the higher occurence. Urban-rural resident distribution also appears to influence the incidence. Floor of the mouth and gingival cancers appear more in urban residents and lip cancer in rural residents.

Cancer of the hard palate has decreased in both sexes, but soft-palate and floor of the mouth cancers have increased mainly in the 45 to 65 age group. The five-year survival rate in the 1929–1958 Toronto group was

TABLE 7-13 SURVIVAL RELATED TO STAGE OF DISEASE IN 37 PATIENTS WITH CARCINOMA OF THE ANTERIOR TWO-THIRDS OF TONGUE*

SURVIVAL TIME (MONTHS)	STAGE I *6 Patients* (%)	STAGE II *15 Patients* (%)	STAGE III *14 Patients* (%)	STAGE IV *2 Patients* (%)	TOTAL *37 Patients* (%)
6	100	100	100	50	97
12	100	100	93	50	95
24	100	100	57	–†	80
36	100	92	36	–	67
48	100	92	22	–	60
60	100	92	22	–	60

*From Trimble, *ibid.*
†The surviving Stage IV patient died of other causes in the eighteenth month, apparently free of cancer.

44.7 per cent for floor and palate cancer, and 44 per cent for buccal mucosa and gingival cancer.[2]

CANADIAN ESKIMOS

Carcinoma of the salivary glands in Eskimos is estimated to be approximately 30 times that of a white population of the same size over the same time span. The majority of malignant tumors observed are carcinomas.[40] Salivary tumors are usually prevalent in Eskimos. Fourteen cases of salivary gland tumors in Canadian Eskimos showed four histologic types (Table 7–14).

The 14 tumors occurred in a population of about 11,500 Canadian Eskimos over a nine-year period. Eleven of the 14 tumors were diagnosed as malignant and constituted about 28 per cent of all the cancers seen. One of the 14 tumors was a poorly differentiated carcinoma that tended to invade locally and invade regional nodes.

The evidence is strong that there is an increase in susceptibility in salivary gland tumors in Eskimos. The incidence in Eskimos is calculated to be approximately 30 times that of the white population of the same size and over the same period of time of Saskatchewan.

TABLE 7–14 SUMMARY OF TUMORS IN 14 CASES*

HISTOLOGICAL TYPE	NO. OF CASES
Mixed tumor salivary gland	3
Adenoid cystic carcinoma	1
Malignant papillary cystadenoma lymphomatosum	1
Carcinoma	9

*From Wallace, A. C., et al.: Salivary gland tumors in Canadian Eskimos. Cancer *16*:1338–1353, 1963.

The increased incidence of salivary gland tumors in Canadian Eskimos may be due to either genetic or environmental factors. Support for a genetic factor is that these Eskimos are such a small, close-knit group. Consideration of the environment of the patients gives no indication of their etiology.[40]

SOUTHWESTERN ALASKA: YUPEK ESKIMOS

During the ten and one-half year period, July, 1957 through December, 1967, there were 45 deaths from cancer in the southwestern Alaska Eskimo with a sex ratio of 1.37:1.0, male to female. In the same

TABLE 7–15 A SUMMARY OF REPORTED CONFIRMED CASES OF CANCER IN ESKIMOS*

SITE	FIBIGER 1923 GREENLAND	GOTTMAN 1960 ALASKA	SCHAEFER 1960 CANADA	THOMAS 1961 LABRADOR	LEDERMAN 1961 CANADA	HURST 1963 ALASKA	S.W. ALASKAN ESKIMOS
Buccal cavity, pharynx	1	–	–	1	1	4	3
Salivary glands	1	–	8†	–	0	1	1
Esophagus	–	2	3	–	–	7	13
Stomach	–	3	–	1	–	3	5
Colon and rectum	–	2	3	4	5	7	12
Other digestive tract	–	3	1	1	–	8	5
Lung	–	2	2	–	3	4	5
Breast	4	1	–	1	2	4	4
Genital tract	1	–	4	3	3	10	7
Urinary tract	–	1	4	1	6	3	11
Skin	1	–	2	–	3	5	2
Thyroid	–	–	–	–	–	5	5
Bone	1	–	–	1	–	1	1
Leukemia and lymphoid	–	1	1	–	2	3	4
Other	–	–	2	–	2	1	3
Unspecified primary	–	–	–	–	1	–	4
Totals	9	15	30	13	37	66	85

*From Fortiune, R.: Cancer *23*:468–474, January–June, 1969.
†Includes several benign tumors, not separated.

period, 82 malignant tumors were found in 82 patients. Forty-six per cent of the 82 malignant tumors originated in the alimentary tract. The most common site was the esophagus.[19] Four cases involved the buccal cavity, pharynx and salivary glands (Table 7–15). One squamous cell carcinoma was thought to have arisen in the submaxillary gland. There was the complete absence of parotid malignancy. These findings are in sharp distinction to those of other investigators who found 14 cases of parotid malignancies.[40]

AUSTRALIA

A total of 30,837 new cases of cancer were registered in Melbourne, Australia (1959–1964). The lip was the most common site of oral cancer in Australia (62.1 per cent) and represented 3.2 per cent of all malignancies reported.[34] The disease was predominant in males as compared to females (3,090 to 484) with a ratio of 64:1, and had a predilection for the lower lip (99:1). In males the lower lip was involved about 15 times more often than the upper lip as compared to a frequency of one and one-half for women.

Histologic types included squamous cell carcinoma, basal cell carcinoma, malignant pleomorphic adenoma, mucoepidermoid carcinoma, adenocarcinoma and mixed salivary gland tumor. The predominant tumors were the squamous cell carcinoma (88.1 per cent) and basal cell carcinoma (9.3 per cent). Cancer of the lip was observed at every decade. However, most cases were found between 50 and 70 years in males and between 55 and 75 years in females. Surgery alone and radiotherapy alone gave comparable five-year survival rates: 87.3 *vs.* 86.4 respectively.[34]

A review of 39 consecutive cases of local recurrence of squamous cell carcinoma of the lip revealed that those patients have more than a 50 per cent chance of survival for five years (Table 7–16).[13] All lesions had originated on the vermillion border; radiotherapy was the initial therapy in 31 cases and excision in eight. The average age of the patients was 66 years (22–88).

TABLE 7–16 SURVIVAL RATE OF PATIENTS WITH ORAL CANCER* IN THE DECADES 1946–1955 AND 1956–1965 IN AUSTRALIA†

LENGTH OF SURVIVAL (YEARS)	DECADES UNDER REVIEW	
	1946–1955	*1956–1965*
One	46%	63%
Three	26%	33%
Five	20%	22%

*Squamous cell cancers of the floor of the mouth and/or of the lower alveolus – 165 consecutive patients.

†From Fleming, W. B.: Cancer of the floor of the mouth: a survey of the problem in Victoria. Med. J. Australia 2:434–436, Sept. 3, 1968.

AFRICA

Tumors of the jaws seem to be more frequent in Africa than in other parts of the world. They formed 3.6 per cent of all tumors seen in Uganda (1952–1957),[12] but only 0.18 per cent of all tumors registered in Denmark (1953–1957).[10] Carcinoma of the jaws usually starts earlier in Africans than in Europeans.

Egypt

The most prevalent oral malignancy in Cairo (United Arab Republic) in 1967 was squamous cell carcinoma. It occurred most frequently in males. The order of decreasing frequency was the tongue (34.6 per cent), gingiva (25.1 per cent), lips (17.3 per cent), buccal mucosa (11.9 per cent), floor of mouth (6.4 per cent) and palate (4.7 per cent).[17]

Bantu Regions

The standardized morbidity for cancer at all sites among Bantu males was one-half that of United States non-whites and one-third that of United States whites. The morbidity among females is approximately one-

TABLE 7–17 COMPARISON OF STANDARDIZED RATES FOR CANCER BY PRIMARY SITE AND SEX IN JOHANNESBURG BANTU RESIDENTS (1953–1955), UNITED STATES WHITES AND NON-WHITES*

	MALE			FEMALE		
ICD	*Johannesburg Bantu*	*U.S. White*	*U.S. Non-White*	*Johannesburg Bantu*	*U.S. White*	*U.S. Non-White*
All Malignant Neoplasms	64.8	172.8	134.2	86.7	192.9	178.1
Buccal Cavity and Pharynx	4.1	10.9	6.1	1.5	3.8	3.9
Lip	10.2	3.1	0.3	–	0.5	0.2
Tongue	1.2	2.0	1.2	0.4	0.6	0.6
Salivary Glands	0.4	1.5	1.6	0.3	1.6	2.0
Floor of Mouth	1.0	–	–	–	–	–
Mouth, Other and Unspecified	0.5	–	–	0.1	–	–

*From Oettle, A. G., and Higginson, J.: Age-specific cancer incidence rates in the South African Bantu: Johannesburg (1953–1955). S. Afr. J. Med. Sci. *31*:21–41, 1966.

half that in United States whites and non-whites (Table 7–17).[24]

Data is presented which suggests that the rates for cancers of the oral cavity are not dissimilar in Bantu children and children of the United States (Table 7–18).

Kampala, Uganda

Between 1953 and 1964, there were 719 children in Kampala, Uganda with malignant disease. The peak age was five to six years. More than 65 per cent of those with malignancies were male. The most frequent malignancy was Burkitt's lymphoma. In descending order, the remaining malignancies were neural (67), embryonal and mixed tumor (60), connective tissue (52), leukemia (36), epithelial tumor (35) and bone tumors (21).[6] The difference in incidence of malignancies in Uganda and the U.S.A. is shown in Table 7–19.

TABLE 7–18 MEAN OF THE QUINQUENNIAL RATES PER 100,000 PER ANNUM FOR CANCERS BY SITE AND SEX IN THE YEARS 0–14, JOHANNESBURG BANTU (1953–1955), U.S. WHITE AND U.S. NEGRO (1947)*

	BANTU		U.S. WHITE		U.S. NEGRO	
	M	*F*	*M*	*F*	*M*	*F*
All Sites	10.0	6.2	17.6	16.3	15.8	9.0
Oral Cavity	0.7	–	0.4	0.3	0.4	0.9

*Modified from Oettle and Higginson, *ibid.*

Ghana

A total of 89 primary bone tumors, 70 of which involved the maxilla and mandible, were found in 7945 surgical and 1159 postmortem examinations in Accra (1962–1965). The jaw tumors fell predominantly in one of the following three groups: odontogenic tumors (22), Burkitt's tumor (27) and carcinoma (13). Twenty of the odontogenic tumors were ameloblastomas.[20]

The peak incidence of patients with Burkitt's tumor with jaw involvement was

TABLE 7–19 TABULAR COMPARISON OF DISTRIBUTION OF TYPES OF MALIGNANCIES IN THE PRESENT STUDY FROM UGANDA CONTRASTED WITH THE DISTRIBUTION FROM A ROUGHLY COMPARABLE AGE GROUP IN THE UNITED STATES*

TUMOR TYPE	UGANDA *1953–1964*	U.S.A.† *1935–1951*
Epithelial	35 = 4.9%	34 = 4.4%
Melanoma	5 = 0.7%	20 = 2.6%
Leukemia	36 = 5.0%	231 = 30.0%
Lymphoma	432 = 60.1%‡	97 = 12.6%
Connective tissue	73 = 10.2%	114 = 14.8%
Neural tumors	67 = 9.3%	180 = 23.4%
Embryonal and mixed	60 = 8.3%	85 = 11.1%
Other tumors	11 = 1.5%	8 = 1.0%
Total	719	769

*From Brown, R. E. and Wright, B. I.: Malignancies in African children. Clin. Pediat. 6(2):106–115, Feb. 1967).
†Adapted from O'Conor and Davies, 1960.
‡Including 61 lymphomas of non-Burkitt type.

TABLE 7-20 FREQUENCY OF AMELOBLASTOMAS*

LOCATION	PERCENTAGE OF ALL MALIGNANCIES	SOURCE	
Ghana	1.9	Edington	1956
Nigeria	1.8	Elmes and Baldwin	1947
French West Africa	2.7	Camain	1954
Uganda	0.8	Dodge	1965
Tanzania	0.7	Slavin and Cameron	1969
Denmark	0.18	Clemmesen	1965
Kampala	0.33	Dodge	1965

*Compiled from data in Slavin and Cameron. Brit. J. Cancer 23(1):31–38, March 1969.

four and five years[20] and is similar to that experienced reported in a series of 260 patients from East Africa.[7] Cases of lymphosarcoma "clinically" and histologically resembling Burkitt's tumor have been described in Caucasian children in the United States.[15, 33]

The ameloblastoma and benign fibro-osseous lesions of the jaw are not uncommon in East Africa.[30] The highest incidence is found in French West Africa (Table 7–20). They occur most often in the mandible (48.6) in the male (34:21) and between 20 and 50 years of age. The ameloblastoma has been seen in children 3½ and 4½ years of age. The tumors were most often cystic, multilocular and either follicular or plexiform. Squamous metaplasia could be shown in 45 per cent of the cases.

LEBANON

During 1950, 1950 newly diagnosed cases of cancer were reported in Lebanon in 1507 resident Lebanese and 443 non-Lebanese, mostly from neighboring Arab countries. An incidence rate of 102.8 for males (1043) and 104.1 for females (1029) per 100,000 population was estimated for all cancers. Fifty-seven cases involved the buccal cavity (Table 8–21). The largest number of cases of buccal cavity cancers was squamous cell carcinoma (56.2 per cent).

In males and females, cancer of the buccal cavity constituted approximately 27 per cent of all confirmed cases of cancer (Table 7–21).[1] Christian males and females had a higher incidence of cancer of the buccal cavity than did Moslem males and females – 15 to 13 and 15 to 11 cases respectively (Table 7–21).

Cancer in Lebanon is diagnosed somewhat more frequently in females than in males. The overall estimated rates of 102.8 for males and 104.1 for females are low compared to the rates in Denmark (258.3 and 289.5) or in other well-developed countries. This may be due to the fact that only 15.2 per cent of the population were over 50 years of age as compared to 25.7 per cent in Denmark.

JAPAN

Squamous cell carcinoma was the most frequent oral neoplasm seen in Japan (1952–1966) (Table 7–22). In descending order of frequency, it involved the gingiva, tongue, palate, floor of the mouth and buccal mucosa (Tables 7–23 and 7–24). The highest frequency was seen in males and in the fifth decade of life (Tables 7–25 and 7–26). Six per cent of oral malignancies involved the salivary glands as adenocarcinoma or malignant epitheliomas (Tables 7–27 and 7–28).[4] Oral carcinomas among Japanese occur earlier than in Europeans and Americans (Table 7–29).

The majority of British patients with oral carcinoma are over 60 years of age, and females have oral carcinoma less frequently than males in a ratio of 1:9.[21]

PAPUA AND NEW GUINEA (BURKITT'S TUMOR)

Two tumors, Burkitt's lymphoma and lymphosarcoma, formed only one-third of 35 cases of the childhood lymphomas diagnosed between 1958 and 1963 in the terri-7–30).[35] Burkitt's lymphoma is more common in children of Papua and New Guinea than is leukemia (Table 7–31).

The histopathologic picture of Burkitt's

TABLE 7-21 MORBIDITY FROM CANCER IN LEBANON

A. Number of Male and Female Cancer Patients by Age Group and Selected Primary Site (Buccal Cavity)

SEX	ALL AGES	10	10–19	20–29	30–39	40–49	50–59	60–69	70–79	80
M	29	–	1	4	3	2	8	8	2	1
F	28	1	–	4	4	8	5	5	2	–

B. Number of Cases of Cancer by Sex, Religion and Primary Site

PRIMARY SITE	CHRISTIAN *Male*	CHRISTIAN *Female*	MOSLEM *Male*	MOSLEM *Female*	OTHER AND UNDETERMINED *Male*	OTHER AND UNDETERMINED *Female*
Buccal Cavity						
Tongue	2	1	1	–	–	–
Salivary glands	–	2	1	–	–	1
Mouth and other	9	10	5	9	1	1
Pharynx	4	2	3	2	–	–
Total	396	437	284	242	80	68

C. Number of Cases of Cancer and Percentage Distribution by Sex, Religion and Selected Primary Site

	MALE				FEMALE			
	Number		*Percentage*		*Number*		*Percentage*	
PRIMARY SITE	*Christian*	*Moslem*	*Christian*	*Moslem*	*Christian*	*Moslem*	*Christian*	*Moslem*
Buccal Cavity	15	13	3.8	4.6	15	11	3.4	4.5
Total – All Sites	396	284	100	100	437	242	100	100

D. Number of Cases of Cancer and Percentage Distribution by Histologic Type and Selected Primary Site*

PRIMARY SITE	NO.	PERCENTAGE ADENO-CARCINOMA	PERCENTAGE TRANSI-TIONAL CELL CARCINOMA	PERCENTAGE BASAL CELL CARCINOMA	PERCENTAGE SQUAMOUS CELL CARCINOMA	PERCENTAGE SARCOMA	PERCENTAGE OTHER AND UNSPECIFIED
Buccal Cavity	57	8.7	5.3	1.7	56.2	7.1	21.0

E. Age-Adjusted Cancer Incidence Rates per 100,000 Population in Lebanon (Estimated) and in Denmark (1953–1957) by Sex and for the Buccal Cavity*†

SITE	MALE *Lebanon*	MALE *Denmark*	FEMALE *Lebanon*	FEMALE *Denmark*
Buccal Cavity	4.4	8.9	5.2	3.2

*Adjusted for age to a combined population of Lebanon (1964) and Denmark (1953–1957).
†Adapted from Abou-Daoud, K. T.: Morbidity from cancer in Lebanon. Cancer *19*:1293–1300, Sept. 1966.

TABLE 7–22 CLASSIFICATION OF TUMOR CASES DURING 14-YEAR BIOPSIES FROM AUGUST 1952 TO DECEMBER 1966 IN THE DEPARTMENT OF PATHOLOGY, NIHON UNIVERSITY SCHOOL OF DENTISTRY*

MALIGNANT TUMORS *Epithelial*	*Case Number*	*Nonepithelial*	*Case Number*	BENIGN TUMORS	*Case Number*
Squamous cell carcinoma	166	Sarcoma	22	Ameloblastoma	35
Carcinoma simplex	2	Leukemia	1	Papilloma	16
Adenocarcinoma or malignant epithelioma of salivary gland	12			Fibroma	16
				So-called mixed tumor of salivary gland	21
				Tumor of salivary gland	5
				Fibromatosis gingivae	5
				Haemangioma	4
				Cementoma	3
				Osteoma	2
				Lymphangioma	1
				Myxoma	1
Total	180		23		109

*From Awazawa, Y., and Moro, I.: On 180 biopsies of oral carcinomas in our department of pathology. Journal of Nihon University School of Dentistry 9:97–106, 1967.

TABLE 7–23 FREQUENCY OF INCIDENCE OF SQUAMOUS CELL CARCINOMA IN ORAL AREA ACCORDING TO SPOT OF ORIGINS*

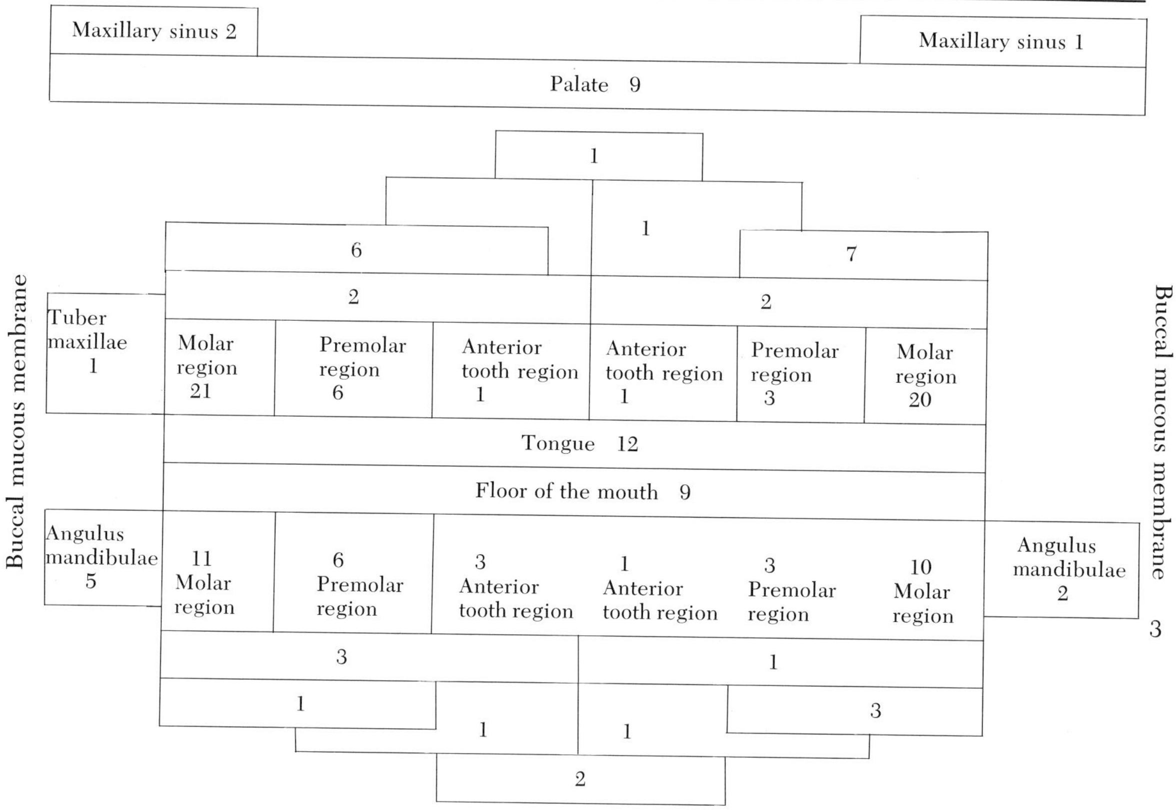

*Each figure in the table indicates case number of incidence. (From Awazawa and Moro, *ibid.*)

TABLE 7–24 RELATIONSHIP BETWEEN AGES AND HISTOLOGIC TYPES REGARDING INCIDENCE OF MALIGNANT EPITHELIOMAS OF SALIVARY GLANDS*

	HISTOLOGIC TYPE						
AGE	*Epidermoid Carcinoma*	*Adeno-carcinoma*	*Mucoepi-dermoid Tumor*	*Adenoid Cystic Carcinoma*	*Clear-Cell Carcinoma*	*Carcinoma Simplex*	TOTAL
10 ~ 19					1		1
20 ~ 29							
30 ~ 39						1	1
40 ~ 49				1			1
50 ~ 59	1	2	1	1			5
60 ~ 69	1	2					3
70 ~ 79		1					1
Total	2	5	1	2	1	1	12

*From Awazawa and Moro, *ibid.*

TABLE 7–25 FREQUENCY OF INCIDENCE OF ORAL CARCINOMAS OWING TO SEX AND AGE*

AGE	MALE	FEMALE	TOTAL
0 ~ 9			
10 ~ 19		1	1
20 ~ 29	1	2	3
30 ~ 39	8	5	13
40 ~ 49	16	14	30
50 ~ 59	40	18	58 (32.2%)
60 ~ 69	33	15	48
70 ~ 79	20	4	24
80 ~ 89	1	1	2
90 ~ 99		1	1
Total	119	61	180
Minimum age	26	18	
Maximum age	80	90	
Average age	56.5	53.8	
Average age of both sexes	55.6		

*From Awazawa and Moro, *ibid.*

TABLE 7–26 FREQUENCY OF INCIDENCE OF SQUAMOUS CELL CARCINOMA IN ORAL REGION OWING TO SEX AND AGE*

AGE	MALE	FEMALE	TOTAL
0 ~ 9			
10 ~ 19			
20 ~ 29	1	2	3
30 ~ 39	7	5	12
40 ~ 49	16	13	29
50 ~ 59	37	16	53 (31.9%)
60 ~ 69	30	13	43
70 ~ 79	19	4	23
80 ~ 89	1	1	2
90 ~ 99		1	1
Total	111	55	166
Minimum age	26	24	
Maximum age	80	90	
Average age	57.5	54.2	

*Keratinized type: 88 cases, non-keratinized type: 75 cases, basal cell carcinoma: 3 cases. (From Awazawa and Moro, *ibid.*)

TABLE 7–27 FREQUENCY OF INCIDENCE OF ADENOCARCINOMA OR MALIGNANT EPITHELIOMA OF SALIVARY GLAND ACCORDING TO SEX AND AGE*

AGE	MALE	FEMALE	TOTAL
10 ~ 19		1	1
20 ~ 29			
30 ~ 39	1		1
40 ~ 49		1	1
50 ~ 59	3	2	5
60 ~ 69	1	2	3
70 ~ 79	1		1
Total	6	6	12
Minimum age	33	18	
Maximum age	73	68	

*From Awazawa and Moro, *ibid.*

TABLE 7–28 FREQUENCY OF INCIDENCE OF ADENOCARCINOMA OR MALIGNANT EPITHELIOMA OF SALIVARY GLAND OWING TO SPOT OF ORIGINS*

Palate	6
Ramus mandibulae	2
Maxillary gingiva	3
Parotid gland	1
Total	12

*From Awazawa and Moro, *ibid.*

tumor and the lymphosarcoma of New Guinea is that of a poorly differentiated lymphocytic lymphosarcoma. However, the cells are uniform but up to three times the size of ordinary lymphocytes. Well-defined nuclei are surrounded by a thin ill-defined rim of slightly basophilic cytoplasm. Nucleoli are usually small, pyknotic and sharply defined. Mitotic figures are plentiful and common. Large, pale phagocytic histiocytes are irregularly interspersed among the sheets of tumor cells, giving a "starry

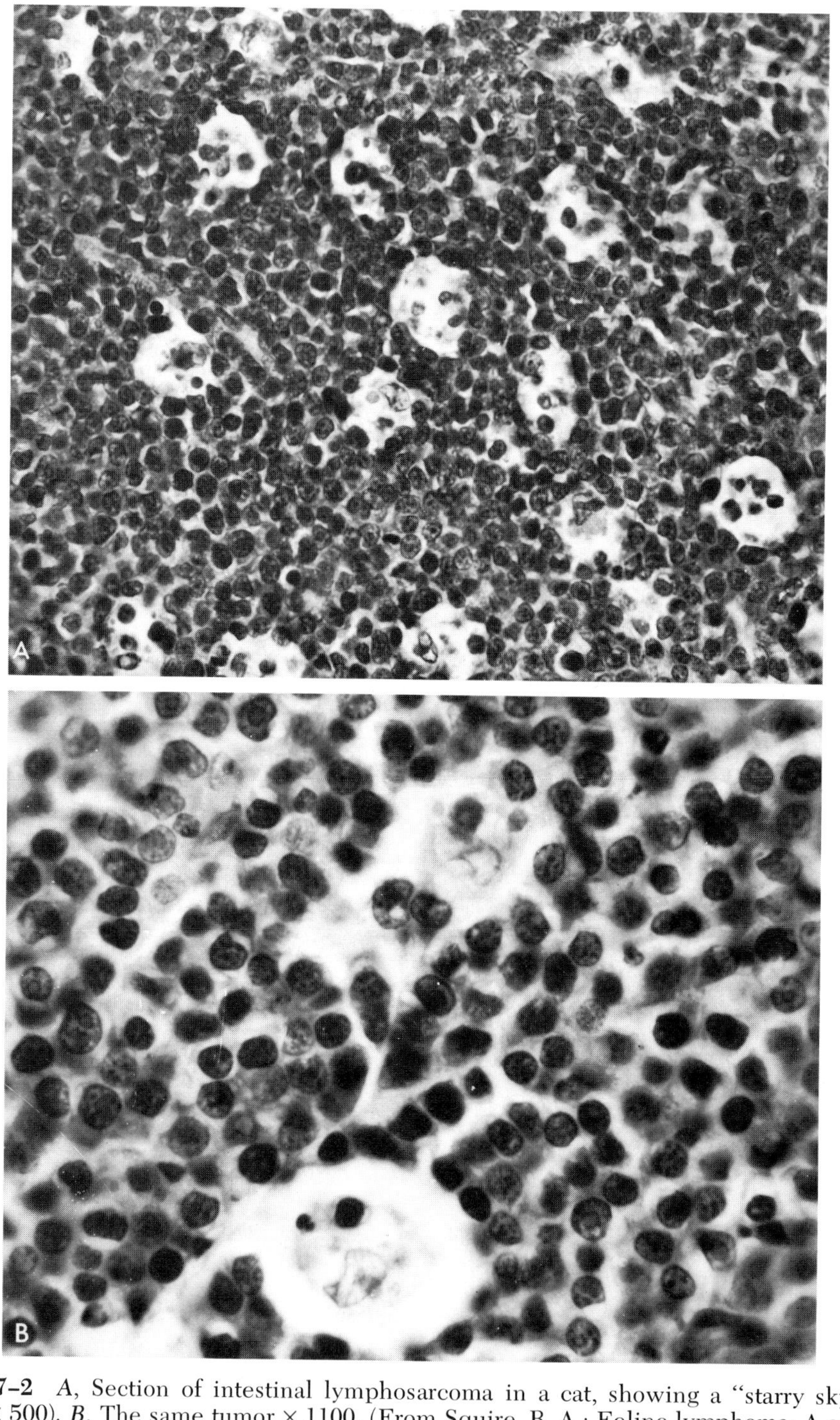

Figure 7–2 *A*, Section of intestinal lymphosarcoma in a cat, showing a "starry sky" pattern (H. and E. × 500). *B*, The same tumor × 1100. (From Squire, R. A.: Feline lymphoma: A comparison with the Burkitt tumor of children. Cancer *19*:447–453, March 1966.)

TABLE 7–29 COMPARISON OF AVERAGE AGES IN HIGHEST ORAL CARCINOMA FREQUENCY*

INVESTIGATORS	AVERAGE AGES GIVEN	YEARS OF SURVEY
Willis	63.9	1953
Tiecke	55.0	1954
Ono	57.3	1959
Otani	54.7, 53.3	1952
Shiota et al.	52.6	1957
Yamada et al.	52.8	1960
Miyazaki et al.	54.0	1958
Awazawa and Moro	55.6	1967

*From Ledlie, F. M., and Harmer, M. H.: Cancer of the mouth; a report on 800 cases. Brit. J. Cancer *4*:6–18, 1960.

TABLE 7–30 CHILDHOOD LYMPHOMA IN PAPUA AND NEW GUINEA (1958–1963 Inclusive)*

ANATOMICAL LOCALIZATION	NO.
Jaw	11
Eye	3
Neck (unspecified)	4
Thyroid	1
Clavicle or shoulder	1
Elbow	1
Axilla	1
Abdominal	
Retroperitoneal	4
Liver	2
Ovaries	1
Kidneys	1
Ileo-cecal	1
Massive	4
Total	35

*From ten Seldam, R. E. J., Cooke, R., and Atkinson, L.: Childhood lymphoma in the territories of Papua and New Guinea. Cancer *19*:437–446, March, 1966.

sky" appearance. Patches of necrosis and a delicate stroma complete the picture.

Evidence provided by histochemistry[41,42] and tissue culture[17,26] strongly support an origin from the reticuloendothelial system. Visceral lymphosarcoma of domestic cats in the United States is also characterized by lack or absence of leukemia with little or no peripheral lymphadenopathy and the "starry sky" histologic appearance (Fig. 7–2).[32]

The geographical distribution of Burkitt's tumor was originally limited to temperature and humidity. No tumors were observed in the equatorial belt above an altitude of about 5000 feet with a suggested minimum temperature of 60° F. with humidity at about 20 inches of annual rainfall. The annual rainfall in the territories of Papua and New Guinea varies from 38 inches to 248 inches; the temperature falls with increasing altitude with the average minimum being above 60° F.

Burkitt's tumor can occur bilaterally, may involve both the maxilla and mandible and occasionally all four quadrants at once. Burkitt's tumor commonly involves the orbit, salivary glands, thyroid and the abdomen.[12, 43]

INDIA

The most common sites of involvement of the oral cavity with cancer in 1916 cases of oral and oropharyngeal carcinomas in India in 1965 was the buccal mucosa (52.3 per cent) and the tongue (26.9 per cent). The anterior two-thirds of the tongue was

TABLE 7–31 MALIGNANCIES OF THE RETICULOENDOTHELIAL SYSTEM IN THE TERRITORIES OF PAPUA AND NEW GUINEA (1958–1963 Inclusive)*

MALIGNANCY	AGE DISTRIBUTION *0–4*	*5–9*	*10–14*	*15–19*	*20–29*	*30–39*	*40*	TOTAL
Lymphosarcoma								
F (14)	2	4	2	1	2	1	2	(9 + 5)
M (42)	6	15	5		8	6	2	(26 + 16)
Reticulosarcoma								
F (11)		1	1		4	2	3	(2 + 9)
M (21)		1			5	6	9	(1 + 20)
Hodgkins								
F (5)			1		4			(1 + 4)
M (11)		2	3	1	3	1	1	(5 + 6)
Leukemia								
F (6)	1				2		3	(1 + 5)
M (29)	3	3	1	3	11	4	4	(7 + 22)

*From ten Seldam, Cooke and Atkinson, *ibid.*

involved four times more frequently than the posterior one-third. The peak incidence was between 50 and 54 years of age. Three cases of carcinoma of the cheek and two cases of palatal carcinoma were in patients under 20 years of age. In males, cancer of the buccal mucosa tended to occur at an earlier age, while malignant tumors of the posterior third of the tongue and palate occurred in advanced age. In females, cancer of the posterior third of the tongue had a tendency to occur late in life (Fig. 7–3). Carcinoma of the buccal mucosa and gingivae was more common in women than in men (Fig. 7–4). At all other sites (lips, tongue, palate and tonsils), the incidence was higher in males than females (Table 7–32).[39]

PUERTO RICO

One hundred fifty-seven cases of carcinoma of the floor of the mouth were seen in Puerto Rico between the years 1950 and 1965. Carcinoma of the floor of the mouth was the second most frequent form of cancer of the oral cavity seen at the I. Gonzales Martinez Oncologic Hospital. The incidence was approximately 1.8 for males

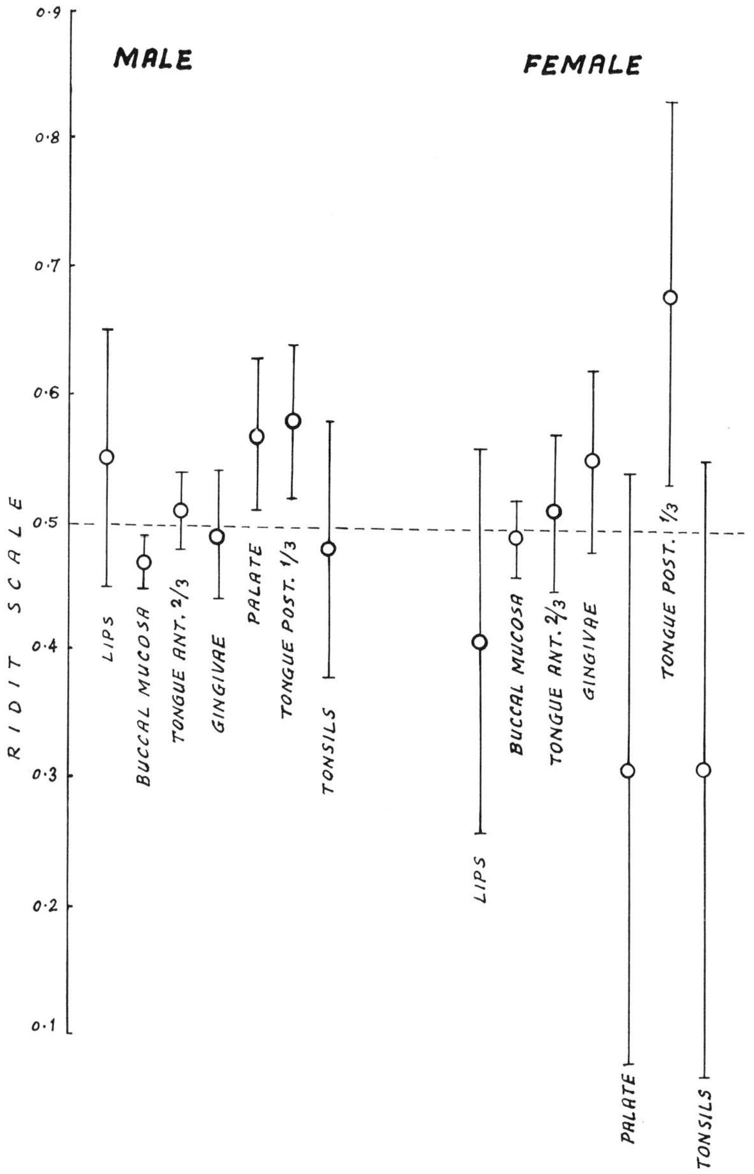

Figure 7–3 Statistical analysis of age. (From Wahi, P. N., Kehar, U., and Lahiri, B.: Factors influencing oral and orpharyngeal cancers in India. Brit. J. Cancer *19*:642–660, 1965.)

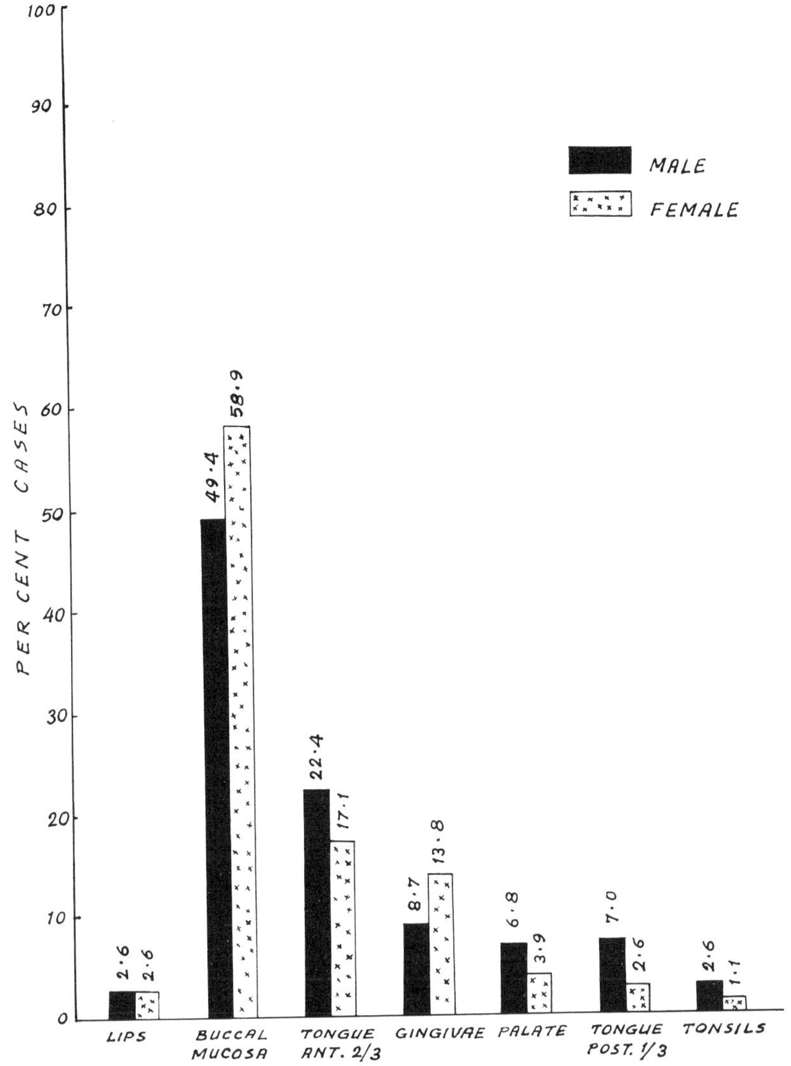

Figure 7–4 Anatomical distribution of oral and oropharyngeal carcinomas in men and women (1916 cases). (From Wahi, Kehar, and Lahiri, *ibid.*)

TABLE 7–32 DISTRIBUTION OF ORAL AND OROPHARYNGEAL CARCINOMAS BY SITE ACCORDING TO SEX AND RELIGION (1909 Cases)*

SITE	HINDU MALE		MOSLEM MALE		HINDU FEMALE		MOSLEM FEMALE	
	Cases	*Per Cent*	*Cases*	*Per Cent*	*Cases*	*Per Cent*	*Cases*	*Per Cent*
Lips	30	2.8	5	1.7	8	2.9	7	2.4
Buccal mucosa	517	48.7	152	53.2	132	47.5	200	70.7
Tongue, anterior two-thirds	266	25.0	42	14.7	63	22.4	32	11.4
Gingivae	84	8.0	33	11.5	44	16.0	31	11.0
Palate	69	6.5	22	7.7	17	6.2	5	1.7
Tongue, posterior one-third	72	6.8	22	7.7	10	3.6	6	2.1
Tonsils	24	2.2	10	3.5	4	1.4	2	0.7
Total	1062	100.0	286	100.0	278	100.0	283	100.0

*From Wahi, P. N., Kehar, U., and Lahiri, B.: Factors influencing oral and oropharyngeal cancers in India. Brit. J. Cancer *19*:642–660, 1965.

TABLE 7–33 CARCINOMA OF THE FLOOR OF THE MOUTH INCIDENCE IN PUERTO RICO*

YEARS	FLOOR OF MOUTH† Male	FLOOR OF MOUTH† Female	TONGUE Male	TONGUE Female	OTHER ORAL CAVITY SITES‡ Male	OTHER ORAL CAVITY SITES‡ Female
1950–1961	1.4	0.5	3.9	1.4	2.3	1.5
1962	2.9	0.9	5.3	1.4	3.3	0.6
1963	1.1	0.5	5.3	1.8	5.3	1.8
1964	2.0	0.8	5.4	1.2	4.3	1.5

*Crude incidence rates per 100,000 population. Data from Puerto Rico Central Cancer Registry. (From Correa, J. N., Bosch, A., and Marcial, V. A.: Carcinoma of the floor of the mouth: Review of clinical factors and results of treatment. Am. J. Roentgenol. Radium Ther. and Nucl. Med. 99(2):302–312, February 1967).

†Includes lower gum.

‡Includes buccal mucosa, upper gum, palate, and oral cavity not otherwise specified.

TABLE 7–34 CARCINOMA OF THE FLOOR OF THE MOUTH FREQUENCY OF ETIOLOGIC FACTORS INCIDENCE AND PER CENT FREQUENCY BY SEX*

	NOT STATED Male	NOT STATED Female	YES Male	YES Female	NO Male	NO Female
Tobacco	18 (15%)	5 (14%)	102 (84%)	26 (70%)	1 (1%)	5 (14%)
Alcohol	40 (33%)	13 (35%)	62 (51%)	7 (19%)	19 (16%)	16 (43%)
Poor oral hygiene (poor teeth)	39 (32%)	12 (33%)	70 (58%)	21 (57%)	12 (10%)	3 (8%)
Leukoplakia	53 (44%)	21 (58%)	14 (12%)	2 (5%)	54 (45%)	13 (35%)
Lues	24 (20%)	11 (30%)	23 (19%)	2 (5%)	74 (61%)	23 (64%)

*Total number of cases: male (121); female (36). (From Correa, Bosch and Marcial, *ibid.*)

and 0.7 for females. The highest form of oral cancer involved the tongue with a sex incidence of 4.97 for males and 1.45 for females (Table 7–33).[11] Those factors most frequently associated with cancer of the floor of the mouth were tobacco, alcohol, poor oral hygiene, leukoplakia and lues (Table 7–34).

Radical surgery was considered best for the treatment of lymph node metastasis and for the management of recurrent and residual primary lesions of carcinoma of the floor of the mouth.

REFERENCES

1. Abou-Daoud, K. T.: Morbidity from cancer in Lebanon. Cancer *19*:1293–1300, Sept. 1966.
2. Anderson, D. L.: Oral cancer incidence in central and western Canada. J. Can. Dent. Assoc. *34*:180–189, 1968.
3. Ashley, D. J.: Sex differences in the incidence of tumors at various sites. Brit. J. Cancer *23*:26–30, March 1969.
4. Awazawa, Y., and Moro, I.: On 180 biopsies of oral carcinomas in our department of pathology. J. Nihon Univ. Sch. Dent. *9*:97–106, 1967.
5. Bolden, T. E., and Smith, R. E.: Hepatoma metastatic to the oral cavity. Q. Natl. Dent. Assoc. *22*:53–55, Jan. 1964.
6. Brown, R. E., and Wright, B. I.: Malignancies in African children. Clin. Pediatr. (Phila.) *6*(2):106–115, Feb. 1967.
7. Burkitt, D.: A Lymphoma Syndrome Dependent on Environment–I. Clinical Aspects in Lymphoreticular Tumors in Africa—A Symposium Organized by the International Union Against Cancer, Paris, 1963 (International Union Against Cancer, Monograph Series, No. 3) F. C. Roulet (ed.), Basel, S. Karger, 1964, pp. 80–93.

7a. Ca-A Journal for Clinicians *26*(1):22–23 Jan.-Feb. 1976. The American Cancer Society.

8. Cawson, R. A.: Leukoplakia and oral cancer. Proc. Roy. Soc. Med. *62*(6):610–615, June 1969.
9. Chomet, B.: Some features of oral carcinoma. (Pres. Address.) Proc. Inst. Med. Chicago *27*:347, Nov. 1969.
10. Clemmessen, J.: Statistical studies in the aetiology of malignant neoplasms—II Basic table. Acta Path. Microbiol. (Scan. Suppl.) *174*:II, 1965.
11. Correa, J. N., Bosch, A., and Marcial, V. A.: Carcinoma of the floor of the mouth: Review of clinical factors and results of treatment. Am. J. Roentgenol. Radium Ther. Nucl. Med. 99(2): 302–312, February 1967.
12. Davies, A. G. M., and Davies, J. N. P.: Tumors of the jaws in Uganda Africans. Acta Un. Int. Cave. *16*:1320–1324, 1960.

13. Dickie, W. R., Colville, J., and Graham, W. J. H.: Recurrent carcinoma of the lip. Oral Surg. *24*(4):449–454, Oct. 1967.
14. Doll, R.: The geographical distribution of cancer. Brit. J. Cancer *23*:1–8, March 1969.
15. Dorfman, R. F.: Childhood lymphosarcoma in St. Louis, Missouri, clinically and histologically resembling Burkitt's tumor. Cancer *18*:418–430, 1965.
16. El-Mofty, S.: Oral cancer in the United Arab Republic. Oral Surg. *24*(2):240–245, August 1967.
17. Epstein, M. A., and Barr, Y. M.: Cultivation in vitro of human lymphoblasts from Burkitt's malignant lymphoma. Lancet *1*:252–253, 1964.
18. Fleming, W. B.: Cancer of the floor of mouth: a survey of the problem in Victoria. Med. J. Aust. *2*:434–436, Sept. 3, 1968.
19. Fortiune, R.: Characteristics of cancer on the Eskimos of southwestern Alaska. Cancer *23*:468–474, Jan.-June, 1969.
20. Kovi, J., and Laing, W. N.: Tumors of the mandible and maxilla in Accra, Ghana. Cancer *19*:1301–1307, Sept. 1966.
21. Ledlie, F. M., and Harmer, M. H.: Cancer of the mouth. A report on 800 cases. Brit. J. Cancer *4*:6–18, 1960.
22. Mackey, E. N., and Sellers, A. H.: The Ontario cancer incidence survey, 1968. A progress report. Can. Med. Assoc. *103*(1):51–52, July 1970.
23. O'Conor, G. T., Rappaport, H., and Smith, E. B.: Childhood lymphoma resembling "Burkitt's tumor" in the United States. Cancer *18*:411–417, 1965.
24. Oettle, A. G., and Higginson, J.: Age-specific cancer incidence rates in the South African Bantu: Johannesburg (1953–1955). S. Afr. J. Med. Sci. *31*:21–41, 1966.
25. Oral Cancer Control. U.S. Department of Health, Education, and Welfare, Public Health Service (Division of Chronic Diseases, Cancer Control Branch). Washington, Government Printing Office, 1966, 10 pp.
26. Pulvertagt, R. J. V.: Cytology of Burkitt's tumor (African lymphoma). Lancet *1*:238–240, 1964.
27. Rowe, N. H., and Kwapis, B. W.: Oral and perioral cancer detection. Dent. Clin. N. Amer. *12*:189–201, March 1968.
28. '71 Cancer Facts and Figures, American Cancer Society.
29. Sisson, G. A., and Goldstein, J. C.: Intraoral carcinoma. Arch. Otolaryngol. *89*:646(108)–651(113), April 1960.
30. Slavin, G., and Cameron, H. MacD.: Ameloblastomas in Africans from Tanzania and Uganda. Brit. J. Cancer *23*(1):31–38, March 1969.
31. Smith, R. R.: Stage Classification and End Result Reporting for Oral Cavity Carcinoma. Sixth National Cancer Conference Proceedings. Philadelphia, J. B. Lippincott Co., 1968, pp. 647–653.
32. Squire, R. A.: Feline lymphoma. A comparison with the Burkitt tumor of children. Cancer *19*:447–453, March 1966.
33. Statistics on Cancer. New York, American Cancer Society, 1967, 11 pp. (p. 5).
34. Tan, K. N.: Cancer of the lip in Australia. Aust. Dent. J. *15*(3):179–184, June 1970.
35. ten Seldam, R. E. J., Cooke, R., and Atkinson, L.: Childhood lymphoma in the territories of Papua and New Guinea. Cancer *19*:437–446, March 1966.
36. Thoma, G. W.: Causes of death in patients with oral cancer. Oral Surg. *30*(6):817–823, Dec. 1970.
37. Trimble, W. M.: Cancer of the oral cavity: Five-year end results in 237 patients. Ann. Otol. Rhinol. Laryngol. *78*:716–723, 1969.
38. Vital Statistics for the United States, 1965. Mortality, Part B. Mortality Figures for Malignant Neoplasms given by Age. U.S. Department of Health, Education, and Welfare, Public Health Service (National Center for Health Statistics), Washington, Government Printing Office, 1967.
39. Wahi, P. N., Kehar, U., and Lahiri, B.: Factors influencing oral and oropharyngeal cancers in India. Brit. J. Cancer *19*:642–660, 1965.
40. Wallace, A. C., MacDougal, J. J., Hildes, J. A., and Lederman, J. M.: Salivary gland tumors in Canadian Eskimos. Cancer *16*:1338–1353, 1963.
41. Wright, D. H.: Cytology and histochemistry of the Burkitt lymphoma. Brit. J. Cancer *17*:50–55, 1963.
42. Wright, D. H.: Cytology and Histochemistry of the Malignant Lymphomas Seen in Uganda. Symposium on Lymphoreticular Tumors in Africa. Basel and New York, S. Karger, 1964, pp. 291–303.
43. Wright, D. H.: Burkitt's tumor—A post mortem study of 50 cases. Brit. J. Surg. *51*:245–251, 1964.

chapter 8

FACTORS RELATED TO ORAL CANCER

by

THEODORE E. BOLDEN, D.D.S., Ph.D.

INTRODUCTION

The use of tobacco, oral habits such as reverse smoking and betel chewing, poor oral hygiene, syphilis, inadequate diets and chronic irritation from rough or broken teeth and ill-fitting dentures are several factors that have been considered responsible for causing oral cancer. Other important etiological factors that have been associated with oral cancer are the consumption of alcohol, viruses, air pollution, sunlight, heredity and anemia.

As a whole, most studies in the United States show a higher frequency of oral cancer in males (Tables 8–1 and 8–2).

There seems to be a higher incidence of cancer of the upper gingiva, palate, buccal cavity and pharynx among Southern white females than in white males or females from other parts of the United States (Table 8–3). Cancer of the lip and pharynx accounted for only nine per cent of oral cancers in females, while cancer in the same two sites accounted for nearly forty per cent of the oral cancers in males (Table 8–3).

The factor that apparently accounts for the excessive frequency of mouth cancers in Southern (American) females is that many are habitual users of *snuff*.

Location studies have shown three major concentration areas for oral cancer: the posterior alveolar-lingual sulcus on either side and the floor of the mouth (Fig. 8–1).[54] The explanation is offered that materials suspended in saliva would have the greatest chance for concentration and pooling in these areas.

SYPHILIS

Clinical experience strongly supports a positive correlation between the incidence of syphilis and the onset of oral cancer. Late stages of syphilis involving the tongue are often complicated with cancer of the tongue.[56] Martin found syphilis in 24 per cent of patients with oral cancer.[47] Vitamin B deficiency and use of tobacco were also related to many of those cases. A positive Wassermann was reported in 18 per cent of Negro patients with oral cancer.[41]

The relationship between syphilis and oral cancer is variable, depending upon the population sample and site of involvement.

TABLE 8–1 AGE-ADJUSTING MORTALITY RATES FOR CANCER OF THE BUCCAL CAVITY AND PHARYNX AMONG THE WHITE POPULATION OF THE U.S. AS A WHOLE AND IN SELECTED REGIONS OF THE U.S. IN 1950*

POPULATION	U.S.	FIVE SOUTHERN STATES	NEW ENGLAND
White Male	5.66	5.54	7.28
White Female	1.41	2.36	1.19
Ratio M:F	4.0	2.3	6.1

*Death rate per 100,000 population. (From Vogler et al.: A retrospective study of etiological factor in cancer of the mouth, pharynx and larynx. Cancer *15*:247–253, 1962).

TABLE 8–2 INCIDENCE RATES FOR CANCER OF THE BUCCAL CAVITY AND PHARYNX IN 10 URBAN AREAS OF THE UNITED STATES IN 1947*

POPULATION	TOTAL *Ten Cities*	SOUTH *Four Cities*	NORTH *Four Cities*	WEST *Two Cities*
White Male	21.1	26.5	18.9	27.4
White Female	6.3	9.4	5.1	8.5
Ratio M:F	3.3	2.8	3.7	3.2

*Incidence per 100,000 population. (From Dorn, H. F., and Cutler, S. J.: Morbidity from Cancer in the United States [Public Health Monograph 56]. Washington, U.S. Government Printing Office, 1959.)

TABLE 8–3 CANCERS OF THE ORAL CAVITY, PHARYNX AND LARYNX: DISTRIBUTION OF PRIMARY SITES BY SEX OF PATIENTS

SITE	ALL PATIENTS		MALE PATIENTS		FEMALE PATIENTS	
	No.	*Per Cent*	*No.*	*Per Cent*	*No.*	*Per Cent*
Lip	49	14.7	46	19.6	3	3.1
Min. saliv. glands	10	3.0	4	2.1	5	5.1
Tongue	55	16.5	39	16.6	16	16.3
Lower gingiva & floor of mouth	32	9.6	18	7.7	14	14.3
Upper gingiva, palate, & buccal mucosa	82	24.6	40	17.0	42	42.9
Oropharynx	16	4.8	14	6.0	2	2.0
Other parts pharynx	36	10.8	26	11.1	10	10.2
Larynx	53	15.9	47	20.0	6	6.1
Total	333	99.9	235	100.1	98	100.0

*From Vogler et al., *op. cit.*

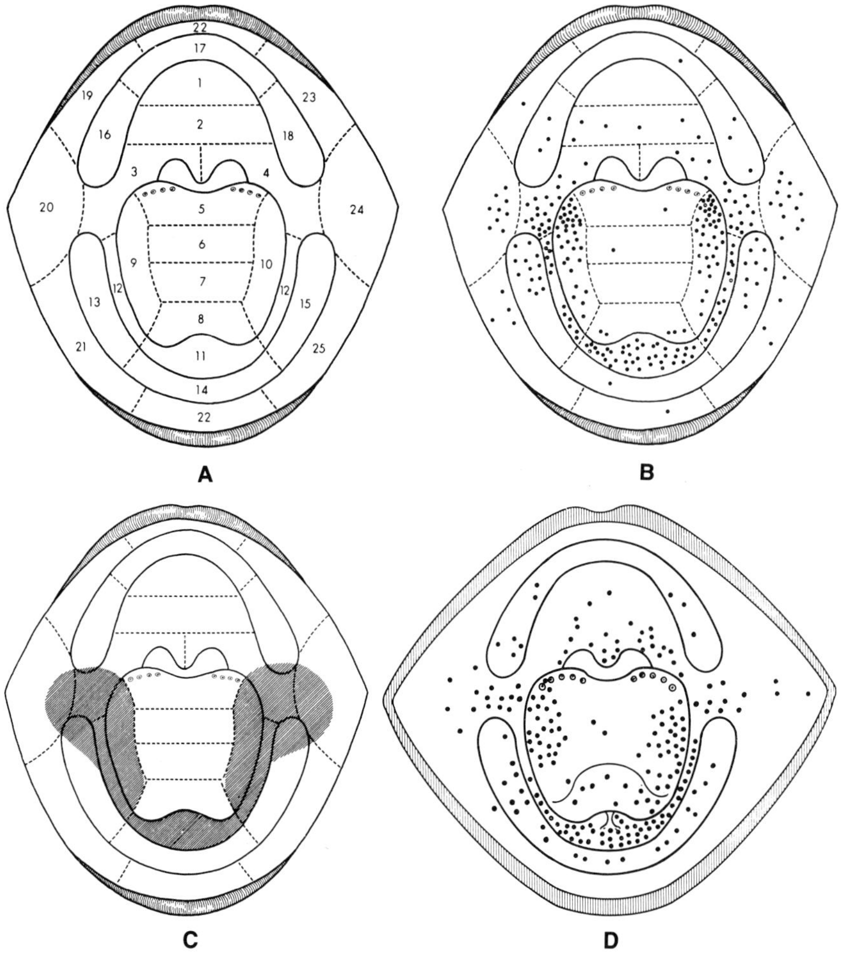

Figure 8–1 Diagrams depicting the anatomic origins and locations of oral cancer. *A*, Segmental division of the oral cavity. *B*, Scattergram of site of origin of 256 cases of oral cancer from the University of Louisville School of Medicine between 1954 and 1965. *C*, Cancer-prone crescent where 75 per cent of cancerous lesions originate. *D*, Site of origin of 209 consecutive cases of mouth cancer from the Memorial Hospital Head and Neck Service between 1962 and 1965. (From Moore, C., and Catlin, D.: Anatomic origins and locations of oral cancer. Am. J. Surg. *114*:510–513, October 1967.)

A high incidence of cancer and syphilis of the tongue has been reported.[45, 21] The involvement varies from eleven per cent in Indians[79] to 13.2 per cent,[22] to 18 per cent,[21] to as high as 33 per cent.[86] Syphilis is least associated with carcinoma of the buccal mucosa.[79]

AIR POLLUTION

Some investigators have suggested that oral cancer may be associated with high degrees of industrialization, atmospheric pollution by coal smoke and exhaust fumes containing benzopyrene and other polycylic hydrocarbons.[55] A paradox is posed by the low incidence of oral cancers in rural area.[23]

SUNLIGHT

The actinic rays of the sun may serve as a causative agent for cancer of the lip.[86] Most labial cancers in the United States are found on the lower lip as squamous cell car-

TABLE 8–4 CASES OF LIP CANCERS AND THEIR MATCHED CONTROLS BY RACE*

	CASES OF LIP CANCERS		GENERAL CONTROLS†	
	No.	*Per Cent*	*No.*	*Per Cent*
Whites	301	99.0	265	87.2
Negroes	3	1.0+	39	12.8‡
Totals	304	100.0	304	100.0

*From Keller, A. Z.: Cellular types, survival, race, nativity, occupations, habits and associated diseases in the pathogenesis of lip cancers. Am. J. Epidemiol. *91*(5):486–499, 1970.
†Males from all diagnostic categories of medical and surgical patients.
‡$p < 0.00001$.

cinomas of white males who are farmers, or sailors or who work out of doors, reside in the South or who emigrate from the South (Tables 8–4 and 8–5).

An increasing number of basal cell tumors appear on the skin and many of them begin in childhood. They appear to be directly related to the carcinogenic effects of actinic radiation on exposed skin. Usually the basal cell carcinoma of the face is a solitary, slowly growing tumor which presents in middle age and beyond in fair-skinned individuals with deficient capacity to produce melanin.

RADIATION

The high rate of leukemia among dentists and physicians is thought to be due to overexposure to irradiation.[12] Ionizing radiations (alpha, beta, gamma) are recognized human environmental carcinogens acting on susceptible cells in the body.[27] Ionizing radiations are among the demonstrated causes of all lymphomas[6, 13, 25] and have been demonstrated to be antigenic for the malignant cells of Burkitt's lymphoma.

Normal mucous glands of the oral cavity frequently undergo squamous metapla-

TABLE 8–5 OCCUPATIONAL CATEGORIES OF CASES OF LIP CANCERS AND THEIR CONTROLS – WHITE MALES ONLY[a]

	CASES OF LIP CANCER		CONTROLS: CANCER[b]		CONTROLS: GENERAL[c]	
	No.	*Per Cent*	*No.*	*Per Cent*	*No.*	*Per Cent*
Professionals	16	5.3	14	4.7	13	4.9
Managerials	9	3.0[d]	13	4.3	20	7.5[d]
Clerical	8	2.7[d, e]	24	7.9[e]	16	6.0[d]
Salesworkers	8	2.7[d]	14	4.7	18	6.8[d]
Craftsmen	68	22.6	90	29.9	69	26.0
Operatives	51	16.9	33	11.0	34	12.8
Service workers	25	8.3[e]	44	14.6[e]	33	12.5
Laborers	28	9.3	40	13.3	27	10.2
Farmers	80	26.6[g]	25	8.3[g]	11	4.2[g]
Unknown	8	2.6[e]	4	1.3[f]	24	9.1[e, f]
Total	301	100.0	301	100.0	265	100.0

[a]From Keller, *ibid.*
[b]Males with squamous cell carcinoma of intra-oral cavity and pharynx.
[c]Males from all diagnostic categories of medical and surgical patients.
[d]$p < 0.05$.
[e]$p < 0.01$.
[f]$p < 0.0001$.
[g]$p < 0.00001$.

sia, with marked hyperplasia incident to irradiation for squamous cell carcinoma with 6000 to 6500 R delivered over a period of 23 to 28 days. Of 64 patients studied, 23 developed this change.[20] A relatively high percentage of patients with cancers of the major salivary glands subsequently developed breast cancer. This suggests the possibility of etiologic factors which are common to both diseases.[7]

ALCOHOL

The accumulated evidence strongly suggests a positive correlation between alcohol consumption and the incidence of oral cancer. Approximately 94 per cent of the 189 patients with oral carcinoma examined by Gardner and associates consumed alcoholic beverages.[22] Thirty-three per cent of the patients with oral cancer examined by Wynder et al. (1957) consumed more than five ounces of alcohol per day.[86]

A positive correlation (r–6.82, t–0.26) appears when mouth cancer death rates[72] are compared with National statistics of per capita alcohol consumption.[18] Per capita consumption of alcohol adjusted for males over 15 years of age is lowest in Israel and the Netherlands and highest in Switzerland and France. Oral cancer death rates are similar.

ALCOHOL PLUS

Alcohol consumption may not function as a single factor but may in fact be related to other habits and other carcinogenic agents. Nearly six per cent of 1916 patients in India with oral and oropharyngeal carcinoma were addicted to tobacco, had poor oral hygiene and gave a history of taking alcohol over a number of years.[79]

One hundred fifty-three cases of epidermoid carcinoma of the mouth (115 in males and 38 in females) were studied in Puerto Rico. Cancer patients tended to use *more* alcohol, tobacco, hot beverages and spices than did their sex-matched controls. Heavy drinkers were usually heavy smokers. The cigarette was the principal use of tobacco.[48]

NITROSAMINES

The presence of diethylnitrosamine in malawi gin and the demonstration that certain nitrosamines are highly selective carcinogens in the induction of esophageal carcinomas in rats suggests the need to screen beverages and foodstuffs for contaminants.[85]

WOOD

Although consumption of alcohol and alcoholic beverages is associated with cancers of the mouth,[15] ethanol has proved negative as a carcinogenic agent in laboratory mice when they are maintained on 20 per cent alcohol for periods up to 15 months.[34] The alcohol did not interfere with the growth and spread of a transplanted tumor or prevent metastatic spread after removal of the tumor. The suggestion has been made that death from the leukemia-lyphoma group of diseases may be directly related to the dissolution of carcinogenic substances out of the *wood* in which alcoholic beverages are contained.[51]

CIRRHOSIS OF THE LIVER

The finding that patients with alcoholic cirrhosis are more likely to develop oral cancers than a similar group of patients with diseases other than alcoholic cirrhosis suggests the influence of alcohol.[32] A study of 706 males with squamous cell carcinoma of the mouth and pharynx with an equal number of controls demonstrated that cirrhosis of the liver is strongly associated at the 0.2 per cent level with cancer of the mouth and pharynx (Table 8–6).[33]

TOBACCO

SMOKING

Smoking has been estimated to increase the likelihood of developing a mouth cancer by two to four times.[86] As early as 1859, the observation was made that out of

TABLE 8-6 PROPORTION WITH CLINICALLY DIAGNOSED LIVER CIRRHOSIS BY ANATOMICAL SITES FOR CASES OF MOUTH AND PHARYNX CANCERS AND THEIR MATCHED CONTROLS*

SITES	No.	CASES No.	CASES Per Cent	CONTROLS No.	CONTROLS Per Cent
Floor of mouth	123	18	14.6†	6	4.9
Tongue	92	7	7.6	8	8.7
Mesopharynx	67	6	9.0	4	6.0
Hypopharynx	108	8	7.4	6	5.6
Other parts of mouth	61	6	9.8	6	9.8
Coexisting sites	46	7	15.2‡	2	4.3‡
Multiple sites	209	22	10.5	12	5.7
Total	706	74	10.5†	44	6.2†

*A control matches its case on age within five years and on a hospital's bed capacity and medical school affiliation status. From Keller, A. Z.: Survivorship with mouth and pharynx cancers and their association with cirrhosis of the liver, marital status and residence. Am. J. Public Health 59(7):1139–1153, July, 1969.
†$p < 0.01$.
‡$p < 0.05$.

68 patients with cancer of the buccal cavity, 66 smoked pipes, one chewed tobacco and one apparently used tobacco in some form.[24] Prior to World War I, tobacco consumption was primarily in the form of snuff, chewing tobacco, pipe tobacco and cigars.[61] Cigarette consumption drastically increased after World War I.[55]

Nearly 36 per cent of the oral cancer patients reported by Mills and Porter gave histories of smoking cigarettes only, while approximately 55 per cent smoked pipes, cigars or some combination.[52] There is an alleged well-established link between tobacco use and cancer of the lower lip and oral cavity.[10] Heavy smoking (40 or more cigarettes daily) has been found to be significant for cases of tongue cancer and cancer of the floor of the mouth. The death rate for heavy smokers (25 grams of pipe or cigar tobacco or more per day) from oral-pharyngeal cancer has been demonstrated to be more than five times that of the light smoker rate.[81]

Recent evidence suggests that acrolein and cyanide, substances present in the gas-vapor phase of tobacco smoke, might contribute to malignant transformation by causing a reduction in cellular respiration.[19] Acrolein has also been shown to produce inhibition of RNA synthesis, loss of RNA, pycnosis and cell destruction within 24 hours after exposure of mouse kidney and slime mold cell cultures to cigarette smoke gas phase.[2, 44]

Ash was able to list nine possible predisposing or etiological factors for oral cancer observed over a 25-year period (Table 8–7). It is interesting to note that in his series trauma (dental, mechanical) and tobacco lead the list at 14 per cent each.[2]

Analysis made of puffs of commercial cigarettes with and without $NaNO_3$ by gas chromatography,[76] showed that the addition of sodium nitrate reduces the components

TABLE 8-7 ORAL CARCINOMA, 1929–1958: RECORDED ETIOLOGICAL FACTORS*

ETIOLOGY	PER CENT	
Trauma (dental, mechanical)	13.8	68.2
Tobacco	13.7	
Leukoplakia	8.7	
Syphilis alone	2.5	
Syphilis with other factor	2.1	
Alcohol	1.8	
Anemia	0.8	
Chronic inflammation	1.0	
Other, or combination	23.8	
Not stated	19.1	31.8
None	12.7	

*From Ash, C. L.: Oral cancer: A twenty-five year study. Am. J. Roentgenol. Radium Ther. Nucl. Med. 87(3):417–430, March 1962.

and properties of cigarette smoke that are associated with tumorigenicity. Cigarettes with $NaNO_3$ added produce smoke that is less tumorigenic and toxic (in mice).[75] The effect is due to thermal decomposition of the nitrate into oxygen and nitrogen oxides; the fumes enhancing combustion of tobacco and later inhibiting free radical reactions leading to formation of *benzo* and pyrine (α)pyrine (Table 8–8).

REVERSE SMOKING

Reverse smoking has been reported as part of the cultural habits of Andhrans (India), Pygmy Negritos (Bantu Peninsula), Sardinians, Jamaicans, Venezuelans, Colombians, Panamanians and South Caribbean islanders. Leukoplakias and cancers of the palate are frequent among the females of Maracaibo and appear to be related to the frequent habit of smoking with the burning end of the cigarette inside the mouth.[43] Women of Visakhapatnam smoke cigars with the burning end inside the mouth and have a high incidence of palatal cancer. The cancer usually appears in the center of the palate where the burning end of the cigar is held. An ulcerated plaque in the center of a wide leukoplakic area is the earliest lesion observed.[66] Chutta cancer is a palatal cancer which is seen in smokers of Chutta (India) and is related directly to the habit of smoking a homemade cigar with the lighted end in the mouth (Fig. 8–2).[35]

Using microminiature thermocouple probes held by a dental plate, it was determined that the maximum internal cigarette temperature in the burning zone for reverse cigarette smoking was 760° C. as compared with 860° C. for conventional smoking. It is significant, however, that radiant energy is apparently transferred from the glowing tip of the cigarette to the oral mucosa in reverse smoking, suggesting the production of a radiation burn. In addition, the time the palatal tissues are exposed to heat and radiant energy is approximately three times longer (18 min.) in reverse smoking than in conventional smoking.[63] It is concluded that heat and volatile tars induce superficial squamous cells to undergo hypercornification.[64]

Whether reverse smoking has a direct relation to the development of *palatal* carcinoma is a moot question.[65] Studies on a group of reverse cigarette smokers from the Netherlands Antilles did not support the relation.[64]

Clinical examination of 250 Caribbean reverse smokers revealed the presence of heavy black tarlike deposits on the teeth, erosion of cementum and leukoplakia most severe on the *hard palate*. Occasionally, smears from *palates* of reverse smokers show leukopenic and hyperkeratotic squamous cells indicative of leukoplakia.[64] Histologic analysis of 21 biopsy specimens from the hard palate of reverse cigarette smokers revealed varying hyperkeratosis, a thick homogenous stratum corneum, occasional acanthosis, rete peg extension, chronic inflammation and the absence of parakeratosis and dyskeratotic changes.[64, 65]

TABLE 8–8 YIELDS OF THE COMPONENTS OF THE VAPOR PHASE OF SMOKE (FIFTH PUFF, 35 ml.) FROM CIGARETTES WITHOUT OR WITH $NaNO_3$ ADDED; AVERAGES OF TEN OR MORE DETERMINATIONS*

COMPONENT	WITHOUT $NaNO_2$	WITH $NaNO_2$
	Mole percentages	
H_2	1.38	1.64
O_2	13.46	12.46
CO	3.00	3.55
CO_2	7.43	7.86
	Micrograms	
$NO + NO_2$	22.9	48.7
N_2O	1.0	11.0
HCN	23.0	23.3
H_2S	4.5	0.3
CH_4	107.5	90.0
C_2H_6	37.8	36.4
CH_3CHO	74.0	146.3
CH_3COCH_3	40.6	55.3
CH_3CN	14.3	29.3
$CH_2 = CHCHO$	9.2	18.4
CH_2O	5.3	5.6

*The method did not distinguish between NO and NO_2; the lower limit of detection of N_2O was 1.0 μg. (From Terrell, J. H., and Schweltz, I.: Cigarettes: Chemical effect of sodium nitrate content. Science *160*(3835):1456, June 1968.)

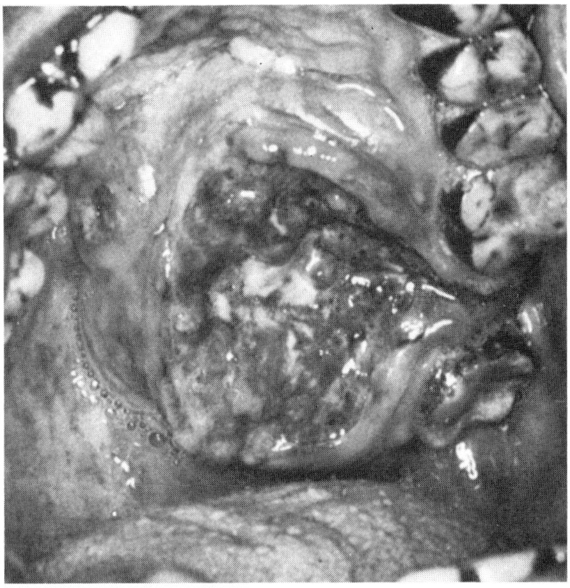

Figure 8–2 Carcinoma of the palate in a reverse smoker. The patient illustrated is a 50-year-old Indian man who, for the past 20 years, had smoked home-made cheroots with the burning end inside the mouth. The result was an extensive palatal squamous cell carcinoma, ulcerated and with leukoplakic patches on the periphery. (From J. J. Pindborg: Atlas of Diseases of the Oral Mucosa. Copyright 1973, by J. J. Pindborg. Original English edition published by Munksgaard, Copenhagen. Distributed in the United States, Canada and Latin America by W. B. Saunders Co., Philadelphia.)

Palatal glands of reverse smokers showed acinar distention and ductal dilatation.[64]

SNUFF DIPPERS

"*Snuff Dippers*" squamous cell carcinoma of the oral cavity has been reported as a disease of males in a ratio 2:1 and as high as 10:1. The sex ratio was reversed in patients with the carcinoma site in the gingivobuccal sulcus. This is where most females place their *quid*. There is evidence that prolonged use of snuff is conducive to the development of squamous cell carcinoma at or near the site of application. These carcinomas are often multicentric with recurrence.

The five-year survival of 84 cases (all females) of snuff users with buccal and gingival squamous cell carcinoma was 44 per cent. Treatment is wide local excision.[69] Carcinomas of the maxillary antrum among rural Africans who insert homemade snuff into their nostrils may be directly related to the presence of high concentrations of nickel, chromium and zinc.[5]

TOBACCO PLUS

In India, tobacco is either chewed alone or with pan (betel leaf, *piperaceae*), betel nut (*areca catachu*), and slaked lime or with lime alone. Tobacco is also used both for chewing and smoking by the same individual. Only 9.62 per cent of cancer cases were not using tobacco.[79] Chewing and smoking were seen in 37.88 per cent, while chewing only was observed in 35.44 per cent of patients with oral cancer. The percentage distribution of various tobacco habits is related to the site of cancer. All female lip cancer cases were tobacco chewers. Oral leukoplakia was frequent to the buccal mucosa, low to the tongue, and was associated with the tobacco habit in approximately 87 per cent of cases of leukoplakia. Khavni cancer, cancer of the lower lip, is extremely low (1 in 100 cases) in Bombay and in most of India except Uttar Pradesh and Bihar. The high incidence observed in the latter two areas is attributed to the habit of placing a mixture of tobacco and lime in the lower gingivolabial groove of the vestibule of the mouth.[36]

Oral cancer shows some ethnic differences. Oral cancer of the inner lining of the cheek is four times more common in Deccani Hindus than in Gujaratis and is probably associated with holding the betel quid against the inner lining of the cheek. On the other hand, cancer of the base of the tongue and tonsil is more than twice as common in Gujaratis and more than 90 per cent of the cases occur in males.[36] Eight hundred seventy-seven of 2000 consecutive cancer patients observed in 11 months at the Tata Memorial Hospital had cancer of the mouth and the adjoining portions of the pharynx and larynx with the following distribution: base of tongue, 25 per cent; buccal mucosa, 13 per cent; tonsil, 13 per cent; extrinsic larynx, 21 per cent.[36]

"Buyo" chewing in the Philippines is comparable to "pan" chewing in India. Spices may be added to the quid. Betel chewing is also common in Taiwan but buccal cancer is rare.[50] No evidence of oral cancer was observed among betel chewers in Guam.[83] Orr (1933) made the observation that when betel nut alone was chewed, oral cancer was rare. However, when individuals chewed tobacco and lime the incidence of oral cancer rose.[60] Malayans who chew betel nut without tobacco seldom develop cancer. However, Indian laborers who include tobacco frequently have oral cancer.[46] Fourteen per cent of people who chewed over five quids (betel, areca nut, chunam and tobacco leaf) a day for over 20 years might show "precancerous" changes.[74]

Experimental studies are equally nonconclusive. Tobacco and betel nut produced carcinomas in the ear of mice.[57] Commercial lime and tobacco produced leukoplakias in the hamster pouch. Lime used alone failed to produce malignant change.[73]

The clinical and the experimental evidence suggests the possibility that tobacco is the carcinogenic agent common to all betel quids.[67]

Betel quid, Nass and coco mixed with quicklime as a base and other plants (Table 8–9) when chewed seem to be associated with damage to the oral mucous membrane.[17]

HEAT

The prevalence of oral cancer among Chinese men is explained by repeated insults to the oral mucosa afforded while eating. The food is eaten while piping hot.[85]

TABLE 8–9 COMPOSITION OF BETEL QUID AND NASS*

BETEL QUID	NASS	COCO
Seed of areca palm	tobacco	1
Leaf of a pepper plant	wood ash	
Tobacco	water	
Spices	oil of cotton seed or sesame	
cardamon		
cloves	lime	lime
cinnamon		
fennel or nutmeg		
Plant substances with tannins		
Lime		

*Data compiled from Dunham, L. J.: A geographic study of the relationship between oral cancer and plants. Cancer Res. 28:2369–2371, November 1968.

Age-adjusted death rates from cancer of the buccal cavity and pharynx correlated negatively (−0.50) for males and positively (+0.50) for females with the temperature index (mean annual temperature plus range) within the United States (Table 8–10).[59]

PLUMMER-VINSON SYNDROME

Several investigators have shown a strong relation between the Plummer-Vinson syndrome and oral cancer. The tendency to develop *multiple* oral cancers has been observed in patients with Plummer-Vinson syndrome.[62] The Plummer-Vinson syndrome is characterized by hypochromic microcytic anemia and hysterical dysphagia.[82, 86] Few American women have the syndrome. However, it is quite prevalent among Swedish women.[1] The incidence of oral cancer among women in the two countries, Sweden and the United States, is strikingly similar. Cancer of the buccal mucosa and tongue is relatively low among American females but is considered to be of high frequency among the women of Scandinavia.

NUTRITION

Avitaminosis may play a role in the etiology of oral cancer.[39] A protracted deficiency of Vitamin B yielded a higher level

TABLE 8-10 CORRELATION COEFFICIENTS FOR AGE-ADJUSTED CANCER MORTALITY BY REGION, FOR WHITE MALES AND FEMALES, UNITED STATES (1959–61)*

SITE	I.C.D. NO.	TEMPERATURE INDEX Male	TEMPERATURE INDEX Female	PER-CAPUT INCOME Male	PER-CAPUT INCOME Female	PHYSICIANS PER 100,000 Male	PHYSICIANS PER 100,000 Female
Buccal cavity and pharynx	104–148	−0.50	0.50	0.43	−0.35	0.53	−0.23
Esophagus	150	−0.80	0.00	0.76	0.16	0.75	0.31
Stomach	151	−0.86	−0.75	0.87	0.77	0.82	0.77
Intestine	152–153	−0.88	−0.90	0.77	0.75	0.72	0.71
Rectum	154	−0.91	−0.89	0.88	0.86	0.83	0.82
Liver and biliary passage	155–156	−0.05	−0.68	−0.14	0.31	−0.17	0.07
Pancreas	157	−0.29	−0.29	0.46	0.43	0.53	0.53
Other digestive	158–159	0.02	0.04	0.01	−0.23	0.17	−0.16
Lung and bronchus	162–163	−0.23	−0.20	0.40	0.58	0.48	0.61
Breast	170	−0.28	−0.92	0.06	0.94	0.26	0.87
Cervix	171	...	0.59	...	−0.73	...	−0.74
Uterus	172–174	...	−0.50	...	0.11	...	0.01
Ovary	175	...	−0.95	...	0.84	...	0.73
Male genital organs	177–179	−0.62	...	0.41	...	0.29	...
Kidney	180	−0.74	−0.63	0.88	0.49	0.78	0.31
Bladder	181	−0.85	−0.59	0.93	0.51	0.87	0.47
Skin	190–191	0.86	0.66	−0.81	−0.83	−0.68	−0.68
Brain	193	−0.53	−0.69	0.35	0.45	0.27	0.27
Thyroid	194	−0.54	−0.41	0.69	0.43	0.61	0.18
Bone	196	−0.24	0.09	−0.17	−0.55	−0.16	−0.57
Connective tissue	197	−0.41	0.25	0.52	0.27	0.55	0.28
Hodgkin's disease	201	−0.81	−0.81	0.67	0.81	0.63	0.89
Lymphoma (except Hodgkin's)	200, 202, 203, 205	−0.78	−0.86	0.94	0.87	0.87	0.81
Leukaemia	204	−0.06	−0.28	−0.10	0.23	−0.13	0.21

*From Newell, G. R., and Waggoner, D. E.: Cancer mortality and environmental temperature in the United States. Lancet *1*(7650):766–767, April 1970.

of susceptibility of the cutaneous tissues of the mouse to the irritating effects of tobacco smoke.[38] However, no significant changes were noted in hamsters under the same experimental regime.[86] Lower Vitamin B excretion level has been found in many patients with oral cancer.[80]

Low serum Vitamin A was found in 76.2 per cent of the series of patients with oral carcinomas and was considered an adjuvant in the carcinogenic process.[79] A diet of rice and tapioca, extremely deficient in protein and Vitamin A, might predispose to oral cancer. This diet was found among the Indian coolie class in Travancore, where oral cancer rates are extremely high.[60, 70]

VIRUSES

Cancer viruses are nucleoprotein macromolecules. They consist mainly of DNA with a covering of protein.[13] The evidence to support the postulate that viruses may play a significant role in the etiology of human oral cancers is non-substantive. Recent studies have related herpes simplex virus to cancer in humans. An association between squamous cell carcinoma of the lip and recurrent infection of the lip by type 1 herpes virus has been postulated. To date, there has been a failure to demonstrate an unequivocal tumor virus in man.[26]

ANIMAL CANCERS

Viruses have been demonstrated as causative agents for various animal cancers such as chicken sarcoma, rabbit Shopes papilloma, frog cancer of the kidney and mouse breast cancer.[68, 86] Virus multiplication has been demonstrated in salivary gland tumors induced by polyoma virus.[37, 40, 71] The polyoma-induced salivary gland tumor is composed predominantly of three types of cells – pleomorphic, fusiform and cells forming small tubules (Figs. 8–3 and 8–4).

Several forms of virus particles have been observed in the polyoma infection: type C (large extracellular particles), intracytoplasmic particles (50–60 mμ. in diameter), type D spherical particles (38 mμ. in diameter),[8] and long filaments. Large particles 42 mμ in diameter have also been shown to be exclusively included in the nuclei of tumor cells.[28] Virus-containing tumor cell nuclei appear to enlarge but do not appear to break down with release of virus into the cytoplasm. Nucleolus and other cytoplasmic organelles appear the same in non-virus-containing tumor cells.

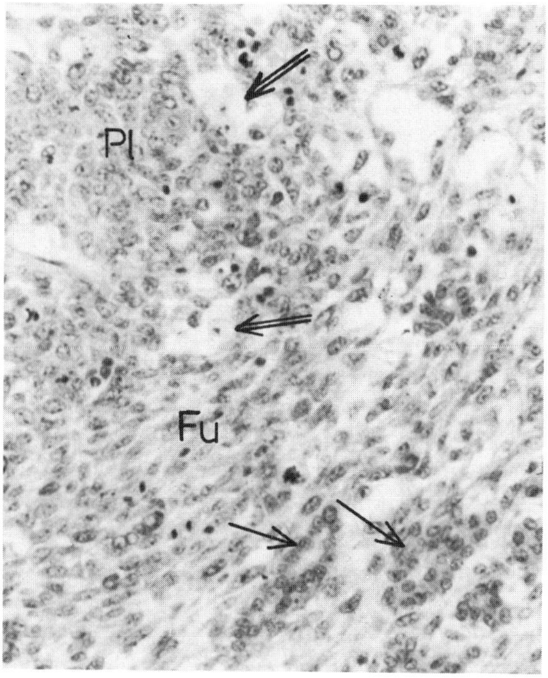

Figure 8–3 Light micrograph showing polyoma-induced salivary gland tumor of a mouse. Three types of cells compose the tumor: pleomorphic (*Pl*), fusiform (*Fu*), and cells forming small tubules (*arrows*). Vacuolated and degenerated cells are also seen (*double arrows*). Hematoxylin and eosin. × 300. (From Imamura, M.: Electron microscope study of polyoma induced salivary gland tumors with special reference to cell virus interaction. J. Natl. Cancer Inst. *41*:1265–1273, December 1968.)

HUMAN DISORDERS AND CANCERS

Chédiak-Higashi Syndrome. The Chédiak-Higashi syndrome is a rare familial disorder characterized by partial albinism, photophobia, nystagmus and anomalous granulations in leukocytes and other cells.[9, 29] Patients suffer recurrent severe infection and death due to malignant lymphoma. The circulating leukocytes of children with the Chédiak-Higashi syndrome have been shown to contain virus-like particles. They are oval with a dense inner nucleoid and a surrounding membrane-like capsule, and are approximately 70 mm. in diameter.[84]

LEUKEMIAS

Structures resembling virus particles (type C murine leukemia particles) and mycoplasma have been found in specimens of blood plasma from acute lymphocytic leukemia and in lymph node biopsy specimens, chiefly from acute lymphocytic leukemia patients, but also from cases of monocytic leukemia. They were not found in chronic lymphocytic or granulocytic leukemias. Bone marrow specimens failed to reveal virus particles (except in one case of reticulum-cell sarcoma). Structures resembling virus particles (type C) have been found in material obtained from tissue culture. Many more patients with different types of leukemia and lymphoma will have to be examined before, during and after treatment before meaningful correlation between the various parameters can be attempted.[53]

BURKITT'S LYMPHOMA

A reovirus, a herpes-type virus,[6] a vaccine virus, a leukovirus and an echovirus are among the several viruses isolated from Burkitt's lymphoma tissue.[58] Virus (EB) has been isolated from cases of infectious mononucleosis and Burkitt's lymphoma.[25] It is interesting to note that the female mosquito (*Aedes aegypti*) is capable of transmitting

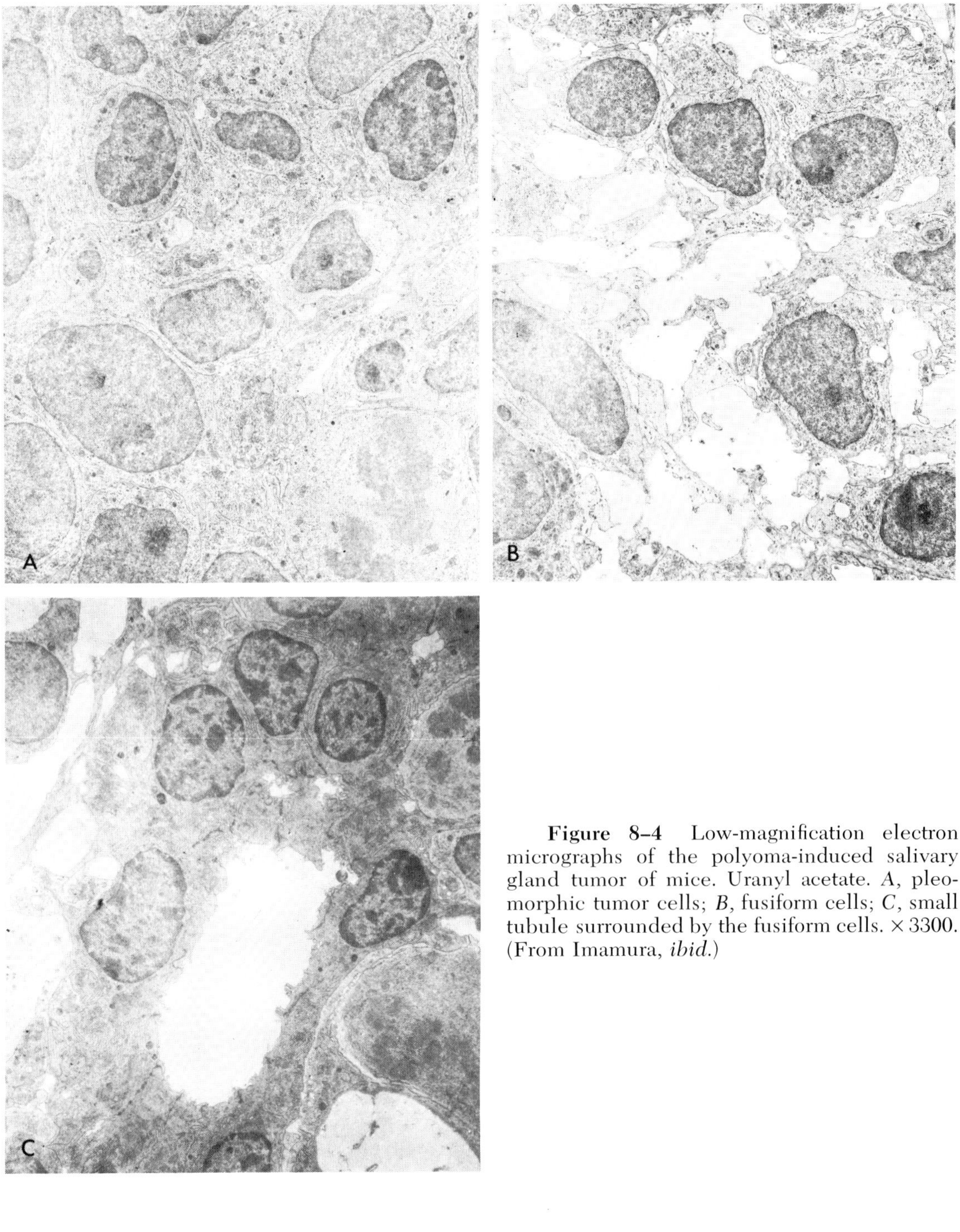

Figure 8–4 Low-magnification electron micrographs of the polyoma-induced salivary gland tumor of mice. Uranyl acetate. *A*, pleomorphic tumor cells; *B*, fusiform cells; *C*, small tubule surrounded by the fusiform cells. ×3300. (From Imamura, *ibid.*)

viable reticulum cell sarcoma cells. However, no responsible insect virus vector has been reported.

SOCIO-ECONOMIC STATUS AND HEREDITY

The majority of patients with oral cancers seem to belong to a low socio-economic group.[78] A general hereditary disposition to cancer as a whole, however, has not been demonstrated.[11] One evidence for heredity as a cancer factor is seen in Gardner's syndrome. Gardner's syndrome is a group of inherited traits with a Mendelian autosomal-dominant inheritance. The onset of symptoms secondary to diffuse polyposis usually does not occur until late childhood or early adult life. The osseous tumors are benign osteomas or exostosis ranging from simple cortical thickening to protuberant bony masses. Although involvement may be almost any of the skeletal system, the mandible is most common. Other sites frequently involved are the maxilla, sphenoid, frontal, ethmoid and temporal bones. These tumors usually attain full size in a few years early in life and remain dormant with slight or no increase in size thereafter.

Another characteristic of Gardner's syndrome is that most patients have poor teeth with numerous caries. The mandible or maxilla may show loss of normal bony trabecular pattern with replacement by irregular dense bone formation throughout. It is also common to have both unerupted and supernumerary teeth. These are some dental abnormalities that accompany Gardner's Syndrome. A characteristic symptom of the syndrome is multiplecolonic polyposis. The incidence of developing carcinoma in the retained rectal or colonic segment after subtotal colectomy was said to be 5.2 per cent.[30]

MULTIPLE CANCER

The available evidence suggests "that the risk of a secondary primary tumor in a person once affected with cancer does not exceed that of other persons not previously affected."[11] Plummer-Vinson's syndrome, however, carries the associated tendency to develop multiple oral cancers.[62] A glandular carcinoma, adenocarcinoma, of accessory salivary gland of the upper lip was reported in the sections of the upper lip of a 70-year-old Caucasian male.[14] The patient presented with multiple submucosal, cystic, movable nodules on the upper lip. The nodules were deep in the stroma and in direct relationship with the accessory glands of the lip. The accessory salivary gland lobules adjacent to the clinical nodules—mucosal surface on left side near midline and on right side approximately one-half cm. in diameter clearly separated from each other—were lined by similar cancer cells. Invasion into the connective tissue by the cancer cells was absent.

RELIGIOUS BELIEFS

Seventh Day Adventists, whose religious beliefs prohibit the use of alcohol and tobacco, experience a 90 per cent decrease in death from mouth cancer as compared to a similarly constituted non-Seventh Day Adventist population.[42] Moslem males and females have greater incidence of carcinoma of the buccal mucosa than do Hindu (Table 7–32, Fig. 7–3).[79] In Lebanon, Moslem males and females have a lower incidence of cancer of the buccal cavity, mouth and pharynx than do Christians. Moslem females have a lower incidence of cancer of the salivary glands (see Table 7–21).

MENTAL STRESS

Mental stress may be a factor in the pathogenesis of cancer.[74] Recent evidence suggests that the five-year cure rates obtained in 306 determinate cases of squamous cell carcinoma of the lip and 74 of the tongue were not related to the protherapeutic duration of the lesion as expressed by the patient.[77]

REFERENCES

1. Ahlbom, H. E.: Simple achlorhydric anemia. Plummer-Vinson syndrome and carcinoma of the mouth, pharynx and oesophagus in women. Brit. Med. J. *2*:331–333, 1936.
2. Ash, C. L.: Oral cancer: A twenty-five year study. Am. J. Roentgenol. Radium Ther. Nucl. Med. *87*(3):417–430, March 1962.
3. Atkinson, L., Chester, I. C., Smyth, F. G., et al: Oral cancer in New Guinea. A study in demography and etiology. Cancer *17*:1289–1298, 1964.
4. Banfield, W. G., Woke, P. A., and Mackay, C. M.: Mosquito transmission of lymphomas. Cancer *19*:1333, 1966.
5. Baumslag, N., Keen, P., and Petering, H. G.: Carcinoma of maxillary antrum and its relationship to trace metal content of snuff. Arch. Environ. Health *23*:1-5, July 1971.
6. Bell, T. M., Massie, A., Ross, M. G. R., and Williams, M. C.: Isolation of a reovirus from a case of Burkitt's lymphoma. Brit. Med. J. *1*:1212, 1964.
7. Berg, J. W., Hatter, R. V. P., and Foot, F. W., Jr.: Unique association between salivary gland cancer and breast cancer. J.A.M.A. *204*:771–774, May 27, 1968.
8. Bernhard, W.: The detection and study of tumor viruses with the electron microscope. Cancer Res. *20*:712–727, 1960.
9. Chédiak, M.: Nouvelle anomalie leucocytaire de caractère constitutionnel et familial. Rev. Hemat. *7*:362–367, 1952.
10. Christen, A. G.: The clinical effects of tobacco on oral tissue. J. Am. Dent. Assoc. *81(6)*:1378–1382, December 1970.
11. Clemmesen Johannes Statistical Studies in Aetiology of Malignant Neoplasms—I. Review and Results. Acta. Pathol. Microbiol. Scand. (Suppl.) *174*, Part 1, 1965.
12. Committee on Genetic Effects of Atomic Radiation: National Academy of Sciences. Science *123*:1157, 1956.
13. Cowdry, E. V.: Etiology and Prevention of Cancer in Man. New York, Appleton-Century-Crofts, 1968.
14. De La Pava, S., Karjoo, R., Mukhtar, F., and Pickreu, J. W.: Multiple carcinoma of accessory salivary gland. A case report. Cancer *19*:1308–1310, Sept. 1966.
15. Doll, R.:The Prevention of Cancer: Pointers from Epidemiology, London, Aldine, 1967.
16. Dorn, H. F., and Cutler, S. J.: Morbidity from Cancer in the United States (Public Health Monograph 56). Washington, U. S. Government Printing Office, 1959.
17. Dunham, L. J.: A geographic study of the relationship between oral cancer and plants. Cancer Res. *28*:2369–2371, November 1968.
18. Efron, V., and Keller, M.: Selected Statistical Tables on the Consumption of Alcohol and on Alcoholism. New Brunswick, N.J., Rutgers Center for Alcohol Studies, 1963.
19. Eichel, B., and Shahrik, H. A.: Tobacco smoke toxicity: Loss of human oral leukocyte function and fluid-cell metabolism. Science *166*:1424–1427, December 1969.
20. Friedman, M., and Hall, J. W.: Radiation induced squamous cell metaplasia and hyperplasia of normal mucous glands of the oral cavity. Radiology *55*:848–851, December 1950.
21. Frieger, N., Ship, I. I., Taylor, G. W., and Weisberger, D.: Cirrhosis and other predisposing factors in carcinoma of the tongue. Cancer N. Y. *11*:357–361, 1958.
22. Gardner, A. F., Hamburger, S., and Love, S.: Oral carcinoma: Analysis of one hundred and eighty-nine cases. J. Am. Dent. Assoc. *66*:456–465, 1963.
23. Hammond, E. C., and Horn, D.: The relationship between human smoking and death rates. J.A.M.A. *155*:1316–1328, 1955.
24. Hammond, E. C.: Effects of smoking. Scient. Am. *207*:39, 1962.
25. Heule, G., Heule, W., and Dilhl, V.: Relation of Burkitt's tumor-associated herpes type virus to infectious mononucleosis. Proc. Nat. Acad. Sci. *59*:94, 1968.
26. Holland, J. J.: Biochemistry of Cell and Virus Multiplications. Sixth National Cancer Conference Proceedings. Philadelphia, J. B. Lippincott Co., 1968, pp. 265–277.
27. Hueper, W. C.: Carcinogens in the human environment. Arch. Pathol. *71*:237, 267, 355, 1961.
28. Imamura, M.: Electron microscope study of polyoma induced salivary gland tumors with special reference to cell virus interaction. J. Natl. Cancer Inst. *41*:1265–1273, December 1968.
29. Itigashi, O.: Congenital gigantism of peroxidase granules—First case ever reported of qualitative abnormality of peroxidase Tohoku. J. Exp. Med. *59*:315–332, 1954.
30. Jones, E. L., and Cornell, W. P.: Gardner's syndrome. Arch. Surg. *92*:287–299, February 1966.
31. Keller, A. Z.: Cellular types, survival, race, nativity, occupation habits and associated diseases in the pathogenesis of lip cancers. Am. J. Epidemiol. *91*(5):486–499, 1970.
32. Keller, A. Z.: The epidemiology of lip, oral and pharyngeal cancers and the association with selected systemic diseases. Am. J. Public Health *53*:1214–1228, 1963.
33. Keller, A. Z.: Survivorship with mouth and pharynx cancers and their association with cirrhosis of the liver, marital status and residence. Am. J. Public Health *59*(7):1139–1153, July 1969.
34. Ketcham, A. S., Wexler, H., and Mantel, N.: Effects of alcohol in mouse neoplasia. Cancer Res. *23*:667–670, 1963.
35. Khanolkar, V. R., and Suryabai, B.: Cancer in relation to usages. Three new types in India. Arch. Pathol. *40*:351–361, 1945.
36. Khanolkar, V. R.: Cancer in India in relation to race, nutrition and customs. Acta Un. Internat. Ctr. Cancrum *7*:51–60, 1951.
37. Kinostuta, H.: Histological and immunofluorescent studies on histogenesis of polyoma induced in AKR mice. Sapporo Med. J. *31*:311–341, 1967.
38. Kreshover, S.: Observations on the effect of tobacco on epithelial tissues of vitamin deficient mice. J. Dent. Res. *34*:789, 1955.
39. Kreshover, S., and Salley, J.: Predisposing factors in oral cancer. J. Am. Dent. Assoc. *54*:509, 1957.
40. Kramer, P. M.: Polyoma virus dose-response stud-

ies in mice. II. Characteristics of induced salivary gland tumors. J. Natl. Cancer Inst. *28*:455–465, 1962.

41. Leffall, L. D., and White, J. E.: Cancer of the oral cavity in Negroes. Surg. Gynec. Obstet. *120*:70–72, 1965.
42. Lemmon, F. R., Walden, R. T., and Woods, R. W.: Cancer of the lungs and mouth in Seventh Day Adventists. Cancer *17*:486–497, 1964.
43. Lepp, H., and Wenger, F.: Leucoplasias y Cancer Buccal por el Habito de Fumar coy el Cigarrillo Invertido. Boletin de la Sociedad de Cirugia *19*:471–481, 1955.
44. Leuchtenberger, C., Schumacher, M., and Haldiman, T.: Z Praeventinied *13*:130, 1968 (cited by Eichel et al. 1969).
45. Lund, C. C.: Epidermoid carcinoma of the buccal mucosa. Surg. Gynec. Obstet. *66*:810–813, 1938.
46. Marsden, A. T.: Betel cancer in Malaya. Med. Malaya *14*:162, 1960.
47. Martin, H.: Mouth cancer and the dentist. J. Am. Dent. Assoc. *33*:845–861, 1946.
48. Martinez, I.: Factors associated with cancer of the esophagus, mouth, and pharynx in Puerto Rico. J. Natl. Cancer Inst. *42*:1069–1094, 1969.
49. Massler, M., Emslie, R., and Bolden, T. E.: Fetor ex Ore. Oral Surg. *4*:110–125, 1951.
50. Maxwell, J. L.: Betel chewing and cancer. Brit. Med. J. *1*:729, 1924.
51. Milham, S., Jr.: Alcohol cancers and wood. Lancet *1*:1059, May 16, 1970.
52. Mills, C. A., and Porter, M. M.: Tobacco smoking habits and cancer of the mouth and respiratory system. Cancer Res. *10*:539–542, 1950.
53. Mochowski, L., Yumoto, T., and Greg, C. E.: Electron microscopic studies of human leukemia and lymphoma. Cancer *20*:760–777, May 1967.
54. Moore, C., and Catlin, D.: Anatomic origins and locations of oral cancer. Am. J. Surg. *114*:510–513, October 1967.
55. Moore, G., and Bock, F.: A summary of research technics for investigating the cigarette smoking–lung cancer problem. Surgery *39*:120–130, 1956.
56. Moertal, C., and Foss, E.: Multicentric carcinomas of the oral cavity. Surg. Gynec. Obstet. *106*:652–654, 1958.
57. Muir, C. S., and Kirk, R.: Betel, tobacco and cancer of the mouth. Brit. J. Cancer *14*:597, 1960.
58. Munube, G. M. R., and Bettl, T. M.: Isolation of echovirus type II from two cases of Burkitt's tumor and three cases of other tumors. Int. J. Cancer 2:613, 1967.
59. Newell, G. R., and Waggoner, D. E.: Cancer mortality and environmental temperature in the United States. Lancet 1:766–767, April 1970.
60. Orr, I.: Oral Cancer in Betel Nut Chewers in Travancore. The Lancet *II*:575–580, 1933.
61. Peacock, E. E. and Brawley, B. W.: An evaluation of snuff and tobacco in the production of mouth cancer. Dent. Abstr. 5:269, May 1960.
62. Pindborg, J. J.: Oral cancer from an international point of view. J. Can. Dent. Assoc. *31*:219–226, 1965.
63. Quigley, L. F., Cobb, C. M., and Hunt, E. E., Jr.: Measurement of oral and burning zone temperatures during conventional and reverse cigarette smoking. Arch. Oral Biol. *10*:35–44, 1965.
64. Quigley, L. F., Cobb, C. M., Schoenfeld, S., Hunt, E. E., and William P.: Reverse smoking and its oral consequences in Caribbean and South American peoples. J. Am. Dent. Assoc. *69*: 427–442, October 1964.
65. Quigley, L. F., Sklar, G., and Cobb, C. M.: Reverse cigarette smoking in Caribbeans: Clinical, histologic and cytologic observation. J. Am. Dent. Assoc. *72*:867–873, April 1966.
66. Reddy, D. G., and Rao, V. K.: Cancer of the palate in Costal Andhra due to smoking cigars with the burning end inside the mouth. Indian J. Med. Sci. *11*(10):791–797, October 1957.
67. Ricafort, E. I.: An investigation of oral cancer and periodontal disease related to environmental factors – Betel nut chewing and reverse smoking in the Philippines. (Unpublished data.)
68. Robinson, H. B.: Practical application of experimental cancer research. J. Am. Dent. Assoc. *54*:524–529, 1957.
69. Rosenfeld, L., and Green, J.: Symposium: Malignant tumors of the alimentary tract: Carcinoma of the oral cavity. J. Tenn. Med. Assoc. *62*:707–710, August 1969.
70. Rowe, N. H.: Epidemiological concepts relative to cancer of the oral cavity. Missouri Med. *65*: 660–664, August 1968.
71. Rowe, W. P., Hartley, J. W., Estes, J. D., and Huebuer, R. S.: Growth curves of polyoma virus in mice and hamsters. J. Natl. Cancer Inst. *4*:189–209, 1960.
72. Segi, M., Kurichara, M., Narai, J., Ito, M., Takano, A., and Matsyama, T.: Cancer mortality for selected sites in 24 countries, No. 3, 1960–61, Sendai, Japan, 1964, Department of Public Health, Tohoku University School of Medicine.
73. Sirsat, S. M., and Kandarkar, S. V.: Histological changes in the oral mucosa of the Wistar rat treated with commercial lime (calcium hydroxide). An optical and submicroscopic study. Brit. J. Cancer *22*:303–315, 1968.
74. Solomon, G. F., and Moss, R. H.: Emotions, immunity and disease. Arch. Gen. Psychiat. *11*:657–674, 1964.
75. Tennekoon, G. E., and Bartlett, G. C.: Effect of betel chewing on the oral mucosa. Brit. J. Cancer *23*(1):39–43, March 1969.
76. Terrell, J. H., and Schweltz, I.: Cigarettes: Chemical effect of sodium nitrate content. Science *160*(3835):1456, June 1968.
77. Sutton, P. R. N.: Prognosis of carcinoma of the lip or tongue in relation to mental stress: Speculation of an anomalous finding. Med. J. Australia 2:312–313, August 17, 1968.
78. Vogler, W. R., Lloyd, J. W., and Milmore, B. K.: A retrospective study of etiological factor in cancer of the mouth, pharynx, and larynx. Cancer *15*:247–253, 1962.
79. Wahi, P. N., Kebar, U., and Lahiri, B.: Factors influencing oral and oropharyngeal cancers in India. Brit. J. Cancer *19*:642–660, 1965.
80. Waravdekar, V. S., Mangaonkar, V. G., and Khanolkar, V. R.: Vitamin B excretion in oral cancer patients. Acta Un. Internat. Ctr. Cancer *6*: 1017–1022, 1950.

81. Weir, J. M., Dunn, J. E., Jr., and Buell, P. E.: Smoking and oral cancer: Epidemiological data, educational responses. Am. J. Public Health *59*(6):959–966, June 1969.
82. Weisburger, D.: Precancerous lesions. J. Am. Dent. Assoc. *54*:507–508, 1957.
83. Wells, C. R.: Betel nut chewing and its effects. U.S. Naval Med. Bull. *22*(4):437, 1925.
84. White, J. C.: Virus-like particles in the peripheral blood cells of two patients with Chédiak Higashi syndrome. Cancer *19*:877–884, June 1966.
85. Wood, D. A.: New concepts in cancer control – preventable and avoidable cancer. Cancer J. Clinicians *20*(3):140–145, May-June 1970.
86. Wynder, E., Bross, I., and Friedman, R. A.: Study of the etiological factors in cancer of the mouth. Cancer *10*:1300–1323, 1957.

chapter 9

NUTRITION AND ORAL DISEASE

by
JUAN M. NAVIA, PH.D.

THE INTERACTION BETWEEN NUTRITION AND ORAL TISSUES

INFLUENCE OF NUTRITION ON THE ETIOLOGY OF ORAL DISEASE

Nutrition is highly influential in the development of host resistance to oral disease. No other factor, aside from the microbial one, can enhance or retard the disease process as much as variations in the quality, quantity, and frequency of foods consumed in the diet. Yet the true magnitude of this component in human oral disease processes has not been sufficiently measured or described.

The science of nutrition deals ultimately with the optimal cell requirements of certain essential elements and compounds during the process of reproduction, growth, maintenance and function. In its broader aspect this science also encompasses the study of the nutritional requirements, reactions, and interactions taking place in tissues, organs, and finally whole organisms. Foods in the diet provide these essential nutrients and so their nutritional composition, the amount and frequency with which they are consumed, and their physical and organoleptic properties are of special importance to the study of nutrition.

To oral tissues nutrition is of special relevance, not only because of their own specific requirements, but because these tissues come in contact with foods twice: once directly, when they are masticated in the oral cavity, and a second time when, after digestion and absorption, the nutrients return by way of the circulatory system to nourish these tissues.

The nutrient composition of foods in the diet can influence teeth at two distinct stages. Preeruptively the structure, chemical composition, and eruption time of teeth may be affected. During this period, nutrients in the diet can also select a pathogenic bacterial flora by enrichment of the environment and thus facilitate later the implantation and colonization of these microorganisms on the enamel surfaces of erupting teeth.

Posteruptively, nutrients in the diet can influence microorganisms on the enamel surface by facilitating plaque formation and stimulating their metabolic activities. Nutrients may also affect the flow and composition of saliva in contact with plaque and enamel, and finally, they can contribute to the composition of the outer enamel surface and to the formation of the acquired pellicle. These different preeruptive and posteruptive effects of dietary nutrients have not been clearly recognized and controlled in experimental situations and epidemiological studies, and have led to misunderstanding as to the true effect of nutrition in the etiology and development of oral disease.

Nutrients in the diet therefore can influence oral disease in the following ways:

1. By changing the chemical environment of cells responsible for the formation of tissues, such as enamel, and changing preeruptively the tooth structure composition and its physicochemical properties.
2. Influencing, either independently or together with hormones, the cellular enzyme systems involved in calcification processes.
3. Altering protein-synthetic reactions and thus modifying the nature of the calcifying organic matrix of mineralized tissues.
4. Modifying the rate of flow, the quantity, or the physical, chemical, or immunological properties of saliva.
5. Enhancing or inhibiting the remineralization process taking place normally on the tooth surface of erupted teeth.
6. Influencing the multiplication, implantation, and metabolism of the plaque flora.

In most oral disease processes the prognosis is usually determined by the interaction of host, microbial, and nutritional factors. When they interact, disease will ensue and when these factors are unbalanced the pathosis may be retarded or even prevented. Host factors involve genetic determinants which affect the quality of enamel, the morphology of teeth, the size ratio of teeth to mandible, degree of salivation, and composition of saliva (lysozyme, IgA, etc.), tissue biochemistry, and other factors. The microbial factor is represented by the bacterial masses in contact with oral tissues. The tooth is normally covered by a dense layer of microorganisms which secrete metabolic products that are in constant contact and interaction with oral tissues. These organisms, under the influence of the nutrient composition of the diet and other unknown factors, may develop such a degree of virulence that disease (caries or periodontal disease) will become rampant if untreated.

Efforts to prevent disease by controlling the etiological microbial agent alone may be frustrating. A total or complete approach to the prevention of disease through modification of all three factors would be most rewarding. In human populations the nutritional factors may be of greater importance than can be surmised from experimental studies. These studies are usually carried out using highly susceptible animals in which a virulent organism is present in the oral cavity. Under these experimental situations studies on the influence of malnutrition usually yield little information, for the virulence of the microorganisms overwhelms and obscures whatever effect this malnutrition may have contributed. The conditions prevailing among human populations are, however, quite different and are described in Figure 9–1. If host conditions are such that they confer a high degree of resistance to the tooth relative to the virulence of the microbial agent, then the disease process resulting from infection will not develop, regardless of the nutritional state during tooth formation. The same would be true if the conditions are reversed, so that if natural or constitutional resistance is very low in relation to the virulence of the microbial agent, then the disease process will develop while being little influenced by nutritional factors during growth and development. Since people and microorganisms have heterogeneous genetic and metabolic backgrounds, nutritional and dietary factors will influence in a great number of cases the course of the disease in humans.

These multifactorial properties of the

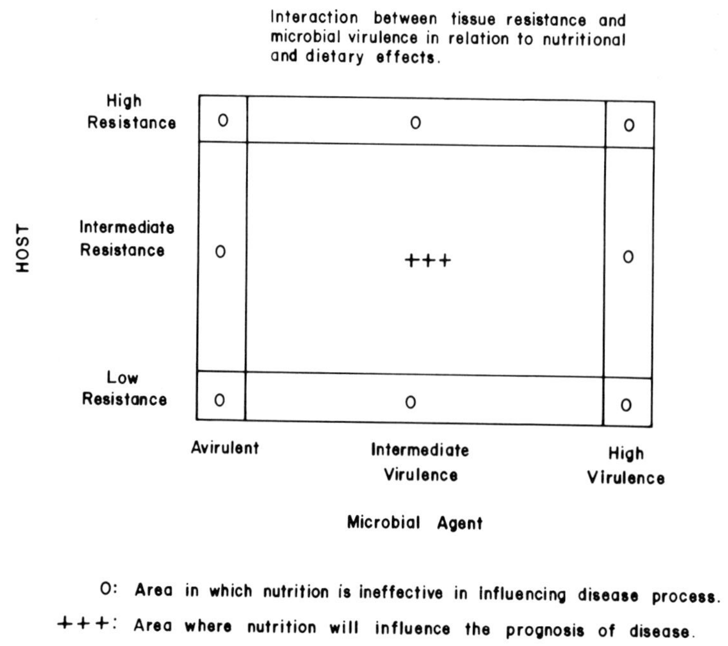

Figure 9–1 Nutritional effects on disease processes will not be seen in extreme cases where the virulence of the microbial agent is high or the resistance of the host is extremely low. However, because of the heterogenous, genetic and metabolic background of humans and microorganisms, nutrition will be able to influence the outcome of human disease in a large number of cases.

etiology of oral disease have made it difficult to evaluate the extent of the contribution of nutritional factors.

EPIDEMIOLOGICAL DATA ON NUTRITION AND ORAL DISEASE

Epidemiological studies relating the incidence of dental caries to nutrition illustrate this point. Russell[36] (1963) has reported on his extensive field work to determine the oral disease prevalence in people from different parts of the world. These findings show that prevalence of caries is not the same around the world, but rather that groups of people living in different areas have a characteristic level of caries activity, thus forming regional patterns (Fig. 9–2). This has enabled Russell to group populations and regions into areas of high, intermediate, and low prevalence of caries (Table 9–1).

Evaluation of the contribution of nutrition to the disease patterns of these people is difficult and confusing due to the multiplicity of factors that enters into the etiology of the disease. Caries prevalence in these different populations is found to be closely related to excessive consumption of refined carbohydrates. People from areas in which fluoride is present in the drinking water, and even sometimes in excess quantities, have been found to have low caries prevalence. Comparisons between the nutritional status of a population at the time when the survey was conducted and its accumulated lifetime total of decayed, missing, or filled permanent teeth have not yielded evidence that optimum nutrition inhibits caries. Despite the widespread consumption of diets low in vitamin A in Alaska or Ethiopia, or diets low in thiamine and riboflavin in Viet Nam and Thailand, the people in these countries exhibit surprisingly low levels of caries prevalence (Russell,[36] 1963). This same pattern has been observed by other investigators and Russell has summarized this concept by stating that "freedom from dental caries commonly observed in primitive peoples cannot be ascribed to any superiority of nutrition."

This interpretation of such data should be made cautiously, as many qualifying factors in the area of nutrition determine the outcome of disease. Two have been mentioned previously: carbohydrate consumption and fluoride level in the diet. The

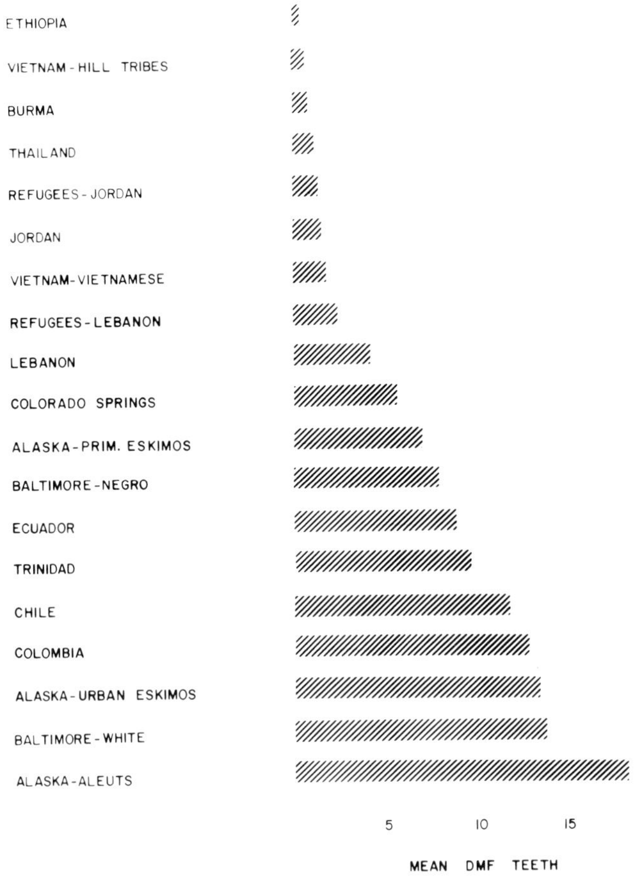

Figure 9–2 Caries prevalence of inhabitants of various parts of the world (Russell, A. L.: J. Dent. Res. *42*:233–244, 1963.)

increased consumption of refined carbohydrates at the expense of proteins is a factor that, when present, will forcibly incline the balance toward disease.[30] Experiments done in our laboratories (Navia[30] et al., 1970) indicate that if rats are undernourished during the time that molars are being formed, and then they are changed at weaning time to a mild caries-promoting diet containing 5 per cent sucrose and 62 per cent cornstarch, they

TABLE 9–1 POPULATIONS AND REGIONS WITH RELATIVELY HIGH, INTERMEDIATE AND RELATIVELY LOW PREVALENCES OF DENTAL CARIES[36]

RELATIVELY HIGH	INTERMEDIATE	RELATIVELY LOW
Most populations in:	Fluoride areas in:	Ethiopia
North America	United States	
South America	Ecuador	
Europe	Bolivia	Burma, Thailand, Viet Nam
New Zealand	Greece	India, China, Taiwan
Australia	Israel	
Tahiti	Lebanon	
Hawaii	Egypt	
		Remote areas of Alaska
Urban Alaska	Malaya	
	Indonesia	Jordan
Trinidad		
		New Guinea

will exhibit 50 per cent higher caries scores than control animals receiving a normal diet during tooth mineralization. Further investigations have clearly shown that the increased caries susceptibility in undernourished rats can also be produced by imposing a specific, marginal protein malnutrition during the time that teeth and salivary glands are actively developing.[25] If a high sucrose (67 per cent) caries-promoting diet is offered at weaning, then all rats will exhibit the same high degree of caries activity regardless of their preeruptive nutritional status. The intensity of the cariogenic potential of sugar has overwhelmed the protective effect of the diet during tooth formation.

Fluoride availability is another factor which has been clearly shown to interfere with the course of the disease. Water drinking patterns and proportions of fluids such as tea, milk, water, or fruit juices consumed by people around the world vary enormously. Whereas in some areas young children are weaned early and start to consume water, fruit juices, or even beverages such as tea, with a high fluoride content, in other parts of the world the consumption of milk is continued for long periods of time to the practical exclusion of water. It is well known that while the nutritional value of milk is outstanding, a child raised on water containing fluoride or tea will obtain the benefit of a higher fluoride intake, while a child who is relatively better nourished on milk will have a lower fluoride intake. A child raised on milk may be better nourished overall, but the protective value of fluoride on caries incidence will be absent. Therefore, total fluoride intakes of diets in different areas should be determined to evaluate the contribution of this parameter to the disease picture.

Two other factors must be considered in order to understand the role of nutrition in a disease such as dental caries. A very important point is the particular distribution of food within the family, depending on sex, economic status, and life style (rural, urban, etc.). Food has strong social and cultural connotations and its distribution within the family unit may vary, depending on the factors listed above, in its influence on the development of teeth and the outcome of the disease and thus obscure the interpretation of the contribution of nutritional status to oral diseases.

A second important consideration is that frequency of consumption of snack foods containing high levels of refined carbohydrate have been clearly known to increase the severity of caries. Malnourished populations not only consume foods with low nutritional quality, but they also eat less frequently. A man working in the field in Latin America may have only one or two meals a day interspaced with consumption of some beverage such as black coffee, while a white-collar worker in an urban economy will have two or three meals together with several snacks during the day. Again, the overall nutritional requirements are better fulfilled in this latter situation, while the incidence of oral disease in these individuals is higher than in their counterparts in the rural Latin American community.

A few years ago, a nutritional survey was carried out in Honduras[18] which included a clinical examination, biochemical evaluation, dietary survey, and oral examination. Figure 9–3 shows that caries prevalence in this rural area is high and increases between five and nine years of age. Young people between 15 and 19 years of age had nearly half of the permanent teeth affected with caries. The DMF for pregnant and lactating women between 15 and 29 years of age was found to be higher than the value for non-pregnant, non-lactating women of the same age. High caries scores were also reported for the deciduous teeth of these children (Tables 9–2 and 9–3).

Dental caries constitutes an important oral problem for people in Honduras and especially those living in rural areas. Evaluation of the diet consumed by the urban and rural populations reveals interesting observations. While the two groups consume nearly the same types of foods, distinct differences are seen in the proportions consumed. Table 9–4 shows the average consumption of foods per person per day for people living in the urban and the rural areas. Foods containing high-quality protein

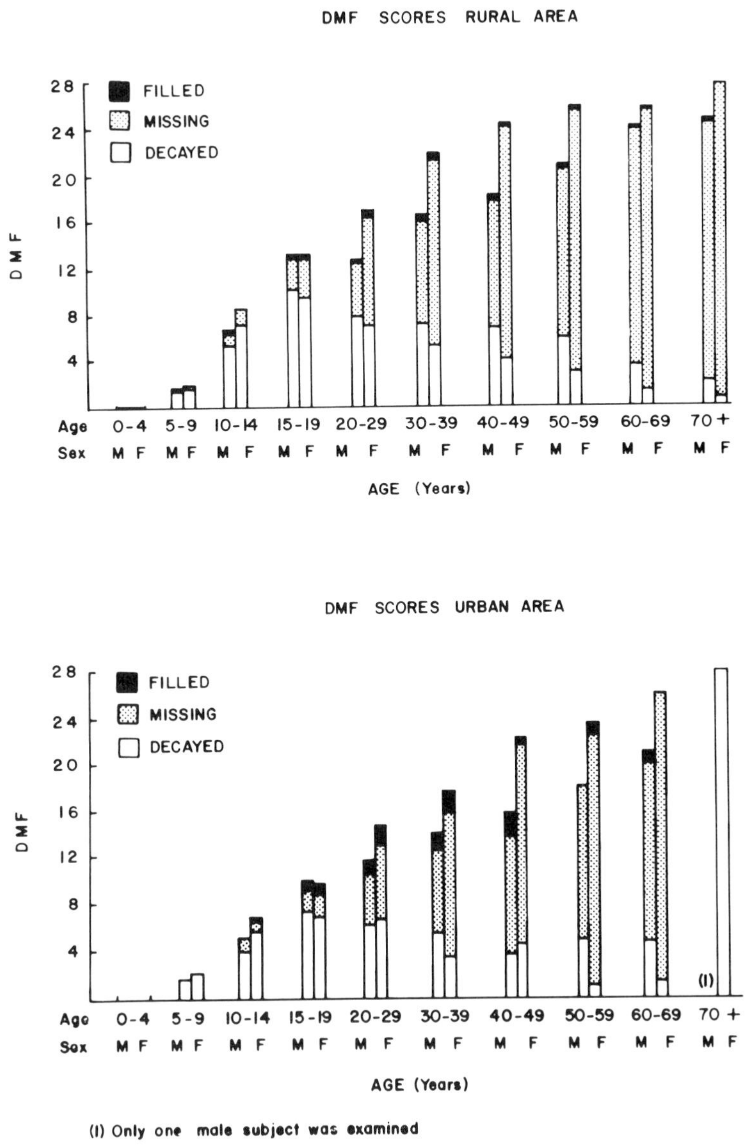

Figure 9-3 Caries prevalence of people living in rural and urban areas in Honduras (INCAP,[14] 1969).

TABLE 9-2 DMF AND df SCORES OF PEOPLE IN RURAL AREAS*

	DMF					*df*		
Age (Yrs.)	*M*	*F*	*Total*	*Pregnant Women*	*Lactating Women*	*M*	*F*	*Total*
0– 4	0	0	0			3.0	3.2	3.1
5– 9	1.8	1.9	1.9			6.8	6.3	6.6
10–14	6.6	8.5	7.6 }			1.5	0.8	1.2
15–19	13.1	13.1	13.1 }	17.9	19.0			
20–29	12.6	16.9	15.1 }					
30–39	16.6	21.9	19.0	21.4	21.3			
40–49	18.2	24.2	21.2	23.6	25.5			
50–59	20.6	25.6	23.1					
60–69	24.1	25.5	24.8					
70 +	24.7	27.5	26.1					

*INCAP,[14] 1969.

TABLE 9-3 DMF AND df SCORES OF PEOPLE IN URBAN AREAS*

	DMF			*df*		
Age (Yrs.)	*M*	*F*	*Total*	*M*	*F*	*Total*
0– 4	0	0	0	2.2	1.3	1.8
5– 9	1.4	1.9	1.6	5.6	4.9	5.3
10–14	5.0	6.9	6.0	0.5	0.7	0.6
15–19	10.1	9.8	9.9	0	0.3	0.2
20–29	11.6	14.6	13.6			
30–39	13.9	17.5	16.2			
40–49	15.7	22.1	19.5			
50–59	18.1	23.5	21.4			
60–69	21.0	26.1	24.4			
70 +	(1)	28.0	28.0			
Total	6.9	10.8	9.2	1.6	1.0	1.2

*INCAP,[14] 1969.
(1) Only one subject was examined.

are consumed more in the urban locality than in the rural. Starchy cereal consumption is somewhat higher in the rural area than in the city, but more sugar is consumed in the urban than in the rural community.

The survey done in Honduras[18] is an interesting example for this discussion for it was found that the most severe nutritional problem in this country was protein deficiency. This was especially true in children who suffered a chronic calorie-protein malnutrition early in life when teeth were being formed. These people showed a high incidence of dental caries, comparable in magnitude to that observed in several areas in the United States where overall nutrition is far superior. A comparison between people living in urban and rural situations in Honduras shows a lower dental caries score in people living in urban communities, with access to a diet which was similar in components but with differences in proportions and nutritional quality. In this case the higher caries scores of rural people may be associated with an inadequate diet, but many other factors not clearly understood could also contribute to the disease pattern.

Dental caries is not the only oral disease or defect associated with nutritional deficiency. Sweeney[45] et al. (1969) reported the presence of a linear hypoplasia of deciduous maxillary incisors which seemed to be correlated with infections during the first month of life and possibly with low serum vitamin A levels. The cause and effect relationship was not clear but infections early in the life of children are common and greatly contribute to the malnourished status of already nutritionally depleted children.

Studies done to ascertain the relationship between nutritional state and oral dis-

TABLE 9-4 AVERAGE FOOD CONSUMPTION PER PERSON PER DAY OF RURAL AND URBAN POPULATIONS IN HONDURAS*

FOODS	RURAL GM	URBAN GM
Dairy Products		
(Expressed as milk)	194	289
Eggs	13	21
Meats	41	87
Legumes	56	47
Fresh Vegetables	51	56
Fruits	40	54
Bananas and plantain	43	49
Roots and Tubercles	22	24
Cereals:		
Tortilla (corn)	338	202
Rice	29	50
Bread (wheat)	12	74
Wheat Flour	8	9
Nacatamal	2	1
Other	5	7
Sugars	39	45
Oils	16	21
Beverages:		
Coffee (beans)	9	9
Carbonated beverages	3	18
Other	–	3

*INCAP,[14] 1969.

ease are complicated by factors such as the ones previously mentioned and their effects are difficult to separate and study independently in human populations. In a study of differences in the occurrence of dental caries between white and black children, it was observed that the former had twice as high a DMF score as the latter. When investigations were made to identify variables that might be associated with the difference in caries score, it was found that (a) specific caries-inducing streptococci of the hamster type were recovered from 30 per cent of the cultures of plaque material from white boys versus 17 per cent obtained from black boys, (b) no differences were observed in mean pH of plaque suspensions from both groups of children, and (c) black boys reported eating sweet foods more often than white boys. These boys, however, reported drinking more milk than black boys (Littleton[21] et al., 1970). No conclusion as to the causative factors of the disease can be drawn from clinical studies of this type.

Differences in the water intake pattern of children may have a profound influence on caries experience, especially if water contains trace elements that may not be present in other beverages such as milk. Curzon[4] et al. (1970) have carried out an epidemiological study comparing 251 children living in an Ohio town that uses water containing a high level of boron and strontium against a control group of 338 children drinking water with low levels of these elements. These authors suggest that the significantly lower caries prevalence in the former group is related to the boron and strontium content of the water. In this case changes in the amount of water consumed and drinking pattern may show a difference in the caries experience of the child. Minerals are extremely important to the development of teeth and their susceptibility to disease (Navia[26], 1970).

The association between malnutrition and dental caries has been difficult to discern in epidemiological studies. High caries incidence has been reported in areas of affluence and in less technologically advanced countries, whereas low caries has been consistently noted in remote areas where inhabitants occasionally show low protein intake. The reasons for these discrepancies may be traced to the following:

1. Caries is an infectious disease produced by one or more types of streptococci and lactobacilli with varying degrees of virulence, which may account, in part, for differences in the incidence and severity of the disease.
2. Diet is highly influential in caries development and can act *preeruptively*, as described for protein, or *posteruptively* by enhancing the implantation and metabolic activity of cariogenic microorganisms. This posteruptive influence of diet can be overwhelming and stimulate rampant caries despite the beneficial effects that may have been contributed preeruptively. In many cases, malnourished populations consume refined carbohydrates infrequently and in small quantities rather than indulging in a nibbling pattern that is customary in some affluent countries. Underfed populations lack adequate nutrition during tooth formation, but they also lack the cariogenic stress that is necessary for the disease to develop and, therefore, their dental caries incidence is low. It is only upon exposure to cariogenic conditions that their teeth seem to melt from such undue stress.

Epidemiological studies are useful in evaluating associations and broad patterns of oral disease and dietary habits but fail if the wrong questions are asked of this research approach. Oral disease is a multifactorial problem which can be influenced in a number of ways at different anatomical and physiological ages of the tissues involved. Nutritional factors are essential to the expression of the genetic information and continue to be important from conception to death. The provision of the right nutrient at the right time and in the proper amount and chemical combination is essential to the growth, development, and function of the tissue. These conditions are characteristic for each tissue and therefore optimum formation and functioning of oral tissues demands that their special nutritional requirements, in the form of proteins, vitamins, minerals and other compounds, be satisfied at the proper time during development. Unfortunately, we know little about the individual requirements of teeth and other oral tissues, but more is being understood of processes which are common to many tissues, such as cell reproduction, protein synthesis, and calcification.

NUTRITIONAL FACTORS IN TISSUE GROWTH, DEVELOPMENT AND FUNCTION

CELL GROWTH AND NUTRITION

Animal studies indicate that growth is a well-ordered series of events which proceed in a sequential manner. During perinatal stages most organs grow by division alone followed by a second stage in which cell size is increased. Thus, for any tissue three distinct phases of growth can be described: hyperplasia, hyperplasia and concomitant hypertrophy, and hypertrophy alone. If a tissue is deprived of nutrients during the first stage in its development, it will show an impaired growth which is due to a diminished cell number. Winick and Noble[48] (1966) have reported that the rate of cell division and the ultimate number of cells within a given organ may be reduced by limiting the number of calories available to experimental animals during their neonatal period.

Some experiments (DiOrio et al.,[7] 1973) indicate that protein, and not calories, is the essential limiting nutrient in these growth stages. Experiments to study the effect of undernutrition in experimental animals during the early stages of growth are usually carried out by manipulations of litter size in which rat dams are given a large number of pups while others are only given a few. The result of these experiments is that pups from large litters have less milk available than those in small litters, as competition for nipples is less for pups in small litters and suckling therefore is carried to complete satisfaction of hunger. Experiments of this type do not separate the effect of calorie deficiency from protein deficiency. In an experiment (DiOrio et al.,[7] 1973) in which all animals were underfed and then given supplements containing either protein or carbohydrates, it was observed that addition of calories alone did not improve growth and development of animals, but when protein was given the growth curve approximated that of animals given a normal diet. In the latter case the protein supplement contributed the necessary building parts and a minimum of energy for cell growth to take place.

These experiments were repeated (Menaker[25] and Navia,[27] 1973) with the modification that pups from all groups were, after weaning, fed a caries-promoting diet to determine their caries susceptibility. In this and in the previous study, feeding the isocaloric protein supplement to the undernourished rats during development allowed the pups to compensate for the loss in body weight. Significantly, it was noted that protein-malnourished pups had higher caries scores than well-nourished controls. In undernourished rats that received isocaloric supplements without protein, caries levels equalled those of control-undernourished rats intubated with distilled water.

Salivary glands and saliva, as well as teeth, were examined in the rats used in the experiments described. These studies indicated that weight, DNA, RNA, and total protein of the submandibular gland were also lower in rats with protein malnutrition. Changes in the protein content or in flow rate of saliva secreted by these affected glands may have an important effect on the caries susceptibility of the tooth.

These experiments clearly illustrate that the number and size of cells in the tissue is governed not only by the genetic information contained in the cell but also by extrinsic factors, such as nutritional status, during critical periods of development. This exerts a profound influence on the growth, development and susceptibility to disease of tissues and organs.

NUTRITIONAL FACTORS INFLUENCING CELL PROTEIN SYNTHESIS

Many cell processes are profoundly influenced by nutritional factors but two have special importance for oral tissues: protein synthesis and calcification. Protein synthesis is constantly being carried out by all cells both during the growth and the maintenance stage. Cell life is therefore dependent on the ability to form proteins of all types. Protein synthesis requires the presence within the cell of different nutrients, such as amino acids, vitamins in the form of cofactors, and minerals which are essential to the process and have to be supplied in the diet. The basic mechanism by which these different amino acids are organized into proteins is fairly well understood. The assembly of a protein depends on having a characteristic messenger RNA which has a code indicating the sequence in which the amino acids are going to be organized into the specific protein being formed. Another group of RNA molecules will transport the amino acids to the messenger strand which is associated with the ribosomes in the cell. Each messenger RNA strand is associated in an aggregate with ribosomes referred to as a polyribosome. The number of ribosomes on a messenger strand is reflective of the protein-synthetic capacity of this organelle. It has been shown that amino acids play an important role in maintaining the integrity of this organelle and therefore regulate to some extent the protein-synthetic activity of the cell. In mammalian cells some polysomes are attached to a system of intracellular membranes, the endoplasmic reticulum, which is usually associated with production of exportable proteins. Free within the cytoplasm, other polysomes are thought to be making proteins intended to remain within the cell.

The regulation of protein synthesis is one of the fundamental aspects of this phenomenon, and in mammalian cells it is carried out partly through regulation of RNA synthesis in the nucleus. The amount of RNA made increases after observable increases in the enzyme RNA polymerase, and also by a change in the availability of its nucleotide substrate or by varying the amount of DNA template exposed to the enzyme. Nutrition can influence the amount of protein in the cell cytoplasm by controlling the amounts of amino acids coming to the tissue and thus in a way regulating the translation by the messenger. In addition, other nutrients can influence the stability of the protein which is formed and thus influence protein synthesis by changing the rate of degradation. The iron-containing protein, ferritin for example, seems to be stabilized by iron and therefore the concentration of this mineral nutrient determines the rate of breakdown of ferritin protein in the cell and hence the absolute amount present at any one time.

Studies performed in gingiva, buccal mucosa, and palate to study the pattern of protein synthesis indicate that these tissues are not different from liver, spleen, and other tissues. Microsomal and polyribosomal preparations from either rabbit or bovine oral tissues require t-RNA, the amino acid activating system and energy source, to synthesize protein in an in vitro system. They are inhibited by puromycin and ribonuclease but not by chloramphenicol. The rate of amino acid incorporation and protein synthesis in oral tissues seems to be high, presumably due to their high rate of tissue turnover.

The biosynthesis of collagen protein, because of its important role in bone, dentin, and the supporting structures of teeth, deserves a closer look. The synthesis of this protein is influenced by nutrition to an even greater extent than other proteins. Collagen contains amino acids, such as hydroxyproline and hydroxylysine, which are incorporated initially into the polypeptide chain as proline and lysine and then subsequently hydroxylated. One of the factors involved in the hydroxylation of particular nutritional interest is ascorbic acid, a vitamin whose role in tissue repair and growth is well documented. Today it is generally accepted that the hydroxylase system belongs to the "mixed-function" oxidases which catalyze a reaction of the type:

$$RH + O_2 + XH_2 \rightarrow ROH + H_2O + X$$

At least three different types of electron donors (XH_2) have been found to function as co-enzymes in different hydroxylating systems: (1) ascorbate, (2) tetrahydropteridines, and (3) NADPH. In the formation of collagen the factors which seem to be involved in the reaction are ascorbate, Fe^{2+}, α-ketoglutarate and O_2.

Gould[10] (1970) has suggested that another nutrient, folic acid, is also involved in the synthesis of the collegen polypeptide. A recent report indicates that folic acid is essential for the maintenance of an intact oral mucosa (Dreizen et al.,[8] 1970). Folic acid-deficient marmosets showed an impaired maturational sequence of the oral mucosal epithelium. Oral target sites included the labial, lingual, buccal, gingival, and pharyngeal mucosa where ulceration and secondary infections are frequently observed. Inclusion of folic acid in the otherwise nutritionally adequate experimental diet offered to marmosets protected them from mucosal ulceration and infection. The authors concluded that this effect of folic acid deficiency might be due either to the effect on collagen synthesis or to the impaired production of DNA which is known to disrupt the production of RNA and prevents the process of cell maturation.

Another nutrient, copper, is also important in the biosynthesis of collagen and of another structural protein, elastin. Collagen is a triple-helical, fibrous structure composed of three chains of about 1000 amino acid residues. The crosslinking of collagen (as well as elastin) is carried out by a copper-dependent oxidase. Much of the evidence for this comes from studies in which β-amino propionitrile, a lathyrogen, is fed to animals. The lathyritic α chains of collagen appear to be normal, however, the ϵNH_2 groups of the lysyl residues which are involved in crosslinkage are not oxidatively deaminated and crosslinking does not occur. Thus normal maturation of collagen does not proceed in the absence of adequate amounts of copper. Other minerals, such as manganese, are essential for the glycosilation reactions essential to the formation of mucopolysaccharides.

CALCIFICATION PROCESSES AND NUTRITION

Collagen, once formed, may undergo another process greatly influenced by nutritional factors. Collagen formed by certain cells, such as osteoblasts and odontoblasts, undergoes a process of mineralization in which a host of vitamins and mineral elements enter to fulfill either a structural or a catalytical role.

For many years it has been observed that dietary systems with low Ca, low phosphate, or deficient in vitamin D are usually associated with the bone deformities referred to as rickets. While identification and synthesis of the antirachitic substances were achieved in the late 1930's, it was not until 30 years later that the metabolism and function of vitamin D were established and this work is still actively being pursued.

As it is understood today, vitamin D undergoes several transformations in the body before forming the final active metabolite. Cholecalciferol from the diet or from irradiation of 7-dehydrocholesterol in the skin is transported in the blood to the liver, where cholecalciferol is transformed to 25-hydroxycholecalciferol (25-HCC). This compound is again transported by blood to the kidney where it is hydroxylated again to form the 1,25-dihydroxycholecalciferol (1,25-DHCC). This metabolite and others such as 24,25 DHCC cause a more rapid enhancement of Ca absorption in rachitic chicks than either vitamin D_3 or 25-HCC. It was also more effective at lower concentrations than these two parent steroids.

Many other nutrients are involved in the process of calcification. Protein, vitamin A, and minerals such as Mg, Mn, Cu, Zn, and F are all involved in the process, but the exact function for all of them is not yet understood in detail. Still, the presence of these factors is essential to the successful formation and maintenance of calcified tissues such as bones and teeth. Severe and even mild deficiencies in these essential elements during the mineralization of teeth may cause the deposition of defective enamel and dentin which may in turn have a deleterious effect on dental health. It should be remembered that enamel, in contrast to bone, has only one opportunity to be formed right. Defects during development cannot be cellularly repaired and constitute irreversible lesions.

NUTRITIONAL REQUIREMENTS OF THE INDIVIDUAL: THE RECOMMENDED DIETARY ALLOWANCES

The evidence presented in the previous section clearly indicates that cells have specific nutritional requirements at different stages in their growth and development. These nutritional requirements also exist for tissues undergoing certain processes, such as calcification, and they have to be met if their different functions are to be completed successfully.

Humans can be considered as a conglomerate of cells, tissues, and organs each with their nutritional requirements which, when considered as a whole, become the nutritional requirements of the individual. Furthermore, these requirements might be considered, collectively, to include the requirements of a group of people with similar genetic backgrounds, living under approximately similar environmental and social conditions. Such values are the recommended dietary allowances (RDA) suggested by the Food and Nutrition Board of the U.S. National Research Council.[35]

The RDA can be used as a guide in planning nutritionally adequate diets for population groups and as a standard reference to interpret the adequacy of nutrient intakes of individuals in dietary surveys of population groups in the U.S.A.

It is important to point out that, although these figures provide a safety margin to allow for individual variations, they cannot be used solely to determine the nutritional adequacy of one individual. This would also require knowledge of the current and past nutrient intake of the individual together with an evaluation of clinical signs and symptoms, and biochemical data on tissue and excretory levels of nutrients. Individuals whose diets meet the RDA are not necessarily free of malnutrition, nor should the ones consuming diets which fail to meet the RDA standards be judged necessarily as undernourished. The evaluation of the nutritional adequacy of an individual must take more into consideration. The RDA figures are given for groups of people, while nutritional requirements of an individual are determined by the needs of cells and tissues to grow and function.

The recommended dietary allowances include nutritional recommendations for 16 categories of men, women, children, and infants, in calories and 17 nutrients: protein; vitamins A, D, E, ascorbic acid, folacin, niacin, riboflavin, thiamine, vitamins B_6 and B_{12}, and the minerals Ca, P, I, Fe, and Mg. The amounts recommended by the RDA are tabulated in Table 9–5.

It should be emphasized that these amounts of nutrients are nutritional goals set for groups of people based on the so-called "reference" man and woman. In the last revision, the reference man is 22 years old and weighs 70 kg. The reference woman is also 22 years old and weighs 58 kg. Both the man and the woman presumably live in an environment with a mean temperature of 20° C and wear clothing which provides thermal comfort. Their physical activity is usually considered "light," involving occupations which are neither sedentary nor overly active. Obviously, adjustments have to be made whenever there is departure from these standard conditions. The RDA table has taken such adjustments into consideration and tabulates requirements for different age groups and for certain physiological states, such as lactation and pregnancy, when nutritional demands are higher. These dietary allowances do not take into consideration nutritional require-

TABLE 9–5 FOOD AND NUTRITION BOARD, NATIONAL ACADEMY OF SCIENCES–NATIONAL RESEARCH COUNCIL RECOMMENDED DAILY DIETARY ALLOWANCES,[1] Revised 1973.

Designed for the maintenance of good nutrition of practically all healthy people in the U.S.A.

	(Years) From Up to	Weight (kg)	Weight (lbs)	Height (cm)	Height (in)	Energy (kcal)[2]	Protein (g)	FAT-SOLUBLE VITAMINS: Vitamin A Activity (RE)[3]	Vitamin A Activity (IU)	Vitamin D (IU)	Vitamin E Activity[5] (IU)	WATER-SOLUBLE VITAMINS: Ascorbic Acid (mg)	Folacin[6] (μg)	Niacin[7] (mg)	Riboflavin (mg)	Thiamin (mg)	Vitamin B_6 (mg)	Vitamin B_{12} (μg)	MINERALS: Calcium (mg)	Phosphorus (mg)	Iodine (μg)	Iron (mg)	Magnesium (mg)	Zinc (mg)
Infants	0.0–0.5	6	14	60	24	kg × 117	kg × 2.2	420[4]	1,400	400	4	35	50	5	0.4	0.3	0.3	0.3	360	240	35	10	60	3
	0.5–1.0	9	20	71	28	kg × 108	kg × 2.0	400	2,000	400	5	35	50	8	0.6	0.5	0.4	0.3	540	400	45	15	70	5
Children	1–3	13	28	86	34	1300	23	400	2,000	400	7	40	100	9	0.8	0.7	0.6	1.0	800	800	60	15	150	10
	4–6	20	44	110	44	1800	30	500	2,500	400	9	40	200	12	1.1	0.9	0.9	1.5	800	800	80	10	200	10
	7–10	30	66	135	54	2400	36	700	3,300	400	10	40	300	16	1.2	1.2	1.2	2.0	800	800	110	10	250	10
Males	11–14	44	97	158	63	2800	44	1,000	5,000	400	12	45	400	18	1.5	1.4	1.6	3.0	1200	1200	130	18	350	15
	15–19	61	134	172	69	3000	54	1,000	5,000	400	15	45	400	20	1.8	1.5	2.0	3.0	1200	1200	150	18	400	15
	19–22	67	147	172	69	3000	54	1,000	5,000	400	15	45	400	20	1.8	1.5	2.0	3.0	800	800	140	10	350	15
	23–50	70	154	172	69	2700	56	1,000	5,000		15	45	400	18	1.6	1.4	2.0	3.0	800	800	130	10	350	15
	51+	70	154	172	69	2400	56	1,000	5,000		15	45	400	16	1.5	1.2	2.0	3.0	800	800	110	10	350	15
Females	11–14	44	97	155	62	2400	44	800	4,000	400	12	45	400	16	1.3	1.2	1.6	3.0	1200	1200	115	18	300	15
	15–18	54	119	162	65	2100	48	800	4,000	400	12	45	400	14	1.4	1.1	2.0	3.0	1200	1200	115	18	300	15
	19–22	58	128	162	65	2100	46	800	4,000	400	12	45	400	14	1.4	1.1	2.0	3.0	800	800	100	18	300	15
	23–50	58	128	162	65	2000	46	800	4,000		12	45	400	13	1.2	1.0	2.0	3.0	800	800	100	18	300	15
	51+	58	128	162	65	1800	46	800	4,000		12	45	400	12	1.1	1.0	2.0	3.0	800	800	80	10	300	15
Pregnant						+300	+30	1,000	5,000	400	15	60	800	+2	+0.3	+0.3	2.5	4.0	1200	1200	125	18+[8]	450	20
Lactating						+500	+20	1,200	6,000	400	15	80	600	+4	+0.5	+0.3	2.5	4.0	1200	1200	150	18	450	25

[1]The allowances are intended to provide for individual variations among most normal persons as they live in the United States under usual environmental stresses. Diets should be based on a variety of common foods in order to provide other nutrients for which human requirements have been less well defined. See text for more-detailed discussion of allowances and of nutrients not tabulated.

[2]Kilojoules (KJ) = 4.2 × kcal.

[3]Retinol equivalents.

[4]Assumed to be all as retinol in milk during the first six months of life. All subsequent intakes are assumed to be one-half as retinol and one-half as β-carotene when calculated from international units. As retinol equivalents, three-fourths are as retinol and one-fourth as β-carotene.

[5]Total vitamin E activity, estimated to be 80 per cent as α-tocopherol and 20 per cent other tocopherols. See text for variation in allowances.

[6]The folacin allowances refer to dietary sources as determined by *Lactobacillus case* assay. Pure forms of folacin may be effective in doses less than one-fourth of the RDA.

[7]Although allowances are expressed as niacin, it is recognized that on the average 1 mg of niacin is derived from each 60 mg of dietary tryptophan.

[8]This increased requirement cannot be met by ordinary diets; therefore, the use of supplemental iron is recommended.

ments under extreme stress or disease conditions in humans, when nutritional demands are even higher.

NUTRITION AND ORAL DISEASE

DENTAL CARIES

Dental caries is an infectious disease which is influenced by the interaction of microbial, dietary and host factors. This disease is ubiquitous and has existed for centuries, for ancient skulls have been found which show some dental decay. The incidence of caries at different time periods in Great Britain indicates that less than 10 per cent of skulls from the second millennium of the Christian Era had caries (Hardwick,[15] 1960). With time a considerable increase in caries incidence has taken place. In Greenland, for example, Pederson[33] (1938) reported that while in ancient times 0.5 per cent of people had caries, in modern times this figure has jumped to 69 per cent and may be even higher today.

This change in the epidemiological pattern could be attributed to increased virulence of the cariogenic bacteria, but diet is the etiological factor considered to be most responsible for this change in the extent and incidence of the disease.

The diet plays an important role in the selection, implantation, colonization, and metabolic activity of the plaque microflora. Nutrients in the diet may retard or promote the formation and activity of a cariogenic plaque, and the understanding of such effects in human caries is extremely important. The dental health status of an individual is thus largely determined by a balance between dietary factors which retard or promote caries (Navia, 1972, 1973; Hartles and Leach, 1975).

Sugar and Sugar-Containing Foods

The carbohydrate component, particularly sucrose, is an important caries-promoting factor in the diet. Sucrose is utilized in the formation of microbial extracellular polysaccharides found in dental plaque and also stimulates the caries potential of the plaque organisms. These effects are enhanced by frequent consumption of sugar-rich foods and are probably further stimulated by other dietary nutrients acting as microbial growth factors.

Studies done with hamsters indicate that caries activity is determined to a large extent by the sucrose content of the experimental diets. Cariogenic streptococci established themselves better on a high sucrose diet than on a high glucose diet. Glucose, when it is available to plaque organisms, is known to induce the synthesis of intracellular polysaccharides, whereas sucrose is capable of producing both the intracellular and extracellular polysaccharides (mostly dextran with some levans which together make up the bulk of plaque matrix). Experiments using monkeys indicated that, when sucrose was restricted in their diet, the amount of plaque on the tooth surfaces was reduced. The numbers of intracellular polysaccharide-forming organisms remained constant and the population of extracellular polysaccharide-forming bacteria fell with the feeding of the low sucrose diet to the monkeys. This has also been found to be true in humans. It should be pointed out that the levans, the intracellular polysaccharide, and to a limited extent the dextrans can be a source of carbon for starved cells. The extracellular polysaccharide can also serve as a support or attachment site for other microorganisms which may later proliferate.

Knowing the caries-promoting properties of sucrose, one question often asked is: Would a substitution of sucrose by other sugars be of any beneficial effect in preventing or reducing dental decay? The results obtained with laboratory animals inoculated with *Streptococcus mutans* point to sucrose as being more cariogenic in comparison with dextrose, fructose, maltose, or starch. However, studies done with rats in which no attempt was made to infect the animals with specific cariogenic microorganisms did not show such a clear difference between different common sugars. Glucose and fructose, for example, were found to be as caries promoting as sucrose.

Experimental designs to test the caries effects of sugars, using streptococcal strains that utilize sucrose to form copious amounts of extracellular polysaccharides, and in which smooth surface lesions are evaluated, may yield different results from those obtained using animal species infected with another type of cariogenic flora and where fissure caries evaluation is used. When the degree of relevance to the human situation is being sought through interpretation of experimental data, careful evaluation of the conditions used to obtain the data is necessary. It seems that while sucrose is an important caries-promoting factor in the diet, its substitution in human foods by glucose or other simple sugars is not going to have a major impact in the prevention of dental caries. Polyols such as sorbitol or xylitol might be an exception to this statement, but their chemical and organoleptical properties make the substitution technologically difficult, although not impossible.

When different types of human foods are evaluated in animal experiments, the conclusion is that foods containing a large proportion of carbohydrate are the ones that give the highest caries scores. The relationship is not constant and direct in all cases, as there are many other factors, such as taste, consistency, and composition, which alter the caries potential of the food tested in this animal model which were not controlled or studied.[31]

Chocolate and Cocoa

When Gustafson and coworkers[13] (1954) evaluated the effect of milk chocolates on caries of human subjects at the Vipeholm Mental Institution, they observed a lower increase in caries activity than the expected one based on the sucrose content of this confection. Several investigators have studied the effect on rat caries of cocoa products and extracts. Stralfors[43] (1966) has done studies which indicate that the defatted cocoa contains some factors that inhibit caries and that these factors can be extracted with water. Hamster caries tests using dialysed water extracts of cocoa point to a high molecular weight compound as having the cariostatic property. Tannin compounds may be responsible for the cariostatic activity observed, but the evidence is as yet not conclusive. These types of tests are difficult to evaluate in terms of their relevance for humans, as the animals were influenced in their growth by the addition of supplements to the diet or the water, and drastic departures from the normal feeding and eating patterns may have taken place, thus confusing the search for the cariostatic compounds in cocoa and chocolates.

Cereals and Bread

Studies on the effect of starch on caries development show that the incidence of caries is low, regardless of whether the starch is cooked or raw.

Konig[20] (1967) has pointed out the differences in cariogenicity between regimes containing flour of different degrees of refinement. Bread made with highly refined flour was less cariogenic than bread made with an unrefined flour. Additions of sucrose or honey made the bread markedly more cariogenic, while addition of fat or cheese decreased its caries potential. These are results with rat experiments and do not necessarily constitute guidelines for humans who have different dietary habits and tooth morphology; however, this observation suggests the possible role of food in the implantation and activity of cariogenic organisms at selected fissure sites.

Grenby[11] (1969a) has attempted to study the stickiness of cereal products by comparing diets containing bread, starch, or gluten. The concomitant changes in chemical composition of these three diets and in their physical properties make their results difficult to interpret. A second report (Grenby,[12] 1969b), in which the investigation of the influence of sticky foods of high sugar content on dental caries in the rat was described, was also found inconclusive. Results obtained with two strains of rats were not consistent and, again, differences in the chemical composition and the level of water between dry powder, a burnt sugar powdery diet (5.0 per cent moisture), and one containing a syrup (16.6 per cent) could be responsible for the lower caries scores obtained with the latter diet. These studies indicate some of the complications and the numerous factors which make tests of this type difficult to interpret.

Breakfast cereals have also been evaluated in rats and found to vary in their caries potential. Those that were sugar coated seemed to be associated with the highest scores. Cereals that were supplemented with 1 per cent NaH_2PO_4 (sodium biphosphate) and offered to rats were found to result in lower caries scores when compared to nonsupplemented controls.

Several investigators have studied the effects of oat and rice hull supplements (5 to 25 per cent) in cariogenic diets fed to rats. These seed hulls reduce caries scores in animals and the effect is thought to be due to certain polyphenols interfering with the oral flora. Since these hulls are not digestible by man, their human use is not visualized in the near future.

Proteins and Protein-Containing Foods

The effects of proteins on tooth development and maintenance must also be considered pre- and postdevelopmentally. Specific essential amino acids are needed by all living tissues and oral tissues are no exception. There has been a tendency to underestimate the importance of proteins and their amino acid units because carbohydrates have been found to be overwhelmingly important in the development of plaque dependent diseases in humans, such as dental caries. Several experimental designs have been used to understand the role of proteins and protein-containing food in oral health, but many experimental approaches have proven inadequate. In some cases the effects of dietary protein have been studied posteruptively when teeth are already formed and in function, and in other cases protein substitutions have been made in cariogenic diets at the expense of the carbohydrate component. In the latter case the incidence of tooth decay has decreased, but this effect is difficult to interpret because changes were made in diet ingredients with opposite caries potential. Sugars are known to foster implantation and activity of cariogenic microorganisms, while proteins do not. The test diet is then unable to support the cariogenic flora and thus one of the etiological factors necessary for the development of the disease is missing, and consequently no pathosis is produced. This in itself is an answer to the question of whether proteins have a caries-inhibitory potential or not. Studies done with cheese and other dairy products, fish flour, and other protein foods indicate that these foods are cariostatic rather than cariogenic. Whether this is done through a modification of the composition or metabolism of the flora, the pellicle, the enamel surface, or all three is not known.

One important role of dietary protein is probably through its systemic effect, which takes place prior to tooth eruption. The evidence for this comes from the understanding we have today of protein synthesis in mammalian cells, from some animal experiments and to a limited extent from epidemiological observations. Essential amino acids have to be present in the proper proportion and at the right time in the cell to be activated and incorporated into the polypeptide being formed on the polysome. Lack of one will alter the polysome pattern and disrupt the formation of the protein. Such impairment results in overall disruption of tissue growth and function and in poor development in the whole organism. If teeth or jaw bones are being formed at this time, they will suffer the effects of such a nutritional insult. In cases where protein malnutrition is severe and is imposed at an early age, the retardation cannot be corrected by subsequent refeeding and the size attained by the organ will be smaller than that for which it has the genetic potential to assume. McCance has described such an effect in young pigs deprived of protein at an early age in which the jaws are so small that overcrowding of teeth results. The effects of protein malnutrition on teeth themselves can also be dramatic. Shaw and Griffith[41] (1963) and Navia et al.[30] (1970) have observed that teeth from experimental rats underfed during lactation and early weaning had smaller teeth, a high incidence of absent cusps, and an increased susceptibility to dental caries. It is not clear at this time whether this is due to a detrimental effect simply on enamel alone or in combination with alterations in salivary gland development and function at a time when this tissue is also rapidly growing.

Protein-containing foods are therefore beneficial to oral health at two distinct times: (1) during the formation of teeth when amino acids are required in the protein synthesis of all cells, including those of oral tissues, and (2) posteruptively, when they compete with carbohydrates for a place in the diet and thus can determine and influence the oral flora by selecting out microorganisms which are not plaque inducers. Some questions still remain unresolved, such as (1) the extent of changes in the nature of the tooth or salivary glands that are induced by a mild degree of protein malnutrition, (2) the extent to which the borderline deficiencies are able to influence human oral health, (3) the influence that proteins and amino acids may have on pellicle formation, and (4) the effect of protein malnutrition on the immune system acting in the oral cavity.

Lipids

The role of dietary lipids in oral tissue health is probably limited to the posteruptive period. Essential fatty acid deficiencies are rare in humans and at the time when teeth are forming, most children have access to the necessary amounts of these nutrients.

Posteruptively, fats may, however, have a cariostatic effect on dental caries. Many investigators agree that adding fats and oils to caries promoting diets reduces the incidence of dental caries. The mechanism of action is not understood, but the limited studies suggest that the presence of oil in the diet is effective, possibly through a change of the surface properties of enamel rather than by interference of sugar solubilization from the diet or by the inhibitory effect of unsaturated fatty acids on streptococci.

Minerals

Because teeth are calcified structures which are anchored in another calcified tissue, bone, the role of minerals such as calcium, phosphate, magnesium, and some of the bone-seeking trace elements such as zinc, manganese, and fluoride have been carefully investigated. Certain vitamins intimately associated with minerals metabolically have also been actively studied for many years in an effort to understand their contribution to the process of calcification.

The first studies in this area involving vitamins were done in the early 1900's by Mellanby, who observed that a fat-soluble vitamin deficiency was associated with poor tooth calcification of experimental dogs. This vitamin was later identified as vitamin D. A hypothesis was then developed stating that teeth that were imperfectly calcified because of a vitamin D deficiency would be more susceptible to caries than those that had calcified normally. Even though the experimental data supported this hypothesis in work done with children, it was not conclusive and in some cases no such relation between vitamin D supplementation and caries was observed. It was unfortunate that such studies were undertaken so early in the history of nutrition and caries, for many of the designs were incomplete, the experimental diets were not nutritionally complete and the dental caries experiments were rudimentary as judged by present standards and knowledge.

Experimental evidence obtained thus far indicates that mineral nutrients involved in calcification, such as Ca and P, are essential to dental health. The role of vitamin D, as explained previously in regard to the metabolism of calcium, is also fundamental. The fallacy, however, is in believing that broad supplementation of diets with nutrients will confer protection against dental caries to everyone. Only those whose nutrition is borderline or clearly impaired (and there are large numbers of these people) will benefit from such a supplementation.

Experimentally, whenever calcium or phosphate is lowered in the posteruptive diet of animals, their caries incidence is increased. This has been shown repeatedly by many investigators. The exact mechanism of this phenomenon is unknown, but seems to be related to the remineralization phenomena taking place at the enamel surface. The concept of Mellanby that imperfections in the enamel surface, due to the impaired calcium metabolism during tooth formation, made these teeth susceptible to caries has not been widely accepted, and in some cases has been rejected, but it is conceivable that such irregularities of enamel could facilitate plaque accumulation and thus make such teeth more caries-susceptible. Further research is needed to elucidate the manner in which these protective effects of calcium and phosphates are brought about.

There is another important effect of phosphates which is not related to preeruptive tooth calcification but rather to the chemical equilibrium of the enamel surface with the acquired pellicle and plaque. During the last 30 years a great deal of interest has been generated by phosphates and their caries-inhibiting properties. Organic phosphates, such as phytates, naturally present in unrefined cereals, and sucrose-phosphate, a man-made derivative, have been found to be cariostatic. Inorganic phosphates, such as the monophosphates (orthophosphate), the linear compounds (pyrophosphate) and the cyclic compounds (sodium trimetaphosphate) have also been found to exert a marked cariostatic effect when supplemented in the diet of experimental rodents. While some clinical studies have confirmed the effects of some of these phosphates in humans, other studies have been inconclusive and further research is required to understand fully the potential that these phosphates have in preventing human caries.

The relation between trace elements and dental caries has been reviewed by Navia[26] (1970). Besides fluoride, which has a definite effect in preventing caries, there are other trace elements in foods and drinking water which can influence caries. Trace elements can be incorporated into tooth enamel preeruptively and posteruptively and change its physiochemical properties. They may also have an effect on the demineralization-remineralization processes at the enamel-plaque interface and influence the implantation and metabolism of cariogenic microorganisms. The evidence to support whether a trace element is cariostatic or cariogenic for humans is in most cases incomplete. A tentative classification would include Mo, V, Li, Sr and B as cariostatic, while Mg and Se are mildly cariogenic. These trace element effects on caries are not clearly established, due to differences in the experimental designs used to study them, which have yielded a confused interpretation of results. The studies, however, suggest that the mineral content of drinking water (which is locally available in contrast to foods which are produced at distant localities) may have a profound effect on dental caries.

Vitamins

Most of the understanding that we have today about vitamins and their relations to dental caries comes from animal studies. The pioneer work as previously indicated on vitamin A and D has been interestingly described in a review by Mellanby and King[24] (1938). Studies on rats and hamsters showed that vitamin A deficiency was associated with a reduction in size of molars and an increased susceptibility to dental caries. This susceptibility could be due to the interference in saliva production, for a reduced number of secretory acini in the major and minor salivary glands is usually seen in vitamin A-deficient animals. Large doses of vitamins, including vitamin A fed to rats posteruptively, have not been found to decrease the number or extent of carious lesions. Addition of fat-soluble vitamins A, D, E, or K to a normal caries-promoting diet at physiological levels has not been found to affect caries in rats.

Two of the water-soluble vitamins, niacin and pyridoxine, have been found to influence dental caries in animals. While the effects of niacin, which increases dental caries, could be mediated through a stimulation of the cariogenic flora, those due to pyridoxine, which seems to reduce caries, may be due to a stimulation of a competitive flora (Strean[44] et al., 1956). In either case the effect seems to be not a systemic one, but a local, pharmacological effect on the enamel surface–plaque interface.

NUTRITION AND PERIODONTAL DISEASE

The relation between nutrition and periodontal disease has been evaluated in epidemiological, animal, and metabolic studies (Hazen[18] 1968). Barros and Witkop[1] (1963) surveyed the prevalence of periodontal disease and related nutritional status in nearly 2000 Chileans. Significant in their findings was the increase in prevalence and severity of the disease with age. Periodontal disease, assessed by pocket depth, was found to be generally severe and widespread in older persons, even though 50 per cent of all persons between 15 and 19 years of age suffered from the disease in a milder form. Periodontal disease was even detected in children nine years old and younger. This same pattern was found in Honduras in 1969,[18] where periodontal index (PI) scores were even higher. The disease was present in young people, although the most severe levels were found among the older persons. In both of these groups of people the oral hygiene status was assessed by the presence or absence of soft debris and dental calculus. A marked, statistically significant correlation was found in each age group between the presence of debris, calculus, or both and the severity of the periodontal disease.

The assumption that nutritional deficiencies may play a major role in the etiology of periodontal disease was tested in the Chilean study by determining serum and urinary vitamin levels and relating these values to the periodontal status of the individual. Persons with acceptable or high vitamin levels showed no less severe disease than persons with deficient or low levels.

Studies done by Russell[36] (1963) in different parts of the world, to evaluate the relation between biochemical findings and periodontal disease in humans, have yielded no significant correlations. The highest correlation was always found to be with a high oral debris index. To conclude from this epidemiological data that nutritional factors do not enter at all into the etiology of the disease is incorrect because:

1. The etiology of the disease is multifactorial and no single factor is solely responsible for its pathological expression in humans.
2. The data have usually been gathered from individuals with a high disease severity. At these late stages nutritional factors have only a minor role. Nutritional effects on periodontal disease, if they are present, should be detected at the initial stages of the disease when the delicate balance between a healthy or a diseased tissue is being established.
3. The evaluation of nutritional status in most surveys is really limited to biochemical determinations carried out on a certain day, and this does not provide adequate understanding about the previous nutritional history of the individual.
4. Periodontal lesions demonstrate several stages of progression which extend from a mild, gingivitis to extensive bone resorption, deep pocket formation, bleeding, and finally, complete disruption of the periodontium with loss of teeth. It is important to understand the relation of nutrition to the various stages of the disease process.
5. Further understanding of the influence of protein malnutrition on the immune system is necessary.

Epidemiological evidence does not support the assumption that broad or specific nutritional deficiencies induce the formation of deep periodontal pockets in the absence of local irritants such as debris or calculus (Ramfjord et al.,[34] 1966). However, this type of information does not indicate whether transient or chronic deficiencies are a factor at the initial stages of the disease (which are poorly diagnosed in most surveys), or whether undernutrition or malnutrition modifies the course and prognosis of the disease.

Animal studies have been useful in studying the relationship between malnutrition and other factors such as infection. These types of studies are relevant to the situation existing in periodontal disease in which one of the etiological components of the disease is bacterial in nature (Socransky,[42] 1970). Studies done on survival of germ-free rats deficient in vitamin A illustrate this point (Bieri[2] et al., 1969). When weanling, germ-free rats were transferred to a conventional animal room and fed a vitamin A-deficient diet, they died in 23 to 54 days. In contrast, their litter mates, kept germ-free and on the same diet, survived for as long as 272 days. The rats kept in germ-free conditions stopped gaining weight after one to four months and developed nervous symptoms, characterized by head wobble and hind-leg weakness, but continued living. These experiments indicate that vitamin A is not essential for prolonged survival of the germ-free rat that has been weaned with low tissue stores of vitamin A. Appearance of the disease symptoms that lead to death of the conventional deficient rats is a direct consequence of bacterial and nutritional interactions.

Studies such as this, and others which have addressed themselves especially to study of the gingival tissue response to local irritations, indicate that malnutrition influences directly the metabolic behavior of the tissue and, indirectly, the course of the disease. Because of the rapid turnover of the connective tissue of the periodontium, nutrients such as protein and ascorbic acid which, as previously seen, intervene in collagen synthesis, have been studied in detail.

Vitamin C deficiency has been reported to be associated with edema, hemorrhage, osteoporosis of alveolar bone, tooth mobility and changes in periodontal fibers. Although inflammation of the gingiva is frequently seen in humans deficient in ascorbic acid, gingivitis in animals is only observed in association with some form of local irritation.

Attempts to show clear relations between ascorbic acid nutriture as determined by blood ascorbic acid levels and severity of periodontitis have not been clear. The same is true for protein malnutrition. Some investigators have found protein supplementation to have a beneficial effect on the health of the periodontium while others have not observed a clear effect.

The study of the factors involved in periodontal disease has been severely handicapped and to a certain point confused by the following experimental limitations:

1. Lack of an appropriate experimental animal model to study periodontal disease.
2. Difficulties in evaluation and objective quantitation of initial stages of gingivitis.
3. Technical limitations in the administration and standardization of the local stress factor in experimental models.

In spite of the limitations outlined above, a definite understanding of the role of nutrition in periodontal disease is emerging today. While nutritional deficiencies do not independently initiate the pathological breakdown of the periodontal tissues, they may set the stage and definitely modify the severity and extent of lesions by influencing the response and repair properties of the tissues. This effect, together with other biochemical changes, such as the ones brought about by aging, determines the outcome of the interaction between pathological stresses and resistance mechanisms. Even aging processes are known to be influenced by nutritional factors, as shown by the general appearance and disease susceptibility of children and young adults in nutritionally deprived areas. Other factors such as hormones, immunological response, and enzymatic activities play a definite role in this disease, but their mode of action and the degree of their contribution to the pathological process varies in different individuals in such a way that their effect is difficult to evaluate clinically. Good animal models are essential to study these interactions.

The influence of nutrition on periodontal disease appears to be exerted mainly at three different levels: (1) on the implantation and metabolism of the gingival crevice-plaque flora, (2) on the repair process in the connective tissue at the local site and, (3) on the immunological response to microbial antigens.

Loesche[22] (1968) has described the importance of microbial nutrition in the definition of the ecology of the gingival crevice. Large numbers of microorganisms colonize and grow in the gingival crevice because in this ecological niche they are able to fulfill their metabolic requirements.

Nutrients for these organisms come from three possible sources: (1) nutrients in food residues collected or impacted in and around the gingival crevice, (2) metabolites liberated by other microbial cells, and (3) preformed biochemical compounds found in the host secretions. The availability of these different products will determine the character and properties of the environment and select the flora which thrive under these conditions and the metabolic products they liberate into the environment. The diet of the individual will determine directly the composition of food residues and indirectly influence, to some extent, the composition of the host fluids. Several studies have indicated that changes in the composition of diet have brought about profound changes in the flora colonizing around teeth. If this is the case, modification of the diet to influence the quantity, the quality or the metabolism of subgingival plaque will contribute to the control of the disease process. In this role, nutritional manipulations would be more useful as a preventive rather than as a therapeutic measure. Once the disease process is so advanced that the tissue integrity is broken and the area is colonized by a multitude of scavenger microorganisms benefiting from the conditions established by the pathosis, then little or no benefit can be derived from nutritional manipulations.

In this last situation the role of nutrition is one which is secondary in the sense that it can only help by facilitating the repair process necessary to reestablish healthy tissue, provided that therapeutic procedures are used to remove the local irritants and the debris interfering with tissue healing. Under these conditions, vitamins such as ascorbic acid, folic acid, and vitamin A; some minerals such as copper and manganese; and the essential amino acids are necessary for protein synthesis and the final reestablishment of tissue integrity.

NUTRITION AND STRESS

The interaction between nutrition and stress agents, such as infections, trauma, surgery, and emotional states is one of the concepts which has been developed within the last decade and which is being actively investigated. This understanding will be used in developing approaches for the prevention and control of disease.

In biological systems the interaction between one or more factors or processes determines the course of a biochemical reaction so that the effect of a factor A may be different in the presence of factor B than in its absence. An example may clarify this concept. If an animal is given a certain level of zinc in the diet, the zinc level in bone may increase to 1000 mg/gm of bone, but if this same level of zinc is fed to an animal which is also receiving a large phosphate supplement, the level of zinc incorporation into bone will be only 60 per cent of that obtained in the absence of phosphate.

Another example may further illustrate the point. Selye[39] (1952) in his works describes the concept of interaction between different stress factors. If rats are given in a diet certain synthetic nitriles such as aminoacetonitrile (AAN), a condition known as osteolathyrism may be produced. The skeletal structures of the rat become tender, the joints swell, the shaft of the femur is thickened, and eventually, major deformities in all bones appear. If threshold doses of AAN are given to the animal, the onset of the disease is delayed and the severity is milder. If these threshold doses are accompanied by other stress factors such as subcutaneous formalin injections or forced immobilization, the syndromes appear rapidly and the bone deformities are more severe.

The understanding of the interactions between nutritional and stress factors is of great importance in the prevention of disease. Among stress factors of importance to oral conditions, two seem to be of major importance: infection and surgical trauma.

Nutrition and Infection

In considering the interactions between nutritional status and infection in the individual, two aspects should be recognized:

1. An infection usually precipitates or aggravates the malnourished state of an individual by a combination of mechanisms to be discussed later.
2. Nutritional status influences the host susceptibility to infections. Scrimshaw[38] et al. (1959) have discussed thoroughly this relationship, pointing out that some of these influences are synergistic in nature. Infections involving bacteria, rickettsiae, and various parasites have been enhanced by nutritional deficiencies as well as nutritional excess, i.e., obesity. Antagonistic interactions have been described in which malnutrition reduces severity of infection. This type of interaction has been observed in animal experiments involving certain viral, protozoan, or helminthic infections.

The effect of stress factors such as infections, including oral infections, is primarily to affect protein metabolism, especially protein catabolism. This effect will in turn affect the maintenance of normal tissue barriers, the production of enzymes essential to repair processes, and production of antibody proteins and phagocytic cells.

The interference with protein synthesis alters the ability of specific cells to initiate, maintain or increase the rate of production of proteins essential to maintain tissue integrity. Clinically, these events determine a wasting of the body. If localized to a certain tissue area, as in the oral cavity, it leads to pathological changes in the tissue which may eventually affect the whole organism. Biochemically, these effects of infectious stress can be detected as an altered metabolic balance of nutrients. Nutrients are on a positive or negative balance depending on whether there is a net gain or a net loss of the nutrient from the body. Infection, trauma, emotional disturbances, and other stresses precipitate a loss of nitrogen from the body, thus producing a negative nitrogen balance. This is produced by the interference with protein synthesis, the increased catabolism and other body reactions, which have been collectively referred to by Selye[39] (1952) as the alarm reaction. This reaction is probably triggered by hormones such as the glucocorticoids and others. The influence of these reactions is not only to increase nitrogen loss but also to induce losses of electrolytes such as sodium and potassium in the urine. This is further compounded by losses of these electrolytes in febrile sweats, vomiting, diarrhea and/or blood loss. Other mineral elements are also affected in these stress situations. In association with fever, surgery, trauma, or bed immobilization, urinary losses of calcium, phosphate, zinc and iron are commonly seen in patients.

At the beginning of the chapter the nutrient requirements of a healthy human were discussed and the importance of fulfilling these needs for growth, development, and maintenance was noted. Most of these allowances, however, do not take into consideration the stressed or the diseased state. If the stress is mild and transiently applied, the nutritional insult will not have lasting consequences for the host, for he will be able to compensate for it from his own stores or from his diet. Supplementation of the losses will not really be necessary, for the reaction to the stress is mild. If, however, the stress is one which is chronically present and of enough severity, then the host will continue to debilitate, with undue prolongation of his diseased state and discomfort. It is especially important under these circumstances to evaluate the losses and supplement the patient's diet with the nutrients which are essential to his defense mechanism and general well-being.

Nutrition and Surgical Stress

The relation between nutrition and surgery, although generally recognized (Navia,[29] 1975) has not received proper attention.[47] Oral surgery is especially stressful to the patient because together with the usual lack of appetite characteristic of disease and depressed emotional status seen in surgery patients, there can be physical disability, pain or discomfort in the oral tissues with which diet must come in contact. This inability to masticate, together with the increased physiological requirements of certain nutrients, and the metabolic losses previously discussed, tend to induce rapid nutritional degradation in surgery patients. It is the surgeon's responsibility to determine when and how to start adequate feeding of seriously ill patients. If surgery is drastic, it is usually not realistic to offer complete nourishment during the first 24 to 72 hours, but soon after this initial period the patient should be offered the full recommended dietary allowance plus any supplements that might be deemed necessary. In cases where the surgical stress is not as severe, soft or liquid diets can be given by tube or conventional means, depending on the condition of the patient.

The evaluation of nutritional requirements of a surgical patient can be determined by evaluating the following:

1. The previous nutritional state of the individual.
2. The nature and severity of the surgery performed.
3. The amount and type of nutrients which are being lost from the body.
4. The anticipated duration of the injury and disease.

One aspect of special consideration in many of these cases is the question of calorie levels in the diet of patients. Table 9–6 tabulates the energy expenditures of a reference man and woman during different types of activity. It is important to note that while the rate of energy expenditure of a person sleeping and reclining is approximately 1 kcal per minute, this rate is three times larger when walking and may increase four- or five-fold during active exercise. The patient confined to bed will have a low energy requirement because of the immobilization, but it should be noted that restlessness in a bed patient may increase requirements by 10 or 20 per cent, and fever increases caloric requirements by approximately 13 per cent for each degree C rise in body temperature (7.2 per cent for each degree F). If large protein losses are known to take place, then a 50–100 per cent increase in calorie require-

TABLE 9–6 EXAMPLES OF ENERGY EXPENDITURES BY REFERENCE MAN AND WOMAN*

		MAN		WOMAN	
ACTIVITY	TIME (*hr*)	*Rate* (*kcal/min*)	TOTAL	*Rate* (*kcal/min*)	TOTAL
Sleeping and reclining	8	1.1	530	1.0	480
Sitting	7	1.5	630	1.1	460
Standing	5	2.5	750	1.5	450
Walking	2	3.0	360	2.5	300
Other	2	4.5	540	3.0	360
			2,810		2,050

*Recommended Daily Allowances, National Acad. Sci. 1968.

ment is in order. In severe disease or trauma, therefore, a calorie requirement of 2500 to 4000 calories per day is not unusual and if such a level cannot be achieved through the diet, parenteral administration should then be considered.

The other nutritional aspect where control is of extreme importance is the nitrogen balance. If a man sustains a fracture of the jaw or undergoes extensive surgery, the first response is an increased urinary N excretion reflecting protein degradation. As indicated previously, this is characteristic of the alarm reaction and reaches a peak in four to seven days and may continue for three to seven weeks, depending on severity or duration of the stress. If immobilized in bed, N losses from immobilization may vary between one and two grams per day. Fracture of a long bone, for example, may lead to a loss of 9 per cent of body protein in one to two weeks. It is essential, therefore, to bring the patient as soon as possible into positive N balance as this will enhance the therapeutic measures and shorten the recovery period.

Among the vitamins, ascorbic acid has a special role in stress conditions such as surgery or trauma. Numerous vitamin C studies have pointed out that besides the role in hydroxylation of proline in the newly formed collagen to be used in repair of tissues, this vitamin is involved in the function of the adrenal cortex. During the alarm reaction the body loses large amounts of vitamin C from the adrenal cortex and probably its rate of utilization is increased two or three times. Administration of vitamin C is recommended in those cases where the demand of the organism for this nutrient is increased.

It is not possible to give definite recommendations for the administration of vitamins to surgical patients but the following guidelines[38] can be used in establishing the best levels for each individual case:

1. A previously healthy patient with a minor illness expected to last less than ten days, ambulatory, and eating well with no history of previous inadequate nutrition, needs to be given no special consideration as to his vitamin requirement.

2. When the foregoing qualifications are not met, the patient is given the maintenance level which is approximately twice the minimum requirement (Table 9–7).

3. When the patient receives his nutrition by the intravenous route, he should be given the maintenance level supplemented with vitamin C.

4. When a serious illness or severe trauma exists, the requirement for the first few days should be supplied at a therapeutic level (Table 9–7). Thereafter, the patient should receive the maintenance level until recovery is complete.

A discussion of nutritional rehabilitation is not really complete without consid-

TABLE 9–7 SUGGESTED DAILY VITAMIN REQUIREMENTS FOR MAINTENANCE OR THERAPY OF SURGERY PATIENTS

	STANDARD DAILY VITAMIN REQUIREMENT		
	Minimum	*Maintenance*	*Therapeutic*
Thiamine HCl	1.4	3	12
Riboflavin (mg)	1.7	3	12
Niacinamide (mg eq)	18	20	80
Ascorbic Acid (mg)	60	120	250
Calcium Pantothenate (mg)	10	20	20
Pyridoxine HCl	2.0	4	10
Folacin (mg)	0.1	0.2	0.4
Vitamin B_{12} (μg)	5.0	10	15
Vitamin A (i.u)	5000	5000	5000
Vitamin D (i.u)	400	400	400
Vitamin E (i.u)	30	60	60
Vitamin K_1 (mg)	2.0	2	2

eration of water, electrolytes, and trace-element requirements. Water accounts for 1/2 to 3/4 of body weight, depending on age and body fat. The multitude of factors determining water loss precludes the setting of a general value for minimal requirement. However, under ordinary circumstances a reasonable allowance is 1 ml/kcal for adults and 1.5 ml/kcal for infants. Special attention to water intake should be paid in situations involving (1) infants being offered high protein diets, (2) comatose patients, and (3) patients with fever, polyuria, diarrhea, or excessive sweating.

The electrolytes such as sodium and potassium should be carefully controlled. Sodium, being an extracellular cation, enters into the maintenance of osmotic equilibrium and body fluid volume, and potassium acts intracellularly to control cellular enzyme function. The adult normal intake of sodium is approximately 100–300 meq per day and that of potassium ranges between 50 and 150 meq per day. Because sweat contains 20–50 meq of sodium per liter, the losses from this source during high fever can be up to 350 meq per day. Supplementation of Na and K is important, therefore, during prolonged intravenous feeding.

Other elements present in low levels in the body, such as magnesium, iron, zinc and manganese, are severely lost in stress conditions of different types. While little is known about the requirements of elements such as zinc and manganese, they are still important and current research suggests that they may play an important role in healing of hard and soft tissues.

NUTRITIONAL AND DIETARY PREVENTIVE MEASURES IN THE CONTROL OF ORAL DISEASE

If a discussion of nutrition and oral disease were to stop at a description of problems, hypothesis, and conditions without suggesting solutions, it would not be complete. Even though there are many areas which have not been sufficiently investigated, enough is understood today to enable the dentist to use dietary manipulations in the preventive or therapeutic procedures used in the office or the hospital. Nutritional and dietary information will not only be useful to the patient but will be carried to the patient's home where it may influence the eating pattern of the whole family. The effectiveness of preventive dentistry relies heavily on patient self-care, a fundamental aspect of disease prevention.

There are three areas in the professional activity of the dentist in which nutritional and dietary knowledge will be required:

1. Clinical diagnosis, where the total health status of the patient is evaluated.
2. Therapeutic procedures, which can be supplemented and made more effective by dietary counseling directed to the clinical problem under consideration.
3. Health education offered to the patient and through the patient to the family unit as a whole. This preventive aspect becomes especially important in the practice of pedodontics, where young patients can be influenced to incorporate into their living pattern those dietary practices that will enable them to maintain not only oral but also general health.

Dental clinicians recognize that even though their treatment may be in the oral cavity, to which they direct their observation and treatment, they still should have enough peripheral vision to evaluate the patient *in toto*. In many cases nutritional deficiencies are manifested in such a way that they are readily available for diagnosis by the dentist rather than by other health professionals. Sandsted et al.[37] (1969) reports the following:

> This happened last summer, when a well-known American adventurer and his wife, bound across the North Atlantic in their 40-foot yawl, sailed into port on the northern coast of Iceland, and the woman went to see a local doctor. She complained of tiredness and lassitude. Her shoes seemed too tight and her teeth ached. The physician apparently did not think women should be making such ocean passages, and quickly concluded there was nothing really wrong that

couldn't be cured if she would only go home where housewives belong. While this advice might have seemed sensible, it was not very helpful. However, the sportswoman accepted the conclusion that she was not really sick and sailed on around the island to the capital, Reykjavik. By the time they got there, she was obviously quite ill. In fact, what alarmed her most was that her gums were bleeding. She immediately sought a dentist instead of a physician. The dentist took one look at her mouth and exclaimed, "Scurvy." Two weeks ashore with plenty of fresh foods and fruit juices and she was cured.

In the United States, nutritional deficiencies are not as common as in technically underdeveloped countries, but recent surveys (Hanes,[14] 1974; Ten-State Nutrition Survey,[46] 1972) indicate that certain economically deprived sectors of our society may show nutritional deficiency syndromes and an even larger sector suffers from overnutritional syndromes (i.e., obesity). Between these two extremes there are groups of people that frequently show borderline and, in some cases, clear malnutrition. These are teenagers with bizarre diets, alcoholics, and elderly persons who, living alone, have neither the motivation nor the facilities to feed themselves properly. In many cases these problems are compounded and made more severe by loss of teeth, inadequate prosthetic appliances, or mucosal lesions which make it difficult for them to masticate and swallow. Children in households where both parents and other members work long and unconventional hours, thus disrupting the management and orderly preparation of foods, are also prime targets for malnutrition.

The dentist is unusual in the sense that in many cases he is the only clinician that has an opportunity to examine such individuals for complaints other than nutritional problems. His understanding of the expression of nutritional deficiencies in the oral cavity can be valuable in the diagnosis of incipient problems before they bloom into overt chronic deficiencies. Some of the lesions are not completely diagnostic of malnutrition but generally indicate a malnourished situation which makes the tissue susceptible to disease. The information obtained by the dentist about nutritional status of the patient can either be used in his own treatment of oral disease, or, if anemia or other severe deficiency states are present, the patient should be prescribed appropriate nutritional supplementation and encouraged to see his physician for further evaluation and treatment if systemic complications are suspected.

ORAL SYMPTOMS ASSOCIATED WITH MALNUTRITION

Some of the oral tissue lesions associated with malnutrition are as follows (Jolliffee[19], 1960):

Lips

The changes in lips are usually observed in the exposed mucosa and the angles of the mouth. Riboflavin, niacin and iron deficiencies are associated with these lesions. Other factors such as environment, exposure to extreme cold, or dry conditions may also produce similar lesions. In certain cases poorly fitting prosthetic appliances, diseases such as herpes, syphilis, or allergic reactions to drugs or cosmetics may also produce similar lesions. The most common lesions are:

1. *Cheilosis.* Edematous, swollen lips; in some cases desquamation and chapping is present with increase in the vertical markings. In *atrophic cheilosis* the exposed mucosa has a parchment-like appearance and vertical fissures disappear.

2. *Angular Lesions.* Pallor and erythema are sometimes associated with monilia infections at the corner of the mouth. The broken or macerated integument in this area can usually be observed bilaterally when the mouth is held half open. Angular scars can sometimes be observed at the angle of lips, sometimes spreading up and down and with a pink or bleached-like color, depending on how recently the lesion was formed.

Teeth

Dental Caries. (See previous discussion.) Microbial breakdown of teeth due to

MILK GROUP . . . Use daily

3 or more glasses milk—children; 4 or more—teenagers (smaller glasses for some children under 8)
2 or more glasses—adults
3 or more glasses—pregnant women
4 or more glasses—nursing women
(a glass—8 ounces or ¼ quart of milk)

Needs of some younger children may be met by smaller servings. That is, a 6-ounce glass may replace an 8-ounce glass.

These quantities of milk provide about ¾ of the day's calcium recommended for good nutrition.

Milk is our main source of calcium in foods. For calcium . . .
1 slice American cheese (1 oz.) = ¾ glass milk
½ cup creamed cottage cheese = ⅓ glass milk
½ cup (¼ pint) ice cream = ¼ glass milk

Milk also contributes fine quality protein, vitamins—especially riboflavin and vitamin A—and many other nutrients.

For children, 3 glasses of milk supply ⅔ to all the protein recommended daily and all the riboflavin.

For adults, 2 glasses of milk supply about ¼ the protein and about ½ the riboflavin.

Skim milk lacks whole milk's fat and vitamin A (unless fortified); other food values are the same, calories less.

One glass of skim milk plus 1 scant tablespoon of butter equals the food values of whole milk.

Butter supplies milk's flavorful and easily digested fat along with its vitamin A.

Use milk as a beverage and in cooking—in hot cereals, milk soups, white sauces, puddings, and custards. Pour on fruit, cereal, and puddings.

The combination of milk with cereal or bread is excellent, especially in meals where little or no meat or eggs are served. The proteins in milk make those in cereals and bread more useful in the body.

MEAT GROUP . . . Use 2 or more servings daily

Meat, fish, poultry, eggs, or cheese—with dry beans, peas, nuts or peanut butter as alternates

Use amounts of these foods to supply *at least* as much protein as that in 4 ounces of cooked lean meat (about ⅓ pound raw).

Good practices to follow are

An egg a day or at least 3 to 5 a week

Liver, heart, kidney, or sweetbread about once a week

Other kinds of meat, fish, poultry, or cheese: 4 to 5 or more times a week

With dried beans, peas, nuts or peanut butter, serve milk or cheese. The animal protein makes the vegetable protein more useful in the body.

Foods in the meat group are counted on to supply about ½ the protein recommended daily for good nutrition.

Two servings for an adult might be, for example . . .
1 medium serving meat (3 ounces, cooked) + 1 egg

Choose combinations from the following which are about equal in amount of protein . . .
1 ounce cooked lean meat, poultry, or fish
1 egg
1 slice cheese, American or Swiss (1 ounce)
2 rounded tablespoons creamed cottage cheese (2 ounces)
2 tablespoons peanut butter (1 ounce)
½ cup cooked dried beans or peas

Eggs and meat, especially liver, are important for iron; also for B-vitamins. Pork supplies large amounts of the B-vitamin, thiamin. The legumes—dried beans, peas, nuts—are good sources of iron and thiamin, but their protein should be supplemented with an animal protein.

VEGETABLES & FRUITS . . . Use 4 or more servings daily

Include a dark green leafy or deep yellow vegetable or yellow fruit at least 3 to 4 times a week for vitamin A; a citrus fruit, or tomatoes, or other good source of vitamin C every day.

Use other vegetables and fruits for variety as well as their minerals, vitamins, and roughage.
Use potatoes frequently for all these food values plus food energy.
Use fresh, canned or frozen vegetables and fruits.
Save food values and flavors of vegetables by cooking quickly in small amount of water.
Dried fruits are valuable for iron.

A serving is ½ cup or more.
Foods in this group should supply over half the vitamin A and all of the vitamin C recommended daily for good nutrition.

Vegetables & fruits high in vitamin A	*These are about equal in vitamin C*
broccoli, chard	1 medium orange, ¾ cup juice
all "greens"	½ grapefruit, ¾ cup juice
kale, spinach	2 medium tomatoes, 2 cups juice
carrots	½ large cantaloupe
sweet potatoes	1 cup strawberries
tomatoes	¾ cup broccoli
cantaloupe, apricots	1½ cups cabbage, raw, shredded

BREADS & CEREALS . . . Use 4 or more servings daily

Use enriched or whole grain products. Check labels!

Choose from breads, cooked and ready-to-eat cereals, cornmeal, crackers, grits, spaghetti and macaroni, noodles, rice, quick breads and other baked goods if made with whole grain or enriched flour.

A serving is 1 slice bread; ½ to ¾ cup cereal.

Foods in this group supply valuable amounts of protein, iron, several B-vitamins, and food energy.

Cereals cooked and/or served with milk and breads made with milk are improved in quality of protein as well as quantity of protein, minerals, and vitamins.

ADDITIONAL FOODS . . . The foods recommended form the foundation for a good diet. In general, use smaller servings for young children; more or larger servings may be needed by teenagers, pregnant and lactating women.

Most nutrient needs are met by the amounts of foods suggested by the Guide. Special attention must be given to food sources of iron for young children, teenagers, and women. Liver, eggs, meat, legumes, dried fruit, dark green leafy vegetables, enriched or whole grain breads and cereals are good iron sources.

More food for energy, calories, is usually required. The amount varies with age, size, and activity. Food from the four groups helps to achieve an adequate diet.

Calorie restricted diets can be pleasing and satisfying when energy comes mostly from foods in these four groups.

Some source of vitamin D should be included for infants and children, pregnant and lactating women, and adults getting little sunshine. Good sources are vitamin D milk, fish liver oils, and direct sunshine.

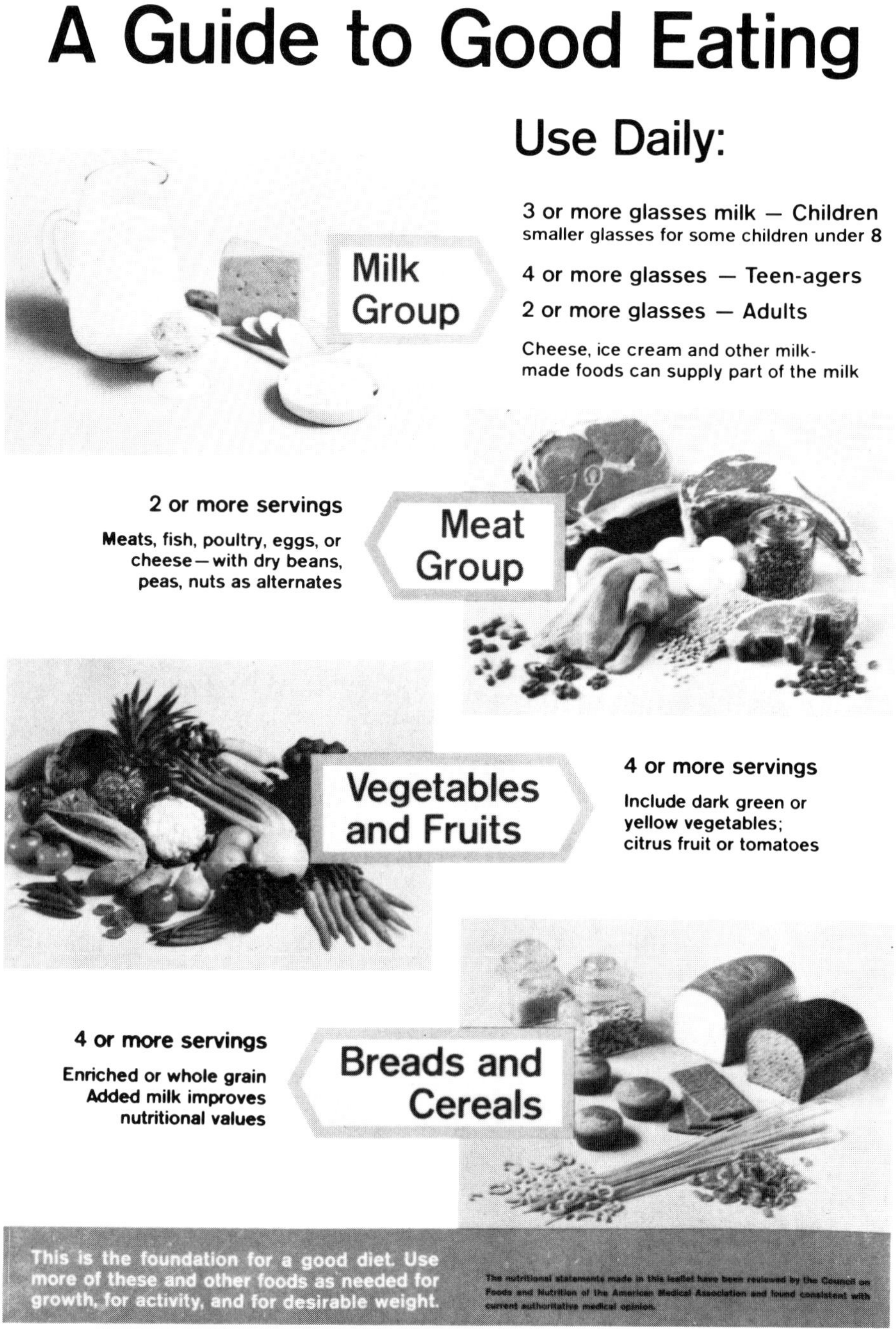

Figure 9–4 A guide to good eating produced by the National Dairy Council (3rd Edition, 1970).

poor dietary habits, such as consumption of large amounts of carbohydrates and frequent intake of snacks, is usually coupled with low fluorine intake.

Mottled Enamel. Stained teeth sometimes associated with aplastic pitted enamel, should not be confused with developmental anomalies and tetracycline stains. This lesion is usually seen in areas where fluoride concentration is overabundant in drinking water and foods.

Linear Hypoplasia. The lesions can be seen in deciduous maxillar incisors. The hypoplastic line stains brown and corresponds in position to the neonatal line. It has been associated with infectious disease attacks which lower the subject's already poor stores of vitamin A.

Melanodontia. Extensive yellowish-brown staining of teeth and high caries susceptibility are characteristics of this condition. Epidemiological data suggest overall undernutrition at critical stages during tooth development as part of its etiology.

Malposition. Crowding and malposition of teeth may have a nutritional origin either due to a lack of protein at an early age that has interfered with jaw development or early loss of deciduous teeth. Genetic factors may be solely responsible and should also be considered.

Gums

Inflammatory changes in the gingival tissues are seen commonly and should be differentiated to ascertain their origin.

Scorbutic Type. This is the classical symptom associated with vitamin C deficiency. Gums are red and spongy, with swollen interdental papillae and spontaneous bleeding. This syndrome is associated with other signs and cannot be seen when teeth are absent.

Gingivitis. This condition has a number of stages from a mild inflammation at the marginal gum tissue to the severe condition in which there is detachment of the gingiva with apical migration of the epithelial attachment and formation of deep periodontal pockets. Although vitamin and protein deficiencies may influence this tissue response, this syndrome commonly results from local bacterial action alone or in association with other factors such as malocclusion, poor restorations, prostheses or calculus.

Hypertrophic Gingivitis. The gingiva enlarges to such an extent that it may cover the teeth in certain non-nutritional manipulations, such as is the case of administration of drugs, i.e., dilantin. This condition, too, probably requires an associated local bacterial action.

Tongue

The tongue has been found to be a sensitive indicator of many pathological conditions through changes in texture and color. Chronic glossitis has been associated with most of the B-complex vitamins, particularly niacin, riboflavin, folic acid, and B_{12}. Chronic iron deficiency is also known to induce glossitis. Certain syndromes, such as the "geographic tongue" or the "furrow tongue," are known to exist in otherwise healthy individuals where no nutritional deficiency is suspected. Infections such as monilia, as well as drug reaction, late syphilis, malignancy, and some of the aphthous lesions may cause a glossitis.

Filiform and/or Fungiform Papillary Atrophy. This is the earliest lesion of chronic glossitis and produces a completely smooth tongue when both types of papillae atrophy. It can change to a red and fissured appearance, depending on whether or not some of the papillae become hypertrophied and fused.

Papillary Hypertrophy or Hyperemia. This may usually be observed by running a tongue depressor over the anterior two-thirds of the tongue. Red dots indicate the presence of hyperemia.

Magenta Tongue. The tongue seems cyanotic and the syndrome is usually related specifically to riboflavin deficiency. It is generally found in association with angular stomatitis and dermatitis.

Scarlet-Red Glossitis. This condition is characteristic of acute niacin deficiency (pellagra) and sprue. In advanced stages the oral mucous membranes also become bright red.

Beefy-Red Glossitis. This condition differs from the previous one in its darker color, which resembles raw beef. It is usually associated with a niacin deficiency, although other B-complex vitamins may contribute to this syndrome.

OTHER POSSIBLE ORAL MANIFESTATIONS OF NUTRITIONAL DEFICIENCIES

Besides the classical signs and symptoms previously described associated with nutritional deficiencies, there are other oral manifestations of malnutrition that can be detected by the dentist better than by any one else. These include ulcerations and keratotic lesions in the mucosa, oral pain and burning sensations, xerostomia or sialorrhea, diminished or absent taste perception (hypogeusia and sometimes also anosmia) and pallor of the oral or lingual mucosa.

Anemias, subclinical B-complex deficiencies, such as folic acid, vitamin A, and zinc deficiencies, have been found to have a part in the causation of these symptoms either directly or indirectly by diminishing the resistance or the function of the tissue. Under the influence of different stresses (i.e., infection, functional stimulation, local irritants), a breakdown takes place and a diseased state is established.

BASIC CONCEPTS IN DIETARY COUNSELING AND DIET THERAPY BY THE DENTIST

The dentist can and should use nutrition in the prevention and cure of oral disease (Shaw,[40] 1972; Enwonwu,[9] 1973, DiOrio and Madsen,[5] 1971). Furthermore, he can provide an inestimable service to the community by guidance of the dietary habits of his patients even after treatment is completed. Some oral diseases such as dental caries can be prevented or controlled if appropriate diets are used consistently and early enough after tooth eruption. In other diseases, as well as in trauma, nutrition can alleviate and shorten the recovery period.

Several approaches have been devised to carry out dietary counseling, such as the ones designed at Tufts University by Dr. A. E. Nizel[32] and at the University of Texas Dental Branch by Drs. L. P. DiOrio and K. O. Madsen.[6, 23] The former approach involves essentially the prescription of normal diet as a base line with modifications to suit the individual's need but keeping in mind the therapeutic goal. The approach used by the University of Texas clinicians involves a personalized approach in which, through a series of organized interviews, the patient is enabled to define his own dental-diet problem. Motivation is elicited by understanding the problem and the preventive measures applied involve dietary and oral hygiene measures. In both approaches there is extensive involvement of the patient in defining his problem and thus facilitating the implementation of the preventive procedures.

Regardless of the approach used, there are some considerations which constitute the basis for successful treatments:

1. A rapport or confidence has to be established between the patient and the dentist to obtain proper communication.

2. Proper clinical and dietary evaluation has to be made of the nutritional status of the patient. This can be done by evaluating the signs and symptoms of malnutrition and by determining the foods consumed and the eating pattern of the patient. In this area we strongly recommend that use be made of a professional dietitian, nutritionist, or dental hygienist trained in this field. This person is an invaluable link between the dentist and the patient. Being technically competent in nutrition, this auxiliary person will effectively evaluate the dietary pattern of the individual.

3. Finally, under the guidance of the dentist, the dietitian will help the patient in finding the diet that will fulfill his nutritional, emotional, economic, and cultural needs, as well as the therapeutic requirements established by the dentist.

GENERAL PRINCIPLES IN DIETARY COUNSELING

Regardless of whether the diet is intended for healthy or for diseased people,[49] it is usually based on the same foods used by a healthy person, with the exception that, in the diseased state, nutrient intake or texture is changed and the food composition of the diet has to be altered to accommodate such requirements. Knowledge about normal diet is thus essential.

In designing a normal diet the following should be kept in mind:

1. For growth and maintenance certain nutrients (approximately 50) are required which cannot be synthesized by the cells and, therefore, have to be provided in the foods consumed daily. These nutrients are especially required for certain body functions and are interrelated in such a way that an excess of one may interfere with the activity of others, so the balance, as well as their presence, is essential to health.

2. The requirements of these nutrients vary with age, sex, activity, climate, physiological status, and health status.[28]

3. Nutrients are present in more than one food in different proportions and degrees of availability. It is important to understand that calcium can be provided by milk in the U.S.A., but it can also be derived from sesame seed in other countries. This concept is also important to explain that *variety of foods* in the diet is essential, as no single food has all the nutrients required for full growth and health. A well-balanced daily diet can only be obtained if many types and combinations of foods are used.

To simplify the preparation of a normal diet, foods have been divided into four basic groups and suggestions for daily servings of these four groups of foods can be used to great advantage in the preparation of diets (Fig. 9–4). This food classification, however, is losing usefulness in the United States owing to the large number of manufactured or prepared foods consumed in the household, which do not clearly fit this classification. Consumers who are nutrition conscious should therefore make frequent use of nutritional information in food labels to guide themselves in making the appropriate dietary choices.

In certain cases, such as the treatment of rampant dental caries, a strict control of the amount of a nutrient such as carbohydrate might be necessary. The dentist can then make use of the food exchange method prepared by committees of the American Dietetic Association and the American Diabetes Association in cooperation with the Chronic Disease Program of the Public Health Service of H.E.W.

In this procedure the foods are divided into six groups of food portions (exchanges) which contribute different amounts of carbohydrate, protein or fat (Tables 9–8 and 9–9) and which can be exchanged in the preparation of a diet.

Nine different diets (Table 9–10) are offered, of which three diets (numbers 5, 6 and 7) are especially intended for children as they contain a higher proportion of milk exchanges. Diet suggestions for children and teen-agers have to take into account their energy requirement so Diet Plan 5 provides 1800 calories and should be used for children around 4 to 6 years of age. Diet Plan 6 provides 2600 calories and is usually appropriate for children 7 to 10 years of age. Diet Plan 7 provides a high intake of calories (3500) and is suggested for very active males between 15 and 22 years of age.

Adult diets and diets for special situa-

TABLE 9–8 COMPOSITION OF FOOD EXCHANGES

LIST	FOOD	MEASURES	GM.	CHO	PROT.	FAT	CAL.
1	Milk Exchanges	½ pint	240	12	8	10	170
2a	Vegetable Exchanges	as desired					
2b	Vegetable Exchanges	½ cup	100	7	2		36
3	Fruit Exchanges	Varies		10			40
4	Bread Exchanges	Varies		15	2		68
5	Meat Exchanges	1 oz.	30		7	5	73
6	Fat Exchanges	1 tsp.	5			5	45

TABLE 9–9

LIST 1. MILK EXCHANGES

Carbohydrate – 12 gm., Protein – 8 gm., Fat – 10 gm., Calories 170

	Meas.	Gm.
* Milk, whole	1 cup	240
Milk, evaporated	½ cup	120
* Milk, powdered	¼ cup	35
* Buttermilk	1 cup	240

* Add 2 fat exchanges if fat free

LIST 2. VEGETABLE EXCHANGES

A. – These vegetables may be used as desired in ordinary amounts. Carbohydrates and Calories negligible.

	"GREENS"	
Asparagus		Lettuce
Broccoli		Mushrooms
Brussels Sprouts	Beet	Okra
Cabbage	Chard	Pepper
Cauliflower	Collard	Radishes
Celery	Dandelion	Rhubarb
Chicory	Kale	Sauerkraut
Cucumbers	Mustard	String Beans, young
Escarole	Spinach	Summer Squash
Eggplant	Turnip	Tomatoes

B. – Vegetables: 1 Serving equals ½ cup equals 100 grams. Carbohydrate – 7 gm., Protein – 2 gm., Calories – 36

Beets	Peas, green	Squash, winter
Carrots	Pumpkin	Turnips
Onions	Rutabaga	

LIST 3. FRUIT EXCHANGES

Carbohydrate – 10 gm., Calories – 40

	Meas.	Gm.
Apple	1 sm. (2″ diam.)	80
Applesauce	½ cup	100
Apricots, fresh	2 medium	100
Apricots, dried	4 halves	20
Banana	½ small	50
Berries: Straw., Rasp., Black.	1 cup	150
Blueberries	⅔ cup	100
Cantaloupe	¼ (6″ diam.)	200
Cherries	10 large	75
Dates	2	15
Figs, fresh	2 large	50
Figs, dried	1 small	15
Grapefruit	½ small	125
Grapefruit Juice	½ cup	100
Grapes	12	75
Grape Juice	¼ cup	60
Honeydew Melon	⅛ (7″ diam.)	150
Mango	½ small	70
Orange	1 small	125
Orange Juice	½ cup	100
Papaya	½ medium	100
Peach	1 medium	100
Pear	1 small	100
Pineapple	½ cup	80
Pineapple Juice	⅓ cup	80
Plums	2 medium	100
Prunes, dried	2 medium	25
Raisins	2 tbsp.	15
Tangerine	1 large	100
Watermelon	1 cup	175

LIST 4. BREAD EXCHANGES

Carbohydrate – 15 gm., Protein – 2 gm., Calories – 63

	Meas.	Gm.
Bread	1 slice	25
Biscuit, Roll	1 (2″ diam.)	35
Muffin	1 (2″ diam.)	35
Cornbread	1 (1½″ cube)	35
Flour	2½ tbsp.	20
Cereal, cooked	½ cup	100
Cereal, dry (flake & puffed)	¾ cup	20
Rice, Grits, cooked	½ cup	100
Spaghetti, Noodles, etc., cooked	½ cup	100
Crackers, graham (2½″ sq.)	2	20
Oyster	20 (½ cup)	20
Saltines (2″ sq.)	5	20
Soda (2½″ sq.)	3	20
Round, thin (1½″ diam.)	6–8	20
Vegetables		
Beans & Peas, dried, cooked (lima, navy, split peas, etc.)	½ cup	90
Baked Beans, no pork	¼ cup	50
Corn	⅓ cup	80
Parsnips	⅔ cup	125
Potatoes,white, baked, boiled	1 (2″ diam.)	100
Potatoes, white, mashed	½ cup	100
Potatoes, sweet, or yams	¼ cup	50
Sponge Cake, plain	1 (1½″ cube)	25
Ice Cream (Omit 2 fat exchanges)	½ cup	70

LIST 5. MEAT EXCHANGES

Protein – 7 gm., Fat – 5 gm., Calories – 73

	Meas.	Gm.
Meat & Poultry (med. fat) (beef, lamb, pork, liver, chicken, etc.)	1 oz.	30
Cold Cuts (4½″ sq., ⅛″ thick)	1 slice	45
Frankfurter	1 (8–9/lb.)	50
Fish: Cod, Mackerel, etc.	1 oz.	30
Salmon, Tuna, Crab	¼ cup	30
Oysters, Shrimp, Clams	5 small	45
Sardines	3 medium	30
Cheese, cheddar, American	1 oz.	30
Cottage	¼ cup	45
Egg	1	50
Peanut Butter*	2 tbsp.	30

*Limit use or adjust carbohydrate.

LIST 6. FAT EXCHANGES

Fat – 5 gm., Calories – 45

	Meas.	Gm.
Butter or Margarine	1 tsp.	5
Bacon, crisp	1 slice	10
Cream, light, 20%	2 tbsp.	30
Cream, heavy, 40%	1 tbsp.	15
Cream Cheese	1 tbsp.	15
French Dressing	1 tbsp.	15
Mayonnaise	1 tsp.	5
Oil or Cooking Fat	1 tsp.	5
Nuts	6 small	10
Olives	5 small	50
Avocado	⅛ (4″ diam.)	25

TABLE 9–10 SAMPLE DIET PLANS

DIET	CARBOHYDRATE GRAMS	PROTEIN GRAMS	FAT GRAMS	CALORIES	CARBOHYDRATE DISTRIBUTION* *Breakfast*	*Lunch*	*Dinner*	*Bedtime*
1	125	60	50	1200	25	37	32	27
2	150	70	70	1500	25	52	47	27
3	180	80	80	1800	40	52	47	42
4	220	90	100	2200	40	67	72	42
5†	180	80	80	1800	37	52	59	27
6†	250	100	130	2600	52	77	74	42
7†	370	140	165	3500	82	122	114	52
8	250	115	130	2600	55	82	72	42
9	300	120	145	3000	70	82	102	42

TOTAL DAY'S FOOD IN SAMPLE MEAL PLANS

DIET	MILK	VEG. A	VEG. B	FRUITS	BREAD EX.	MEAT EX.	FAT EX.
1	1 pt.	as desired	1	3	4	5	1
2	1 pt.	as desired	1	3	6	6	4
3	1 pt.	as desired	1	3	8	7	5
4	1 pt.	as desired	1	4	10	8	8
5†	1 qt.	as desired	1	3	6	5	3
6†	1 qt.	as desired	1	4	10	7	11
7†	1 qt.	as desired	1	6	17	10	15
8	1 pt.	as desired	1	4	12	10	12
9	1 pt.	as desired	1	4	15	10	15

*In these meal plans the total carbohydrate has been divided approximately into fifths. About one-fifth is allotted for breakfast and the other four-fifths distributed between lunch, dinner, and bedtime snack. The division of the carbohydrate is flexible and can be varied to meet the patient's needs. For example, it may be desirable for some patients to take a part of the food from each meal for mid-morning or afternoon snacks.

†These diets contain more milk and are especially suitable for children.

tions can be easily developed with this approach by consulting the table of recommended allowances, depending as indicated previously on age, sex, activity, height and weight, and other special considerations.

This valuable therapeutic approach to diet counseling when used with understanding of the nutrition principles and awareness of the patient's preferences it can be an effective way for the dentist to help the patient in the control of disease as well as in the maintenance of overall health.

OTHER FOOD INGREDIENTS AND BEVERAGES

The following seasonings may be used freely, if desired:

Chopped Parsley	Mint
Garlic	Onion
Celery	Nutmeg
Mustard	Cinnamon
Pepper and other spices	Saccharin
Lemon	Vinegar

These foods may be used as desired:

Coffee	Rennet tablets
Tea	Pickles, sour
Clear broth	Pickles, unsweetened dill
Bouillon (without fat)	
Gelatin, unsweetened	Cranberries

If the patient requires other diet modifications involving the diet consistency, reference should be made to handbooks on diet therapy, such as the one by Goodhart and Shils[49] and others which describe the formulation and preparation of such diets.

Because foods not only provide nutrients for the host but also for the bacterial flora in the different parts of the oral cavity, the dentist has to pay attention to two more factors with which other clinicians are not normally concerned: (1) frequency with which foods are consumed and (2) texture of foods.

Dentists interested in caries control understand that high frequency of food intake, especially foods containing large amounts of carbohydrates, is probably the most likely means of inducing heavy plaque formation which can lead to dental decay or periodontal disease. Several investigations have clearly shown that increased frequency of snack consumption is definitely associated with caries increase. Diet planning therefore should take into account this important factor by advising not only on the composition of the diet, but also on the manner and frequency with which it is consumed.

The second fundamental point has been fully discussed by Caldwell[3] (1970) and involves the question of the physical properties of foods and their caries-promoting potential. Even though a few clinical studies have been conducted to explore the relation between such physical properties of food as adhesiveness, solubility, viscosity, hardness, etc., and their caries-promoting potential, there are indications that these properties do influence the amount of residues left on and around teeth. This is an area which is important to understand in order to select appropriate foods for diet counseling and eventually may have application in the manufacture of foods of low caries-promoting potential.

REFERENCES

1. Barros, L., and Witkop, C. J., Jr.: Oral and genetic study of Chileans. III. Periodontal disease and nutritional factors. Arch. Oral Biol. 8:195–206, 1963.
2. Bieri, J. G., McDaniel, E. G., and Rogers, W. E.: Survival of germfree rats without vitamin A. Science *163*:574–575, 1969.
3. Caldwell, R. C.: Physical properties of foods and their caries-producing potential. J. Dent. Res. *49*:1293–1298, 1970.
4. Curzon, M. E. J., Adkins, B. L., Bibby, B. G., and Losee, F. L.: Combined effect of trace elements and fluorine on caries. J. Dent. Res. *49*:526–528, 1970.
5. DiOrio, L'.P., and Madsen, K. O.: Patient education—a health service for the prevention of dental disease. Dent. Clin. North Am. *15*:905–917, 1971.
6. DiOrio, L. P., and Madsen, K. O.: A personalized program: Educating the patient in the prevention of dental disease. Chicago, Ill., March Publishing Co., Inc., 1972.
7. DiOrio, L. P., Miller, S. A., and Navia, J. M.: The separate effects of protein and calorie malnutrition on the development and growth of rat bones and teeth. J. Nutr. *103*:856–865, 1973.
8. Dreizen, S., Levy, B. M., and Bernick, S.: Studies on the biology of the periodontium of marmosets. VII. The effect of folic acid deficiency on the marmoset oral mucosa. J. Dent. Res. *49*:616–620, 1970.
9. Enwonwu, C. O.: Elements of dietetics for the general practitioner. Int. Dent. J. *23*:317–327, 1973.
10. Gould, B. S.: Possible folate-ascorbate interaction in collagen formation. *In* Balazs, E. A.: Chemical and Molecular Biology of the Intercellular Matrix. New York and London, Academic Press, 1970.
11. Grenby, T. H.: The stickiness of cereal products and the composition of cereal diets as factors in their cariogenicity in the rat. Arch. Oral Biol. *14*:1253–1258, 1969a.
12. Grenby, T. H.: The influence of sticky foods of high sugar content on dental caries in the rat. Arch. Oral Biol. *14*:1259–1265, 1969b.
13. Gustafsson, B., Quensel, C., Lanke, L., Lundqvist, C., Grahnen, H., Bonow, B., and Krasse, B.: The Vipeholm dental caries study: The effect of different levels of carbohydrates intake on caries activity in 436 individuals observed for five years. Acta Odontol. Scan. *11*:232–252, 1954.
14. HANES: First Health and Nutrition Examination Survey United States 1971–72: Dietary intake and biochemical findings. Rockville, Md., U.S. Dept. H.E.W. (D.H.E.W. Publication No. [HRA] 74-1219-1), Jan. 1974.
15. Hardwick, J. L.: The incidence and distribution of caries throughout the ages in relation to the Englishman's diet. Br. Dent. J. *108*:9–17, 1960.
16. Hartles, R. L., and Leach, S. A.: Effect of diet on dental caries. Br. Med. Bull. *31*:137–141, 1975.
17. Hazen, S. P.: The role of nutrition in periodontal disease. J. Ala. Med. Sci. 5(No. 3):328–335, 1968.
18. INCAP: Evalucion Nutricional de la Poblacion de Centro America y Panama: Honduras. INCAP, Guatemala City, Guatemala, Pub. V-29, 1969, p. 6.
19. Jolliffee, N.: The physical signs of malnutrition. *In* The Control of Malnutrition in Man. New York, Am. Public Health Assoc., 1960, p. 8.
20. Konig, K. G.: Caries induced in laboratory rats. Posteruptive effect of sucrose and of bread of different degrees of refinement. Br. Dent. J. *123*:585–589, 1967.
21. Littleton, N. W., Kabehashi, S., and Fitzgerald, R.: Study of differences in the occurrence of dental caries in Caucasian and Negro children. J. Dent. Res. *49*:742–751, 1970.
22. Loesche, W. J., and Gibbons, R. J.: Influence of nutrition on the ecology cariogenicity of the oral microflora. *In* A. E. Nizel: The Science of Nutrition and Its Application in Clinical Dentistry. Philadelphia, W. B. Saunders Co., 1966.

23. Madsen, K. O.: Nutritional Basis of Oral Health in Dental Biochemistry. Philadelphia, Lea and Febiger, 1968, pp. 158–212.
24. Mellanby, M., and King, J. D.: Vitamins and dental caries. Ergebnisse der Vitamin- und Hormonforschung 2:1–54, 1939.
25. Menaker, L., and Navia, J. M.: The effect of undernutrition during the perinatal period on caries development II, III, IV. J. Dent. Res. *52*:680–687, 688–691, 692–697, 1973.
26. Navia, J. M.: Effect of minerals on dental caries *In* Dietary Chemicals vs. Dental Caries. Washington, D.C., Amer. Chem. Series, No. 94, A.C.S., 1970, pp. 123–160.
27. Navia, J. M.: Prospects for prevention of dental caries: Dietary factors. Special issue, J. Am. Dent. Assoc., *87*:1010–1012, 1973.
28. Navia, J. M.: Prevention of dental caries: Agents which increase tooth resistance to dental caries. Int. Dent. J. *22*:427–440, 1972.
29. Navia, J. M.: Nutrition and wound healing. *In* L. Menaker (Ed.): Biologic Basis of Wound Healing. New York, Harper and Row, 1975.
30. Navia, J. M., DiOrio, L. P., Menaker, L., and Miller, S.: Effect of undernutrition during the perinatal period on caries development in the rat. J. Dent. Res. *49*:1091–1098, 1970.
31. Navia, J. M.: Evaluation of nutritional and dietary factors that modify animal caries. J. Dent. Res. *49*:1213–1228, 1970.
32. Nizel, A.: The Science of Nutrition and Its Application to Clinical Dentistry. Philadelphia, W. B. Saunders Co., 1966.
33. Pedersen, P. O.: Investigations into dental conditions of about 3,000 ancient and modern Greenlanders. Dent. Rec. *58*:191–198, 1938.
34. Ramfjord, S. P., Kerr, D. A., and Ash, M. M.: World Workshop in Periodontics, Ann Arbor, Michigan, 1966.
35. Recommended Dietary Allowances. (8th Ed.) Food and Nutrition Board National Council, National Academy of Sciences, Washington, D.C., 1974.
36. Russell, A. L.: International Nutrition Surveys: A summary of preliminary dental findings. J. Dent. Res. *42*:233–244, 1963.
37. Sandstead, H. D., Carter, J. P., and Darby, W. J.: How to diagnose nutritional disorders in daily practice. Nutrition Today *4*:20–26, 1969.
38. Scrimshaw, N. W., Taylor, C. F., and Gordon, J. E.: Interactions of nutrition and infection. Am. J. Med. Sci. *237*:367–403, 1959.
39. Selye, H.: The story of the adaptation syndrome. Montreal, Acta Medical Publishers, 1952.
40. Shaw, J. H.: Nutritional guidance in the prevention of oral disease. Dent. Clin. North Am. *16*:733–746, 1972.
41. Shaw, J. H., and Griffith, D.: Dental abnormalities in rats attributable to protein and deficiency during reproduction. J. Dent. Res. *80*(No. 2):123–141, 1963.
42. Socransky, S. S.: Relationship of bacteria to the etiology of periodontal disease. J. Dent. Res. *49*:203–222, 1970.
43. Stralfors, A.: Inhibition of hamster caries by cocoa. The effect of whole and defatted cocoa in the absence of activity in cocoa fat. Arch. Oral. Biol. *11*:149–161, 1966. (See also *11*:323–328, 1966; *11*:609–615, 1966; and *12*:959–962, 1967.)
44. Strean, L. P., Gilfillan, E. W., and Emerson, G. A.: Suppressive effect of pyridoxine as a dietary supplement on dental caries in Syrian hamsters. N.Y. State Dent. J. *22*:325–327, 1956.
45. Sweeney, E. A., Cabrera, J., Urrutia, J., and Mata, L.: Factors associated with linear hypoplasia of human deciduous incisors. J. Dent. Res. *48*:1275–1279, 1969.
46. Ten-State Nutrition Survey in the United States 1968–1970. Washington, D.C., U.S. Dept. H.E.W. Health Services and Mental Health Administration (D.H.E.W. Publ. No. [HSM] 72–8134). 1972.
47. Therapeutic Nutrition. National Academy of Sciences, National Research Council, Publication No. 234, 1951.
48. Winick, M., and Noble, A.: Cellular response during malnutrition at various ages. J. Nutr. *89*:300–305, 1966.
49. Goodhart, R. S., and Shils, M. E.: Modern Nutrition in Health and Disease (5th Ed.) Philadelphia, Lea & Febiger, 1973.

ADDITIONAL REFERENCES ON NUTRITION

HISTORY

McCollum, E. V.: A History of Nutrition. Boston, Houghton Mifflin Co., 1957.

NUTRIENTS AND BIOCHEMISTRY

Beaton, G. H. and E. W. McHenry: Nutrition: A Comprehensive Treatise. New York, Academic Press, 1969.

Lehninger, A. L.: Biochemistry: The Molecular Basis of Cell Structure and Function. 2nd Ed., New York, Worth Publishers, Inc., 1975.

McGilvery, R. W.: Biochemistry, A Functional Approach. Philadelphia, W. B. Saunders, 1970, Chap. 27.

Munro, H. N., and J. B. Allison: Mammalian Protein Metabolism. New York, Academic Press, 1964, Vols. I–II.

Sebrell, W. H. and R. S. Harris: The Vitamins. (2nd Ed.) New York, Academic Press, 1967–1968, Vols. I–II.

Sipple, H. L., and McNutt, K. W.: Sugars in Nutrition. New York, The Nutrition Foundation, Academic Press Inc., 1974.

Underwood, E. J.: Trace Elements in Human and Animal Nutrition. New York, Academic Press, 1971.

NUTRITION: ANIMAL AND EXPERIMENTAL NUTRITION

Albanese, A. A.: Newer Methods of Nutritional Biochemistry. New York, Academic Press, 1965, Vols. I–IV.

Committee on Animal Nutrition: Nutrient Requirements of Domestic Animals. (Nos. 1, 3 (1966); 4 (1963); 5, 7 (1968); 8 (1962); 9 (1966); 10 (1972). National Academy of Sciences, Washington, D.C.

Navia, M. M.: Animal Models in Dental Research. Birmingham, University of Alabama Press, 1976.

NUTRITION: HUMAN NUTRITION AND DIETETICS

Human Nutrition (Formerly Heinz Handbook of Nutrition). New York, McGraw-Hill Book Co., 1976.

Nizel, A. E.: The Science of Nutrition and Its Application in Clinical Dentistry. Philadelphia, W. B. Saunders Co., 1968.

Goodhart, R. S., and Shils, M. E.: Modern Nutrition in Health and Disease. (5th Ed.) Philadelphia, Lea and Febiger, 1973.

Present Knowledge in Nutrition. (4th Ed.) New York, The Nutrition Foundation, Inc., 1976.

DISORDERS AND DISEASES

Hsai, Y. D.: Inborn Errors of Metabolism. Chicago, Year Book Medical Publishers, 1966.

Stanbury, J. B., Wyngaarden, J. B., and Fredrickson, D. S.: The Metabolic Basis of Inherited Disease. New York, Blakiston Division, McGraw-Hill Book Company, 1966.

FOOD SCIENCE, TOXICANTS, AND ADDITIVES

Borgstrom, G.: Principles of Food Science. New York, Macmillan Company, 1968, Vols. I–II.

Food Protection Committee, Food and Nutrition Board: Chemicals Used in Food Processing. Pub. 1274, National Academy of Sciences, Washington, D.C., 1965.

Food Protection Committee, Food and Nutrition Board: Toxicants Occurring Naturally in Foods. Pub. 1354, National Academy of Sciences, Washington, D.C., 1966.

Frazier, W. C.: Food Microbiology. (2nd Ed.) New York, McGraw-Hill Book Company, 1967.

Harris, R. S., and Karmas, E.: Nutritional Evaluation of Food Processing. 2nd ed., Westport, Conn., Avi Publishing Co. 1975.

Riemann, H.: Food-Borne Infections and Intoxications. New York, Academic Press, 1969.

Watt, B. K. and A. L. Merrill: Composition of Food—Raw, Processed, Prepared. Agriculture Handbook No. 8, U.S. Department of Agriculture, Washington, D.C., 1963.

Food. The Yearbook of Agriculture, U.S. Department of Agriculture, 1959.

chapter 10

WATER FLUORIDATION AND SYSTEMIC FLUORIDE THERAPY

by
ROBERT C. CALDWELL, D.M.D., PH.D.
and DANIEL C. NORNOO, B.D.S., M.Sc.D.

HISTORICAL ASPECTS

One of the most interesting and best-documented chapters in the history of dentistry is the story of fluoridation. Detailed information about it can be found in the excellent historical review of the relationship among fluorides, dental fluorosis, and dental caries in Cox's chapter in *A Survey of the Literature of Dental Caries*. Prior to that, collections of papers edited in 1942 and 1946 by Moulton, serve as useful review material. The most recent text on the subject, *Water Fluoridation, the Search and the Victory*, by McClure, is also of historical and contemporary value. These references provide the entrée to a fascinating aspect of dental history which students of preventive dentistry and public health should find entertaining and instructive. The review of the history of fluoridation in this chapter is limited to mentioning some of the most notable highlights of the past century and a half.

In 1802, le compte Morozzo published his findings of a "gros animal"—a fossilized elephant—near Rome. Apparently, this caused considerable interest in the scientific community, and the following year, Morichini analyzed a tooth of the animal and observed that it was rich in fluorine. He also found fluorine present in human tooth enamel. These reports created widespread scientific interest, so that in the next five years, several important scientists, including Gay-Lussac and Berzelius, examined various hard tissues and confirmed that fluorine was present in fossil teeth and in fresh bone and tooth structure in somewhat low concentrations.

By 1850, it was well established in the European literature that fluorine occurred in varying quantities in water and food. Also, it had been confirmed that the ubiquitous fluorine was present in mammalian blood and in various body tissues and organs. Drinking water was suspected of being the source of the fluorine present in the body, and studies in Germany and France showed that the fluorine content of drinking water varied in different communities. In 1845, Middleton observed that fluorine was in the city of London's water supply and could be detected in the piped water. Other European reports confirmed the variability of fluoride concentration in drinking water. It is therefore surprising that it was not until almost fifty years later that the same finding was made in the United States. These observations plus the well known reactivity of fluorine with bone, led Carnot to the discovery that bone could be used to extract fluorine from water.

The great French investigator, Magitot, seems to have been the first to relate fluorides to resistance to decalcification by acid. He postulated that fluorine was responsible for his finding that tooth enamel was resistant to attack by 1:100 acetic acid and stated, "As to the integrity preserved by the enamel, it is owing perhaps to a smaller proportion of the phosphates, and doubtless also to the minute quantity of fluoride of calcium it contains, or perhaps to certain combinations of these substances of a nature calculated to resist all alteration."* Many years later, after the advent of radioactive fluoride, it was shown by Volker, Sognnaes, and Bibby at the University of Rochester that the fluoride ion was rapidly deposited in bone and could be adsorbed by enamel exposed to a fluoride solution.

Prior to the turn of the century, some scattered reports drew attention to a discoloration of the teeth which was endemic in nature. In Mexico, it was considered that the condition might be due to manganese. In Naples, the condition of "denti neri," "denti de Chiaie," or "denti scritti" was well known to the local populace, but it was not until Eager's report of the condition in 1901 that dentists began to pay attention to this unusual appearance of the teeth. Reports of the same condition, known in the Rocky Mountain area as "Colorado brown stain," came to the attention of Black, who made several important studies of the condition with McKay. In 1916, they suggested the term "mottled enamel" and investigated the chemistry of the altered enamel and the relation of mottled enamel to freckles. Finding no such correlation, McKay continued extensive epidemiological studies and gradually came to the conclusion that mottling did not cause the teeth to be more susceptible to dental caries. In 1925 he wrote, "Why is it then, if the integrity of the enamel is held to be the determining factor in caries, that mottled enamel, which is so obviously defective, is able to escape carious attack with not more than average frequency of incidence?" The following year, Hannan, a Canadian chemist, postulated that mottling was due to a lack of fluoride in the drinking water. However, this suggested link between water fluoride concentration and mottled enamel was not followed up by dental scientists.

In 1931, Petrey, working in Churchill's laboratory at the Aluminum Company of America, performed an analysis of water from Bauxite, Arkansas. Subsequently, Churchill reported that the mottling of enamel which occurred in that town seemed to be related to the fluoride concentration in the water. Analyses of water from several other communities soon revealed that the higher the fluoride concentration, the more severe the mottling (Fig. 10–1, A, B, C and D). Around the same time, Smith showed that a fluoride solution given to rats caused their teeth to become mottled. This discovery of the relationship of fluoride to mottling (chronic dental fluorosis) immediately led to efforts to remove all fluoride from the water with no regard for the potential benefits of fluoride. The communities of Oakley, Idaho, Bauxite, Arkansas, and Andover, South Dakota, abandoned their existing water supplies and obtained water from nearby areas where the teeth of the children were free from mottling. In areas such as Arizona and Texas, where dental fluorosis was common, various procedures for the removal of fluorine from water were tried, including the use of bone, ashed bone, and synthetic apatite.

During the nineteenth century, various fluoride concoctions such as fluoride tooth cleaning powders, lozenges, and pastilles were recommended for the care of the teeth. The general opinion was that fluorides were

*Chandler translation, 1878.

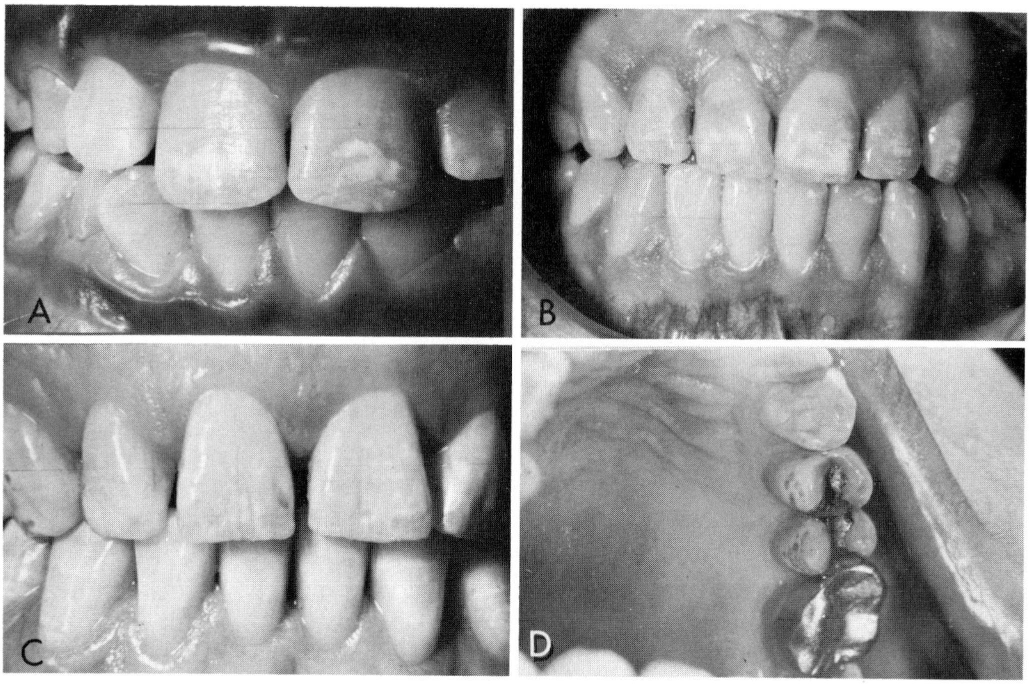

Figure 10–1 Various degrees of mottled enamel can be seen in this series of clinical photographs. The three individuals were born and raised in areas of high natural fluoride content in the drinking water. *A*, Mild mottling can be observed as simple white spots without any morphologic alterations in the tooth structure in this patient. *B*, The severity of the mottling is greater in this patient. The white areas are to such an extent as to create a mild aesthetic problem. *C*, The high level of fluoride ingested by this individual created not only white areas within the enamel but also actual defects in enamel formation. The surface of the tooth structure is rough and pitted. *D*, The pitting observed in the enamel in *C* can be observed clearly on the two bicuspids.

beneficial, and in 1892, Crichton-Browne suggested, "I think it well worthy of consideration whether the re-introduction into our diet, and especially the diet of child-bearing women and of children, of a supply of fluorine in some suitable form . . . might not do something to fortify the teeth of the next generation." However, now that fluoride had been shown to cause mottling of teeth, the seeds of antifluoridation were sown. Effective antifluoridation arguments retarded public acceptance of water fluoridation, and the following thirty years were marked by scientific, legal, sociological, religious, and moral arguments over the merits of fluoridation.

There is still some opposition to water fluoridation, but much of the sting has been removed from the antifluoridation arguments. The simple fact is that time and research have shown that fluoridation does not cause mongolism, poisoning, left-handedness, loss of moral fiber, or any of the other bizarre effects which were forecast by some individuals. The almost universal acceptance of the value of fluorides in dental health is largely due to the work and dedication of a large number of scientists who should be recognized as pioneers in the advancement of dental health and preventive dentistry.

WATER FLUORIDATION

The first study of caries in an area of endemic dental fluorosis was by Bunting and his coworkers in 1928. They observed that the caries pattern in the children was unusual, the extent of lesions and activity of the process being "remarkably limited," and they postulated that the drinking water was responsible for the inhibition of caries activity. Ten years later, Dean demonstrated an inverse relationship between dental fluorosis and dental caries in a series of classic epidemiological studies with accompanying water analyses by Elvove. These studies laid the groundwork for the first experimental addition of fluoride to the drinking water. Dean's findings in a study of over seven thousand 12- to 14-year-old children in 21 cities in four states in the United States clearly demonstrate that there were fewer caries in communities with higher fluoride levels in their water. Of fundamental significance was the observation that a reduction in caries was obtained in many instances without accompanying mottling of the teeth. This led to the concept of an "optimal concentration." In the part of the country where the epidemiological studies were carried out, it seemed that the preferred concentration was one part fluoride per million parts water (1 ppm.). Table 10–1 shows the correlation Dean observed between water fluoride content and endemic dental fluorosis.

Cox had shown that young rats receiving a submottling dosage of fluoride during gestation and lactation had fewer caries. He recommended that fluoride be added to fluoride-deficient water as a caries-preventive measure. Since no deleterious effects were known to be caused by the 1 ppm. fluoride, data available from various sources now seemed to justify the clinical trial of water fluoridation.

From clinical studies it was shown that the total number of decayed, missing, and filled teeth decreased markedly as the amount of fluoride in the water increased; however, most of the caries reduction was achieved at 1 ppm. At 2 or 3 ppm., there was only slightly more protection. On the other hand, no noticeable mottling of the teeth occurs at 1 ppm. fluoride, and it is not until the concentration is considerably higher that the undesirable effects of mottling become an esthetic problem (Figure 10–2).

In 1945, controlled fluoridation studies were started at Newburg, New York, and Grand Rapids, Michigan. In the same year, another study was started in Canada at Brandtford, Ontario, and two years later, a fourth city, Evanston, Illinois, began controlled fluoridation. In each of these studies, a control immunity (C) with a low level of fluoride in the communal water supply was chosen for comparison with the

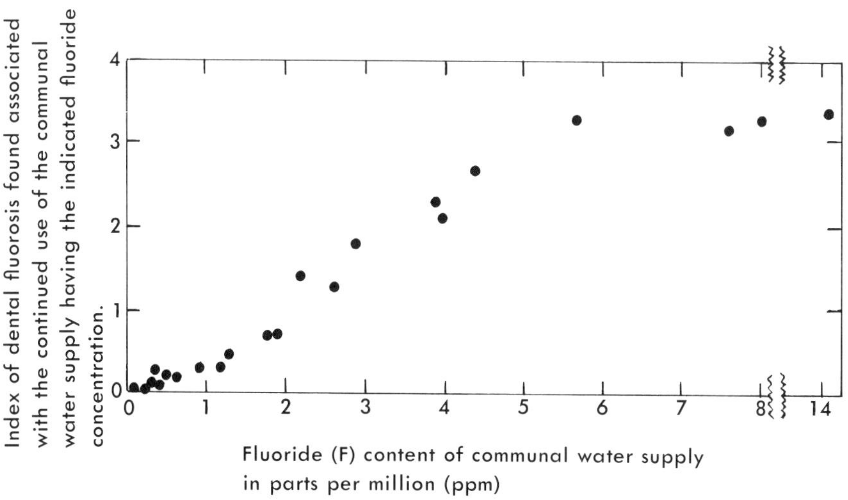

Figure 10–2

TABLE 10–1 VARIATION IN THE EFFECTS OF FLUORIDE INGESTION ASSOCIATED WITH THE CONTINUOUS USE OF DOMESTIC WATERS OF DIFFERENT FLUORIDE CONCENTRATION
(Observations on 5824 white children of 22 cities of 10 states)

					PERCENTAGE DISTRIBUTION						
					SIGNS ABSENT		WHITE OPAQUE SPOTS		BROWN STAINS AND PITTING		
PLACE	*Number examined*	*Per cent affected*	*Index of fluorosis***	*Fluoride concentration*[1] *(ppm)*	*Normal*	*Questionable*	*Very mild*	*Mild*	*Moderate*	*Severe*	AGE GROUP OR SCHOOL GRADE
Waukegan, Illinois	423	0.2	0.01	0.0	97.9	1.9	0.2	0.0	0.0	0.0	12–14 yrs.
Michigan City, Indiana	236	0.0	0.01	0.1	97.5	2.5	0.0	0.0	0.0	0.0	12–14 "
Zanesville, Ohio	459	1.5	0.08	0.2	85.4	13.1	1.5	0.0	0.0	0.0	12–14 "
Lima, Ohio	454	2.2	0.09	0.3	84.1	13.7	2.2	0.0	0.0	0.0	12–14 "
Marion, Ohio	263	6.1	0.25	0.4	57.4	36.5	5.3	0.8	0.0	0.0	12–14 "
Elgin, Illinois	403	4.2	0.22	0.5	60.5	35.3	3.5	0.7	0.0	0.0	12–14 "
Pueblo, Colorado	614	6.5	0.17	0.6	72.3	21.2	6.2	0.3	0.0	0.0	12–14 "
Kewanee, Illinois	123	12.2	0.31	0.9	52.8	35.0	10.6	1.6	0.0	0.0	12–14 "
Aurora, Illinois	633	15.0	0.32	1.2	53.2	31.8	13.9	1.1	0.0	0.0	12–14 "
Joliet, Illinois	447	25.3	0.46	1.3	40.5	34.2	22.2	3.1	0.0	0.0	12–14 "
Elmhurst, Illinois	170	40.0	0.67	1.8	28.2	31.8	30.0	8.8	1.2	0.0	12–14 "
Galesburg, Illinois	273	47.6	0.69	1.9	25.3	27.1	40.3	6.2	1.1	0.0	12–14 "
Clovis, New Mexico	138	71.0	1.4	2.2	13.0	16.0	23.9	35.4	11.0	0.7	9–11 "
Colorado Springs, Colorado	404	73.8	1.3	2.6	6.4	19.8	42.1	21.3	8.9	1.5	12–14 "
Plainview, Texas	97	87.6	1.8	2.9	4.1	8.3	34.0	26.8	23.7	3.1	9–12 "
Amarillo, Texas	289	90.3	2.3	3.9*	3.1	6.6	15.2	28.0	33.9	13.2	9–12 "
Conway, South Carolina	59	88.2	2.1	4.0	5.1	6.7	20.4	32.2	23.7	11.9	9–11 "
Lubbock, Texas	189	97.8	2.7	4.4	1.1	1.1	12.2	21.7	46.0	17.9	9–12 "
Post, Texas	38	100.0	3.3	5.7†	0.0	0.0	0.0	10.5	50.0	39.5	4–6 grades
Chetopa, Kansas	65	100.0	3.2	7.6†	0.0	0.0	9.2	21.5	10.8	58.5	3–12 "
Ankeny, Iowa	21	100.0	3.3	8.0†	0.0	0.0	0.0	9.5	47.6	42.8	2–12 "
Bauxite, Arkansas	26	100.0	3.4	14.1†	0.0	0.0	3.9	3.9	38.5	53.8	14–19 yrs.

[1]All fluoride determinations were made by Senior Chemist Elias Elvove, Division of Chemistry.

*Subject to possible correction to 4.2 ppm during susceptible period of age group examined.

†Single determination; all others, arithmetical mean of 12 consecutive monthly samples.

**For public health administrative guidance an index of dental fluorosis of 0.4 or less is of no concern from the standpoint of mottled enamel *per se;* when, however, the index rises above 0.6 it begins to constitute a public health problem warranting increasing consideration. It is highly important to note that an index of fluorosis as low as about 0.3 has been found associated with remarkably low dental caries experience rate. (From Dean, H. T., et al.: Fluorine and Dental Health, Washington, DC, American Association for the Advancement of Science, 1942.)

fluoride community (F). The paired cities were as follows:

Newburg, New York (F) and Kingston, New York (C)

Grand Rapids, Michigan (F) and Muskegon, Michigan (C)

Brandtford, Ontario (F) and Sarnia, Ontario (C)

Evanston, Illinois (F) and Oak Park, Illinois (C).

Additional useful comparisons were made in cities such as Aurora, Illinois, and Stratford, Ontario, where the water supply naturally contained approximately 1.2 ppm. fluoride.

In the intervening years, many reports have been published demonstrating the caries reduction obtained by natural or artificial fluoridation. Even antifluoridationists have gradually conceded the truth of the overwhelming evidence that fluoridation protects the teeth. In more recent years, similar findings have been made in various countries throughout the world.

To demonstrate the dental effects of discontinuing water fluoridation, Lemke *et al.* (1970) instituted controlled fluoridation in Antigo, Wisconsin. Dental examinations made in 1960 in Antigo—before the removal of fluorides—showed DMF rates comparable to those characteristic of other fluoridated areas in Wisconsin. Dental exams made in 1964, four years after fluoridation was stopped, and in 1970, just after fluoridation was reinstituted, showed increased DMF rates characteristic of those found in nonfluoridated areas.

Children in kindergarten showed a 92 per cent increase in the DMF rate, and children in the second and fourth grades showed 18.3 per cent and 41 per cent increases in DMF rates as compared with the 1960 survey findings, respectively. This substantiated previous studies regarding the withdrawal of fluoride from the water supply and the ineffectiveness of fluoride as a prenatal therapeutic measure.

In Britain, Lucas *et al.* observed that children who had lived in Launton since 1942 when the fluoride content was 0.8 ppm., showed no dental mottling, and the appearance of their teeth was not harmed by the fluoride in the water supply. Twenty-eight per cent of these children had a zero DMF, as compared to only 10.8 per cent of those who had moved to Launton from other nonfluoridated areas.

About five years later, Beal *et al.* (1971) observed reductions of 62.5 per cent and 50.1 per cent in the mean number of DMF of children living in the fluoridated districts of Birmingham, thereby providing more evidence of the effect of the fluoride ion on dental caries. A controlled group, consuming unfluoridated water, maintained a fairly constant level of dental caries prevalence over the same period.

In Australia, Bruder (1971) reported that all school children of Mallnitz (1.0 ppm. fluoride), Silz (1.5 ppm. fluoride), and Umhausen (1.8 ppm. fluoride) were re-examined after ten years; the fluoride content of the drinking water had remained nearly the same in all ten years. The difference between the DMF values of the test groups and the control groups was significant now and ten years ago, but caries frequency increased in all groups. Caries reduction, and frequency and severity of mottling seem to depend not only on the quantity of ingested fluoride, but also on other environmental factors.

An epidemiologic survey was undertaken by Baume *et al.* (1970) among French Polynesians whose drinking water contains practically no fluoride, but who have a staple diet of sea food rich in fluoride. Epidemiological evidence of an average fluoride concentration of 45.17 ppm. in the enamel of caries-free Polynesians remains unmatched so far in the literature. The remarkable feature of the high topical and systemic absorption of fluorides from food lies in the fact that it occurs under physiological conditions with no known untoward effects on general health, such as might occur in a correspondingly high water-borne fluoride of 5 to 10 ppm. which had the same topical effect.

The physiology of dietary fluoride appears to have many features in common with that of fluoridated water. However, from the point of view of toxicology, it shows that some new aspects, such as the

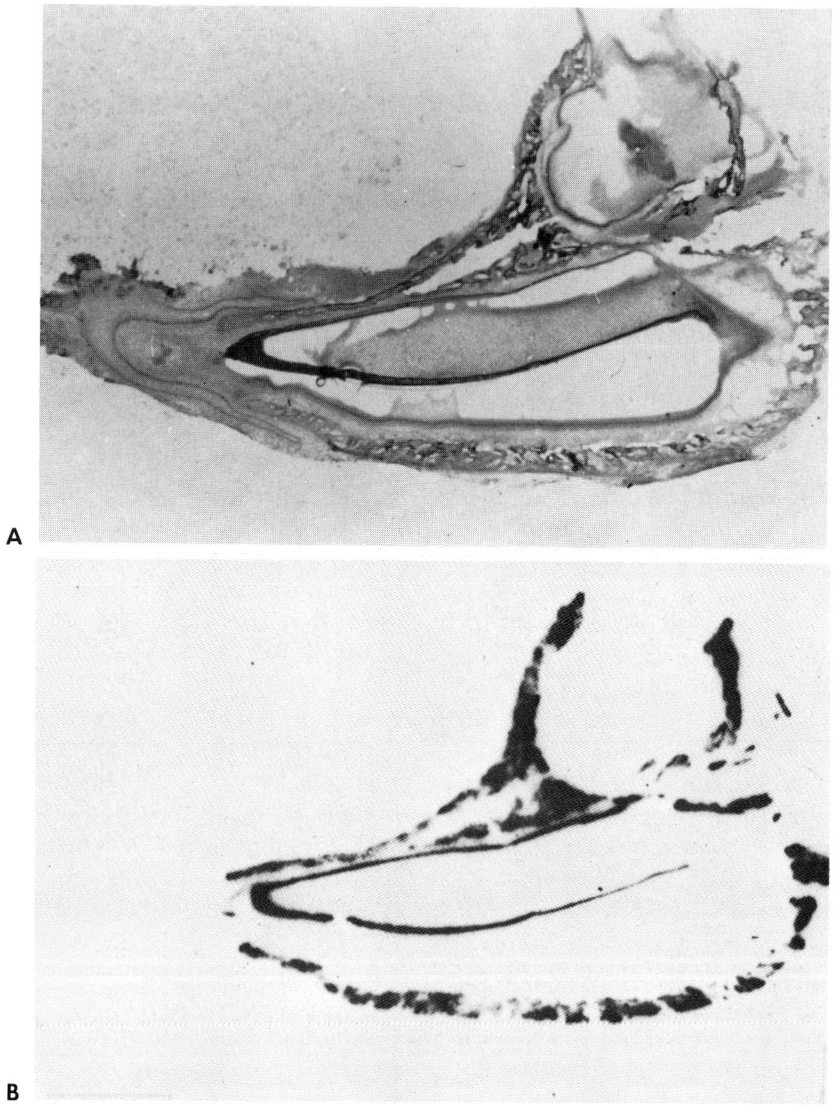

Figure 10–3 The affinity of fluoride for developing bone and teeth is clearly shown in this series of photomicrographs taken from a young rat injected with radioactive fluoride (F^{18}). *A*, Photomicrograph of a section which was covered with a film sensitive to nuclear radiation; *B*, resultant autoradiograph;

possibility of a very high topical enrichment of enamel with no untoward esthetic and systemic effects, may be of particular assistance in devising prophylactic measures to ensure a lifelong resistance to caries.

Utilizing F^{18}, Buzzi and Stallard were able to localize the uptake of radioactive fluoride by the mineralizing bone, dentin, and enamel matrix in a qualitative and semiquantitative way over a period of one hour after intraperitoneal injection of the isotope (Figure 10–3 A, B and C). It was shown that the distribution, as well as the initial uptake of the tracer, was extremely rapid. The intensity of the label increased continuously over a 30 minute interval; thereafter any further intensity increment became small.

Improved resolution led to the observation of radioactivity over the ameloblasts and odontoblasts. The significance of this finding in regard to possible mechanisms of

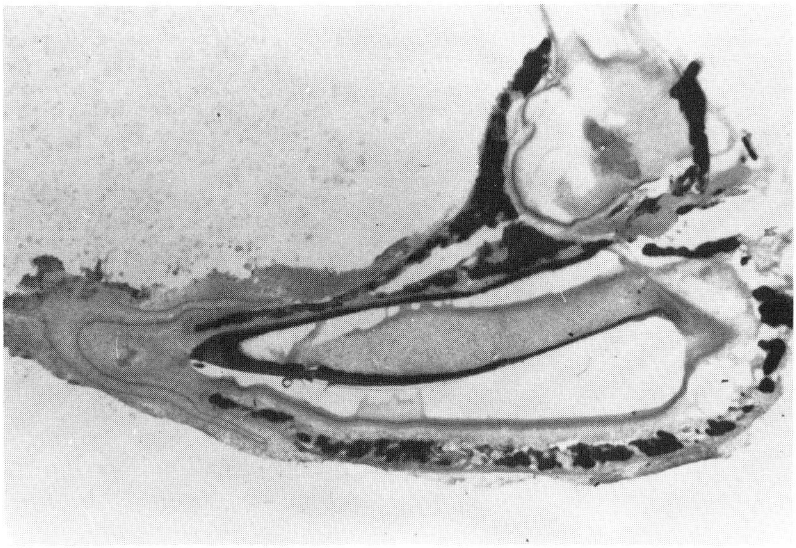
C

Figure 10–3 (*Continued*). *C*, composite of the two. Note the localization of the radioactive fluoride in the developing hard structures.

mineralization is important. In regard to the cells, there appeared to exist a closer correlation of the cellular uptake of fluoride to the developmental state of these cells, or the layer of mineralizing tissue between them, than to the time elapsed between the injection of the isotope and the sacrifice of the animals.

From a concomitant histochemical evaluation on the state of mineralization, it is suggested that the uptake of the radioactive fluoride by the developing dentin coincides approximately with a change in staining (v. Kossa Method) of the organic matrix towards mineralization.

The observation of the presence of fluoride within the ameloblasts and odontoblasts appears challenging and may hold the key to the actual role of fluoride in mineralization of the teeth.

REFERENCES

Baud, C. A., and Bang, S.: Electron probe and x-ray diffraction microanalysis of human enamel treated *in vitro* by fluoride solution. Caries Res. *4*:1–13, 1970.

Baume, L. J., and Vulliemoz, J. P.: Dietary fluoride uptake into the enamel of caries-susceptible yellow permanent teeth, caries-resistant permanent teeth of Polynesians. Arch. Oral Biol. *15*:431–443, 1970.

Cox, G. J.: An annotated bibliography of the literature on the pharmacology and toxicology of fluoride and its compounds. Revised. Including unabridged V. Univ. of Rochester Atomic Energy Project. Health and Biology UR-154.

Dean, H. T., *et al.*: Fluorine and dental health. Am. Assoc. Adv. Sci., Washington, 1942, No. 19, p. 26.

Forest, R. M.: Fluorine and dental health. Am. Assoc. Sci., Washington, 1942, No. 19, p. 29.

Lemke, C. W., Doherty, J. M., and Arra, M. C.: Controlled fluoridation: The dental effects of discontinuation in Antigo, Wisconsin. J.A.D.A. *80*:782–786, 1970.

Lucas, T.: Mottling of tooth enamel in Launton. An investigation. Brit. Dent. J. *121*:183–184, 1966.

RECOMMENDED READING

Buzzi, R. A., and Stallard, R. E.: Uptake of Radioactive Fluoride by Developing Teeth. Monograph, Group Health J. Dent. Res. Jan. 1977.

Cox, G. J., Finn, S. B., and Ast, D. B.: Effect of fluoride ingestion on the size of the cusp of Carabelli during tooth formation. J. Dent. Res. *40*:393–395, 1961.

Dean, H. T., Arnold, F. A., and Elvove, E.: Domestic water and dental caries. V. Additional studies of the relation of fluoride domestic waters to dental caries experience in 4425 white children aged 12 to 14 years, of 13 cities in 4 States. Public Health Rep., *57*:1155–1179, 1942.

Ericsson, Y.: The distribution of simultaneously administered fluoride and molybdate studied with F-18 and MO-99 in the rat. Acta Odont. Scand. *24*:405–417, 1966.

Ericsson, Y., and Ullberg, S.: Autoradiographic investigations of the distribution of F-18 in mice and rats. Acta Odont. Scand. *16*:363–381, 1958.

Ericsson, Y., Ullberg, S., and Appelgren, L. E.: Autoradiographic localization of radioactive fluorine (F-18) in developing teeth and bones. Acta Odont. Scand. *18*:253–361, 1960.

Hammarstrom, L.: Different Distribution of Fluoride-18 and Calcium-45 in Developing Rat Enamel. Int. Assoc. Dent. Res., 48th General Meeting, Abstract No. 591, p. 196, 1970.

Pindborg, J. J., and Weinmann, J. P.: Morphologic and functional correlations in the enamel organ of the rat incisor during amelogenesis. Acta Anat. *36*: 367–381, 1959.

Traves, D. R.: Normal human serum fluoride concentrations. Nature (London) *211*:192–193, 1966.

Volker, J.: Introduction to a symposium on recent clinical advances in the use of fluorides for controlling caries. Bull. Acad. Med. N.J., *14*:4; 206–209, 1960.

chapter 11

TOPICAL FLUORIDE THERAPY

by
DANIEL C. NORNOO, B.D.S., M.Sc.D.
and RICHARD E. STALLARD, D.D.S., PH.D.

In the pioneer clinical studies undertaken by Bibby (1942), Cheyne and Rice (1942), and Knutson and Armstrong (1943), topical application of alkaline fluoride solutions to dental enamel reduced caries. The physiochemistry of enamel underlying fluoride therapy has also been studied by several researchers, including Brudevold and Soremark (1967). They showed that the unit cell, or smallest repeating, can be expressed by the formula, $Ca_{10}(PO_4)_6(OH)_2$. The crystal lattice has the capacity to substitute other ionic species of appropriate size and charge. Sodium, magnesium, or strontium may replace calcium; vanadium or carbonate may replace phosphate; and fluoride may replace hydroxyl groups. There are many ionic forms that may be located at the crystal surface.

The ability to retain foreign ions is further enhanced by the ability of hydroxyapatite crystals to bind water and hydrated ions. Apparently electrical asymmetry on the crystal surface sets up a powerful electrical field which pulls in charged ions and water molecules. Layers of water (the hydration shell) adjacent to the crystals must be considered part of the crystal, from a chemical point of view.

Exchange of ions between apatite and surrounding fluids probably may be effected by the hydration shell, the crystal surface, or the body of the crystal. It has been suggested that H^+ in the form of H_3O can replace up to two Ca^{++} in the crystal lattice of hydroxyapatite in the presence of acid (Brudevold and Soremark, 1967).

The surface of enamel, compared to the subsurface, is harder, less reactive to fluoride, less acid soluble, more resistant to the carious process, and has a higher concentration of minerals and a lower concentration of water. There is a great deal of unresolved controversy regarding the underlying mechanism of reduced enamel solubility when enamel is fluoridated. Van der Lugt, *et al.* (1970) found, by nuclear magnetic resonance determination of fluoride position in mineral hydroxyapatite, that the fluoride ions form part of the linear chains of hydroxyl ions in one of the configurations OH—F vacancy or OH—F—HO. A fluoride ion in this position will block diffusion along these chains. A fluoride ion is more strongly bound to its lattice site than is a hydroxyl ion. This analysis shows how a very small amount of fluoride could have a large effect on inhibiting diffusion. The principal theory of enamel caries involves the concept of the dissolution of enamel by acids. If diffusion of hydroxyl ions within the apatite structure is an important factor in controlling the rate of dissolution, then the diffusion blocking system described here affords a satisfactory explanation for the reduction in this rate when small amounts of fluoride are present.

The mechanism of fluoride acquisition by enamel is thought to be accomplished by diffusion and exchange with anions in the tightly held water adjacent to the enamel crystal, by migration into the body of the crystal, and incorporation into the interior lattice structure. The permeability of human enamel has been researched by Tarbet and Fosdick, who used ultraviolet microscopy to follow the penetration of acriflavine and the increased resistance to acid etching following potassium fluoride penetration. The results indicated that the prism boundary is the permeable structure of the enamel. Acriflavine diffuses more rapidly into enamel than does potassium fluoride, and each diffuses more rapidly *in vivo* than *in vitro*. After six hours of diffusion, the dye penetrates almost the entire thickness of the enamel in a diffuse fashion. The dye appears to be localized in the interprismatic area, specifically, in the prism boundary of the enamel rod (similar to potassium fluoride). This supports the assumption that penetration of substances should be along the channels of least calcification. Subsurface decalcification without cavitation is usually located in the outer 600 microns of the enamel; establishment of an acid-resistant layer in this outer susceptible region should markedly reduce the progress of decalcification, especially soon after the eruption of permanent teeth.

About the same time as Tarbet and Fosdick, Joyston-Bechal, *et al.* devised a method for studying the passage of radioactive ions into fragments of enamel taken from different depths, from the enamel surface to the dento-enamel junction. The rate at which ^{18}F and ^{24}Na pass into an enamel fragment varied according to the depth of the fragment in the enamel surface and, by inference, can be related to the quantity of loosely bound water present. Dehydration at 110° and 200° C., followed by immersion in water for more than 24 hours, significantly reduced the uptake of ^{18}F, while no significant change was apparent after heating at 70° C. The mechanism of uptake in each case was still diffusion controlled. The conclusion is that diffusion of ions into enamel is influenced by the volume of water, loosely bound to the organic material of enamel. Iso-ionic exchange of ^{18}F and ^{19}F at higher concentrations was obtained.

Several factors enhance the uptake of fluoride. Studying the mechanism of fluoride uptake of hydroxyapatite, Spinelli, Brudevold, and Moreno (1971) suggested that prolonged reaction of fluoride with enamel surfaces enhances fixation of fluoride. Recrystallization was enhanced by decreasing the pH, a fact which explains the well known greater retention of fluoride from acid than from neutral solutions used in topical application.

Uptake of fluoride from dentrifices is diffusion controlled, and therefore, uptake rate depends on the viscosity of the dentrifice. The incorporation of fluoride by human enamel from topical application was viewed by Stearns (1971) to be an exothermic chemical process, especially when acidulated phosphate-fluoride topical solution is used. This agrees with the calculation of the heat of reaction of the conversion of HA to FA. The reaction is suppressed by increasing the temperature of reaction; thus, if some topical fluoride applications, using agents other than the acidulated-phosphate fluoride solution (e.g., SnF_2) result in higher fluoride deposits as the temperature is increased, it is to be concluded irrefutably that an endothermic reaction is involved.

Etching of the enamel prior to fluoride application was found by Caslavska, Brudevold, Vrbic, and Moreno (1971) to enhance its uptake. *In vivo* uptake of fluoride by intact enamel from 0.62 M. solution of NH_4F was greater than that from NaF at low pH, but it was similar at nearly neutral or alkaline pH. Fluoride contents in enamel biopsies taken two weeks after a three-minute topical treatment with the acid solution were also higher for the NH_4 fluoride treatment. The *in vivo* and *in vitro* uptake from each solution was enhanced by penetrating the enamel for one minute with 0.05 M. phosphoric acid. Examination by electron microscope of enamel exposed to fluoride ion, before and after washing, revealed that the deposit from NH_4F was more tenaciously retained than that formed from NaF. X-ray diffraction patterns showed formation of CaF_2 when ground enamel was treated with either of the two acid fluoride solutions. The CaF_2 in the case of NH_4F was slowly released, thus increasing its beneficial effects.

Trace elements of the polyvalent metals such as aluminum, titanium, zirconium, boron, and strontium were found by McCann (1969) to enhance fluoride uptake. Maximum fluoride retention was obtained when enamel was treated first with the aluminum salt. This finding was substantiated by Vrbic and Brudevold (1970) when aluminum salt was used in a prophylaxis paste prior to topical fluoride application.

According to McCann, the aluminum can form dual bonds with fluoride and enamel mineral and thus, serve as a mechanism for fluoride fixation. Through animal experimentation, Konig, Muhlemann, *et al.* (1965) found that the less matured or mineralized enamel took up more fluoride than matured enamel. The level of natural fluoride concentration of human tooth enamel also affected fluoride uptake. Muhler (1960) and Saunders and Weidmann (1969) correlated fluoride uptake and the degree of mineralization of the dental structures. They concluded that despite the choice of agent and technique, fluoride uptake by enamel has been found to be inversely proportional to both the natural fluoride content of the enamel and the age of the teeth being treated.

COMPARISON OF THE VARIOUS MAJOR AGENTS IN EFFECTIVENESS

AMINE FLUORIDES

It has been reported that amine fluorides give greater resistance to enamel solubility than any agent, but little research on these agents has been done thus far. Recently, Caslavska, and Brudevold, *et al.* (1971) showed that *in vivo* uptake of fluoride by intact enamel from 0.62 M. solutions of NH_4F was greater than that from NaF at low pH. Examination by electron microscope of fluoride ion, exposed before and after washing, revealed that the deposit from NH_4F was more tenaciously retained than that formed from NaF.

SODIUM HEXAFLUOROSTANNATE

Optimistic claims are made for this compound, which has been shown by Von der Fehr (1970) to give a 40 per cent reduction in new DMFS, as compared to a 30 per cent reduction in a group treated with sodium fluoride.

SODIUM FLUORIDE

Sodium fluoride has been applied prophylactically in various forms. As a topical aqueous solution, Bibby (1942) obtained about 50 per cent DMFT reduction in children aged 10 to 13 years. Kutler and Ireland (1953), using 2 per cent NaF solution, however, found no significant caries reduction in 147 students with an average age of 24.6 years. This finding demonstrates the benefits that different age groups derive from topically applied NaF. Harris (1959) achieved caries incidence reduction of 33.4 per cent using 2 per cent NaF on 6.11 year old children. When incorporated in a gel and applied by custom-fitted mouthpieces, reductions of 67 per cent DMFT and 80 per cent DMFS were obtained by Englander, *et al.* (1967). With acidulated sodium fluoride phosphate gel, reductions of 64 per cent DMFT and 75 per cent DMFS were obtained in 500 children aged 11 to 14.

Using 0.2 per cent sodium fluoride mouthwash applied weekly, Horowitz, *et al.* (1971) observed reductions of 25 per cent DMFT and 16 per cent DMFS in 493 Grade 1 children and 52 per cent DMFT and 44 per cent DMFS in 381 Grade 5 children after 20 months' clinical trial. As a dentifrice, Bibby and Winkler, *et al.* (1953) observed no inhibition of caries. Peterson and Williamson (1968) observed caries reduction of between 14 and 22 per cent after two years of permissive tooth brushing. After three years, Koch (1970) reported 20 per cent caries reduction in the first year, 34 per cent in the second, and 48 per cent in the third year, thus showing the cumulative effect of topical application of fluorides.

STANNOUS FLUORIDE

By far the greatest number of publications is concerned with the use of stannous fluoride. The increased effectiveness of stannous fluoride led to a loss of interest in the use of sodium fluoride as a topical agent. Muhler (1958, 1960) found that a single annual application of 10 per cent SnF_2 solution reduced DMFT by 24 per cent, and DMFS by 16 per cent in adults aged 17 to 38. He also observed that semiannual application of 8 per cent SnF_2 solution was superior to 2 per cent NaF solution as a topical agent.

With a single application of 8 per cent SnF_2, a reduction of 49 per cent DMFT and 80 per cent DMFS of teeth erupting during the study, was observed in children residing in an optimal communal fluoride area. The multiple principle of preventive dentistry is effected here. Horowitz (1969), however, observed as low as a 21 per cent reduction in both DMFT and DMFS in a similar situation.

With a 0.1 per cent SnF_2 mouthwash, Swerdloff, *et al.* (1969) observed 33 per cent less DMFT and 30.5 per cent less DMFS. Stannous fluoride is very effective when used concurrently as a prophylactic paste, aqueous solution, and dentifrice. Scola and Ostrom (1968) found that 70 per cent of naval personnel using the three-agent SnF_2 treatment had no new DMFT after 24 months.

Used as a dentifrice, Muhler (1953, 1962) obtained 71 per cent less DMFS after 6 months and 49 per cent less DMFT after 12 months. After three years, the reduction was 22.4 per cent DMFS. Horowitz, *et al.*, (1966) after 3 years of supervised brushing, obtained 16.3 per cent DMFT and 20.9 per cent DMFS reduction, both significant at less than probability level 0.01. Adeeb and Homer (1966) obtained better results: 37 per cent less DMFS during two years' clinical trial with Crest toothpaste. Gish and Muhler (1966), as two independent examiners, found dental caries reductions of 30 per cent and 35 per cent DMFS among children who used stannous fluoride-calcium pyrophosphate dentifrice and whose teeth calcified in a natural fluoride area. This is further evidence that the use of stannous fluoride adds to the caries-reducing effect of near optimum levels of fluoride in the water supply. Slack, *et al.* (1967) obtained a reduction of 36 per cent DMFS after three years. James and Anderson (1967) observed a lower score of DMFS (reduction of 49 per cent) in girls.

A few comparative studies of SnF_2 and other fluoride compounds have been done. In a majority of these studies, the investigators have reported the relative superiority of SnF_2 as an anticariostatic agent. Muhler, *et al.* (1953) showed the superiority of SnF_2 in its cariostatic properties by obtaining a 56 per cent reduction in DMFT with SnF_2 as compared with a mere 23 per cent reduction in DMFT with NaF solution. Howell, *et al.* (1955) obtained for SnF_2 a DMFS reduction of 58.8 to 65.5 per cent and a 36 per cent DMFS reduction with NaF after two years of application. McDonald and Muhler (1957) observed a DMFT reduction of 57 per cent for SnF_2 and a 21 per cent DMFT reduction for NaF. The SnF_2 was significantly superior to NaF at the 0.05 level of confidence.

By using inhibition of enamel demineralization by repeated treatments with sodium fluoride and stannous fluoride, Fisher (1962) found SnF_2 superior to NaF when each was applied twice daily. Recently Mercer and Muhler (1972), by a single application of 8 per cent SnF_2 and 2 per cent NaF every six months, observed a reduction of 54.7 per cent in DMFT for SnF_2 and 28 per cent in DMFT for NaF, after 24 months. The superiority of SnF_2 was evident when each compound was used at suggested optimum concentration. The difference in the anticariostatic properties of SnF_2 and NaF is quite marked when dentifrices containing these compounds are compared. Muhler, *et al.* (1955) observed a DMFS reduction of 9.9 per cent for NaF dentrifice and 36 per cent for SnF_2 dentifrice. Naylor and Emslie (1967) reported in their clinical test of SnF_2 and sodium monofluorophosphate (MFP) dentifrices in London school children that MFP dentifrice was slightly superior to SnF_2 dentifrice. They observed DMFS reduction of 18.1 per cent with MFP dentifrices and 14.5 per cent with SnF_2 dentifrice.

ACID PHOSPHATE FLUORIDE

Several research findings resulted in the use of the agent acid phosphate fluoride. Pameijer and Brudevold, *et al.* (1963) added phosphate (0.15 M. orthophosphoric acid) to 2 per cent sodium fluoride and observed a further decrease of the increment of dental caries by about 50 per cent of the decrease obtained with neutral 2 per cent NaF alone. In a study by Wellock and Brudevold (1963), 113 children (third, fourth, and fifth grade) who received single topical applications of an acidic fluoride and phosphate solution once a year for two years, had approximately 70 per cent fewer carious surfaces than 113 children who served as controls.

Considerably less reduction in DMFS was observed by Averill, *et al.* (1967) when 2 per cent acidulated phosphate fluoride was compared with 2 per cent aqueous NaF, 4 per cent aqueous SnF_2, and 2 per cent acidulated phosphate-buffered sodium fluoride. A reduction of 12 per cent in DMFS was reported for acidulated phosphate-buffered sodium fluoride, 16 per cent for NaF, and 8 per cent for SnF_2. The magnitude of the difference in caries reduction failed to demonstrate conclusively the superiority of any of those agents, although the 2 per cent NaF solution produced consistently greater reductions in DMFS.

Used in a prophylaxis paste, Mellberg and Nicholson (1968) observed an *in vitro* uptake of fluoride from acidulated phosphate fluoride of 1745 ppm., compared to 1311 ppm. of untreated blocks of enamel. There was no fluoride uptake with SnF_2-compatible pumice paste. Peterson, *et al.* (1969) in a two-year study with acidulated phosphate fluoride pumice, found consistently smaller DMFT, DMFS, and proximal surface increments in the treated groups. The only difference significant at the 0.05 level, however, was that in the nonfluoride community.

Varying degrees of caries reduction are claimed for acidulated phosphate fluoride chewable tablets and mouthwashes. Depaola and Lax (1968) observed a 20 to 23 per cent caries reduction in permanent teeth at the end of two school years. Marthaler (1969) obtained approximately a 41 per cent reduction in carious teeth at the end of eight years. This is evidence that the longer the fluoride therapy, the greater the benefit derived from it.

SODIUM MONOFLUOROPHOSPHATE (MFP)

The use of 6 per cent solutions by means of a daily toothbrush application has shown a significant 52 per cent reduction of DMFS (Groaz, *et al.*, 1966). With MFP dentifrice, Moller, *et al.* (1968) obtained 19 per cent fewer new DMFS over a 30-month period. In 1970, Thomas observed a DMFS decrease of 30 per cent using MFP dentifrice on children 8 to 16 years old.

SURFACE EFFECTS OF SOME TOPICAL FLUORIDES

Very little data are available on the effects on surface topography and depth of penetration of the various topical flourides. In a recent study by Nornoo and Stallard, enamel surfaces treated with sodium fluoride (Theraflur) showed little effect

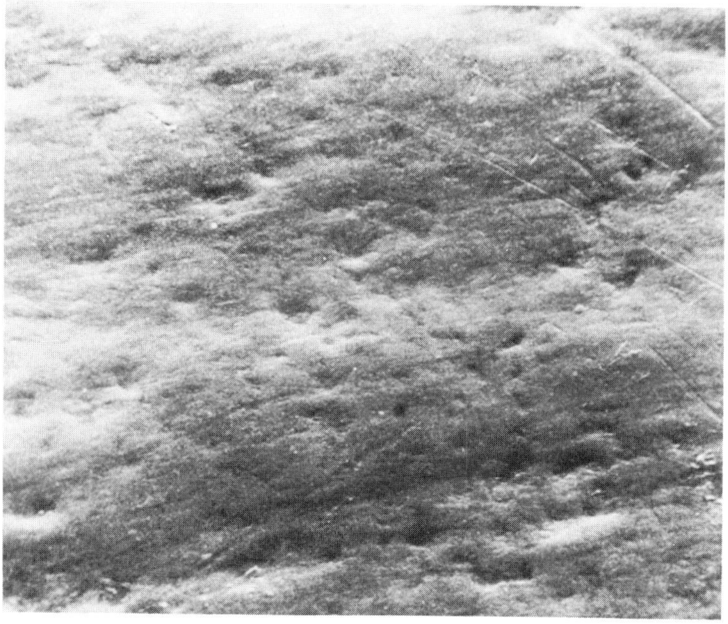

Figure 11–1 Enamel surface treated with Thera-Flur. Note the smooth textured, amorphous, non-crystalline, matlike substance overlying the enamel surface interrupted by perikymata. Magnification × 1050.

owing to the topical application. The surface topography in the scanning electron microscope was similar to that of a sound enamel surface. There were distinct perikymata; however, a smooth textured, amorphous, noncrystalline, matlike substance appeared to be overlying the enamel surface (Fig. 11–1). In the stannous fluoride

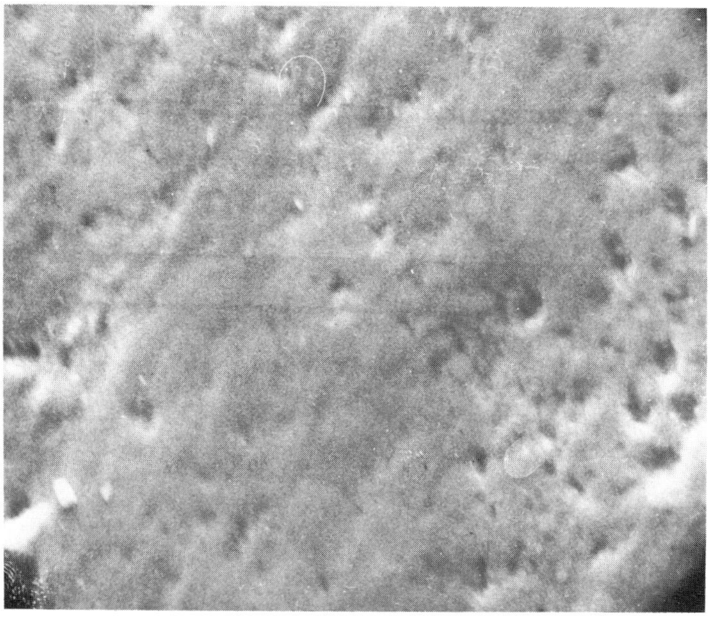

Figure 11–2 Enamel surface treated with stannous fluoride gel. Note the demineralizing effect of the fluoride treatment as the enamel surface is pitted. Magnification × 1050.

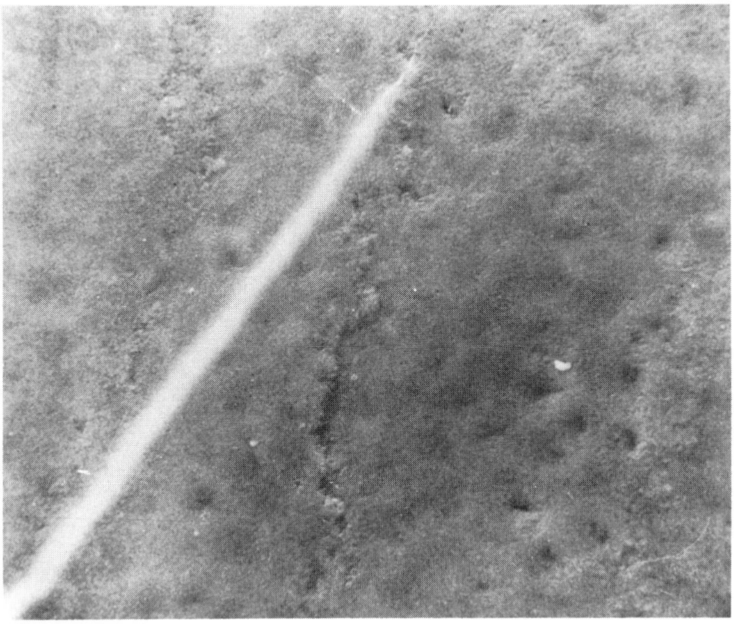

Figure 11–3 Enamel surface treated with phosphate fluoride paste. Note the smooth surface imparted by the abrasive nature of the paste and shallow discrete depressions covering the entire field. The bright diagonal line is an artifact as a result of surface charging. Magnification × 1000.

treated enamel surface (Fig. 11–2), transitioned changes were apparent. Pits appeared in linear groups along the slopes of crest of the imbrication lines and again, the enamel surface appeared to be covered with amorphous matlike material. Enamel surfaces treated with phosphate fluoride prophylaxis paste seem to have lost the characteristic

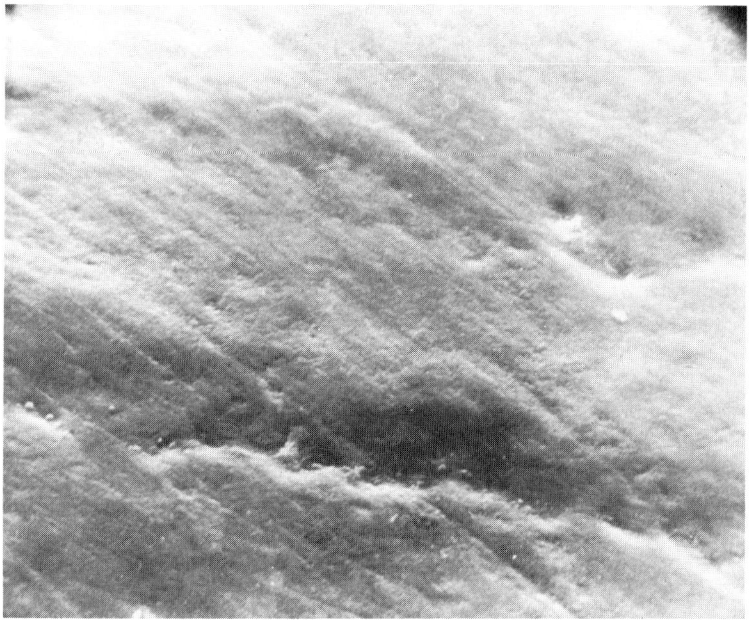

Figure 11–4 Enamel surface given 3M brand caries preventive treatment. The smooth and glossy surface is produced by the sealant. Etching by the pretreatment solution appears to have been filled in by the sealant. Magnification × 1025.

TABLE 11-1 UPTAKE AND PENETRATION OF TOPICAL FLUORIDES*

DEPTH OF ENAMEL SURFACE	THERAFLUR	3M BRAND CARIES PREVENTIVE TREATMENT	PHOSPHATE FLUORIDE PROPHYLAXIS PASTE	STANNOUS FLUORIDE GEL	CONTROL
Surface	6403	7369	7231	1958	237
15 μ	6107	7078	7089	289	282
30 μ	5119	7065	7354	176	211

*The figures shown are raw readings obtained from the energy dispersive x-ray analyzer of the scanning electron microscope assembly.

features described for sound enamel. The abrasive effect of the prophylaxis paste imparted a smooth amorphous surface to the enamel (Fig. 11–3). Minnesota Mining's (3M) caries-preventive treatment of enamel showed an interesting surface topography. In spite of the etching the surface exhibited a glossy appearance with a few depressions filled with the sealant (Fig. 11–4).

FLUORIDE UPTAKE

The figures presented in Table 11–1 indicate the relative uptake and penetration of fluoride in treated and control teeth. With the fluoridated paste and 3M treatment the uptake was the greatest, and equal amounts of fluoride were observed on the surface and at a depth of 30μ, giving a greater penetration than stannous fluoride. The uptake from the stannous fluoride gel was the smallest of all the fluoride preparations used. The drop in fluoride content in the stannous fluoride treated enamel was sharp, showing the least penetration. The fluoride content at depths 15μ and 30μ was similar to that of the control tooth.

REFERENCES

Bergman, G.: Microscopic demonstration of liquid flow through human dental enamel. Arch. Oral Biol. *8*:233–234, 1964.

Bibby, B. G.: Preliminary report on the use of sodium fluoride applications in caries prophylaxis. J. Dent. Res. *21*:314, 1942.

Brudevold, F., McCann, H. G., and Gron, P.: An enamel biopsy for determination of fluoride in human teeth. Arch. Oral Biol. *13*:877–885, 1968.

Brudevold, F., McCann, H. G., Nilson, R., *et al.*: The chemistry of caries inhibition problems and challenges in topical treatments. J. Dent. Res. Suppl. to No. 1, 1967.

Caslavska, V., Brudevold, F., Vrbic, V., and Moreno, E. C.: Response of human enamel to topical application of ammonium fluoride. Arch. Oral Biol. *16*:1173–1180, 1971.

Cheyne, W. D., and Rice, T. B.: Effects of topically applied fluoride on human dental caries, including a method for its application. J. Dent. Res. *21*:341, 1942.

Depaola, P. F., and Lax, M.: The caries-inhibiting effect of acidulated phosphate-fluoride chewable tablets: A two-year double-blind study. J.A.D.A. *76*:554–557, 1968.

Englander, H. R., Sherrill, L.T.T., Miller, B. G., Carlos, J. P., and Mellberg, J. R.: Incremental rates of dental caries after repeated topical sodium fluoride applications in children with lifelong consumption of fluoridated water. J.A.D.A. *82*:354–358, 1971.

Fischer, E. E.: Inhibition of enamel demineralization by repeated treatments with sodium and stannous fluoride solutions. J. Dent. Res. *41*:392–397, 1962.

Harris, R.: Observations on the effect of topical NaF on caries incidence in children. Austr. Dent. J. *4*:257–260, 1959.

Horowitz, H. S.: Evaluation of topical applications of SnF_2 to teeth of children born and reared in a fluoridated community. Final report. J. Dent. Child. *36*:355–361, 1969.

Horowitz, H. S., Creighton, W. E., and McClendon, B. J.: The effect on human dental caries of weekly oral rinsing with NaF mouthwash. A final report. Arch. Oral Biol. *16*:609–616, 1971.

Joyston-Bechal, S., Duckworth, R., and Braden, M.: Diffusion of radioactive ions into human dental enamel. Arch. Oral Biol. *16*:375–384, 1971.

Koch, G.: Long-term study of effect of supervised toothbrushing with a sodium fluoride dentifrice. Caries Res. *4*:149–157, 1970.

Marthaler, T. M.: The value in caries prevention of other methods of increasing fluoride ingestion, apart from fluoridated water. Int. Dent. J. *17*:606–618, 1967.

Marthaler, T. M., and Zilio, R.: Enamel solubility studies *in vivo*; method, error and effect of topi-

cally applied fluorides. Helv. Odont. Acta *4*:27, 1960.
McDonald, R. E., and Muhler, J. C.: The superiority of topical application of SnF_2 on primary teeth. J. Dent. Child. *24*:84–86, 1957.
Mellberg, J. R., and Nicholson, C. R.: *In vitro* evaluation of an acidulated phosphate fluoride prophylaxis paste. Arch. Oral Biol. *13*:1223–1234, 1968.
Mellberg, J. R., and Nicholson, C. R.: *In vitro* fluoride uptake by erupted and unerupted tooth enamel. (Research annotations) J. Dent. Res. *47*:176, 1968.
Mercer, V. H., and Muhler, J. C.: Comparison of single topical applications of sodium fluoride and stannous fluoride. J. Dent. Res. *51*:1325–1330, 1972.
Moller, I. J., Holst, J. J., and Sorensen, E.: Caries reducing effect of a sodium monofluorophosphate dentifrice. Brit. Dent. J. *124*:209–213, 1968.
Muhler, J. C.: Effect of a stannous fluoride dentifrice on caries reduction in children during a three-year study period. J.A.D.A. *64*:217, 1962.
Muhler, J. C.: The anticariogenic effectiveness of a single application of SnF_2 in children residing in an optimal communal fluoride area. II. Results at the end of 30 months. J.A.D.A. *61*:431–438, 1960.
Muhler, J. C., Nebergall, W. H., and Day, M. G.: Preparations of SnF_2 compared with sodium fluoride for the prevention of dental caries in the rat. J.A.D.A. *46*:290, 1953.
Mulher, J. C., Radike, A. W., and Nebergall, W. H.: Comparison between the anticariogenic effects of dentifrices containing SnF_2 and NaF. J.A.D.A. *51*:415–556, 1955.
Naylor, M. N., and Emslie, R. D.: Clinical testing of stannous fluoride and sodium monofluorophosphate dentifrices in London school children. Brit. Dent. J. *123*:17–23, 1967.
Pameijer, J.H.N., Brudevold, F., and Hunt, E. E.: A study of acidulated fluoride solutions. III. The cariostatic effect of repeated topical NaF applications with and without PO^-_4—A pilot study. Arch. Oral Biol. *8*:183, 1963.
Scola, F. P., and Ostrom, C. A.: Clinical evaluation of stannous fluoride when used as a constituent of a compatible prophylactic paste, as a topical solution, and in a dentifrice in naval personnel. II. Report of findings after two years. J.A.D.A. *77*:594–597, 1968.
Spinelli, M. A., Brudevold, F., and Moreno, E.: Mechanism of fluoride uptake by hydroxyapatite. Arch. Oral Biol. *16*:187–203, 1971.
Stearns, R. I.: Incorporation of fluoride by human enamel. II. An exothermic chemical process. J. Dent. Res. *50*:1575–1579, 1971.
Thomas, A. E.: Effect of a combination of two cariostatic agents in children: two-year clinical study of supervised brushing in children's home. J.A.D.A. *81*:118–124, 1970.
Van der Lugt, W., Knottnerus, D.I.M., and Young, R. A.: Nuclear magnetic-resonance determination of fluoride position in mineral hydroxyapatite. Caries Res. *4*:89–95, 1970.
Von der Fehr, F. R.: The caries inhibiting effect of topically applied sodium hexafluorostannate on dentine and enamel. Caries Res. *4*:269–282, 1970.
Wellock, W. D., and Brudevold, F.: A study of acidulated fluoride solutions. II. The caries inhibiting effect of single annual topical applications of an acidic fluoride and phosphate solution. A 2 year experience. Arch. Oral Biol. *18*:179–182, 1963.

RECOMMENDED READING

Brudevold, F., and Soremark, R.: Chemistry of the mineral phase of enamel: Structural and chemical organization of teeth. A. E. Miles, Vol. 2, N.Y. and London, Academy Press, 1967.
Brudevold, F., Chilton, N. W., and Wellock, W. D.: A preliminary comparison of a dentifrice containing fluoride and soluble phosphate and employing calcium-free abrasive with other types of fluoride dentifrices. J. Oral Therap. *1*:1–6, 1965.
Englander, H. R., Keyes, P. H., and Gestwicki, M.: Clinical anticaries effect of repeated topical sodium fluoride applications by mouthpieces. J.A.D.A. *75*:638–644, 1967.
Gish, C. W., and Muhler, J. C.: Effectiveness of a SnF_2-$Ca_2P_2O_2$ dentifrice on dental caries in children whose teeth calcified in a natural fluoride area. II. Results at the end of 24 months. J.A.D.A. *73*:853–855, 1966.
Groaz, P. W., McElwaine, L. P., Biswell, H. A., and White, W. E.: The anticariogenic effect of sodium monoflurophosphate solution in children after 21 months of use. J. Dent. Res. *45*:286–290, 1966.
Horowitz, H. S., Law, F. E., Thompson, M. B., and Chamberlain, S.: Evaluation of a SnF_2 dentifrice for use in dental public health programs. I. Basic findings Grades 1–3. J.A.D.A. *72*:408–422, 1966.
Howell, C. L., Gish, C. W., Smily, R. E., and Muhler, J. C.: Effect of topically applied SnF_2 on dental caries experience in children. J.A.D.A. *50*:14–17, 1955.
König, K. G., Muhlemann, H. R., Shait, A., and Schmid, H. R.: The effect of post-eruptive fluoride uptake and enamel maturation on dental caries in Osborne-Mendel rats. Helv. Odont. Acta *9*:135, 1965.
Kutler, B., and Ireland, R. L.: The effect of NaF application on the dental caries experience in adults. J. Dent. Res. *32*:458, 1953.
Kutson, J. W., and Armstrong, W. D.: The effect of topically applied NaF on dental caries experience. Public Health Rep. *58*:1701, 1943.
Mellberg, J. R., and Loertscher, K. L.: Fluoride acquisition *in vitro* by sound human tooth enamel from sodium fluoride and ammonium silicofluoride-phosphate solution. Arch. Oral Biol. *17*:1107–1116, 1972.
Mellberg, J. R., Nicholson, C. R., and Miller, B. G.: Acquisition of fluoride *in vivo* by enamel from repeated topical NaF applications in a fluoridated area. A preliminary report. J. Dent. Res. *47*:733–736, 1968.
Muhler, J. C.: The effect of a single topical application of SnF_2 on the incidence of dental caries in adults (17–38 years). J. Dent. Res. *37*:415–416, 1958.
Muhler, J. C.: Topical treatment of teeth with SnF_2 single application technique. J. Dent. Child. *25*:306, 1958.
Muhler, J. C., Radike, A. W., Nebergall, W. H., and Day, M. G.: Effect of a SnF_2 containing dentifrice on caries reduction in children. II. Caries experience after one year. J.A.D.A. *50*:163, 1955.
Peterson, J. K., and Williamson, L.: Field test of a so-

dium fluoride dentifrice containing acid orthophosphate and an insoluble metaphosphate abrasive—second year report. J. Oral Therap. *4*:1–4, 1968.
Saunders, M., and Weidmann, S. M.: Uptake and retention of fluoride by teeth of dogs of different ages. Arch. Oral Biol. *14*:365–372, 1969.
Swerdloff, F., *et al.*: Feasibility of the use of SnF_2 mouthwash in a school system. J. Dent. Child. *36*:363–368, 1969.
Tarbet, W. J., and Fosdick, L. S.: Permeability of human dental enamel to acriflavine and potassium fluoride. Arch. Oral Biol. 951–961, 1971.
Thomas, A. E., and Jamison, H. C.: Effect of SnF_2 dentifrices on caries in children: Two year clinical study of supervised brushing in children's homes. J.A.D.A. *73*:844–852, 1966.
Vrbic, V., and Brudevold, F.: Fluoride uptake from treatment with different fluoride prophylaxis pastes and from the use of pastes containing a soluble aluminum salt followed by topical application. Caries Res. *4*:158–167, 1970.

chapter 12

DENTIFRICES AND MOUTH RINSES

by
ANTHONY R. VOLPE, D.D.S., M.S.

PART ONE • DENTIFRICES

RELATIONSHIP OF DENTIFRICES TO A PREVENTIVE DENTISTRY PROGRAM

A successful dental office preventive dentistry program consists of at least two important elements. First, the dental practitioner should provide the patient with the most advanced and efficiently administered treatment in the areas of restorative dentistry and preventive dentistry. Additionally, he should educate the patient in respect to the nature of proper oral hygiene procedures and stress the importance of the continuous and habitual home use of these procedures.

The most important aspect of a patient's home-care oral hygiene program involves the efficient and thorough cleaning of the dentition. In order to achieve this objective, the patient requires both a cleaning substance (dentifrice) and a cleaning device (toothbrush).

DEFINITION AND FUNCTIONS OF A DENTIFRICE

Traditionally, a dentifrice has been defined as a substance used with a toothbrush for the purpose of cleaning the accessible surfaces of the teeth (Accepted Dental Therapeutics,* Gershon, Pokras and Rider, 1957). This definition primarily concerned the cosmetic functionality of a dentifrice and involved the removal of *materia alba*, "film," food debris and stain from the tooth surfaces. Thus, one obtained a cosmetically clean dentition and a fresher breath.

It was further indicated that the use of a dentifrice also provided "secondary beneficial effects" upon the incidence of dental caries and gingival disease. These secondary beneficial effects, in contra-

*The 36th Edition (1975/1976) of Accepted Dental Therapeutics is currently available.
Gershon and Pader, 1972, is the revised and updated version of the original 1957 reference.

distinction to an actual therapeutic effect obtainable by the incorporation of a drug substance into a dentifrice, were based primarily upon two considerations. The first consideration was the axiom that "a clean tooth does not decay," which was extensively expounded. The second factor was the results obtained from a two-year clinical study which indicated that brushing the teeth with a neutral (nontherapeutic) dentifrice immediately after the ingestion of food provided a substantial reduction (approximately 50 per cent) in the incidence of dental caries (Fosdick, 1950).

Knowledge that has been obtained in the past decade concerning the important role of dental plaque in the onset of oral disease has provided substantiation for these secondary beneficial effects. Dental plaque, which is a deposit that is primarily composed of microorganisms and which forms rapidly on tooth surfaces, has been shown to be the primary etiological factor in the initiation of dental caries, dental calculus and gingival disease. In addition to the classic animal experiments which established a definite cause-effect relationship between caries and specific microorganisms (Keyes, 1960; Fitzgerald and Keyes, 1960), direct clinical evidence also has been obtained by numerous investigators regarding the relationship between plaque, calculus and gingivitis.

In one clinical study (Löe, Theilade and Jensen, 1965), it was shown that the withdrawal of toothbrushing in young persons with excellent oral hygiene and clinically normal gingiva resulted in the accumulation of plaque on the teeth. Clinical gingivitis developed after 10 to 21 days, and was closely correlated with the degree of plaque accumulation. When toothbrushing was reinstituted, clinically normal conditions were reestablished in about one week. Another clinical study (Villa, 1968) has indicated that the rate of early calculus formation on lower central incisor teeth was about 50 per cent lower in persons performing their habitual and individual toothbrushing than in persons who were instructed not to brush this area of the dentition.

Thus, a cosmetic dentifrice can be considered to be providing a "therapeutic effect" to the oral cavity when it is utilized in the efficient and thorough physical-mechanical removal of dental plaque from the tooth surfaces.

Additionally, the past decade has also provided substantiation for the therapeutic (or actual drug) effect that can be chemically or pharmacologically provided by a dentifrice. A variety of clinical studies conducted in many areas of the world, and by many different investigators, has confirmed the caries-reducing therapeutic effect of some dentifrices containing various fluoride compounds in compatible and stable formulations.

The functions of a dentifrice could thus be threefold (cosmetic, cosmetic-therapeutic and therapeutic) and described as follows:

1. Cosmetic. This function involves the use of a cosmetic dentifrice (not containing a drug substance) in a routine, nonspecific manner in an attempt to remove materials such as *materia alba*, film (pellicle and plaque), food debris and stain from the tooth surfaces. The net effect of this dentifrice function would include the providing of a "cosmetically clean and healthy dentition" and a fresher breath.

2. Cosmetic-Therapeutic. This function involves the use of a cosmetic dentifrice (not containing a drug substance) in such a manner as to provide for the efficient and thorough physical-mechanical removal of dental plaque. The net effect of this dentifrice function would include, in addition to those already associated with the use of a cosmetic dentifrice, a "therapeutic" effect upon the incidence of caries, calculus and gingival disease.

3. Therapeutic. This function involves the use of a therapeutic dentifrice (containing a drug substance) so as to transport the drug substance to the tooth surface or the tooth environment (plaque, saliva, gingival tissues, etc.). Thus, the net effect of this dentifrice function would be the providing of the specific chemical or pharmacological action of the drug substance, as manifested clinically by a reduction in the incidence of plaque, calculus, caries and/or gingival disease. Additionally, depending upon the efficiency of the toothbrushing procedure, secondary cosmetic or cosmetic-therapeutic effects could be provided.

The previous discussion has been utilized as a basis for an expanded definition of a dentifrice. The revised definition is as follows:

> A dentifrice is a substance used with a toothbrush to clean the accessible surfaces of the teeth so as to provide one or more of the following effects: (1) primarily cosmetic, including cleaning, polishing and breath freshening, (2) cosmetic-therapeutic, through the efficient and thorough physical-mechanical removal of dental plaque and (3) therapeutic or pharmacological, by means of conveying a drug substance to the tooth surfaces or the tooth environment.

INGREDIENTS AND COMPOSITION OF DENTIFRICES

Although dentifrices are available in various physical forms (paste, powder and liquid) throughout the world, the predominant physical form is the paste. This is especially true in the United States, and thus, this discussion of the ingredients and composition of dentifrices will basically concern dentifrices that are in a paste form (commonly referred to as toothpaste).

Dentifrices are composed of a variety of materials, each of which has a specific function. These materials include cleaning and polishing agents, detergents (or surface-active agents), binding agents, flavoring agents, sweetening agents, preservatives, water and, in the case of therapeutic dentifrices, a drug substance. Additionally, miscellaneous ingredients, such as coloring materials, corrosion inhibitors and whitening agents, are often utilized in the dentifrice formulation. The approximate amounts of these ingredients that are present in typical dentifrice formulations are shown in Table 12–1.

TABLE 12–1 APPROXIMATE RANGES OF BASIC INGREDIENTS IN DENTIFRICE FORMULATIONS

INGREDIENT	APPROXIMATE PER CENT OF FORMULATION
Cleaning and Polishing Agents	25 to 60%
Detergents (Surface-Active Agents)	Up to 2%
Humectants	20 to 40%
Binding Agents	Up to 2%
Flavoring Agents	Up to 1.5%
Water	15 to 50%
Colors, Preservatives, Sweeteners, Stabilizers, etc.	Up to 3%
Therapeutic (or Drug) Substance	Up to 2%

CLEANING AND POLISHING AGENTS

The largest component in a dentifrice is the cleaning and polishing agent, which accounts for approximately 25 to 60 per cent of the entire formulation. Substances that clean or polish the tooth surfaces are also commonly referred to as abrasives. Dentifrice cleaning and polishing agents may be defined as solid substances which have a twofold purpose: (1) to remove debris, stain and plaque from tooth surfaces, and (2) to polish, or impart a luster to the tooth surfaces.

Most persons must use a dentifrice containing a cleaning and polishing agent several times daily in order to keep their teeth reasonably clean and healthy. The cleaning and polishing agent is required to assist in the removal of the following accumulations:

(1) *plaque*, which is potentially pathologic to the teeth and periodontium and which accumulates very rapidly on a clean tooth surface;
(2) *debris*, which constantly accumulates on the tooth surfaces due to the ingestion and mastication of foodstuffs; and
(3) *stain*, which continuously forms on the tooth surfaces of most individuals due to substances such as food, beverages and tobacco.

Additionally, it is estimated that approximately 90 per cent of the population would form a "brown pellicle" on their teeth if they did not use a dentifrice that contained a cleaning and polishing agent. The occurrence of this cosmetically undesirable brown-black pellicle in persons using either nonabrasive dentifrices (such as the "liquid" dentifrices that do not contain conventional cleaning and polishing agents) or mildly abrasive dentifrices, has been reported by several investigators (Manly, 1943; Vallotton, 1945; Kitchin and Robinson, 1948; and Gerdin, 1970).

Ideally, cleaning and polishing agents should provide a maximum of cleaning with a minimum of abrasion, so as not to damage the tooth surfaces or the surrounding structures. Also, it is essential that the cleaning and polishing agent be chemically and physically compatible with the other dentifrice ingredients. This is especially important in formulations which contain therapeutic substances, such as fluoride compounds, where it has been shown that certain cleaning and polishing agents have the capability to inactivate some fluoride compounds.

The dentifrices currently available in the United States are largely based on various grades of one or more of the following cleaning and polishing agents:

- Calcium carbonate, precipitated ($CaCO_3$)
- Dicalcium phosphate, dihydrate ($CaHPO_4 \cdot 2H_2O$)
- Dicalcium phosphate, anhydrous ($CaHPO_4$)
- Sodium metaphosphate, insoluble $(NaPO_3)_x$
- Calcium pyrophosphate ($Ca_2P_2O_7$)

In general, the dihydrate form of dicalcium phosphate is the least inherently abrasive compound, while the anhydrous form is the most abrasive. The remaining materials hold some intermediate position between these two extremes. Other cleaning and polishing agents that are less commonly used include tricalcium phosphate, hydrated alumina and various silica and silicate compounds. Thermoplastic resins, such as polymethylmethacrylate, are currently being used as the principal cleaning and polishing agents in some European dentifrices.

Although the vast majority of currently available dentifrices are of an opaque nature, recent trends have demonstrated an increased popularity for transparent/translucent products. These are the so-called clear gel dentifrices, and they are produced by carefully matching the refractive indices of the abrasive and humectant systems. Abrasives particularly suited for this purpose include a synthetic amorphous silica zerogel and a synthetic amorphous complex aluminosilicate salt.

It should be emphasized that the cleaning and polishing characteristics of a particular substance could vary considerably depending upon such factors as the source of the material, the physical or chemical treatment that the material has received, and the particle size of the material. This is especially true in the case of calcium carbonate.

Some cleaning and polishing agents are excellent cleaning substances but have only limited polishing ability and thus tend to leave a dull finish on the tooth surfaces. Conversely, other cleaning and polishing agents have excellent polishing characteristics but are less efficient in reference to their cleaning properties. Thus, manufacturers often combine different agents in an effort to take advantage of the cleaning ability of one material and the polishing ability of another material. When such a combination of materials is utilized, the dentifrice is said to contain an "abrasive system."

Many *in vitro* methods and technics have been used to investigate the comparative cleaning and polishing abilities of various materials and formulations. These procedures are reviewed in detail in a number of excellent publications (Gershon, Pokras and Rider, 1957; Harry, 1962; Manly, Wiren, Manly and Keene, 1965; Bouchal, 1966; Wright and Stevenson, 1967; Stookey and Muhler, 1968; Swartz and Phillips, 1968; Gershon and Pader, 1972; and Bogle, 1974). In general, abrasion is achieved in a relatively short period of time by exposing the materials to be abraded to a large number of brushing strokes with the substance or formulation under investigation. Spe-

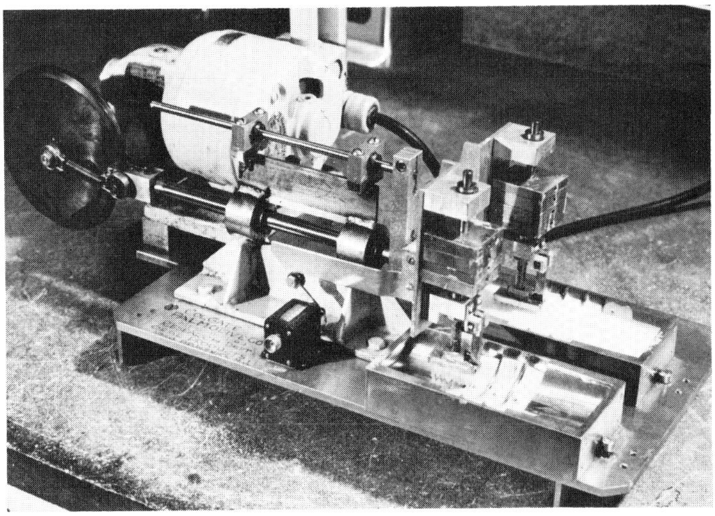

Figure 12–1 This photograph shows a two-brush model abrasion machine which is used in *in vitro* dentifrice abrasion studies. (Reproduced from Bouchal, A. W.: Proc. Scient. Sect. TGA *45*:2–5, 1966.)

cially constructed laboratory toothbrushing devices have been used for this purpose (Fig. 12–1).

The comparative abrasiveness of a particular substance or formulation has been estimated by the use of such techniques as determination of weight loss (Tainter and Epstein, 1943), measurement of the cross-sectional area of loss with shadowgraphs and a planimeter (Manly, 1944), determination of loss of material by use of a radioactive dentin abrasion procedure (Grabenstetter, Broge, Jackson, and Radike, 1958), and determination of relative abrasion through use of a dentin section-shadowgraph procedure (Cordon, 1971). Since dental enamel is a relatively difficult substance to abrade, dentin has been the material most frequently used in these procedures.

The Council on Dental Therapeutics of the American Dental Association has conducted a series of laboratory investigations to determine the comparative abrasiveness of some dentifrices commercially available in the United States. The laboratory procedure utilized to measure the abrasiveness of these dentifrices was the basic Radioactive Dentin Abrasion (RDA) procedure, which had been slightly modified.

This procedure involves the use of the accelerated tooth-brushing apparatus and dentin sections that contain radioactive phosphorus. The American Dental Association standard was set at 100, which corresponds to an RDA value of 475. The comparative abrasiveness of some representative dentifrices, as determined in this evaluation, are presented in Table 12–2.

Unfortunately, it is often difficult to correlate results obtained from *in vitro* technics with the actual abrasiveness of these dentifrices on similar structures in the oral cavity. Two factors that make this correlation difficult are (1) the difference between the normal conditions of dentifrice use and employment of the accelerated toothbrushing apparatus, and (2) the effect of the oral environment (saliva, pellicle, plaque, diet, etc.) on a particular tooth surface.

A number of *in vivo* technics have been developed in an effort to evaluate the comparative cleaning and polishing ability of substances or formulations directly on the tooth surfaces. These methods, in general, were specially designed to measure one particular characteristic, such as ability to polish enamel surfaces, capacity to prevent or remove stain, ability to remove interproximal plaque, and capacity to abrade acrylic surfaces of veneer crowns.

One technic used a tooth reflectance

TABLE 12–2* COMPARATIVE ABRASIVENESS OF SOME COMMERCIALLY AVAILABLE DENTIFRICES AS DETERMINED BY A RADIOACTIVE DENTIN PROCEDURE†

DENTIFRICE	MANUFACTURER	PRINCIPAL ABRASIVE	ABRASIVITY INDEX
Sensodyne	Block Drug Co.	Silica	157
Vote	Bristol-Myers Co.	Silica	134
Plus White Plus	Bishop Industries, Inc.	Dicalcium Phosphate (anhydrous)	132
Plus White	Bishop Industries, Inc.	Dicalcium Phosphate (anhydrous)	110
Gleem II	Procter and Gamble Co.	Calcium Pyrophosphate	106
Macleans (old formulation)	Beecham Products, Inc.	Calcium Carbonate	93
Crest (Mint and Regular)	Procter and Gamble Co.	Calcium Pyrophosphate	88
Close-Up	Lever Brothers Co.	Silica	87
Pearl Drops	Carter-Wallace, Inc.	Alumina and Dicalcium Phosphate (dihydrate)	72
Macleans (new formulation)	Beecham Products, Inc.	Dicalcium Phosphate (dihydrate)	68
Ultra Brite	Colgate-Palmolive Co.	Dicalcium Phosphate (dihydrate)	64
Colgate with MFP	Colgate-Palmolive Co.	Insoluble Sodium Metaphosphate	51
Pepsodent	Lever Brothers Co.	Dicalcium Phosphate (dihydrate)	26
Thermodent	Chas. Pfizer and Co.	Magnesium Carbonate (basic) and Calcium Carbonate	24

*The data presented in this table was reproduced from Accepted Dental Therapeutics, 1971/1972 Edition.
†The American Dental Association standard is set at 100, which corresponds to a Radioactive Dentin Abrasion (RDA) value of 475. The abrasivity index values presented are averages; the lower the index value, the lower the abrasivity of the particular dentifrice, and vice versa.

meter to measure cleaning effectiveness of dentifrice materials (Schiff and Shaver, 1971). The reflectance meter measures directly from the tooth surfaces (in a reproducible manner) both the diffuse and specular components of reflected light, which are believed to be related to both the degree of tooth whiteness and tooth polish (Fig. 12–2).

Another technic utilized a specially

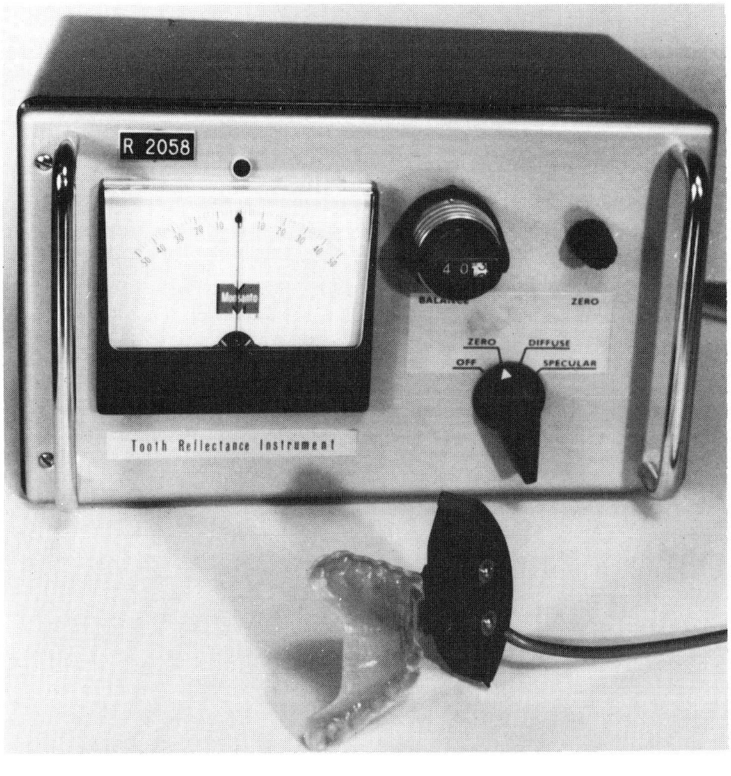

Figure 12–2 This photograph shows a tooth reflectometer and the intraoral positioning device whereby specular and diffuse readings are obtained in a reproducible manner. (Courtesy of Dr. Thomas Schiff, Monsanto Chemical Co., St. Louis, Missouri.)

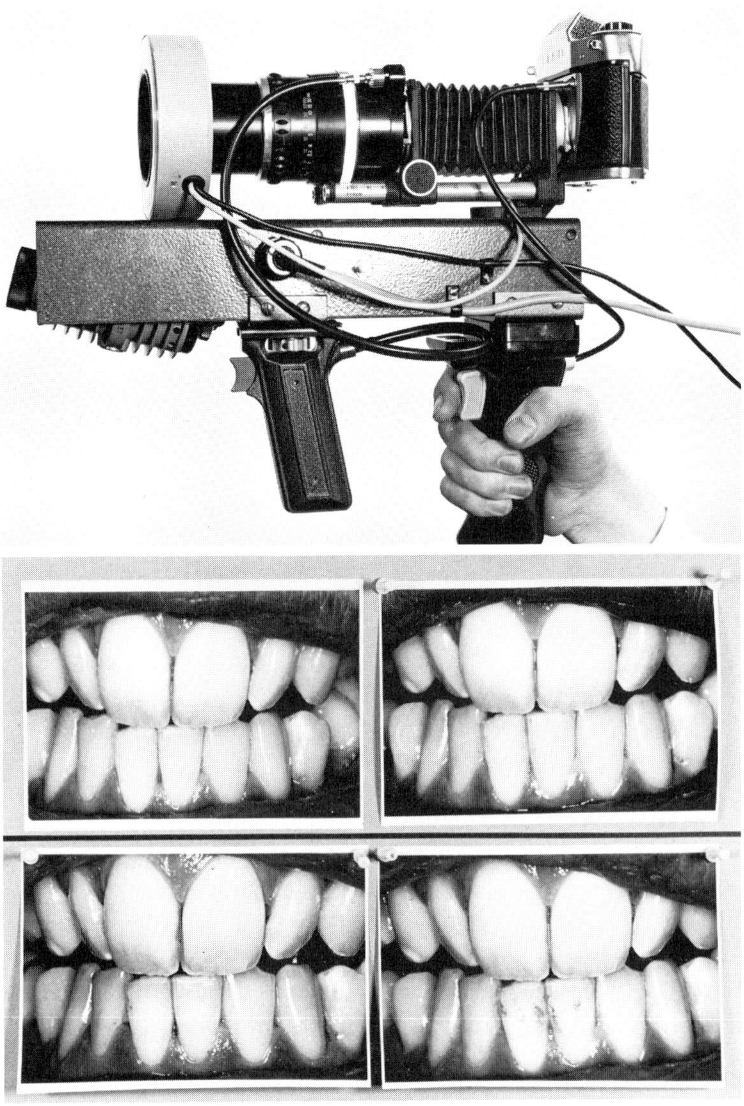

Figure 12–3 The upper portion of this photograph shows the camera that is used for intraoral photography. The lower portion depicts a representative series of photographs arranged for assessment. (Reproduced from Bull, W. H., Callendar, R. M., Pugh, B. R., and Wood, G. D.: Br. Dent. J. *124*:331–337, 1968.)

constructed intraoral photography apparatus to obtain reproducible pictures which were subsequently compared and assessed for the amount of stain that was present (Bull, Callender, Pugh and Wood, 1968). The camera equipment employed and some representative photographs are shown in Figure 12–3.

The effect of dentifrices on tooth stain has been evaluated *in vivo* through the use of a reproducible technic which subjectively assigns numerical values which represent equal increments of stain intensity (Lobene, 1968).

The *in vivo* clearance and removal of interproximal plaque have been evaluated through the use of specially constructed removable tooth slabs inset in full gold crowns (Henden, Keller and Manson-Hing, 1969; Keller and Manson-Hing, 1969).

An *in vivo* technic has been recently developed to investigate the actual abrasiveness of dentifrices by determining the effect of dentifrices against acrylic surfaces

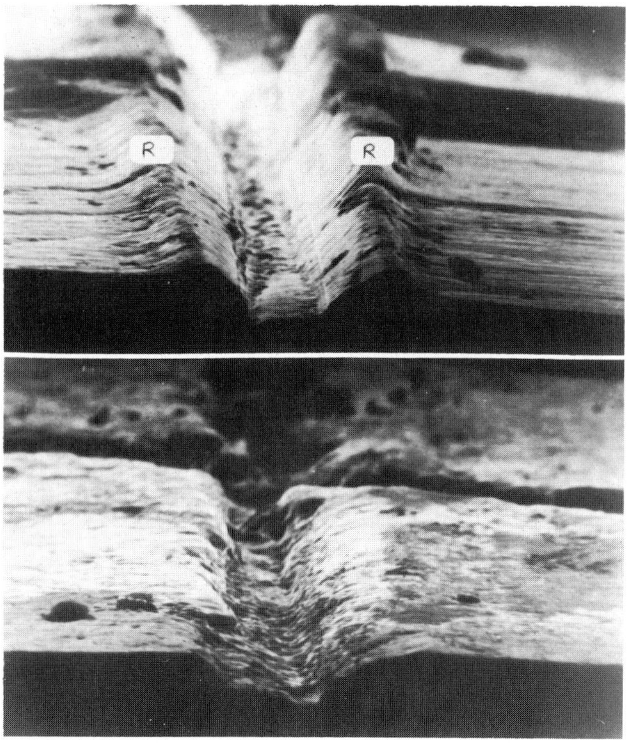

Figure 12–4 This photograph shows a cross-sectional view of the measurable arm of an indentation line in the acrylic surface of a veneer crown (500×). The upper photograph is before use of a dentifrice (R refers to the acrylic ridges created by the carving instrument). The lower photograph is after using a dentifrice for three weeks. Depth of indentation line in upper photograph is 12 microns; depth in lower photograph is 10 microns, indicating a loss of 2 microns due to the use of the dentifrice. (Reproduced from Facq, J. M., and Volpe, A. R.: J. Am. Dent. Assoc. *80*:317–323, [Feb.] 1970.)

of veneer crowns (Fig. 12–4). The technic consists of a tooth surface replication procedure and an evaluation of the obtained replica with a scanning electron microscope (Facq and Volpe, 1970).

Other *in vivo* tooth cleaning methods reported have included the use of tracer foods (Cobb, Hay and Schram, 1961; and Pinsent, 1962), standardized tooth surface replicas (Brasch, Lazarou, Van Abbé and Forrest, 1969), standardized photos (Wilkinson and Pugh, 1970) and a modified Lobene subjective scoring system (Van Abbé, Bridge, Ribbons, Dean and Lazarou, 1971).

The question constantly arises as to what is the optimal level of abrasiveness that a dentifrice should possess. This is a difficult question to answer because the abrasive needs of individuals vary to such a great extent. For example, persons with exposed cementum and dentin, or who have just undergone dental treatment procedures such as a gingivectomy, have need of a very mildly abrasive dentifrice. On the other hand, persons with healthy dentitions, periodontium and mucosal tissues can safely utilize much more abrasive dentifrices.

It is probably much more meaningful to define a minimum level of dentifrice abrasiveness rather than attempt to establish a maximum limit. The minimum dentifrice abrasive level for a particular person could be defined as that level which allowed for the efficient and thorough removal of dental plaque and which did not permit "brown pellicle" (or other similar type stains) to accumulate.

Probably the most realistic and meaningful approach to dentifrice abrasiveness is that which assigns the dentist the responsibility for determining the particular level of abrasiveness that a particular person requires (Robinson, 1969). This approach is referred to as "Individualizing dentifrices—the dentist's responsibility."

DETERGENTS (SURFACE-ACTIVE AGENTS)

Detergents are basically cleaning agents and when present in dentifrices probably exert their cleaning effect by the following actions: (1) lowering the surface tension, (2) penetrating and loosening surface deposits, and (3) emulsifying and suspending the debris, which the dentifrice then removes from the tooth surfaces. Additionally, detergents provide dentifrices with the foaming (or sudsing) characteristic that is so popular (and expected) by almost all dentifrice purchasers.

In the early days of dentifrice manufacture, soap was the most commonly used detergent. However, soap-containing dentifrices had a relatively high alkaline pH and thus were sometimes irritating to the oral soft tissues. Also, the use of soap as a detergent greatly limited the selection of cleaning and polishing agents that could be used in the dentifrice.

All dentifrices currently available in the United States use synthetic detergents. Synthetic detergents have the following major advantages in comparison to soap: (1) compatability with many cleaning and polishing agents, thus permitting greater flexibility in the formulation of the dentifrice, (2) lack of the characteristic soapy taste, and (3) provision for the formulation of a dentifrice with a more neutral pH, resulting in no alkaline irritation to the oral soft tissues. The three most commonly used synthetic detergents are:

Sodium lauryl sulfate
$$\left(CH_3(CH_2)_{10}CH_2OSO_3Na\right)$$

Sodium N-lauroyl sarcosinate
$$\left(CH_3(CH_2)_{10}CON(CH_3)CH_2COONa\right)$$

Sodium cocomonoglyceride sulfonate
$$\left(RCOOCH_2CH(OH)CH_2SO_3Na\right)$$

Sodium lauryl sulfate is probably the most widely used dentifrice detergent. In addition to its excellent detergent properties, sodium lauryl sulfate (and other detergents) possesses some antibacterial characteristics.

Sodium N-lauroyl sarcosinate, another widely used detergent, is, in addition to having excellent detergent properties, an effective enzyme inhibitor. Dentifrices containing this inhibitor have been evaluated in several human caries clinical studies which are discussed in the Therapeutic Dentifrices section of this report.

HUMECTANTS

The primary function of a humectant in a dentifrice is to retain moisture and thus provide for a paste that is chemically and physically stable, even if the cap on the tube is not closed and the dentifrice is exposed to air. Honey was the original humectant used, but this was gradually replaced by more satisfactory materials. The most commonly utilized dentifrice humectants are glycerin, sorbitol and propylene glycol. Both glycerin and sorbitol have a sweet taste, and thus also function to some extent as sweetening agents in the dentifrice. Since aqueous solutions of some glycols can permit bacterial or mold growth, preservatives such as sodium benzoate are often added to the humectant solution.

BINDING AGENTS

The physical blending or mixing of the liquid and solid phases of a dentifrice may be inadequate to prevent separation, particularly during storage. The function of the binding agent in the dentifrice formulation is to prevent separation by providing a stable suspension. Basically, all binders are hydrophilic colloids which appear to dissolve but actually disperse, swell or absorb water to form viscous liquid phases. Thus, the binder stabilizes the dentifrice against separation by increasing the consistency of the mixture of liquid and solid phases.

The first binder used in dentifrices was starch. Natural tree exudations such as gum arabic and tragacanth then became prominent as binders. Since 1940, seaweed colloids, such as Irish moss extract, and the sodium alginates have been widely used. Additionally, the synthetically prepared water-dispersible derivatives of cellulose, such as sodium carboxymethylcellulose, and a complex colloidal magnesium aluminum silicate are also in wide use as dentifrice binders.

The binder of choice depends upon the composition of the dentifrice and the desired ease of dispersion of the dentifrice in the oral cavity. It must also be chemically stable toward the other ingredients. As is the case with humectants, aqueous dispersions of the binders require preservation against microbial or mold contamination.

FLAVORING AGENTS

The taste of a dentifrice is probably one of the most important factors in reference to the purchase and continuous use of a particular product. Market research and experience have shown that the majority of consumers will not re-purchase and continue to use a particular dentifrice solely because it will provide a therapeutic (or drug-related) benefit. The product must also be pleasant to use and refreshing to the taste. This may be referred to as the "cosmetic aspects of a therapeutic dentifrice" and is of great importance to the dentifrice manufacturers.

At times, some patients are advised to clean their dentition with mildly abrasive substances such as sodium chloride or sodium bicarbonate, rather than through use of conventional dentifrices. Although the use of these mildly abrasive substances is justifiably warranted in special situations and will be of some value in cleaning the dentition, it is extremely unlikely that a person will continuously utilize these relatively bland materials over a long period of time.

This was shown quite convincingly in a clinical study conducted to determine patients' reactions to brushing their teeth with either water, a powder composed of table salt and baking soda, or a conventional dentifrice (Dudding, Dahl and Muhler, 1960). The general reaction of the participants who used either water or the salt/soda powder was most unfavorable. By contrast, in the group using a conventional flavored dentifrice, the great majority of the participants stated that they preferred this method.*

The development of an acceptable flavor for a dentifrice is both an art and a science. Some of the most commonly used essential flavoring oils include spearmint, peppermint, wintergreen, cinnamon and anise. Most dentifrices are produced by blending the various essential oils. It is interesting to note that flavor preferences vary considerably from country to country.

MISCELLANEOUS DENTIFRICE INGREDIENTS AND PACKAGING

Water is the most important of the remaining ingredients. Deionized or distilled water is utilized. As previously mentioned, preservatives such as one of the parahydroxy benzoates are common dentifrice ingredients. In addition to naturally sweet humectants, such as glycerin and sorbitol, sodium saccharin is also used as a sweetening agent.

The dentifrice formulation may also contain tube-corrosion inhibitors, such as sodium silicate, approved food colors and traces of titanium dioxide, which is used as a whitening agent. In the case of dentifrices containing dicalcium phosphate as the principal cleaning and polishing agent, tetrasodium pyrophosphate is often used as a stabilizer to prevent hardening.

Oxygen salts, such as hydrogen peroxide, sodium perborate and magnesium peroxide, are sometimes used to enhance the stain-removing properties of dentifrices. The efficacy of these materials, however, has not been established, and it has been

*Recently, a standard type toothpaste product (Peak), which has sodium bicarbonate as the principal cleaning and polishing agent and a conventional dentifrice flavor, has become available. This represents an attempt by the manufacturer to combine the mildly abrasive properties of sodium bicarbonate with conventional dentifrice characteristics, such as form, flavor and foaming ability.

suggested that their long-term effect on the oral soft tissues may be injurious.

In regard to packaging, most dentifrices are placed into either plain or epoxy-lined, fully collapsible aluminum tubes. One major manufacturer uses a semicollapsible polylaminate (plastic) tube.

OTHER PHYSICAL FORMS

The previous discussion has been primarily concerned with dentifrices in their most common form, that is, toothpaste. As previously stated, other physical forms of dentifrices include power and liquid.

Toothpowders contain essentially the same ingredients as toothpaste, with the exception of water, humectants or binders. Their capacity to clean or polish teeth (abrasivity) would depend, to a great extent, on the degree of dilution (essentially water) that is used with them.

Liquid dentifrices, such as some "tooth polishers," also contain ingredients similar to those in toothpaste. However, they have a lesser amount of binder and thus flow more freely. Some liquid dentifrices have been formulated without detergents and thus lack conventional foaming characteristics. In general, liquid dentifrices may not be sufficiently abrasive to maintain tooth cleanliness, especially if they do not contain conventional quantities of cleaning and polishing agents.

THERAPEUTIC (OR DRUG-CONTAINING) DENTIFRICES

DEFINITION AND IMPLICATIONS

A therapeutic dentifrice may be described as one that contains a drug substance which has been incorporated into the formulation in an effort to produce a beneficial effect upon the oral tissues. This beneficial effect can be produced upon either the hard tissues (tooth surfaces) or the soft tissues (gingiva) and can be achieved by chemical, physiological or pharmacological means. The two most important and beneficial oral health effects that can be attributed to a therapeutic dentifrice are (1) the prevention or reduction of the incidence of dental caries formation, and (2) the prevention or reversal of gingival disease.

When a manufacturer is considering the incorporation of a drug substance into a dentifrice formulation for the purpose of obtaining a therapeutic claim, the nature of the particular drug substance to be utilized is very important. If the drug substance is one that would be generally regarded as safe and efficacious by experts (in respect to a particular formulation and a particular therapeutic claim), then the marketing of this dentifrice probably can be accomplished within a reasonable period of time and with a reasonable financial expenditure.

However, if the drug substance of interest is one that would not be generally regarded as safe and efficacious by experts, then the material is classified as a "new drug substance." As such, the manufacturer is required to comply with stringent Food and Drug Administration regulations in an effort to establish and document the safety and efficacy of the dentifrice containing the new drug substance.

The Food and Drug Administration regulations require that extensive laboratory and clinical evaluations be conducted and the results submitted as part of a New Drug Application. This New Drug Application must be approved by the Food and Drug Administration prior to the marketing of the dentifrice. In the case of a therapeutic dentifrice with a caries-reducing claim (which is the major therapeutic claim utilized with current dentifrices), this could be a very long and very costly procedure. This situation occurs because caries clinical studies are usually conducted over a 2 to 3 year period of time, and several such studies may be required.

DEVELOPMENT OF A THERAPEUTIC DENTIFRICE

The development of a therapeutic (containing a new drug) dentifrice, in general, is a very expensive and lengthy endeavor. When a material is either obtained from a natural source or synthesized, and is suspected to be of oral disease preventive value, it is generally subjected to the following evaluation sequence:

1. Laboratory *in vitro* screening procedures to determine the specific activity of the material (for example, antimicrobial, enzymatic, enamel solubility reducer, etc.).
2. Animal *in vivo* experiments to determine the ability of the material to reduce or prevent oral disease (such as caries or gingivitis) in an experimental animal model system.
3. Animal *in vivo* investigations to ascertain the relative toxicity of the material so as to determine at an early stage whether any serious problems exist or can be anticipated.
4. Short-term (carefully monitored and supervised) *in vivo* human studies to determine the pharmacological and metabolic pattern of the material.
5. Laboratory experiments to produce an acceptable and stable formulation (dentifrice, mouth rinse, etc.).
6. Short-term *in vivo* human clinical studies to evaluate a specific activity, such as the ability of the formulation to reduce dental plaque formation, to reduce the solubility of enamel, to prevent plaque pH decreases, to inhibit specific microorganisms, etc.
7. Short-term *in vivo* human clinical studies to evaluate the effect of the formulation on a specific oral disease parameter, such as gingivitis.
8. Additional (and long-term) animal *in vivo* toxicological evaluations so as to determine whether more extensive clinical investigations can be safely conducted in humans.
9. Long-term *in vivo* human clinical studies to establish and document the safety and efficacy of the formulation.

The Food and Drug Administration (FDA) is notified of a sponsor's intention to conduct *in vivo* human clinical investigations with a new drug substance by means of a formal submission referred to as a Notice of Claimed Investigational Exemption for a New Drug (IND). The IND contains the complete details concerning the new drug substance and the clinical study to be conducted. At the completion of each human investigation, the sponsor submits a complete report to the FDA providing the results obtained from the study.

The regulations concerning the components and preparations of an IND are published in the United States Code of Federal Regulation (C.F.R. 21, Part 130). This publication also includes a complete description of the FDA's classification of clinical studies (Phase I—pharmacology, Phase II—pharmacology and therapeutics, and Phase III—extensive use studies).

The laboratory and animal screening procedures currently employed in the evaluation of oral disease preventive materials are discussed in detail in an excellent publication, Evaluation of Agents Used in the Prevention of Oral Disease, 1968. The fundamentals of well-designed and well-executed human clinical studies are also discussed, to some extent, in this publication. The conductance of caries clinical studies is discussed in four additional and equally excellent reports (American Dental Association, 1955, 1960 and 1968; Backer-Dirks, Baume, Davies and Slack, 1967; and Horowitz, 1972).

*AMERICAN DENTAL ASSOCIATION CLASSIFICATION**

The Council on Dental Therapeutics of the American Dental Association will consider for evaluation dentifrices and mouth rinses which make a therapeutic claim. Commercial products are examined either upon the request of the manufacturer

*The material in this section has been reproduced from *Accepted Dental Therapeutics*, 1975/1976 Edition.

or distributor or upon the initiative of the Council. Any firm may submit its appropriate products to the Council for consideration for acceptance. Products will be listed in Accepted Dental Therapeutics and described in suitable reports in the Journal of the American Dental Association if they meet standards of acceptance with respect to usefulness, composition, advertising and labeling. Products are usually accepted for three years. Acceptance is renewable and may be reconsidered at any time. After consideration of a new product has been completed, the Council will classify the product as *accepted, provisionally accepted* or *unaccepted.*

Accepted products include those for which there is adequate evidence of safety and effectiveness. They will be listed in *Accepted Dental Therapeutics* and may use the Seal of Acceptance.

Provisionally accepted includes those products for which there is reasonable evidence of usefulness and safety, but which lack sufficient evidence of dental usefulness to justify being *accepted.*

Unaccepted products include those for which the Council has determined that no substantial evidence of usefulness exists and those for which a question of safety exists.

NON-FLUORIDE THERAPEUTIC DENTIFRICES

Chlorophyll-Containing Dentifrices. The water-soluble derivatives have been used in dentifrices as caries-preventive materials, as well as gingival disease-preventive agents. Their use was based primarily on the ability of chlorophyll to reduce bacterial growth and to reduce the acid formed in dental plaque. The specific compound utilized is sodium copper chlorophyllin. Although human clinical caries studies have not been conducted with this compound, several animal (hamster) studies have indicated that it may have some anticaries potential.

Four clinical studies have been conducted to ascertain the effect of a dentifrice containing 0.1 per cent sodium copper chlorophyllin against gingival disease (Costich and Hein, 1952; McDonnell and Domalakes, 1952; Kutscher and Chilton, 1953; and Hein, 1954). Only one of these studies indicated that the material was of benefit against gingival disease.

The Council on Dental Therapeutics of the American Dental Association has previously indicated that the evidence available concerning chlorophyll-containing dentifrices is so limited or inconclusive that such products cannot accurately be evaluated. These dentifrices are not currently classified.

Antibiotic-Containing Dentifrices. A basic theory for the incorporation of antimicrobial substances into dentifrices is to destroy or inactivate the microorganisms that are associated with oral disease. Five clinical studies have been conducted to evaluate the anticariogenic effect of dentifrices and tooth powders containing penicillin, and one clinical study was conducted to evaluate a tyrothricin-containing dentifrice. The majority of the penicillin studies utilized a tooth powder, with the level of antibiotic ranging from 100 to 1000 units per gram of product. A summary of these clinical studies is presented in Table 12–3.

The results from these six studies (of which four provided a reduction in the incidence of caries) indicates that certain antibiotics are probably effective anticariogenic agents. However, there are two major deterrents to the routine use of antibiotics. They are as follows: (1) the possibility of allergic sensitization, and (2) the possibility of the development of resistant or cross-resistant strains of microorganisms.

The Council on Dental Therapeutics of the American Dental Association has indicated that because of the overwhelming disadvantages of the topical application of penicillin, its use for the local treatment of oral disease is contraindicated (Accepted Dental Therapeutics, 1975/1976). The use of antibiotics is also closely regulated by the Food and Drug Administration, who have expressed considerable opposition to the regular use and general availability (with-

TABLE 12–3* CLINICAL ANTICARIES STUDIES CONDUCTED UTILIZING ANTIBIOTIC-CONTAINING TOOTH POWDERS OR DENTIFRICES

INVESTIGATOR(S)	ANTIBIOTIC EVALUATED	DURATION OF STUDY	AGE RANGE	PER CENT REDUCTION IN CARIES
Hill and Kniesner, 1949	Penicillin	12 Months	8–15	None
Zander, 1950	Penicillin	24 Months	6–16	42 (DMFT) 56 (DMFS)
Walsh and Smart, 1951	Penicillin	12 Months	5–15	None
Hill, Sims and Newman, 1953†	Penicillin	12 Months	6–12	10 (DMFT) 16 (DMFS)
Lunin and Mandel, 1955	Penicillin	18 Months	School Children	14 (DMFT)
Shiere, 1957†	Tyrothricin	24 Months	7–14	26 (DMFS)

*Adapted from Wallace, 1962.
†These studies used a conventional dentifrice (toothpaste), while the other studies utilized a tooth powder.

out prescription) of all antibiotic-containing preparations.

The possibility exists that other antimicrobial agents may be able to accomplish the same purpose (destroy or inactivate microorganisms related to caries and gingival disease) and not have the undesirable characteristics of penicillin, mainly sensitization and resistance. Clinical investigations are currently being conducted in this area (discussed in the Mouth Rinse section).

Ammonium Containing Dentifrices. Urea and dibasic ammonium phosphate have been of considerable interest as anticariogenic materials since the late 1940's. Products containing these compounds were often referred to as "ammoniated dentifrices." Initially, it had been theorized that ammonia and urea might provide an anticariogenic effect by neutralizing the acid that was produced by the bacteria in dental plaque. Also, urea could function as an enzyme inhibitor by virtue of its protein-denaturant properties.

Many clinical studies were conducted with dentifrices containing either urea, dibasic ammonium phosphate or combinations of these substances. A summary of these clinical studies is presented in Table 12–4. As is apparent from the data, the majority of the studies, especially with the high-urea formulations, provided a beneficial anticariogenic effect. It has been indicated that a preliminary recommendation of a high urea-containing dentifrice would be consistent with the available data (Mandel and Cagan, 1964). The Council on Dental Therapeutics of the American Dental Association has not classified preferentially any dentifrice containing urea or urea and ammonium compounds as the active ingredients, since the evidence for the usefulness of these products is so contradictory that they cannot be accurately evaluated (Accepted Dental Therapeutics, 1975/1976).

Enzyme Inhibitor-Containing Dentifrices. In the late 1940's, a theory was presented which suggested that dental plaque might serve as a medium for the retention of enzyme inhibitors on the tooth surfaces, where they would be available to prevent the enzymatic conversion of sugar into acid. An *in vitro* procedure employing casein in a saliva-glucose medium was developed and used to screen many potential enzyme inhibitors, of which sodium N-lauroyl sarcosinate was discovered to be extremely effective (King, 1950; King, Manahan and Russell, 1957).

A modification of this procedure (artificially developed plaque being substituted for the casein) was used to evaluate ten compounds, of which only penicillin was retained in a sufficient concentration to inhibit acid production (Fosdick, Ludwig and Schantz, 1951). Further investigations substantiated the sarcosinate effect and suggested that sodium dehydroacetate was also effective (Fosdick, Calandra, Blackwell and Burrill, 1953).

The *in vivo* duration of the effectiveness of sodium N-lauroyl sarcosinate has been evaluated using various procedures to measure changes that occurred in the

TABLE 12–4* CLINICAL ANTICARIES STUDIES CONDUCTED UTILIZING AMMONIUM-CONTAINING DENTIFRICES

INVESTIGATOR(S)	AMMONIUM COMPOUNDS(S)	DURATION OF STUDY	AGE RANGE	PER CENT REDUCTION IN CARIES
Stephan and Miller, 1944	45% Urea (Liquid Dentifrice)	16 Months	12–25	80–100 (DMFS)
Henschel and Lieber, 1949	22.5% Urea and 5% DBAP†	34 Months	17–55	38 (Lesions)
and 1952		49 Months		44 (Lesions)
Kerr and Kesel, 1951	3% Urea and 5% DBAP	24 Months	10–11	11 (DMFT)
Davies and King, 1951‡	3% Urea and 5% DBAP	8 Months	12–31	None
Gale, 1951	12% Urea and 5% DBAP	21 Months	Preschool	33 (DMFT)
Lefkowitz and Venti, 1951	High Urea	18 Months	5–19	60 (DMFT)
Backer-Dirks, Winkler and Van Aken, 1953	3% Urea and 5% DBAP	18 Months	10–14	None
Hawes and Bibby, 1953‡	12% Urea and 1% Urease	12–15 Months	7–13	None
Cohen and Donzanti, 1954	13% Urea and 3% DBAP	24 Months	9–13	25 (DMFT)
Vogel and Hess, 1957	13% Urea and 3% DBAP	14 Months	11–12	28 (Lesions)

*Adapted from Wallace, 1962 and Mandel and Cagan, 1964.
†DBAP refers to dibasic ammonium phosphate.
‡These studies used tooth powders, while the other (except Stephan and Miller) used a conventional dentifrice.

pH of plaque material that formed on proximal surfaces of non-carious teeth (Forscher and Hess, 1954; Brudevold, Little and Rowley, 1955; Hein, 1955; and Hassell and Mühlemann, 1971). There is general agreement that acid production is effectively inhibited immediately after use of sodium N-lauroyl sarcosinate, but results in reference to duration of effectiveness have ranged from 2 to 12 hours.

The retention of sodium N-lauroyl sarcosinate has also been demonstrated by other techniques, including the use of C^{14} labeled sarcosinate (Allison and Nelson, 1958), and the use of a dentin chip placed into a removable prosthetic device (Tomlinson and Davies, 1962). Although this compound has been shown to reduce caries formation in animals, the results have not always been comparable (Rosenthal, Marson and Abriss, 1954; Zipkin and McClure, 1955; Volker, Apperson and King, 1956; and Keyes and White, 1959).

One clinical study has been conducted to evaluate the caries inhibitory effect of a dentifrice containing a combination of 0.75 per cent sodium dehydroacetate and 0.5 per cent sodium oxalate (Sulser, Fosket and Fosdick, 1958). The two-year results indicated an approximately 50 per cent reduction in new carious lesions.

Dentifrices containing 2.0 per cent sodium N-lauroyl sarcosinate as the anticaries agent have been evaluated in several human clinical studies. A summary of five long-term studies comparing this dentifrice to a control dentifrice is presented in Table 12–5A. As is apparent from the data, the sarcosinate-containing dentifrice provided a reduction in caries in a majority of the studies. Another clinical study conducted over a two-year period of time indicated that a combination of sodium N-lauroyl sarcosinate and sodium N-palmitoyl sarcosinate provided a 17 per cent reduction in caries (Emslie, 1963).

Five long-term clinical studies in which a dentifrice containing 2.0 per cent sodium N-lauroyl sarcosinate was compared with a positive control dentifrice (0.4 per cent stannous fluoride in a calcium pyrophosphate formulation) are summarized in Table 12–5B. In the majority of these studies, there was no statistically significant difference between the two dentifrices. A one-year clinical study has also been reported which indicated that the positive control was significantly better than the sarcosinate dentifrice (Muhler, 1970).

The data from the caries clinical studies evaluating a dentifrice containing 2.0 per cent sodium N-lauroyl sarcosinate indicate some effectiveness in reducing the incidence of new carious surfaces. Further evaluation of the data on an individual tooth surface basis has indicated that the denti-

TABLE 12–5 CLINICAL ANTICARIES STUDIES CONDUCTED UTILIZING SODIUM N-LAUROYL SARCOSINATE-CONTAINING DENTIFRICES

A. Comparisons with a Control Dentifrice

INVESTIGATOR(S)	DURATION OF STUDY	SPECIAL CONDITIONS	AGE RANGE	PER CENT REDUCTION IN CARIES (DMFS)
Fosdick, 1956	24 Months		17–35	47*
Frasher and Hein, 1958	27 Months	Fluoridated Water	4–12	43*
Backer-Dirks, Kwant and Starmans, 1959	20 Months	Supervised Brushing and Controlled Diet	10–13	4
Mergele, 1968A	36 Months	Fluoridated Water	9–13	4
Zacheral, 1970	24 Months	5–10 Bite Wing X-rays	Elem. School	−15
B. Comparisons with a Stannous Fluoride–Calcium Pyrophosphate Dentifrice				
Finn and Jamison, 1963	24 Months	Supervised Brushing and Controlled Diet	8–15	−2
Frankl and Alman, 1968	36 Months		8–14	3
Mergele, 1968A	36 Months	Fluoridated Water	9–13	−10
Homan and Messer, 1969	20 Months		7 13	0 to −2 −12 to −16
Zacherl, 1970	24 Months	5–10 Bite Wing X-rays	Elem. School	−39*

*Difference is statistically significant at the 95% level of confidence.

frice is more effective on pit and fissure surfaces than on smooth surfaces. This effect would be anticipated, since the sarcosinate is probably better retained (and not so readily washed away) in the pits and fissures as on the smooth surface areas.

The Council on Dental Therapeutics of the American Dental Association has indicated that evidence in support of anti-enzyme dentifrices is controversial and that the usefulness of these dentifrices in caries control has not been adequately established (Accepted Dental Therapeutics, 1975/1976).

*FLUORIDE-CONTAINING THERAPEUTIC DENTIFRICES**

Sodium Fluoride Dentifrices. As a result of the success achieved in reducing the incidence of dental decay through the use of fluoride compounds in communal water supplies and as topical solutions applied to the teeth, it was only natural that fluoride compounds be incorporated into dentifrices. The first such fluoride compound to be used in a dentifrice formulation was sodium fluoride.

The initial clinical studies conducted to evaluate dentifrices containing 0.22 per cent sodium fluoride indicated that the dentifrices were ineffective in reducing the incidence of dental caries (Bibby, 1945; Winkler, Backer-Dirks and Van Amerongen, 1953; Muhler, Radike, Nebergall, and Day, 1955; and Kyes, Overton and McKean, 1961). It has been theorized that these sodium fluoride clinical studies may have provided negative results because of the two following reasons: (1) basic incompatibilities in the dentifrice formulations, particularly the presence of calcium containing cleaning and polishing agents which rendered the fluoride compound inactive by forming insoluble calcium fluoride, and

*Three excellent review publications are available which contain discussions concerning the subject of fluoride-containing therapeutic dentifrices (Peterson, 1968; Duckworth, 1968; and Heifetz and Horowitz, 1970).

(2) basic inadequacies in the design and conduction of the clinical studies (Grøn and Brudevold, 1967).

During the past decade, however, a number of clinical studies have been reported which indicate that dentifrices containing 0.22 per cent sodium fluoride may be effective anticaries materials when properly formulated and evaluated in properly designed and conducted clinical studies. A summary of these more recent clinical studies is presented in Table 12–6. The cleaning and polishing agents used in the different dentifrice formulations were all selected because of their compatibility with sodium fluoride.

The Council on Dental Therapeutics of the American Dental Association currently states that the early evidence to justify the inclusion of sodium fluoride in commercially available dentifrices is not convincing. They further indicate, however, that more recent reports of clinical studies with dentifrices containing sodium fluoride suggest that incompatibility is an important factor and that formulation modification can be made to provide products which will reduce the incidence of caries (Accepted Dental Therapeutics, 1975/1976).

A government notice has been issued which indicates that dentifrices containing sodium fluoride (as well as chlorophyllins, anti-enzymes and urea) lack substantial evidence of effectiveness in reference to therapeutic claims (Federal Register, 1970). This notice was based on a review conducted by the National Academy of Sciences–National Research Council (Drug Efficacy Study Group) of certain commercially available dentifrices that were the subject of approved New Drug Applications obtained prior to the enactment of the New Drug Relations of 1962, which required efficacy substantiation as well as safety data.

Stannous Fluoride Dentifrices. Stannous fluoride-containing dentifrices have been subjected to extensive clinical investigation. The most well-known stannous fluoride dentifrice contains 0.4 per cent stannous fluoride and calcium pyrophosphate as the cleaning and polishing agent. Calcium pyrophosphate was selected because it was found to be more compatible with stannous fluoride; that is, it did not inactivate the

TABLE 12–6 RECENT CLINICAL ANTICARIES STUDIES CONDUCTED UTILIZING SODIUM FLUORIDE-CONTAINING DENTIFRICES

INVESTIGATOR(S)	TYPE OF FORMULATION	DURATION OF STUDY	AGE RANGE	PER CENT REDUCTION IN CARIES (DMFS)
Torell and Ericsson, 1965A	Sodium bicarbonate	24 Months	10–11	18
Brudevold and Chilton, 1966	Dicalcium phosphate Dihydrate			6
	Insoluble sodium metaphosphate (IMP) and sodium orthophosphate	24 Months	10–19	19
Koch, 1967 and 1970*	Plastic abrasive (methacrylate polymer)	36 Months	8–10	40
			11–12	48
Peterson and Williamson, 1968	IMP and sodium orthophosphate	36 Months	9–15	20
Zacherl, 1968	Calcium pyrophosphate	20 Months	7–14	28
Reed and King, 1970	Calcium pyrophosphate	24 Months	8–13	30
Weisenstein and Zacherl, 1972	Calcium pyrophosphate	21 Months	5–15	11–38

*Supervised brushing once per day.

TABLE 12-7 CLINICAL ANTICARIES STUDIES CONDUCTED UTILIZING A STANNOUS FLUORIDE-CALCIUM PYROPHOSPHATE DENTIFRICE

INVESTIGATOR(S)	DURATION OF STUDY	SPECIAL CONDITIONS	AGE RANGE	PER CENT REDUCTION IN CARIES (DMFS)
Muhler and Radike, 1957	24 Months		17–36	34
Jordan and Peterson, 1959	24 Months	Supervised School Brushing	8–12	21
Hill, 1959	24 Months		9–16	15
Peffley and Muhler, 1960	24 Months	Supervised Brushing–Military School	10–19	46
Kyes, Overton and McKean, 1961	24 Months	Naval Academy	17–24	8
Muhler, 1962	36 Months		6–18	21
Bixler and Muhler, 1962	24 Months	Supervised School Brushing	11–18	32
Henriques, Frankl and Alman, 1964	24 Months		5–12	13
Mergele, Jennings and Gasser, 1964	24 Months	Supervised School Brushing Fluoridated Water	8–15	9
Zacherl and McPhail, 1965	18 Months		Grades 1, 2, 7	40
Torell and Ericsson, 1965A	24 Months		10–11	23
Horowitz, Law, Thompson and Chamberlin, 1966	36 Months	Home Use Supervised School Brushing	6–10	17 21
Thomas and Jamison, 1966	24 Months	Supervised Brushing	7–16	36
Brudevold and Chilton, 1966	24 Months		10–19	4
Bixler and Muhler, 1966A	19 Months	Oral Hygiene Motivation Military and Boarding Schools	11–23	54
Jackson and Sutcliffe, 1967	36 Months		11–12	None (Males) 18 (Females)
James and Anderson, 1967	36 Months		11–12	16–24
Slack, Berman, Martin and Hardie, 1967	36 Months		11–13	None (Clinical) 36 (Radiographic)
Onishi, et. al., 1967	24 Months		Grade 1	13 (DMFT)
Peterson and Williamson, 1968	36 Months		9–15	25
Zacherl, 1968	20 Months		7–14	28
Zacherl, 1970	24 Months		Elem. School	30
Zacherl, 1972	20 Months	Fluoridated Water High-Beta Phase Abrasive	7–14	28
Zacherl, 1972A	24 Months	Dentifrice Aged One Year at Room Temperature	Grades 2–6	22

stannous fluoride as readily as did commonly used polishing agents such as calcium carbonate or dicalcium phosphate dihydrate. Extensive laboratory and clinical investigations were conducted by scientists from both the manufacturing company and Indiana University in an effort to develop this dentifrice. These investigations are discussed in three excellent publications (Radike, 1960; Muhler, 1965; and Accepted Dental Therapeutics, 1971/1972).

Many clinical studies have been published concerning 0.4 per cent stannous fluoride-calcium pyrophosphate dentifrices. A summary of some of the longer-term clinical studies comparing stannous fluoride-calcium pyrophosphate dentifrices with a control dentifrice is presented in Table 12–7. It is readily apparent that such dentifrices are effective in reducing the incidence of new carious surfaces. The variations in the magnitude of reductions are most likely due to different degrees of usage, different criteria of examiners and to the relative incidence between caries of smooth surfaces and pit or fissure surfaces. It is generally agreed that effectiveness is greater on smooth surfaces.

In addition to the studies listed in Table 12–7, several short-term studies (less than 18 months) have been conducted and show positive reductions compared to a control dentifrice (Muhler, Radike, Nebergall and Day, 1954, 1955 and 1956). There are also several clinical studies reported in which the stannous fluoride-calcium pyrophosphate dentifrice was evaluated in conjunction with other forms of fluoride therapy, such as prophylaxis pastes, topical solutions and fluoridated water (Muhler, 1959; Gish and Muhler, 1966; Bixler and Muhler, 1966; Muhler, Spear, Bixler and Stookey, 1967; and Scola and Ostrom, 1968). Such combined therapy has been shown to be effective, but it is generally difficult to assess the precise contribution of the fluoride dentifrice.

The Council on Dental Therapeutics of

the American Dental Association classified one stannous fluoride-calcium pyrophosphate dentifrice (Crest) as *provisionally*

Since 1960, three other stannous fluoride dentifrices have been classified as *provisionally accepted* by the Council on Dental Therapeutics of the American Dental Association (Cue, Fact and Super Stripe). *accepted* in August, 1960. In 1964, this classification was changed to *accepted,* which is the present classification. Thus, this was the first therapeutic dentifrice to receive the American Dental Association's Seal of Acceptance.
These dentifrices all contained 0.4 per cent stannous fluoride and utilized insoluble sodium metaphosphate as the principal cleaning and polishing agents. Stannous fluoride-insoluble sodium metaphosphate dentifrices are extremely stable, maintaining high soluble fluoride levels for relatively long periods of time.

Even though all three of these dentifrices were effective in regard to reducing caries and had been developed and clinically tested at considerable cost, they were removed from the market by their respective manufacturers because of an inability to promote them successfully to the consumer.

Clinical studies demonstrating the effectiveness of 0.4 per cent stannous fluoride-insoluble metaphosphate dentifrices, as compared to a control dentifrice, are summarized in Table 12–8. Also, five clinical studies have compared stannous fluoride-insoluble sodium metaphosphate dentifrices to a stannous fluoride-calcium pyrophosphate dentifrice (Henriques, Frankl and Alman, 1964; Mergele, Jennings and Gasser, 1964; Thomas and Jamison, 1966; Brudevold and Chilton, 1966; and Homan and Messer, 1969). The results suggest that the stannous fluoride-insoluble sodium metaphosphate dentifrice may be slightly more effective than the stannous fluoride-calcium pyrophosphate dentifrice.

The National Academy of Sciences–National Research Council also reviewed stannous fluoride dentifrices (with approved New Drug Applications) that were commercially available prior to the New Drug Regulations of 1962. The only such dentifrice available at that time was the stannous fluoride-calcium pyrophosphate dentifrice. The government (in the same notice previously referred to – Federal Register, 1970) indicated that there is substantial evidence that a dentifrice containing 0.4 per cent stannous fluoride in a suitable formulation is effective as an aid in reducing the incidence of dental caries.

The notice further states that because

TABLE 12–8 CLINICAL ANTICARIES STUDIES CONDUCTED WITH STANNOUS FLUORIDE-INSOLUBLE SODIUM METAPHOSPHATE-CONTAINING DENTIFRICES

INVESTIGATOR(S)	DURATION OF STUDY	AGE RANGE	MINOR AMOUNT OF CALCIUM COMPOUND	SPECIAL CONDITIONS	PER CENT REDUCTION IN CARIES (DMFS)
Henriques, Frankl and Alman, 1964	24 Months	5–12	Yes		17
Mergele, Jennings and Gasser, 1964	24 Months	8–15	Yes	Fluoridated Water/Supervised Brushing	16
Slack and Martin, 1964	24 Months	11–13	Yes	No Radiographs	None (Clinical)
Thomas and Jamison, 1966	24 Months	7–16	Yes	Supervised Brushing/ Controlled Diet	37
Brudevold and Chilton, 1966	24 Months	10–19	No		25
Segal, Stiff, George and Picozzi, 1966	24 Months	7–12	Yes	Supervised Brushing	25 (DFS)
Fullmer, Volpe, Apperson and Kiraly, 1966	36 Months	8–10	Yes		30
Naylor and Emslie, 1967	36 Months	11–13	Yes		15
Slack, Berman, Martin and Young, 1967	36 Months	11–13	Yes	Supervised Brushing	None (Clinical) 28 (Radiographs)
Fanning, Gotjamanos and Vowles, 1968	24 Months	11–13	No		22
Mergele, 1968	22 Months	7–21	No	Supervised Brushing	9

the other ingredients in a stannous fluoride dentifrice may have a role in modifying the effectiveness of the products in reducing the incidence of dental caries, the usefulness of a specific formulation must be determined on the basis of adequate data. Adequate data is defined as data to assure that, in the formulation to be marketed, the fluoride ion is available for incorporation into the structure of the teeth or other data providing substantial evidence of clinical effectiveness.

Sodium Monofluorophosphate Dentifrices. Sodium monofluorophosphate-containing dentifrices have been extensively evaluated in laboratory and clinical investigations. The most well-known dentifrice (and the only one currently available throughout the United States) contains 0.76 per cent sodium monofluorphosphate and insoluble sodium metaphosphate as the cleaning and polishing agent.

Sodium monofluorophosphate (Na_2PO_3F) could be considered a more advantageous fluoride agent than stannous fluoride (SnF_2) because of the following factors:

1. Na_2PO_3F has a more neutral pH than SnF_2 (Na_2PO_3F dentifrices have an approximate pH range of 5.5 to 6.5, while SnF_2 dentifrices have a pH of approximately 4.8).
2. Na_2PO_3F has greater stability to oxidation and hydrolysis than SnF_2.
3. Na_2PO_3F has greater compatibility with calcium-containing cleaning and polishing agents used in dentifrices (as indicated by the clinical studies presented in Table 12–9).
4. Na_2PO_3F-containing dentifrices do not stain teeth as do SnF_2 dentifrices (Naylor and Emslie, 1967; Fanning, Gotjamanos, Vowles and Van Der Wielen, 1968A).
5. Na_2PO_3F dentifrices have been shown to reduce the incidence of tooth hypersensitivity (Bolden, Volpe, and King, 1968; Hazen, Volpe and King, 1968; Kanouse and Ash, 1969; Shapiro, Kaslick, Chasens and Weinstein, 1970; and Hérnandez, Mohammed, Shannon, Volpe and King, 1972).
6. Some clinical studies suggest that a Na_2PO_3F-insoluble sodium metaphosphate dentifrice may provide more caries protection than a SnF_2-calcium pyrophosphate dentifrice (Finn and Jamison, 1963; Frankl and Alman, 1968; and Mergele, 1968A).

Sodium monofluorophosphate is especially unique in that its calcium salt is relatively soluble as compared with calcium fluoride, which is almost completely insoluble and inert. Calcium fluoride is the insoluble and inactive salt that is found when either stannous fluoride or sodium fluoride are in the presence of calcium ions. This property of not being readily inactivated by calcium permits sodium monofluorophosphate to be used in a variety of dentifrice-abrasive formulations without loss of efficacy. In contrast, stannous fluoride and sodium fluoride are incompatible with such common cleaning and polishing agents as calcium carbonate and dicalcium phosphate because of the formation of insoluble and inactive calcium fluoride. A summary of the clinical studies conducted with various sodium monofluorophosphate-containing dentifrices is presented in Table 12–9.

In 1969, the Council on Dental Therapeutics of the American Dental Association classified a sodium monofluorophosphate-insoluble sodium metaphosphate dentifrice (Colgate Dental Cream with MFP) as *accepted,* which is its present classification. Thus, this dentifrice, too, has received the American Dental Association's Seal of Acceptance.

Additionally, the Food and Drug Administration approved a New Drug Application submitted in reference to this same sodium monofluorophosphate-insoluble sodium metaphosphate dentifrice in 1967. This approval was granted on the basis of an extensive review of the laboratory and clinical data that was submitted to the Food and Drug Administration to substantiate and

TABLE 12-9 CLINICAL ANTICARIES STUDIES CONDUCTED UTILIZING SODIUM MONOFLUOROPHOSPHATE-CONTAINING DENTIFRICES*

INVESTIGATOR(S)	CLEANING AND POLISHING AGENT	DURATION OF STUDY	AGE RANGE	PER CENT REDUCTION IN CARIES (DMFS)
Finn and Jamison, 1963†	Insoluble Sodium Metaphosphate	24 Months	8–15	27**
Torell and Ericsson, 1965B	Calcium Carbonate	24 Months	11	15
			10	6
Naylor and Emslie, 1967	Dicalcium Phosphate (dihydrate)	36 Months	11–12	18
Fanning, Gotjamanos and Vowles, 1968	Insoluble Sodium Metaphosphate	24 Months	11–13	20
Møller, Holst and Sørensen, 1968	Insoluble Sodium Metaphosphate	30 Months	10–12	19
Thomas, 1968†	Insoluble Sodium Metaphosphate	24 Months	8–16	34
Mergele, 1968†	Insoluble Sodium Metaphosphate	22 Months	7–21	21
Mergele, 1968A‡	Insoluble Sodium Metaphosphate	36 Months	8–14	17
Frankl and Alman, 1968	Insoluble Sodium Metaphosphate	36 Months	6–15	11**
Takeuchi, Schimizu, Kawasaki and Kizu, 1968	Dicalcium Phosphate (dihydrate)	12 Months	Grades 3 and 4	24
Kinkel and Stolte, 1968	Insoluble Sodium Metaphosphate	24 Months	6–13	25–33
Torell, 1969	Calcium Carbonate	20 Months	Grade 4	29
Patz and Naujoks, 1969	Insoluble Sodium Metaphosphate	24 Months	18–28	22 (Maxillary Pre-molars)
				8 (Overall)
Onisi and Tani, 1970	Dicalcium Phosphate (dihydrate)	12 Months	Elem. School	16 (Pits and Fissures)
				41 (Smooth Surfaces)
Zacherl, 1972‡	Calcium Pyrophosphate	20 Months	7–14	23
Gerdin, 1972	Calcium Carbonate	24 Months	12	5 (Compared to a NaF Dentifrice)
Kinkel and Raich, 1972	Dicalcium Phosphate (dihydrate)	36 Months	School	37–46
and 1974		48 Months	Children	32–38
Lind, Møller, Von Der Fehr and Larsen, 1974‡§	Aluminum Oxide	36 Months	8–11	32 (Clinical plus X-ray)
Hargreaves and Chester, 1973 and 1974§	Aluminum Oxide	36 Months	5	23
			8	8
			11	23
Kinkel, Stole and Weststrate, 1974	Dicalcium Phosphate (dihydrate) (Also contained 2% Sodium Trimetaphosphate)	36 Months	School Children	17–38 (Unsupervised)
				35–43 (Supervised)
Andlaw and Tucker, 1975	Aluminum Oxide	36 Months	11–12	19 (Overall)
Mainwaring and Naylor, 1975	Calcium Carbonate	24 Months	11–12	31 (X-ray)
Peterson and Williamson, 1975‡	Calcium Carbonate	32 Months	8–12	23
Downer, Holloway and Davies, 1975	Calcium Carbonate (Also AFP topical and prophy paste)	36 Months	11	56 (Erupting teeth)

*Adapted from Volpe, 1968.
**These two particular reductions were obtained versus a stannous fluoride-calcium pyrophosphate dentifrice (positive control dentifrice).
†Supervised brushing and controlled diet.
‡Fluoridated water.
§These two studies evaluated 2% sodium monofluorophosphate dentifrices. All the other studies evaluated dentifrices containing approximately 0.76% of the fluoride compound.

document the safety and anticaries efficacy of this dentifrice. Since the safety and efficacy of this particular dentifrice were established under the New Drug Regulations of 1962, it was not necessary for it to be reviewed by the National Academy of Sciences—National Research Council (as were sodium fluoride- and stannous fluoride-containing dentifrices).

Other Fluoride Dentifrices. A dentifrice containing an organic fluoride compound has been investigated in at least two clinical studies thus far. The dentifrice (Elmex) contains amine fluorides, and the principal cleaning and polishing agent is insoluble sodium metaphosphate. These fluoride compounds were selected for clinical evaluation because laboratory and animal investigations had indicated that they might provide better anticaries protection (fluoride plus antibacterial activity) than sodium fluoride. This comparison of fluoride compounds is discussed in an excellent publication (König and Mühlemann, 1961).

The dentifrice contains 0.125 per cent fluoride, which is provided by the following materials:

1. diethanol aminoprophyl-N-ethanol octa-decylamine-dihydrofluoride (1.51 per cent of this compound equals 0.1 per cent fluoride), and
2. cetylamine hydrofluoride (0.40 per cent of this compound equals 0.025 per cent fluoride).

The results reported thus far from two long-term clinical studies are very encouraging. In the first study, which progressed for seven years, the amine fluoride dentifrice provided a 23 to 35 per cent reduction in caries (Marthaler, 1968). In the second study, which was a six-year investigation, the dentifrice provided a 33 per cent reduction in caries (Marthaler, 1974).

Several recent three-year clinical studies have been reported, wherein a dentifrice (Magnaforte) containing 0.45 per cent potassium fluoride and 0.14 per cent manganese chloride (formulated with a methacrylate abrasive) has been shown to be slightly superior to a dentifrice containing 0.22 per cent sodium fluoride (Gerdin, 1972; Koch, 1972). Further studies are necessary in order to determine the actual caries-inhibiting potential of this combination of agents.

DENTIFRICES FOR PERIODONTAL DISEASE

Thus far, the discussion of dentifrices has been primarily concerned with their effect on the incidence of caries. As stated, dentifrices can have a beneficial effect on caries, either through removal of bacterial plaque (cosmetic/therapeutic function), or through the application of drug substances, such as various fluoride compounds (therapeutic function).

Since plaque accumulation is also associated with the onset of such entities as calculus and gingivitis, its thorough and efficient removal by a dentifrice (cosmetic/therapeutic function) can also have a beneficial effect on calculus formation and gingival health.

In this regard, the Council on Dental Therapeutics of the American Dental Association recognizes the importance of home care in the control of dental plaque and indicates that the brushing of the teeth and gingiva has been the home care procedure most widely recommended to promote their cleanliness. The Council further states that the basic purpose of toothbrushing is to remove oral accumulations of plaque and debris, and thereby assist in the prevention of dental disease (Accepted Dental Therapeutics, 1975/1976).

At the present time, no commercially available dentifrice in the United States makes a direct drug-related (therapeutic function) claim in regard to the prevention of plaque, calculus or gingivitis. However, many agents are currently under investigation with regard to their effect on these parameters. These agents, some of which are very promising, include quaternary ammonium compounds, antibiotics, biguanides, enzymes, organic fluorides, etc. Although these materials are evaluated to some extent in dentifrices, they are, for the most part, initially evaluated in mouth rinse formulations, since this vehicle provides the fewest problems concerning ingredient compatibility and overall product stability.

For this reason, a more complete discussion of drug substances which have been shown to affect plaque, calculus and gingivitis is presented in the Therapeutic Mouth Rinse section of this report.

DENTIFRICES FOR HYPERSENSITIVE TEETH

Two dentifrices have been available which specifically claim to have a beneficial effect on hypersensitive teeth. One dentifrice (Sensodyne) contains 10 per cent strontium chloride as the active agent, and the other dentifrice (Thermodent) contains 1.4 per cent formalin as the active agent. In either case, the precise mechanism of action is not known. Both of these dentifrices have been evaluated in a variety of clinical studies, many of which have indicated that they do provide a desensitizing effect.

The Council on Dental Therapeutics of the American Dental Association indicates that it has not seen adequate evidence to justify claims for dentifrices that are promoted to provide relief from hypersensitive teeth (Accepted Dental Therapeutics, 1975/1976).

It should also be mentioned that a dentifrice (Colgate Dental Cream with MFP) containing 0.76 per cent sodium monofluorophosphate has also been clinically shown to have desensitization properties, in addition to its well-known anticaries effect.*

DENTIFRICES WITH SPECIALIZED FUNCTIONS

A specialized ingestible dentifrice has been developed in response to the specific needs of astronauts while on space missions. This ingestible dentifrice, designed to assist in maintaining oral hygiene during prolonged periods of chamber confinement, was developed at the United States Air Force School of Aerospace Medicine (Brooks Air Force Base, San Antonio, Texas) under the direction and supervision of Col. Ira L. Shannon.†

The ingestible dentifrice was formulated within the following imposed limitations: (1) no volatile oils, (2) no detergent (or foaming agent), and (3) low calcium content. The ingestible dentifrice contains the following ingredients: insoluble sodium metaphosphate (40 per cent), dicalcium phosphate dihydrate (2.6 per cent), glycerin (32 per cent), carboxymethylcellulose (1.3 per cent), saccharin (0.1 per cent), and distilled water (24 per cent). The specific method of preparation of this ingestible dentifrice is provided in a separate report (Shannon, 1966).

*These clinical studies have previously been referred to in the Sodium Monofluorophosphate section of this report.

†Dr. Shannon is Chief, Special Laboratory for Research in Oral Physiology, Veterans Administration Hospital, 2002 Holcombe Boulevard, Houston, Texas, 77031.

A clinical study was conducted which indicated that this ingestible dentifrice was equivalent to a commercially available dentifrice in reference to patient acceptance and cleaning performance (Terry and Shannon, 1968). This study also indicated that the ingestible dentifrice has potential for employment not only by isolated subjects, but also for hospital use in the maintenance of oral hygiene in the physically or mentally handicapped patients.

DENTIFRICES AND THE ORAL TISSUES

From time to time, questions are raised concerning the possible adverse effects of dentifrices on the dentition and mucosal tissues.

EFFECTS ON DENTITION

In regard to the dentition, this subject has been discussed to some extent in the section concerning cleaning and polishing agents. As stated previously, it is very difficult to predict with any accuracy the degree of abrasivity that a dentifrice will exhibit under actual *in vivo* use conditions. This is because of the great extent of variation from person to person—especially with regard to degree of exposed cementum and dentin, frequency and method of toothbrushing, type of toothbrush, diet characteristics, masticatory forces and other such factors.

Nor is it feasible to directly correlate laboratory data (such as RDA values) to the actual clinical situation. In one long-term clinical study (54 months), two groups of 60 subjects each used dentifrices which ranged from an RDA of 260 to an RDA of 460. The study was supervised, and each subject's dentition was exposed to his respective dentifrice for a total of approximately 45 hours during the course of the study. Careful clinical examinations at three-month intervals indicated that neither of the dentifrices caused any adverse reactions of the oral mucosal tissues and that both groups of subjects had similar patterns and levels of cervical abrasion and/or erosion (Volpe,

Mooney, Zumbrunnen, Stahl and Goldman, 1974).

Also, these same two dentifrices (RDA of 260 and RDA of 460) were studied in another long-term clinical investigation (24 months) to determine their comparative effect on selected dental materials. Again, careful periodic clinical examinations indicated that neither dentifrice produced any abnormal or unusual effect on the surface characteristics of either acrylic or silicate anterior restorations, or the acrylic surfaces of veneer crowns (Schiff and Volpe, 1975).

To further complicate the matter, evidence is now coming forth that strongly suggests that the toothbrush used, as well as the duration and method of toothbrushing employed, may play as important a role in regard to tooth wear as the dentifrices themselves (Workshop Conference on the Physical Functionality of Dentifrices, 1974).

As previously mentioned, this author feels that the most realistic and meaningful approach to dentifrice abrasivity is that which assigns the dentist responsibility for determining the particular level of abrasiveness that a particular person requires. At the same time, dentifrice manufacturers should continue to strive to produce more efficient products which have the least potential for producing adverse effects upon the dentition.

EFFECTS ON MUCOSA

In regard to the mucosal tissues, at one time or another just about every commercially available dentifrice and mouth rinse has been reported to be associated with some type of reaction (Shea, 1967; Smith, 1968; Hutchins, Whitehurst and Barnes, 1971; Stec, 1972; Guarnieri, 1970; Millard, 1973; Kowitz, Lucatorto and Bennett, 1973; Kowtiz, Lucatorto and Cherrick, 1974; and Guarnieri, 1974).

Similarly, at one time or another almost all dentifrice ingredients (cleaning and polishing agents, detergents, flavoring oils, fluoride compounds, etc.) have been reported to be associated with some particular reaction that occurred in a particular person. In this regard, dentifrices are thus behaving in a manner identical to all other cosmetic products, including soaps, shampoos, shaving creams, deodorants, antiperspirants, facial cosmetics and so on.

In a recent study, an exhaustive attempt was made to determine the relationship between various oral habits (use of specific toothbrushes, dentifrices, mouth rinses, tobacco, alcohol, foods, beverages, etc.) and the status of the oral mucosal tissues, as determined by clinical, microscopic and cytologic evaluation. A population of approximately 450 persons was included in the investigation, and the results indicated that there was no association between the various factors considered and the status of the mucosal tissues (Bolden, Lemeh, Stewart and Volpe, 1974).

In fact, all of the ingredients used in today's dentifrices either have a substantial amount of data available concerning their utilization, or they are thoroughly tested prior to use in a product. Also, it is important to indicate that the incidence of mucosal reactions to today's dentifrices is incredibly small—especially when one considers the hundreds of millions of people who use these products on a daily basis throughout their lives.

If a dentist suspects that a particular dentifrice may be associated with a mucosal reaction in a particular person, he should advise the person to discontinue the use of the present product and use another brand. In most cases, the reaction will subside and not recur with the second brand. If the person continues to experience the reaction with the new product, then a more generalized allergic-type response should be suspected, and the person should be referred to a dermatologist for further evaluation and examination. In all probability, that person will exhibit a similar response with other cosmetic products.

CURRENT TRENDS IN DENTIFRICES

Although the majority of the dentifrices are currently being sold in the United States on the basis of an anticaries therapeutic claim, it would appear that a definite trend has appeared in the past several years that indicates a consumer acceptance of purely cosmetic dentifrices (Pader, 1971). It may be recalled that cosmetic dentifrices were defined as dentifrices which did not contain a drug substance or make a therapeutic claim. When used in a routine, non-specific manner, cosmetic dentifrices will provide a "cosmetically clean and healthy dentition and a fresher breath."

The success of five particular dentifrices (Ultra Brite, Close-Up, Macleans, Pearl Drops* and Gleem II), all of which were primarily cosmetic in nature, has substantiated this trend. In general, the cosmetic dentifrices that are commercially available are all utilizing similar types of approaches to the consumer, including "whiter teeth," "brighter teeth," "extra-strength cleaning," high-impact flavors, a combination of dentifrice and mouth rinse properties and a combination of cosmetic and therapeutic properties.

In regard to cosmetic/therapeutic combinations, Gleem II contains sodium fluoride, and Aim toothpaste, a clear gel product similar to Close-Up, contains stannous fluoride. Macleans contains sodium monofluorophosphate.

It would appear that although efforts to develop dentifrices with therapeutic claims (prevention or reduction of the formation of dental plaque, caries, calculus, gingivitis, etc.) will continue, the manufacturers will also be very interested in the development of cosmetic dentifrices which, in addition to appealing to the consumer, make no therapeutic claims, and thus do not require extensive clinical testing prior to marketing.

*A tooth polish in liquid form.

PART TWO • MOUTH RINSES

DEFINITION OF A MOUTH RINSE

A mouth rinse may be defined simply as a substance that is swished around the oral cavity and then expectorated in order to freshen the mouth and breath. Thus, its purpose is primarily cosmetic. The most popular form is a liquid, although mouth rinse troches, lozenges, concentrates and sprays are also available. In the case of the liquid mouth rinses, the material may be introduced into the oral cavity in either a full-strength or diluted form.

By these criteria, water and saline solution could be considered to be the simplest mouth rinses. However, the most widely purchased and utilized mouth rinses in the United States are flavored formulations that contain a variety of specialized ingredients and characteristic flavors, such as cinnamon, clove, peppermint and wintergreen. Mouth rinses are also often referred to by other names, such as mouthwashes, oral antiseptics and gargles.

COMPOSITION OF MOUTH RINSES

The basic ingredients in a liquid mouth rinse formulation are water, alcohol, flavoring oils and coloring materials. Other components may include humectants, astringents, emulsifiers, antimicrobial agents, sweeteners and therapeutic substances. These ingredients are described in detail in three excellent publications (Rosenthal, 1957 and 1972; Darlington, 1968).

Although water makes up the greatest part of any mouth rinse formulation, ethyl alcohol is also present in fairly high concentrations (approximately 15 to 30 per cent). Alcohol is primarily present to enhance the solubility of flavoring oils and other compounds of low solubility in water.

The humectants utilized include glycerin and sorbitol, and the astringents, when present, are usually either zinc or aluminum salts. Emulsifiers, such as polyoxyethylene sorbitan fatty acid esters and block copolymers consisting of polyoxyethylene and polyoxypropylene, are used to reduce surface tension and assist in the stabilization of other ingredients. Saccharin is a widely used sweetening agent. Common anesthetics (used mainly in the troches or lozenges) are benzocaine and benzyl alcohol.

An important ingredient in the mouth rinse formulation is the antimicrobial agent. This is due to the fact that one of the means by which mouth rinses can exert their "deodorizing" effect is by inhibiting bacterial activity in the oral cavity. Although such materials as certain flavoring oils and alcohol can exert some antimicrobial effect, their action is minor compared to that of the specific antimicrobial ingredients.

The most commonly used antimicrobial agents are the quaternary ammonium compounds, such as cetylpyridinium chloride, benzethonium chloride and domiphen bromide, and the phenolic compounds, such as phenol, thymol, betanaphthol and hexylresorcinol. Miscellaneous antimicrobial agents include povidone-iodine, hexetidine and certain organic mercurial compounds.

At one time, hexachlorophene was a widely used antimicrobial agent in many cosmetic products, including mouth rinses. However, federal regulations now prohibit its use in any such formulations, except possibly in trace amounts as a preservative.

Oxygen liberating agents, such as sodium perborate and urea peroxide, have also been used to some extent, even though they have limited capabilities as antimicrobial agents.

Some newer and very promising antimicrobial mouth rinse ingredients are currently being subjected to clinical investigation and are discussed in detail in the Therapeutic Mouth Rinse section of this report.

FUNCTIONS OF A MOUTH RINSE

COSMETIC FUNCTION

As previously mentioned, the primary objective in using a mouth rinse is a cosmetic one, whereby the mouth and breath are freshened. In this respect, mouth rinses could be considered to serve a social function.

Substantiation of the effect of mouth rinses on the incidence of objectionable breath odor (and other oral parameters) has generally been obtained through the use of four types of investigations, which may be described as follows:

1. *In vitro* microbiological evaluations, whereby the antimicrobial spectrum of the mouth rinse has been determined. These laboratory tests are described in three excellent publications (Rosenthal, 1957; Wedderburn, 1963; and Gucklhorn, 1969).
2. *In vivo* clinical microbiological sampling procedures (such as the "buccal scrapings" obtained from the inside of the cheeks) which indicate the reduction in microorganisms that occurs as a result of using the mouth rinse for specific periods of time (Vinson and Bennett, 1958; Manhold, Parker and Manhold, 1962; Manhold and Manhold, 1963; Alderman, 1965; and Robinson, 1970).
3. *In vivo* clinical investigations which have determined the beneficial effect of certain mouth rinses on such specific parameters as high-speed drill bacterial aerosol contamination (Mohammed, Manhold and Manhold, 1964; Litsky, Mascis and Litsky, 1970; and Mohammed and Monserrate, 1970) and oral debris clearance (Manhold, Manhold and Weisinger, 1967). Also, the use of mouth rinses (containing such materials as iodine, hexetidine and phenol) in the area of pre-surgical and post-surgical care has been investigated and

found to be of some value (Keosian, Weinman and Rafel, 1956; Sackler, Rockoff and Rockoff, 1956; Blum, 1960; Simring, 1963; Pinson and Stanback, 1964; Ball and Ball, 1967; and Batten and Collings, 1970).

4. *In vivo* clinical investigations which measure the direct effect of mouth rinses on objectionable breath odor, either through the use of organoleptic procedures (direct nose-mouth evaluation) employing the Fair-Wells osmoscope (Morris and Read, 1949) or through the use of recently developed microcoulometric-chromatographic instrumental procedures (Tonzetich, 1971; Solis and Volpe, 1973).

Some mouth rinses, in addition to performing a cosmetic function, also claim to provide relief for sore throats and to reduce the occurrence of the common cold. These claims have been, for the most part, substantiated by *in vitro* microbiological data, although in some instances human clinical studies have been conducted. However, claims of this nature are considered to be therapeutic, and regulatory agencies have indicated their concern in reference to the adequacy of the substantiating data.

Indeed, the Food and Drug Administration, based on a review of mouth rinse data that was conducted by the National Academy of Sciences—National Research Council, has questioned the effectiveness of mouth rinses in regard to preventive or therapeutic claims (Federal Register, 1970A).

The Council on Dental Therapeutics of the American Dental Association refers to mouth rinses as liquids with pleasant taste and odor, used to rinse the mouth. The Council further states: "Unfortunately, mouth rinses are often advertised to the public with claims or implications of value in preventing or treating diseases of the mouth and upper respiratory tract. The Council on Dental Therapeutics does not presently recognize any substantial contribution to oral health in the unsupervised use of medicated mouthwashes by the general public. The need for a truly therapeutic mouthwash and the degree of its usefulness must be ascertained by a dentist or physician."*

The Council on Dental Therapeutics of the American Dental Association has classified as unacceptable medicated mouth rinses which are marketed for unsupervised use by the public (Accepted Dental Therapeutics, 1975/1976).

THERAPEUTIC FUNCTION

As was the case with dentifrices, a therapeutic mouth rinse can be defined as a formulation containing a drug substance and used to transfer this drug substance to the hard and soft tissues of the oral cavity. This drug substance then imparts a chemical, physiological or pharmacological action which clinically is manifested as a reduction in the incidence of plaque, caries, calculus and gingival disease.

As previously mentioned, claims in reference to the relief of sore throats and the prevention of the common cold would also be considered therapeutic, but primarily from a medical aspect, rather than a dental aspect.

Many therapeutic mouth rinse formulations (containing drug substances) have been evaluated with regard to their effect on plaque, calculus, caries or gingival disease. These clinical investigations can be summarized as follows.

Fluoride-Containing Mouth Rinses.† In the early 1940's it was shown that fluoride treatment could make the teeth more resistant to caries formation (Volker, Hodge, Wilson and Van Voochis, 1940; Volker, Sognnaes and Bibby, 1941). A clinical study conducted with a 0.1 per cent acidulated sodium fluoride mouth rinse did not produce a caries reduction in a group of 31 dental students (Bibby, Zander, McKelleget and Labunsky, 1946). The authors indicated that the small number of subjects and their age were the probable causes of failure to obtain a significant caries reduction.

*Accepted Dental Therapeutics, 1975/1976.

†The subject of fluoride-containing mouth rinses is reviewed in several excellent publications (McCormick, 1968; Horowitz, 1973; and Torell and Ericsson, 1974).

Three subsequent studies did, however, provide significant caries reductions with a neutral 0.2 per cent sodium fluoride mouth rinse (Weisz, 1960; Fjaestad-Seger, Norstedt-Larsson and Torell, 1961; and Torell and Siberg, 1962).

Since that time, many clinical studies have been conducted with fluoride mouth rinses. For the most part, sodium fluoride has been the most widely utilized and investigated substance. A summary of some of these clinical studies is presented in Table 12–10. The data indicate that mouth rinses containing sodium fluoride (at various concentrations and frequencies of use) are safe and effective with regard to reducing the incidence of caries.

This conclusion was also substantiated at an International Workshop on Fluorides and Dental Caries Reductions (1974), where the recommendations indicated that sodium fluoride rinses, in either neutral or acidulated form, were safe and efficacious. Furthermore, the committee stated that sodium fluoride rinses should be used by individuals of age six and above who reside in either water-fluoridated or nonfluoridated areas. The committee indicated that the recommendation of mouth rinses containing other fluoride compounds, such as stannous fluoride, potassium fluoride, ferric fluoride, and potassium and sodium fluoride with manganese would not be in order until further clinical data became available, even though, in some cases, the data already available were encouraging.

A government notice also attests to the safety and effectiveness of sodium fluoride mouth rinses (Federal Register, 1974). The notice indicates that:

1. Aqueous solutions of 0.2 per cent sodium fluoride with a pH of approximately 7.0 are safe and effective in reducing the incidence of dental caries when applied to the teeth as a rinse once a week or once every two weeks.
2. Aqueous solutions of 0.05 per cent sodium fluoride with a pH of approximately 7.0 are safe and effective in reducing the incidence of dental caries when applied to the teeth once daily as a rinse.
3. Aqueous solutions of acidulated phosphate sodium fluoride with a pH of approximately 4.0 that yield a fluoride ion concentration of approximately 0.02 per cent, are safe and effective in reducing the incidence of dental caries when applied to the teeth once daily as a rinse.

Also, the Council on Dental Therapeutics of the American Dental Association has classified as "Accepted" both neutral sodium fluoride and phosphate acidulated fluoride solutions as effective agents for use in reducing the incidence of dental decay. The Council announcement also lists the specific sodium fluoride mouth rinse products that are classified as "Accepted" (Report of Councils and Bureaus, American Dental Association, 1975).

Antimicrobial-Containing Mouth Rinses. As previously mentioned, quaternary ammonium compounds are common mouth rinse ingredients and have been included primarily because of their antimicrobial properties. Several clinical studies have been conducted which indicate that substances such as benzethonium chloride, cetylpyridinium chloride and the combination of cetylpyridinium chloride and domiphen bromide have a moderate effect (about 30 to 40 per cent reduction) on the formation of dental plaque (Arnim, 1963; Volpe, Kupczak, Brant, King, Kestenbaum and Schlissel, 1969; Sturzenberger and Leonard, 1969; Bergenholtz, Hugoson, Lundgren and Östgren, 1969; and Beiswanger, Sturzenberger and Bollmer, 1974).

Other compounds with antimicrobial properties that have shown a moderate degree of effectiveness in mouth rinses with regard to plaque, calculus and gingivitis include thymol and eucalyptol (Gomer, Holroyd, Fedi and Ferrigno, 1972), hexetidine (Bergenholtz and Hänström, 1974), alexidine (Lobene and Soparkar, 1973), various peroxides (Shipman, Cohen and Kaslick, 1971; and Rundegren, Fornell and

TABLE 12–10 CLINICAL INVESTIGATIONS CONDUCTED WITH MOUTH RINSES CONTAINING FLUORIDES

INVESTIGATOR(S)	MATERIAL UTILIZED*	CONCLUSIONS
McCormick and Koulourides, 1965	NaF (3–40 ppm F^-) plus calcium and phosphate	Daily rinsing for one year produced significantly less interproximal caries in Grade 1 and 2 children
Torell and Ericsson, 1965A	NaF (226 ppm F^-)	Daily rinsing for two years produced a 50% DMFS caries reduction in 10 year old children
	NaF (904 ppm F^-)	Rinsing every two weeks for two years produced a 21% DMFS caries reduction in 10 year old children
Kasakura, 1966	NaF (452 ppm F^-)	Daily rinsing for two years produced a 60% DMFT caries reduction in Grade 4 children
Koch, 1967	NaF (2260 ppm F^-)	Rinsing every two weeks for three years produced a 23% DMFS caries reduction in 10 year old children
Torell, 1969	NaF (904 ppm F^-) plus $CaCO_3$/0.8% sodium monofluorophosphate dentifrice used daily at home	Rinsing every two weeks for 2½ years in conjunction with daily use of the fluoride dentifrice produced significantly less caries than use of the fluoride rinse alone
Gerdin and Torell, 1969	0.2% KF + Mn Cl_2 0.2% NaF + Mn Cl_2 0.2% NaF	Weekly rinsing for four years indicated that the KF/Mn Cl_2 rinse produced significantly less caries than the other two rinses in 9–13 year old children
Swerdloff and Shannon, 1969	0.1% SnF_2 (250 ppm F^-)	Daily rinsing for five months established the feasibility of using this rinse and produced a non-significant DMFT caries reduction in school children
Horowitz, Creighton and McClendon, 1971	NaF (904 ppm F^-)	Weekly rinsing for 20 months produced a 44% DMFS caries reduction in Grade 5 children and a 16% reduction in Grade 1 children
Frankl, Fleisch and Diodati, 1972	NaF (200 ppm F^-) pH 4.0	Daily rinsing for two years produced a 25% DMFS caries reduction in 14 year old children
Aasenden, DePaola and Brudevold, 1972	NaF (200 ppm F^-) NaF (200 ppm F^-) pH 4.0	Daily rinsing for three years produced a 27% DMFS caries reduction (neutral rinse) and a 30% reduction (acidulated rinse) in 8–10 year old children
Brandt, Slack and Waller, 1972	NaF (904 ppm F^-)	Twice weekly rinsing for two years produced a 36% DMFS caries reduction in 11 year old children
Moreira and Tumang, 1972	NaF (452 ppm F^-)	Weekly rinsing for two years produced a 35% DMFS caries reduction and three times weekly rinsing produced a 36% reduction in 7 year old children
Radike, Gish, Peterson, King and Segreto, 1973	0.1% SnF_2 (250 ppm F^-) Fluoridated Water	Daily rinsing for two years produced a 33–43% DMFS caries reduction in 8–13 year old children
Rugg-Gunn, Holloway and Davies, 1973	NaF (226 ppm F^-)	Daily rinsing for three years produced a 35% DMFS caries reduction in 11–12 year old children
Gallagher, Glassgow and Caldwell, 1973	NaF (1808 ppm F^-)	Weekly rinsing for two years produced a 27% DMFT caries reduction in 11–13 year old children
Heifetz, Driscoll and Creighton, 1973	NaF (0.3% F^-) NaF (0.3% F^-) pH 4.0	Weekly rinsing for two years produced a 38% DMFS caries reduction (neutral rinse) and a 27% reduction (acidulated rinse) in Grade 7 and 9 children
Forsman, 1974	NaF (113 ppm F^-) NaF (904 ppm F^-)	Weekly rinsing for two years produced significant caries reductions for both rinse groups, with the lower level of fluoride providing a somewhat better effect

*All rinses are essentially neutral, unless otherwise indicated.

Ericson, 1973), zinc phenolsulfonate and zinc tribromsalan (Fischman, Picozzi, Cancro and Pader, 1973), sodium hypochlorite (Lobene, 1972) and amine fluoride (Lobene, 1974).

Antibiotic compounds that have also shown effectiveness in clinical investigations include vancomycin (Mitchell, Holmes, Martin and Sakurai, 1967), erythromycin (Lobene, Brion and Socransky, 1969) and kanamycin (Loesche, Green, Kenney and Nafe, 1971).

In recent years, two antimicrobial substances have been subjected to clinical evaluation and have been shown to have a marked effect on the incidence of plaque, calculus and gingival disease.

The first substance is chlorhexidine, which is effective against gram-positive and gram-negative microorganisms as well as yeasts. Initial clinical investigations indicated that a mouth rinse containing 0.1 per cent chlorhexidine (numerically coded as Z7y) was an effective calculus-preventive material (Schroeder, Marthaler and Mühlemann, 1962; Renggli, 1966). This material has been subjected to many clinical investigations, and it has been shown that a mouth rinse containing 0.2 per cent chlorhexidine is very effective against plaque and calculus formation as well as gingival disease (Löe and Schiött, 1970; Löe and Schiött, 1970A; Rölla, Löe and Schiött, 1970; Davies, Jensen, Schiött and Löe, 1970; Löe, Mandell, Derry and Schiött, 1971; Gjermo and Rölla, 1971; Flötra, Gjermo, Rölla and Waerhang, 1972; Gjermo, Rölla and Arsbaug, 1973; and Gjermo and Eriksen, 1974).

Chlorhexidine continues to be the subject of extensive laboratory and clinical investigations and still appears to be a very promising agent. One problem that has emerged concerns the formation of a brown-black extrinsic tooth stain that occurs with the continuous use of chlorhexidine dentifrices or mouth rinses (Flötra, Gjermo, Rölla and Waerhang, 1971). Although this stain is readily removed by an oral prophylaxis, attempts are being made to prevent its formation.

The second antimicrobial substance is a macrolide antibiotic, numerically designated as CC 10232.* It is the natural product obtained from the fermentation of a novel strain of *Streptomyces caelestis*, NRRL-2821. CC 10232 shows strong activity against a variety of gram-positive microorganisms, including staphylococci, streptococci, enterococci, corynebacteria and bacilli. Gram-negative bacteria, yeasts and molds are not readily inhibited.

A series of clinical investigations have been conducted with a mouth rinse containing 0.01 per cent CC 10232. This mouth rinse has been shown to be effective against plaque and calculus formation (supra-gingival as well as sub-gingival) and gingival disease. A summary of some of these studies is presented in Table 12–11. Although these results are extremely encouraging, it should be emphasized that this substance is an antibiotic and thus must be subjected to further evaluation to determine whether its utilization causes the development of resistant microorganisms or allergic hypersensitivity reactions.

Miscellaneous Therapeutic Mouth Rinses. A variety of other substances (in mouth rinses) have been clinically evaluated for their effect on plaque, calculus or gingivitis formation. These substances include sodium ricinoleate, urea, polyvinylpyrrolidone, lysosyme, Victamine C,† Ascoxal,‡ etc. These materials all show some degree of effectiveness and are discussed in detail in several excellent publications (Weinstein and Mandel, 1964; Mühlemann, 1968; Belting, 1968; Schroeder, 1969; McNeal, 1969; Parsons, 1974; Gjermo, 1974; and Volpe, 1974).

Several clinical studies have been conducted with a tablet mouth rinse containing a proteolytic enzyme obtained from a mutant strain of *Bacillus subtilis* (Shaver and Schiff, 1970; Schiff, 1970). This enzyme-containing preparation was very effective in reducing plaque formation and is being subjected to further investigation. Conversely, mouth rinses containing the

*This antibiotic was provided by Abbott Laboratories, North Chicago, Illinois and is the subject of U.S. Patent No. 3,342,687 (Colgate-Palmolive Co.).

†A surface-active organophosphorous compound.

‡A mixture of ascorbic acid, sodium percarbonate and copper sulfate.

TABLE 12-11 CLINICAL INVESTIGATIONS CONDUCTED WITH A MOUTH RINSE CONTAINING 0.01 PER CENT OF A MACROLIDE ANTIBIOTIC (CC 10232)

INVESTIGATOR(S)	PARAMETER EVALUATED	RESULTS
Volpe, Kupczak, Brant, King Kestenbaum and Schlissel, 1969	Supragingival plaque and calculus	Approximately 70–77% reduction in plaque Approximately 75% reduction in calculus
Stallard, Volpe, Orban and King, 1969	Supragingival plaque, calculus and gingivitis	11–23% reduction in plaque 70–91% reduction in calculus 55–72% reduction in gingivitis
Volpe, Schulman, Goldman, King and Kupczak, 1970	Supragingival calculus	38% reduction at 3 months 50% reduction at 6 months 33% reduction at 9 months
Kovaleski and Ash, 1970	Supragingival plaque, calculus and gingivitis	Beneficial effect on plaque up to 60 days.
Rokita, Hazen, Millen and Volpe, 1975	Subgingival plaque and calculus	Less deposit, less mineralization and less Spirochetes.

enzyme dextranase have not demonstrated a similar degree of efficacy (Caldwell, Sandham, Mann, Finn and Formicola, 1971; Lobene, 1971; and Keyes, Hicks, Goldman, McCabe and Fitzgerald, 1971).

Another interesting compound is ethane-1-hydroxy-1,1 diphosphonate-hexahydrate, which has been shown to reduce calculus formation when evaluated in a mouth rinse (Mühlemann, Bowels, Schaitt and Bernimoulin, 1970) and a dentifrice (Sturzenberger, Swancar and Reiter, 1971; and Suomi, Horowitz, Barbano, Spolsky and Heifetz, 1974).

FUTURE TRENDS IN MOUTH RINSES

Although a reduction in objectionable breath odor will probably always remain an important consideration in the formulation of mouth rinses, it is obvious that the future trend is toward the development of therapeutic mouth rinses. The function of these therapeutic mouth rinses will be to have a beneficial effect upon the oral hard and soft tissues, including the formation of dental plaque, calculus, caries and gingival disease.

As of now, however, there are no over-the-counter mouth rinses commercially available in the United States which make a therapeutic (or drug related) claim in regard to these parameters. Mouth rinses containing sodium fluoride are available for use on a prescription basis for the reduction of dental caries.

PART THREE • SOME GENERAL CONSIDERATIONS

FLUORIDE DENTIFRICES AND MOUTH RINSES IN A FLUORIDATED WATER AREA

Fluoride-containing dentifrices and mouth rinses are not intended to be used as substitutes for water fluoridation. First, they produce a topical effect on erupted teeth, while water fluoridation acts systemically during the pre-eruptive stage of tooth development. Second, clinical studies indicate that the cariostatic effect obtained from either fluoride dentifrices or mouth rinses is approximately one half that provided by water fluoridation.

Several clinical studies have, however,

indicated that the use of either fluoride-containing dentifrices or mouth rinses in a community with optimal water fluoridation can provide some degree of *additive* cariostatic benefit over and above that which is provided by the water fluoridation itself.

Since there are no known contraindications to the use of fluoride-containing dentifrices and mouth rinses in a fluoridated water community, their use should be recommended and encouraged.

ADULT USE OF FLUORIDE DENTIFRICES AND MOUTH RINSES

Although the majority of the caries clinical studies conducted with fluoride-containing dentifrices and mouth rinses have utilized children and teen-age populations because of the greater incidence of the disease in these groups, there is no evidence to indicate that these products would not also be beneficial to an adult population.

On the contrary, there are two factors which would indicate that fluoride-containing dentifrices and mouth rinses should be recommended for use by adults. First, fluoride-containing products have been shown in many clinical studies to have a beneficial effect on tooth hypersensitivity, which is a condition most prevalent in adults. Second, recent information (Hazen, Chilton and Mumma, 1974) indicates that adults, although not very prone to conventional pit and fissure caries, are very susceptible to a special phenomenon called "root surface" caries.

GUIDELINES FOR DRUG INGREDIENTS IN DENTIFRICES AND MOUTH RINSES

The government has recently convened panels and advisory groups of scientific experts to review the available safety and efficacy data pertaining to drug ingredients used in all dental products, including dentifrices and mouth rinses. As this chapter is being written, these panels are in the midst of carefully analyzing this material. These reviews will culminate in the issuance of monographs which will provide guidelines for regulation of the use of all drug ingredients in all dental products.

ACKNOWLEDGMENTS

The author wishes to express his deep appreciation to Dr. William J. King and to Dr. Lester D. Apperson of the Colgate-Palmolive Research Center for their valuable comments and assistance in the preparation and editing of this manuscript.

REFERENCES

Aasenden, R., DePaola, P. F., and Brudevold, F.: Effects of daily rinsing and ingestion of fluoride solutions upon dental caries and enamel fluoride. Arch. Oral Biol. *17*:1705–1714, 1972.

Accepted Dental Therapeutics, 34th Ed., 1971/1972; 36th Ed., 1975/1976; published by the American Dental Association, 211 East Chicago Avenue, Chicago, Illinois, 60611.

Alderman, E. J.: An *in vivo* study of the effect of prolonged use of a specific mouthwash on the oral flora. Chron. Omaha Dist. Dent. Soc. Vol. 28, pp. 284–289, 1965.

Allison, J. B., and Nelson, M. F.: The distribution of C^{14} from sodium n-lauroyl sarcosinate in the rat (unpublished data), Bureau of Biological Research, Rutgers University, and Colgate-Palmolive Company Radioisotope Laboratory, 1958.

American Dental Association, Clinical testing of dental caries preventives – Report of a conference to develop uniform standards and procedures in clinical studies of dental caries, published by the American Dental Association, 1955.

American Dental Association, Conference on clinical trials of drugs used in dentistry, published by the American Dental Association, 1960.

American Dental Association, Proceedings of the conference on the clinical testing of cariostatic agents, published by the American Dental Association, 1968.

Andlaw, R. J., and Tucker, G. J.: A three-year clinical trial of a dentifrice containing 0.8 per cent sodium monofluorophosphate in an aluminum oxide trihydrate base. Brit. Dent. J. *138*:426–432, 1975.

Arnim, S. S.: The use of disclosing agents for measuring tooth cleanliness, J. Periodontol. *34*:227–245, 1963.

Backer-Dirks, O., Winkler, R. C., and Van Aken, J. A.: A reproducible method for caries evaluation, III. Test in a therapeutic experiment with an ammoniated dentifrice. J. Dent. Res. *32*:18–26, 1953.

Backer-Dirks, O., Baume, L. J., Davies, G. N., and Slack, G. L.: Principal requirements for controlled clinical trials. Int. Dent. J. *17*:93–103, 1967.

Backer-Dirks, O., Swant, G. W., and Starmans, J. L.: Effect of a sodium lauroyl sarcosinate dentifrice: A clinical investigation. J. Dent. Belge. *50*:163–175, 1959.

Ball, D. M., and Ball, E. L.: Comparative effectiveness of two mouthwashes used after gingivectomy. J. Periodontol. *38*:395–397, 1967.

Batten, J. R., and Collings, C. K.: The evaluation of an anesthetic mouthrinse on four hundred periodon-

tal surgery patients. J. Periodontol. *41*:654–656, 1970.
Beiswanger, B. B., Sturzenberger, O. P., and Bollmer, W.: Clinical effect of an antibacterial mouthwash on dental plaque and gingivitis. International Association for Dental Research. Preprinted Abstract No. 367, p. 146, 1974.
Belting, C. M.: Design of clinical studies on dental calculus. Ann. N.Y. Acad. Sci. (Evaluation of agents used in the prevention of oral disease). *153*: (Art. 1) 307–313, Dec. 23, 1968.
Bergenholtz, A., Hugoson, A., Lundgren, D., and Östgren, A.: The plaque-inhibiting property of some mouthwashes and their effect on the oral mucosa, Sven. Tandlak, Tidskr. *62*:7–14, 1969.
Bergenholtz, A., and Hänström, L.: The plaque-inhibiting effect of hexitidine (Oraldene) mouthwash compared to that of chlorhexidine. Community Dent. Oral Epidemiol. 2:70–74, 1974.
Bibby, B. G.: Test of the effect of fluoride-containing dentifrices on dental caries. J. Dent. Res. *24*:297–303, 1945.
Bibby, B. G., Zander, H. A., McKelleget, M., and Labunsky, B.: Preliminary reports on the effect on dental caries of the use of sodium fluoride in a prophylactic cleaning mixture and in a mouthwash. J. Dent. Res. *25*:207–211, 1946.
Bixler, D., and Muhler, J. C.: Experimental clinical human caries test design and interpretation. J. Am. Dent. Assoc. *65*:482–490, 1962.
Bixler, D., and Muhler, J. C.: Effect on dental caries in children in a nonfluoride area of combined use of three agents containing stannous fluoride: A prophylactic paste, a solution, and a dentifrice, II: Results at the end of 24 and 36 months. J. Am. Dent. Assoc. 72:392–396, 1966.
Bixler, D. and Muhler, J. C.:Effectiveness of a stannous fluoride-containing dentifrice in reducing dental caries in children in a boarding school environment. J. Am. Dent. Assoc. *72*:653–658, 1966A.
Blum, B.: Clinical evaluation of an anesthetic mouthwash. N.Y. Dent. J. *26*:419–421, 1960.
Bogle, G. C.: Abrasivity of dentifrices and toothbrushes. Periodontal Abstracts *22*:7–13, 1974.
Bolden, T. E., Volpe, A. R. and King, W. J.: The desensitizing effect of a sodium monofluorophosphate dentifrice. Periodontics, *6*:112–114, 1968.
Bolden, T. E., Lemeh, D., Stewart, E. B., and Volpe, A. R.: A comparison of oral soft tissue cytologic findings and oral habits. Quart. Nat. Dent. Assoc. *33*:4–17, 1974.
Bouchal, A. W.: The abrasiveness of dentifrices. Proceedings of the Scientific Section of the Toilet Goods Association. No. 45, pp. 2–5, 1966.
Brandt, R. S., Slack, G. L., and Waller, D. F.: The use of a sodium fluoride mouthwash in reducing the dental caries increment in eleven year old English school children. Proc. Brit. Paedodont. Soc. 2:23–25, 1972.
Brasch, S. V., Lazarou, J. A., Van Abbé, N.J., and Forrest, J. O.: The assessment of dentifrice abrasivity *in vivo*. Brit. Dent. J. pp. 119–124, 1969.
Brudevold, F. and Chilton, N. W.: Comparative study of a fluoride dentifrice containing soluble phosphate and a calcium-free abrasive: Second year report. J. Am. Dent. Assoc. 72:889–894, 1966.
Brudevold, F., Little, M. F. and Rowley, J.: Acid reducing effects of "antienzymes" in the mouth. J. Am. Dent. Assoc. *50*:18–22, 1955.
Bull, W. H., Callender, R. M., Pugh, B. R., and Wood, G. D.: The abrasion and cleaning properties of dentifrices. Br. Dent. J. *124*:331–337, 1968.
Caldwell, R. C., Sandham, H. J., Mann, W. V., Finn, S. S. and Formicola, A. J.: The effect of a dextranase mouthwash on dental plaque in young adults and children. J. Am. Dent. Assoc. *82*:124–131, 1971.
Cobb, A. B., Hay, D. I., and Schram, C. J.: A method of measuring tooth-cleaning. Brit. Dent. J. pp. 249–253, 1961.
Cohen, A., and Donzanti, A.: Two-year clinical study of caries control with high-urea ammoniated dentifrice. J. Am. Dent. Assoc. *49*:185–190, 1954.
Cordon, M.: A method for measuring the abrasion of dentin by dentifrices. J. Dent. Res. *50*:491–497, 1971.
Costich, E. R., and Hein, J. W.: Clinical study of the effect of a tooth paste containing sodium copper chlorophyllin on oral bacteria and gingival disease. J. Dent. Res. *31*:474 (Abstract), 1952.
Darlington, R. C.: O-T-C topical oral antiseptics and mouthwashes. J. Am. Pharm. Assoc. *NS8*:484–496, 1968.
Davies, G. N., and King, R. M.: The effectiveness of an ammonium ion tooth powder in the control of dental caries. J. Dent. Res. *30*:645–655, 1951.
Davies, R. M., Jensen, S. B., Schiött, C. R., and Löe, H.: The effect of topical application of chlorhexidine on the bacterial colonization of the teeth and gingiva. J. Periodont. Res. *5*:96–101, 1970.
Downer, M. C., Holloway, P. J., and Davies, T. G. H.: Clinical testing of a multiple therapeutic agent caries preventive program. International Association for Dental Research, Preprinted Abstract L303, p. L76, 1975.
Duckworth, R.: Fluoride dentifrices, a review of clinical trials in the United Kingdom. Br. Dent. J. *124*:505–509, 1968.
Dudding, N. J., Dahl, L. O., and Muhler, J. C.: Patient reactions to brushing teeth with water, dentifrice or salt and soda. J. Periodontol. *31*:386–392, 1960.
Emslie, R. D.: Clinical trial of a toothpaste containing sarcosinate. J. Dent. Res. *42*:1079–1086, 1963.
Evaluation of agents used in the prevention of oral disease. Ann. N.Y. Acad. Sci. (Ward Pigman, Consulting Ed.) *153*:1–388, Dec. 23, 1968.
Facq, J. M., and Volpe, A. R.: *In vivo* abrasiveness of three dentifrices against acrylic surfaces of veneer crowns. J. Am. Dent. Assoc. *80*:317–323, 1970.
Fanning, E. A., Gotjamanos, R., and Vowles, N. J.: The use of fluoride dentifrices in the control of dental caries: Methodology and results of a clinical trial. Aust. Dent. J. *13*:201–206, 1968.
Fanning, E. A., Gotjamanos, T., Vowles, N. J., and Van Der Weilen, I.: The effects of fluoride dentifrices on the incidence and distribution of stained tooth surfaces in children. Arch. Oral Biol., *13*:467–469, 1968A.
Federal Register, Tues., July 21, 1970, Vol. 25, No. 140, pp. 11643–11645, Notice from the Dept. of Health, Education and Welfare (Food and Drug Administration) in Reference to the Efficacy of Certain Dentifrices.
Federal Register, Tues., Aug. 4, 1970 (A), Vol. 35, No. 150, pp. 12411–12412 and 12423–12424, Notice from the Department of Health, Education and Welfare (Food and Drug Administration) in Reference to the Efficacy of Certain Mouthwash and Gargle Preparations.
Federal Register, Tuesday, May 14, 1974. Vol. 39, No.

94, p. 17245, Notice from the Department of Health, Education and Welfare (Food and Drug Administration) in reference to Topical Fluoride Preparations for Reducing Incidence of Dental Caries. (A correction to this notice appears in the Federal Register, Wednesday, June 26, 1974. Vol. 39, No. 124, p. 23081; an amendment to this notice appears in the Federal Register, Thursday, November 7, 1974. Vol. 39, No. 216, p. 39488).

Finn, S. B., and Jamison, H. C.: A comparative clinical study of three dentifrices. J. Dent. Child. *30*:17–25, 1963.

Fischman, S. L., Picozzi, A., Cancro, L. P., and Pader, M.: The inhibition of plaque in humans by two experimental oral rinses. J. Periodontol. *44*:100–102, 1973.

Fitzgerald, R. J., and Keyes, P. H.: Demonstration of the etiologic role of streptococci in experimental caries in the hamster. J. Am. Dent. Assoc. *61*:9–19, 1960.

Fjaestad-Seger, M., Norstedt-Larsson, K., and Torell, P.: Forsok Med Enkla Metoder for Klinisk Fluorapplication. Sver. Tandlakarforb. Tidn. *53*:169–178, 1961.

Flötra, L., Gjermo, P., Rölla, G., and Waerhang, J.: Side effects of chlorhexidine mouthwashes. Scand. J. Dent. Res. *79*:119–125, 1971.

Flötra, L., Gjermo, P., Rölla, G., and Waerhang, J.: A four-month study on the effect of chlorhexidine mouthwashes on 50 soldiers. Scand. J. Dent. Res. *80*:10–17, 1972.

Forscher, B. K., and Hess, W. C.: The validity of plaque pH measurements as a method of evaluating therapeutic agents. J. Am. Dent. Assoc. *48*:134–139, 1954.

Forsman, B.: The caries preventing effect of mouth rinsing with an 0.025% sodium fluoride solution in Swedish children. Community Dent. Oral Epidemiol. *2*:58–65, 1974.

Fosdick, L. S.: The reduction of the incidence of dental caries, I. Immediate toothbrushing with a neutral dentifrice. J. Am. Dent. Assoc. *40*:133–143, 1950.

Fosdick, L. S.: Clinical experiment on the use of sodium n-lauroyl sarcosinate in the control of dental caries. Science *123*:988–989, 1956. (A more detailed description of this study has also been written by L. S. Fosdick and published as a report from Northwestern University Dental School. It is entitled: A Report of Some Clinical Experiments on the Use of Sodium N-Lauroyl Sarcosinate in the Control of Dental Caries.)

Fosdick, L. S., Ludwick, W. E., and Schantz, C. W.: Absorption of enzyme inhibitors and antibiotics on dental plaque. J. Am. Dent. Assoc. *43*:26–31, 1951.

Fosdick, L. S., Calandra, J. C., Blackwell, R. W., and Burrill, J. H.: A new approach to the problem of dental caries control. J. Dent. Res. *32*:486–496, 1953.

Frankl, S. N., and Alman, J. E.: Report of a three-year clinical trial comparing a toothpaste containing sodium monofluorophosphate with two marketed products. J. Oral Therap. Pharm. *4*:443–450, 1968.

Frankl, S. N., Fleisch, S., and Diodati, R. R.: The topical anticariogenic effect of daily rinsing with an acidulated phosphate fluoride solution. J. Am. Dent. Assoc. 85:882–886, 1972.

Frasher, L. A., and Hein, J. W.: Sodium n-lauroyl sarcosinate dentifrice: Effect on dental caries in children. J. Dent. Res. *37*:75 (Abstract), 1958.

Fullmer, J., Volpe, A. R., Apperson, L. D., and Kiraly, J.: Unpublished data, Colgate-Palmolive Company, 1966.

Gale, J. A.: A controlled experiment on pre-school children with an ammoniated dentifrice. Dent. Rec. *71*:184–185, 1951.

Gallagher, S. J., Glassgow, I., and Caldwell, R.: Self-application of fluoride by rinsing. J. Pub. Health Dent. *34*:13–21, 1973.

Gerdin, P.: Studies in dentifrices. I. Abrasiveness of dentifrices and removal of discoloured stains. Swed. Dent. J. *63*:275–282, 1970.

Gerdin, P. O., and Torell, P.: Mouth rinses with potassium fluoride solutions containing manganase. Caries Res. *3*:90–107, 1969.

Gerdin, P.: Studies in dentifrices, VI: The inhibiting effect of some grinding and nongrinding fluoride dentifrices on dental caries. Swed. Dent. J. *65*: 521–532, 1972.

Gershon, S. D., and Pader, M.: Dentifrices, Cosmetics-Science and Technology. (M. Balsam and E. Sagarin, Eds.) New York: John Wiley and Sons, pp. 423–531, 1972.

Gershon, S. D., Pokras, H. H., and Rider, T. H.: Dentifrices (Chapter 15), Cosmetics-Science and Technology. (E. Sagarin, Ed.) New York: Interscience Publishers, Inc., pp. 296–360, 1957.

Gish, C. W., and Muhler, J. C.: Effectiveness of a SnF_2-$Ca_2P_2O_7$ dentifrice on dental caries in children whose teeth calcified in a natural fluoride area, II. Results at the end of the 24 months. J. Am. Dent. Assoc. *73*:853–855, 1966.

Gjermo, P.: Some aspects of drug dynamics related to oral soft tissues. Presented at Sixth International Conference on Oral Biology, Toronto, 1974. J. Dent. Res. In press, 1974.

Gjermo, P., and Eriksen, H. M.: Unchanged plaque inhibiting effect of chlorhexidine in human subjects after two years of continuous use. Arch. Oral. Biol. *19*:317–319, 1974.

Gjermo, P., and Rölla, G.: The plaque-inhibiting effect of chlorhexidine-containing dentifrices. Scand. J. Dent. Res. *79*:126–132, 1971.

Gjermo, P., Rölla, G., and Arskang, L.: E53ct on dental plaque formation and some *in vitro* properties of 12 bis-biguanides. J. Periodont. Res. *12*:81–88, 1973.

Gomer, R. M., Holroyd, S. V., Fedi, P. F., and Ferrigno, P. D.: The effects of oral rinses on the accumulation of dental plaque. J. Am. Soc. Preventive Dent., pp. 6–9, March-April, 1972.

Grabenstetter, R. J., Broge, R. W., Jackson, F. L., and Radike, A. W.: The measurement of the abrasion of human teeth by dentifrice abrasion: A test utilizing radioactive teeth. J. Dent. Res. *37*:1060–1068, 1958.

Grøn, P., and Brudevold, F.: The effectiveness of NaF dentifrices. J. Dent. Child. *34*:122–127, 1967.

Guarnieri, L. J.: Effect of dentifrice components on guinea pig oral tissue. International Association for Dental Research. Preprinted Abstract No. 661, p. 220, 1974.

Guarnieri, L. J.: The effect of dentifrice components on the oral tissues of humans and guinea pigs. Thesis, University of Indiana, 1970.

Gucklhorn, I. R.: Antimicrobials in cosmetics. Toilet Goods Assoc. Cosmetic J. *1*:15–32, Fall, 1969.

Hargreaves, J. A., and Chester, C. G.: Clinical trial among Scottish children of an anticaries dentifrice

containing 2% sodium monofluorophosphate. Community Dent. Oral Epidemiol. *1*:47–57, 1973.
Hargreaves, J. A., Chester, C. G., and Wagg, B. J.: Assessment of children in active and placebo groups, one year after termination of a clinical trial of a 2% sodium monofluorophosphate dentifrice. ORCA (Europen Organization for Caries Research). Preprinted Abstract, 1974.
Harry, R. G.: The tooth and oral hygiene (chap. 15) and dentifrices (chap. 16), The principles and practice of modern cosmetics. Modern Cosmeticology, Chemical Publishing Company, New York, *1*:239–290, 1962.
Hassell, T. M., and Mühlemann, H. R.: Effects of sodium n-lauroyl sarcosinate on plaque pH *in vivo*. Helv. Odontol. Acta. *15*:52–53, 1971.
Hawes, R. R., and Bibby, B. B.: Evaluation of a dentifrice-containing carbamide and urease. J. Am. Dent. Assoc. *46*:280–286, 1953.
Hazen, S. P., Chilton, N. W., Mumma, R. D.: The problem of root caries. I. literature review and clinical description. J. Am. Dent. Assoc. *86*:137–144, 1973.
Hazen, S. P., Volpe, A. R., and King, W. J.: Comparative desensitizing effect of dentifrices containing sodium monofluorophosphate, stannous fluoride and formalin. Periodontics. *6*:230–233, 1968.
Heifetz, S. B., and Horowitz, H. S.: An appraisal of therapeutic dentifrices. J. Public Health Dent., *30*:206–211, 1970.
Heifetz, S. B., Driscoll, W. S. and Creighton, W. E.: The effect on dental caries of weekly rinsing with a neutral sodium fluoride or an acidulated phosphate-fluoride mouthwash. J. Am. Dent. Assoc. *87*:364–368, 1973.
Hein, J. W.: Present status of chlorophyll derivatives as dental therapeutic agents. J. Am. Dent. Assoc. *48*:14–20, 1954.
Hein, J. W.: Effect of sodium n-lauroyl sarcosinate on the fall of pH of tooth surface films and plaques. J. Dent. Res. *34*:755 (Abstract No. T21), 1955.
Hendon, G. E., Keller, S. E., and Manson-Hing, L. R.: Clearance studies of proximal tooth surfaces – Part I. Ala. J. Med. Sci. *6*:213–227, 1969.
Henriques, B. L., Frankl, S. N., and Alman, J. E.: Cited in evaluation of Cue tooth paste. J. Am. Dent. Assoc. *71*:197–198, 1964.
Henschel, C. J., and Lieber, L.: Caries incidence reduction by unsupervised use of a 27.5 per cent ammonium therapy dentifrice. J. Dent. Res. *28*: 248–257, 1949.
Henschel, C. J., and Lieber, L.: High urea ammoniated dentifrice: Caries reduction through four years home use. Oral Surg. *5*:155–169, 1952.
Hernandez, F., Mohammed, C., Shannon, I., Volpe, A. R., and King, W. J.: Clinical study evaluating the desensitizing effect and duration of two commercially available dentifrices. J. Periodontol., *43*: 367–372, 1972.
Hill, T. J.: Fluoride dentifrices. J. Am. Dent. Assoc. *59*:1121–1127, 1959.
Hill, T. J., and Kniesner, A. H.: Penicillin dentifrice and dental caries experience in children. J. Dent. Res. *28*:263–266, 1949.
Hill, T. J., Sims, J., and Newman, M.: The effect of penicillin dentifrice on the control of dental caries. J. Dent. Res. 32:696–702, 1953.
Homan, B. T., and Messer, H. H.: The comparative effect of three fluoride dentifrices on clinical caries in Brisbane school children – Preliminary report. J. Dent. Res. *48*:1094 (Abstract), 1969.
Horowitz, H. S.: Clinical trials of preventives for dental caries. J. Pub. Health Dent. *32*:229–233, 1972.
Horowitz, H. S.: The prevention of dental caries by mouth rinsing with solutions of neutral sodium fluoride. Int. Dent. J. *23*:585–590, 1973.
Horowitz, H. S., Creighton, W. E., and McClendon, B. J.: The effect on human dental caries of weekly oral rinsing with a sodium fluoride mouthwash: A final report. Arch. Oral Biol. *16*:609–616, 1971.
Horowitz, H. S., Law, F. E., Thompson, M. B., and Chamberlin, S. R.: Evaluation of a stannous fluoride dentifrice for use in dental public health programs, I. Basic findings. J. Am. Dent. Assoc. *72*: 408–422, 1966.
Hutchins, D. W., Whitehurst, V. E., and Barnes, G. P.: Evaluation of tissue response to commercially available dentifrices: Clinical and laboratory results. International Association for Dental Research. Preprinted Abstract No. 280, p. 122, 1971.
International workshop on fluorides and dental caries reductions, University of Maryland School of Dentistry (Chairman: Dr. Donald Forrester), 1974.
Jackson, D., and Sutcliffe, P.: Clinical testing of a stannous-fluoride-calcium pyrophosphate dentifrice in Yorkshire school children. Br. Dent. J. *123*:40–48, 1967.
James, P. M. C., and Anderson, R. J.: Clinical testing of a stannous fluoride-calcium pyrophosphate dentifrice in Buckinghamshire school children. Br. Dent. J. *123*:33–39, 1967.
Jordan, W. A., and Peterson, J. K.: Caries-inhibiting value of a dentifrice containing stannous fluoride: Final report of a two-year study. J. Am. Dent. Assoc. *58*:42–46, 1959.
Kanouse, M. C., and Ash, M. M.: The effectiveness of a sodium monofluorophosphate dentifrice on dental hypersensitivity. J. Periodontol. *40*:38–39, 1969.
Kasakura, T.: Dental observation on school feeding. Part 3 – Effect of dental caries prevention by oral rinsing with a sodium fluoride solution. Shigaker Odontology. *54*:22–39, 1966.
Keller, S. E., and Manson-Hing, L. R.: Clearance studies on proximal tooth surfaces, Parts III and IV. *In vivo* removal of interproximal plaque. Ala. J. Med. Sci. *6*:399–405, 1969.
Keosian, J., Weinman, I., and Rafel, S.: The effect of aqueous diatomic iodine mouthwashes on the incidence of postextraction bacteremia. Oral Surg. *9*:1337–1341, 1956.
Kerr, D. W., and Kesel, R. G.: Two-year caries control study utilizing oral hygiene and an ammoniated dentifrice. J. Am. Dent. Assoc. *42*:180–188, 1951.
Keyes, P. H.: The infectious and transmissable nature of experimental dental caries – Findings and implications. Arch. Oral Biol., *1*:304–320, 1960.
Keyes, P. H., and White, C. L.: Dental caries in the molar teeth of rats, III. Bio-assay of sodium fluoride and sodium lauroyl sarcosinate as caries-inhibiting agents. J. Am. Dent. Assoc. *58*:43–55, 1959.
Keyes, P. H., Hicks, M. A., Goldman, B. M., McCabe, R. M., and Fitzgerald, R. J.: Dispersion of dextranous bacterial plaques on teeth with dextranase. J. Am. Dent. Assoc. *82*:136–141, 1971.
King, W. J.: Unpublished data, Colgate-Palmolive Company, 1950.
King, W. J., Manahan, R. D., and Russell, K. L.: Laboratory methods for screening possible inhibitors of dental caries. J. Dent. Res. *36*:307–313, 1957.
Kinkel, H. J., and Raich, R.: Die Karieshemmung einer

Na_2FPO_3-Zahnpaste nach 3 Jahren Applikation. Schweiz. Mschr. Zahnheilk. *82*:1240–1244, 1972.

Kinkel, H. J., and Raich, R.: Die Kariesheimmung einer Na_2FPO_3-Zahnpaste nach 4 Jahren Applikation. Schweiz. Mschr. Zahnheilk. *84*:226–229, 1974.

Kinkel, H. J., and Stolte, G.: On the effect of a sodium monofluorophosphate- ,and bromochlorophene-containing toothpaste in a chronic animal experiment and on caries in children during a two-year period of unsupervised use. Dtsch. Zahnaerstb. *22*:455–460, 1968.

Kinkel, H. J., Stolte, G., and Westrate, J.: Etude de l'efficacite d'une pâte dentifrice au fluorophosphate sur la denture des enfants. Schweiz. Mschr. Zahnheilk. *84*:577–589, 1974.

Kitchin, P. C., and Robinson, H. B.: How abrasive need a dentifrice be? J. Dent. Res. *27*:501–505, 1948.

Koch, G.: Comparison and estimation of effect on caries of daily supervised toothbrushing with a dentifrice containing potassium fluoride and manganese chloride. Odont. Revy *23*:341–354, 1972.

Koch, G.: Effect of sodium fluoride in dentifrice and mouthwash on incidence of dental caries in school children. Odont. Revy *18*: (Suppl. 12) 1–125, 1967.

Koch, G.: Long-term study of effect of supervised toothbrushing with a sodium fluoride dentifrice. Caries Res. *4*:149–157, 1970.
children. Odont. Revy *18*: (Suppl. 12) 1–125, 1967.

König, K. G., and Mühlemann, H. R.: Caries-inhibiting effect of amine fluoride-containing dentifrices tested in an animal experiment and in a clinical study. Caries Symposium Zürich, The present status of caries prevention by fluoride-containing dentifrices. Hans Huber Publishers, Berne, Switzerland, pp. 126–132, 1961.

Kovaleski, W. C., and Ash, M. M.: Clinical evaluation of a macrolide antibiotic as a plaque preventing agent. Thesis, University of Michigan, 1970.

Kowitz, G., Lucatorto, F., and Bennett, W.: Effects of dentifrices on soft tissues of the oral cavity. J. Oral Med. *28*:36–40, 1973.

Kowitz, G., Lucatorto, F., and Cherrick, H.: Effect of mouthwashes on the oral soft tissues. International Association for Dental Research. Preprinted Abstract No. 660, p. 219, 1974.

Kutcher, A. H., and Chilton, N. W.: Observations on the clinical use of a chlorophyll dentifrice. J. Am. Dent. Assoc. *46*:420–429, 1953.

Kyes, F. M., Overton, N. J., and McKean, T. W.: Clinical trials of caries-inhibitory dentifrices. J. Am. Dent. Assoc. *63*:189–193, 1961.

Lefkowitz, W., and Venti, V. I.: A preliminary clinical report on caries control with a high urea ammoniated dentifrice. Oral Surg. *4*:1576–1580, 1951.

Lind, O. P., Möller, I. J., von der Fehr, F. R., and Larsen, M. J.: Caries-preventive effect of a dentifrice containing 2% sodium monofluorophosphate in a natural fluoride area in Denmark. Community Dent. Oral Epidemiol. *2*:104–113, 1974.

Litsky, B. Y., Mascis, J. D., and Litsky, W.: Use of an antimicrobial mouthwash to minimize the bacterial aerosol contamination generated by the high-speed drill. Oral Surg. *29*:25–30, 1970.

Lobene, R. R.: A clinical study of the effect of dextranase on human dental plaque. J. Am. Dent. Assoc. *82*:132–135, 1971.

Lobene, R. R.: Effect of dentifrices on tooth stain with controlled brushing. J. Am. Dent. Assoc. *77*:849–855, 1968.

Lobene, R. R., and Soparkar, P. M.: The effect of an alexidine mouthwash on human plaque and gingivitis. J. Am. Dent. Assoc. *87*:848–851, 1973.

Lobene, R. R., and Soparkar, P. M.: The effect of amine fluorides on human plaque and gingivitis. International Association for Dental Research. Preprinted Abstract No. 369, p. 147, 1974.

Lobene, R. R., Brion, M., and Socransky, S. S.: Effect of erythromycin on dental plaque and plaque forming microorganisms in man. J. Periodont. *40*:287–291, 1969.

Lobene, R. R., Soparkar, P. M., Hein, J. W., and Quigley, G. A.: A study of the effects of antiseptic agents and a pulsating irrigating device on plaque and gingivitis. J. Periodont. *43*:564–568, 1972.

Löe, H., and Schiött, C. R.: The effect of suppression of the oral microflora upon the development of dental plaque and gingivitis. *In* Dental Plaque. (W. D. McHugh, ed.) D. C. Thomson and Company, Ltd., Dundee, Scotland, pp. 247–256, 1970.

Löe, H., and Schiött, C. R.: The effect of mouthrinses and topical applications of chlorhexidine on the development of dental plaque and gingivitis in man. J. Periodont. Res. *5*:79–83, 1970A.

Löe, H., Theilade, E., and Jensen, S. B.: Experimental gingivitis in man. J. Periodont. Res. *36*:177–189, 1965.

Löe, H., Mandell, M., Derry, A. W., and Schiött, C. R.: The effect of mouthrinses and topical application of chlorhexidine on calculus formation in man. J. Periodont. Res. *6*:312–314, 1971.

Loesche, W. J., Green, E., Kenney, E. B., and Nafe, D.: Effect of topical kanamycin sulfate on plaque accumulation. J. Am. Dent. Assoc. *83*:1063–1069, 1971.

Lunin, M., and Mandel, I. D.: Clinical evaluation of a penicillin dentifrice. J. Am. Dent. Assoc. *51*:696–702, 1955.

Mainwaring, P., and Naylor, M. N.: The clinical testing of an MFP toothpaste and A.P.F. gel. International Association for Dental Research. Preprinted Abstract No. L304, p. L76, 1975.

Mandel, I. D., and Cagan, R. S.: Pharmaceutical agents for preventing caries—A review, Part I. Dentifrices. J. Oral Therap. Pharm. *1*:218–227, 1964.

Manhold, B. A., Manhold, J. H., and Weisinger, E. A.: A study of total oral debris clearance, J. N.J. State Dent. Soc. pp. 1–14, 1967.

Manhold, J. H., and Manhold, B. A.: Further *in vivo* study of commercial mouth wash efficacy. N.Y. J. Dent. *33*:383–386, 1963.

Manhold, J. H., Parker, L. A., and Manhold, B. A.: Efficacy of a commercial mouth wash: *In vivo* study. N.Y. J. Dent. *32*:165–171, 1962.

Manly, R. S.: A structureless recurrent deposit on teeth. J. Dent. Res. *22*:479–486, 1943.

Manly, R. S.: Factors influencing tests on the abrasion of dentin by brushing with dentifrices. J. Dent. Res. *23*:59–72, 1944.

Manly, R. S., Wiren, J., Manly, P. J., and Keene, R. C.: A method for measurement of abrasion of dentin by toothbrush and dentifrice. J. Dent. Res. *44*: 533–540, 1965.

Marthaler, T. M.: Caries-inhibition by an amine fluoride dentifrice—Results after six years in children with low caries activity. Helv. Odont. Acta *18*:35–44, 1974.

Marthaler, T. M.: Karieshemmung durch Aminfluoridzahnpasten nach sieben jähriger Studiendauer (Results after seven years' use of an amine fluoride dentifrice). Schweiz. Monatsschr. Zahnheilkd. 78:134–147, 1968.

McCormick, J.: A critical review of the literature on mouthwashes. Ann. N.Y. Acad. Sci. (Evaluation of agents used in the prevention of oral disease). *153*:374–385, Dec. 23, 1968.

McCormick, J., and Koulourides, T.: A study of neutral calcium, phosphate, and fluoride remineralizing mouthwashes. International Association for Dental Research, Abstract No. 402, p. 138, 1965.

McDonnell, C. H., and Domalakes, E. F.: The effects of toothbrushing with dentifrices containing chlorophyllin on gingivitis, J. Periodont. 23:219–236, 1952.

McNeal, D. R.: Anticalculus agents for the treatment, control and prevention of periodontal disease. J. Public Health Dent. 29:138–152, 1969.

Mergele, M.: Report I. A supervised brushing study in state institution schools. Bull. Acad. Med. N.J. *14*: 247–250, 1968.

Mergele, M.: Report II. An unsupervised brushing study on subjects residing in a community with fluoride in the water. Bull. Acad. Med. N.J. *14*: 251–255, 1968A.

Mergele, M., Jennings, R. E., and Gasser, E. B.: Cited in evaluation of Cue tooth paste. J. Am. Dent. Assoc. *69*:197–198, 1964.

Millard, L.: Acute contact sensitivity to a new toothpaste. J. Dentistry *1*:168–170, 1973.

Mitchell, D. F., Holmes, L. A., Martin, P. W., and Sakurai, E.: Topical antibiotic maintenance of oral health. J. Oral. Ther. Pharm. *4*:83–92, 1967.

Mohammed, C. I., and Monserrate, V.: Preoperative oral rinsing as a means of reducing air contamination during use of air turbine handpieces. Oral Surg. *20*:291–294, 1970.

Mohammed, C. I., Manhold, J. H., and Manhold, B. A. Efficacy of preoperative oral rinsing to reduce air contamination during use of air turbine handpieces. J. Am. Dent. Assoc. *69*:715–718, 1964.

Möller, I. J., Holst, J. J., and Sörensen, E.: Caries-reducing effect of a sodium monofluorophosphate dentifrice. Br. Dent. J. *124*:209–213, 1968.

Moreira, B. W., and Tumang, A. J.: Prevencão da cárie dentária através de bochechos com solucões de fluoreto de sodio a 0.1% – Resultados após dois anos de estudos. Rev. Bras. Odont. Nr. *173*:37–42, 1972.

Morris, P. P., and Read, R. R.: Halitosis: Variations in mouth and total breath odor intensity resulting from prophylaxis and antisepsis. J. Dent. Res. *28*: 324–331, 1949.

Mühlemann, H. R.: *In vivo* measurements of calculus. Ann. N.Y. Acad. Sci. (Evaluation of agents used in the prevention of oral disease) *153*:164–196, Dec. 23, 1968.

Mühlemann, H. R., Bowles, D., Schaitt, A., and Bernimoulin, J. P.: Effect of diphosphonate on human supragingival calculus. Helv. Odontol. Acta *14*: 31–35, 1970.

Muhler, J. C.: A clinical comparison of fluoride and antienzyme dentifrices. J. Dent. Child. *37*:501–514, 1970.

Muhler, J. C.: The combined anticariogenic effect of a single stannous fluoride treatment and the unsupervised use of a stannous fluoride dentifrice. J. Dent. Res. *38*:994–1007, 1959.

Muhler, J. C.: Effect of a stannous fluoride dentifrice on caries reduction in children during a three-year study period. J. Am. Dent. Assoc. *64*:216–224, 1962.

Muhler, J. C.: Fifty-two pearls and their environment (Chapter 12 – Dentifrices and Oral Hygiene). Bloomington, Indiana University Press, pp. 124–143, 1965.

Muhler, J. C., and Radike, A. W.: Effect of a dentifrice containing stannous fluoride on dental caries in adults, II. Results at the end of two years of unsupervised use. J. Am. Dent. Assoc. *55*:196–198, 1957.

Muhler, J. C., Radike, A. W., Nebergall, W. H., and Day, H. G.: The effect of a stannous fluoride-containing dentifrice on caries reduction in children. J. Dent. Res. *33*:606–612, 1954.

Muhler, J. C., Radike, A. W., Nebergall, W. H., and Day, H. G.: A comparison between the anticariogenic effect of dentifrices containing stannous fluoride and sodium fluoride. J. Am. Dent. Assoc. *51*:556–559, 1955.

Muhler, J. C., Radike, A. W., Nebergall, W. H., and Day, H. G.: The effect of a stannous fluoride-containing dentifrice on adults. J. Dent. Res. *35*:49–53, 1956.

Muhler, J. C., Spear, L. B., Bixler, D., and Stookey, G. K.: The arrestment of incipient dental caries in adults after the use of three different forms of SnF_2 therapy: Results after 30 months. J. Am. Dent. Assoc. *75*:1402–1408, 1967.

Naylor, M. N., and Emslie, R. D.: Clinical testing of stannous fluoride and sodium monofluorophosphate dentifrices in London school children. Br. Dent. J. *123*:17–23, 1967.

Onisi, M., and Tani, H.: Clinical test on the caries-preventive effect of two kinds of fluoride dentifrices. Jap. J. Dent. Health *20*:105–111, 1970.

Onishi, E., Okada, S., Hinoide, M., Akada, H., Kon, K., Sugano, N., Sakakibara, Y., Morita, J., and Imamura, Y.: Effect of stannous fluoride dentifrice on the reduction of dental caries in school children. Jap. J. Dent. Health, *17*:68–74, 1967.

Pader, N.: Dentifrices: Problems of growth. Drug and cosmetic industry *108*: Part I (from p. 36) June, 1971; and *109*: Part II (from p. 36) July, 1971.

Parsons, J. C.: Chemotherapy of dental plaque – A review. J. Periodont. *45*:177–186, 1974.

Patz, J., and Naujoks, R.: Clinical investigation of a fluoride-containing dentifrice in adults, Results of a two-year unsupervised study. Dtsch. Zahnaertztl. Z. 7:614–621, 1969.

Peffley, G. E., and Muhler, J. C. The effect of a commercially available stannous fluoride dentifrice under controlled brushing habits on dental caries incidence in children: Preliminary report. J. Dent. Res. *39*:871–875, 1960.

Peterson, J. K.: The current status of therapeutic dentifrices. Ann. N.Y. Acad. Sci. (Evaluation of Agents Used in the Prevention of Oral Disease) *153*:334–349, Dec. 23, 1968.

Peterson, J. K., and Williamson, L.: Three-year caries inhibition of a sodium fluoride acid orthophosphate dentifrice compared with a stannous fluoride and a non-fluoride dentifrice. International Association for Dental Research, Preprinted Abstract No. 255, p. 101, 1968.

Peterson, J., and Williamson, L. D.: Caries inhibition with MFP–calcium carbonate dentifrice in fluoridated area. International Association for Dental Research, Preprinted Abstract No. L 338, p. L 85, 1975.

Pigman, Ward (ed.): Evaluation of agents used in the prevention of oral disease. Ann. N.Y. Acad. Sci. *153*:1–388, Dec. 23, 1968.

Pinsent, B. R. W.: Methods of assessing the efficiency of tooth-cleaning products. Cosmetic Science. (A. W. Middleton, Ed.) 1962.

Pinson, T. J., and Stanback, J.: Evaluation of chloraseptic solution as an anesthetic mouth wash. Q. Natl. Dent. Assoc. *22*:49–52, 1964.

Radike, A. W.: Current status of research on the use of a stannous fluoride dentifrice. J. Indiana Dent. Assoc. *39*:82–92, 1960.

Radike, A. W., Gish, C. W., Peterson, J. K., King, J. D., and Segreto, V. A.: Clinical evaluation of stannous fluoride as an anticaries mouth rinse. J. Am. Dent. Assoc. *86*:404–408, 1973.

Reed, M. W., and King, A. D.: A clinical evaluation of a sodium fluoride dentifrice. International Association for Dental Research, Preprinted Abstract No. 340, p. 133, 1970.

Renggli, H.: Zahnbelage und Gingivale Entzündung unter dem Einfluss eines antibakteriellen Mundspülmittels (Effect of antimicrobial mouthwash on dental deposits and gingival inflammation). Medical Thesis, University of Zürich, Zürich, Switzerland, 1966.

Report on Councils and Bureaus–Council on Dental Therapeutics. Council classifies fluoride mouthrinses. J. Am. Dent. Assoc. *91*:1250–1252, Dec. 1975.

Robinson, H. B. G.: Individualizing dentifrices: The dentist's responsibility. J. Am. Dent. Assoc. *79*: 633–636, 1969.

Robinson, R. G.: The effect of a quaternary ammonium compound on oral bacteria: An *in vivo* study using cetylpyridinium chloride. J. Dent. Assoc. S. Afr. *25*:68–74, 1970.

Rokita, J. R., Hazen, S. P., Millen, D., and Volpe, A. R.: An *in vivo* study of an antimicrobial mouth rinse on supragingival and subgingival plaque and calculus formation. Pharm. Therap. Dent. *2*:1–11, 1975.

Rölla, G., Löe, H., and Schiött, C. R.: The affinity of chlorhexidine for hydroxyapatite and salivary mucins. J. Periodont. Res. *5*:90–95, 1970.

Rosenthal, M. W.: Mouthwashes (Chapter 16), Cosmetics-Science and Technology. (E. Sagarin, Ed.) New York: Interscience Publishers, Inc., pp. 361–379, 1957.

Rosenthal, M. W.: Mouthwashes, Cosmetics-Science and Technology. (M. Balsam and E. Sagarin, Eds.) New York: John Wiley and Sons, pp. 533–563, 1972.

Rosenthal, M. W. Marson, L. M., and Abriss, A.: Some laboratory observations on the chemical, bacterial and enzymatic properties of sodium n-lauroyl sarcosinate. J. Dent. Child. *21*:194–199, 1954.

Rugg-Gunn, A. J., Holloway, P. J., and Davies, T. G. H.: Caries prevention by daily fluoride mouth rinsing. Brit. Dent. J. *135*:353–360, 1973.

Rundegren, J., Fornell, J., and Ericson, T.: *In vivo* and *in vitro* studies on a new peroxide-containing toothpaste. Scand. J. Dent. Res. *81*:543–547, 1973.

Sackler, A. M., Rockoff, S. C., and Rockoff, H. S.: Evaluation of chlorpactin WCS 60 as an adjunct in periodontal therapy. N.Y. J. Dent. *26*:199–201, 1956.

Schiff, T.: Clinical study to evaluate a proteolytic enzyme in plaque retardation. International Association for Dental Rsearch, Preprinted Abstract No. 706, p. 225, 1970.

Schiff, T., and Shaver, K.: The comparative effect of two commercially available dentifrices on tooth surfaces as determined by a tooth reflectance meter. J. Oral Med. *26*:127–133, 1971.

Schiff, T., and Volpe, A. R.: A two-year clinical study comparing the effect of dentifrices on selected dental materials. J. Oral Rehab. *2*:407–412, 1975.

Schroeder, H. E.: Formation and Inhibition of Dental Calculus. Hans Huber Publishers, Berne, Switzerland, 1969 (available in the U.S.A. from International Medical Press, 130 East 59th Street, New York, N.Y.).

Schroeder, H. E., Marthaler, T. M. and Mühlemann, H. R.: Effect of some potential inhibitors on early calculus formation. Helv. Odontol. Acta *6*:6–9, 1962.

Scola, F. P., and Ostrom, C. A.: Clinical evaluation of stannous fluoride when used as a constituent of a compatible prophylactic paste, as a topical solution, and in a dentifrice in naval personnel, II. Report of findings after two years. J. Am. Dent. Assoc. *77*: 594–597, 1968.

Segal, A. H., Stiff, R. H., George, W. A., and Picozzi, A.: Caries-inhibiting effectiveness of a stannous fluoride-insoluble sodium metaphosphate (IMP) dentifrice in children, Two-year results. International Association for Dental Research, Preprinted Abstract No. 250, p. 101, 1966.

Shannon, I. L.: Preparation and use of stannous fluoride solutions and ingestible dentifrice. Aeromedical Reviews (USAF School of Aerospace Medicine, Aerospace Medical Division, Brooks Air Force Base, Texas), Review 2–66, pp. 1–11, May, 1966.

Shapiro, W. B., Kaslick, R. S., Chasens, A. I., and Weinstein, D.: Controlled clinical comparison between a strontium chloride and a sodium monofluorophosphate toothpaste in diminishing root hypersensitivity. J. Periodontol. *41*:523–525, 1970.

Shaver, K. J., and Schiff, T.: Oral clinical functionality of enzyme AP used as a mouthwash. J. Periodontol. *41*:333–336, 1970.

Shea, J. J.: Allergy to fluoride. Ann. Allergy *25*:388–391, 1967.

Shiere, F. R.: The effectiveness of tyrothrycin dentifrice in the control of dental caries. J. Dent. Res. *36*:237–244, 1957.

Shipman, B., Cohen, E., and Kaslick, R. S.: The effect of a urea peroxide gel on plaque deposits and gingival status. J. Periodont. *42*:283–285, 1971.

Simring, M.: Deodorization and healing: Hexetidine in periodontal surgery. Oral Surg. *16*:1432–1442, 1963.

Slack, G. L., and Martin, W. J.: The use of a dentifrice containing stannous fluoride in the control of dental caries. Br. Dent. J. *117*:275–280, 1964.

Slack, G. L., Berman, D. S., Martin, W. J., and Young, J.: Clinical testing of a stannous fluoride-insoluble metaphosphate dentifrice in Kent school girls. Br. Dent. J. *123*:9–16, 1967.

Slack, G. L., Berman, D. S., Martin, W. J., and Hardie, J. M.: Clinical testing of a stannous fluoride-calcium pyrophosphate dentifrice in Essex school girls. Br. Dent. J. *123*:26–33, 1967.

Smith, I. L. F.: Acute allergic reaction following the use of toothpaste. Brit. Dent. J. *33*:304–305, 1968.

Solis, M. C., and Volpe, A. R.: Determination of sulfur volatiles in putrefied saliva by a gas chromatography-microcoulometric system. J. Periodont. *44*:775–778, 1973.

Stallard, R. E., Volpe, A. R., Orban, J. E., and King, W. J.: The effect of an antimicrobial mouth rinse on

dental plaque, calculus and gingivitis. J. Periodontol. *40*:683–694, 1969.
Stec, I. P.: A possible relationship between desquamation and dentifrices–A clinical study. J. Am. Dent. Hygienists Assoc. *46*:42–45, 1972.
Stephan, R. M., and Miller, B. F.: Effectiveness of urea and synthetic detergents in reducing activity of human dental caries. Proc. Soc. Exp. Biol. Med. *55*:101–104, 1944.
Stookey, G. K., and Muhler, J. C.: Laboratory studies concerning the enamel and dentin abrasion properties of common dentifrice polishing agents. J. Dent. Res. *47*:524–532, 1968.
Sturzenberger, O. P., and Leonard, G. J.: The effect of a mouthwash as an adjunct in tooth cleaning. J. Periodontol. *40*:299–302, 1969.
Sturzenberger, O. P., Swancar, J. R., and Reiter, G.: Reduction of dental calculus in humans through use of a dentifrice containing a crystal-growth inhibitor. J. Periodont. *42*:416–519, 1971.
Sulser, G. F., Fosket, R. R., and Fosdick, L. S.: Use of a sodium dehydroacetate-sodium oxalate dentifrice in the control of dental caries. J. Am. Dent. Assoc. *56*:368–375, 1958.
Suomi, S. D., Horowitz, H. S., Barbano, J. P., Spolsky, V. W., and Heifetz, S. B.: A clinical trial of a calculus inhibitory dentifrice. J. Periodont. *45*:139–145, 1974.
Swartz, M. L., and Phillips, R. W.: Cleansing, polishing and abrasion techniques (*in vitro*). Ann. N.Y. Acad. of Sci. (Evaluation of Agents Used in the Prevention of Oral Disease) *153*:120–136, 1968.
Swerdloff, G., and Shannon, I. L.: A feasibility study of the use of a stannous fluoride mouthwash in a school preventive dentistry program. SAM-TR-67-52, June, 1967.
Tainter, M. L., and Epstein, S.: Use of metal plates for testing the abrasiveness of dentifrices. J. Dent. Res. *22*:381–387, 1943.
Takeuchi, M., Schimizu, T., Kawasaki, T., and Kizu, T.: A field study on the effect of a dentifrice containing sodium monofluorophosphate in caries prevention. J. Soc. Oral Hygiene *18*:26–57, 1968.
Terry, J. M., and Shannon, I. L.: Clinical evaluation of an ingestible dentifrice. J. Oral Therap. Pharm. *4*:426–430, 1968.
Thomas, A. E., and Jamison, H. C.: Effect of SnF_2 dentifrices on caries in children: Two-year clinical study of supervised brushing in children's homes. J. Am. Dent. Assoc. 73:844–852, 1966.
Thomas, A. E., and Jamison, H. C.: Effect of a combination of two cariostatic agents on caries in children: Two-year clinical study of supervised brushing in children's homes. Bull. Acad. Med. N.J. pp. 241–246, 1968. (Also published in J. Am. Dent. Assoc. *81*:118–124, 1970.)
Tomlinson, K., and Davies, T. G. H.: Unpublished data, Colgate-Palmolive Company, 1962.
Tonzetich, J.: Direct gas chromatographic analysis of sulphur compounds in mouth air in man. Arch. Oral Biol. *16*:587–597, 1971.
Torell, P.: Bruk av fluortandkräm i samband nud fluorsköloljning varannan vecka. (The use of fluoride toothpaste confined with fluoride rinsing every two weeks.) Sveriges Tandläk. Tidning. *61*:873–875, 1969.
Torell, P., and Ericsson, Y.: Two-year clinical tests with different methods of local caries-preventive fluorine application in Swedish school-children (Part I: The Göteberg study). Acta Odontol. Scand. *23*: 287–312, 1965A.
Torell, P. and Ericsson, Y.: Two-year clinical tests with different methods of local caries-preventive fluorine application in Swedish school-children (Part II: The Södertälje study). Acta Odontol. Scand., *23*:313–321, 1965B.
Torell, P., and Ericsson, Y.: The potential benefits to be derived from fluoride mouth rinses. International workshop on fluorides and dental caries reductions, University of Maryland School of Dentistry, 1974.
Torell, P., and Siberg, A.: Mouthwash with sodium fluoride and potassium fluoride. Odont. Revy *13*: 62–72, 1962.
United States Code of Federal Regulations, Title 21, Part 130.
Vallotton, C. F.: An acquired pigmented pellicle of the enamel surface I. Review of the literature. J. Dent. Res. *24*:161–169, 1945.
Van Abbé, N. J., Bridge, A. J., Ribbons, J. W., Dean, P. M., and Lazarou, J. A.: The effect of dentifrices on extrinsic tooth stain. J. Soc. Cosmetic Chemists *22*:457–476, 1971.
Villa, P.: Degree of calculus inhibition by habitual toothbrushing. Helv. Odontol. Acta *12*:31–36, 1968.
Vinson, L. J., and Bennett, H. G.: Evaluation of oral antiseptic products on buccal epithelial tissue. J. Am. Pharm. Assoc. (Scientific Ed.). *47*:635–639, 1958.
Vogel, P., and Hess, W.: Clinical evaluation of caries-reducing effect of a dentifrice containing 13% carbamide and 3% dibasic ammonium phosphate. J. Dent. Child. *24*:237–242, 1957.
Volker, J. F., Sognnaes, R. F., and Bibby, B. G.: Studies on the distribution of radioactive fluoride in the bones and teeth of experimental animals. Am. J. Physiol. *132*:707–712, 1941.
Volker, J. F., Apperson, L. D. and King, W. J.: The influence of certain protein adsorbed agents on hamster caries. Antiobiot. Chemother. *6*:56–62, 1956.
Volker, J. F., Hodge, H. C., Wilson, H. J., and Van Voochis, S. M.: The adsorption of fluorides by enamel, dentin, bone and hydroxyapatite as shown by the radioactive isotope. J. Biol. Chem. *134*:543–548, 1940.
Volpe, A. R.: Indices for the measurement of hard deposits in clinical studies of oral hygiene and periodontal disease. J. Periodont. Res. 9:31–60, 1974.
Volpe, A. R.: Summary of clinical findings with a monofluorophosphate dentifrice. Bull. Acad. Med. N.J. *14*:256–260, 1968.
Volpe, A. R., Kupczak, L. J., Brant, J. H., King, W. J., Kestenbaum, R. C., and Schlissel, H. J.: Antimicrobial control of bacterial plaque and calculus and the effects of these agents on the oral flora. J. Dent. Res. *48*:832–841, 1969.
Volpe, A. R., Mooney, R., Zumbrunnen, C., Stahl, D., and Goldman, H. M.: A long-term clinical study evaluating the effect of two dentifrices on oral tissues. J. Peridont. *46*:113–118, 1975.
Volpe, A. R., Schulman, S. M., Goldman, H. M., King, W. J., and Kupczak, L. J.: The long-term effect of an antimicrobial formulation on dental calculus formation. J. Periodontol. *41*:464–467, 1970.
Wallace, D. A.: Therapeutic dentifrices, A review of

the literature on clinical investigations. Dent. Prog. *2*:242–248, 1962.
Walsh, J. P., and Smart, R. S.: Clinical trial of a penicillin tooth powder, N. Z. Dent. J. *47*:118–122, 1951.
Wedderburn, D. L.: The use of antiseptics and germicides in toilet preparations (Chap. XXI), Handbook of Cosmetic Science. (H. W. Hibbott, Ed.) Oxford University Press, Fairlawn, New Jersey, pp. 445–472, 1963.
Weinstein, E., and Mandel, I. D.: The present status of anticalculus agents. J. Oral Therap. Pharm. *1*:327–343, 1964.
Weisenstein, P. R., and Zacherl, W. A.: A multiple-examiner clinical evaluation of a sodium fluoride dentifrice. J. Am. Dent. Assoc. *84*:621–623, 1972.
Weisz, W. S.: The reduction of dental caries through use of a sodium fluoride mouthwash. J. Am. Dent. Assoc. *60*:438–443, 1960.
Wilkinson, J. B., and Pugh, B. R.: Toothpastes – Cleaning and abrasion. J. Soc. Cosmetic Chemists *21*: 595–605, 1970.
Winkler, K. C., Backer-Dirks, O., and Van Amerongen, J.: Reproducible method for caries evaluation, Test in a therapeutic experiment with a fluorinated dentifrice. Br. Dent. J. *95*:119–127, 1953.
Workshop conference on the physical functionality of dentifrices (abrasion-cleaning-polishing). American Dental Association (Chairman: Dr. John Hefferen), 1974.
Wright, K. H. R., and Stevenson, J. I.: The measurement and interpretation of dentifrice abrasiveness. J. Soc. Cosmetic Chemists *18*:387–411, 1967.
Zacherl, W. A.: A clinical evaluation of sodium fluoride and stannous fluoride dentifrices, International Association for Dental Research, Preprinted Abstract No. 253, p. 101, 1968.
Zacherl, W. A.: Clinical evaluation of a sarcosinate dentifrice, International Association for Dental Research, Preprinted Abstract No. 339, p. 133, 1970.
Zacherl, W. A., and McPhail, C. W. B.: Evaluation of a stannous fluoride-calcium pyrophosphate dentifrice. J. Can. Dent. Assoc. *31*:174–180, 1965.
Zacherl, W. A.: Clinical evaluation of neutral sodium fluoride, stannous fluoride, sodium monofluorophosphate and acidulated fluoride-phosphate dentifrices. J. Can. Dent. Assoc. *1*:35–38, 1972.
Zacherl, W. A.: Clinical evaluation of an aged stannous fluoride-calcium pyrophosphate dentifrice. J. Can. Dent. Assoc. *4*:155–157, 1972A.
Zander, H. A.: Effect of a penicillin dentifrice on caries incidence in school children, J. Am. Dent. Assoc. *40*:569–574, 1950.
Zipkin, I., and McClure, F. J.: The effect of sodium lauroyl sarcosinate, sodium lauryl sulfate and dehydroacetic acid on occlusal and smooth surface caries in the rat. J. Dent. Res. *34*:768–773, 1955.

RECOMMENDED READING

COMPOSITION OF DENTIFRICES AND CLEANING AND POLISHING ASPECTS

Accepted Dental Therapeutics, 34th Ed., 1971/1972; 36th Ed. 1975/1976; published by the American Dental Association, 211 East Chicago Avenue, Chicago, Illinois 60611.
Bouchal, A. W.: The abrasiveness of dentifrices. Proc. of the Scient. Section of the Toilet Goods Assoc. No. 45, pp. 2–5, 1966.
Gershon, S. D., and Pader, M.: Dentifrices, Cosmetics-Science and Technology. Vol. 1, 2nd Ed. (M. Balsam and E. Sagarin, Eds.) New York: John Wiley and Sons, pp. 423–531, 1972.
Gershon, S. D., Pokras, H. H., and Rider, T. H.: Dentifrices (Chapter 15), Cosmetics-Science and Technology. (E. Sagarin, Ed.) New York: Interscience Publishers, Inc., pp. 296–360, 1957.
Harry, R. G.: The tooth and oral hygiene and dentifrices, The principles and practice of modern cosmetics. (Vol. 1). Modern Cosmeticology, Chemical Publishing Co., New York, pp. 239–290, 1962.
Hendon, G. E., Keller, S. E., and Manson-Hing, L. R.: Clearance studies of proximal tooth surfaces, Part I. Ala. J. Med. Sci. *6*:213–227, 1969.
Jefopoulos, T.: Dentifrices, 1970, published by Noyes Data Corporation, Park Ridge, New Jersey (also Zug, Switzerland and London, England).
Manly, R. S., Wiren, J., Manly, P. J., and Keene, R. C.: A method for measurement of abrasion of dentin by toothbrush and dentifrice. J. Dent. Res. *44*:533–540, 1965.
Robinson, H. B. G.: Individualizing dentifrices: The dentist's responsibility. J. Am. Dent. Assoc. *79*: 633–636, 1969.
Stookey, G. K., and Muhler, J. C.: Laboratory studies concerning the enamel and dentin abrasion properties of common dentifrice polishing agents. J. Dent. Res. *47*:524–532, 1968.
Swartz, M. L., and Phillips, R. W.: Cleansing, polishing and abrasion techniques (*in vitro*). Ann. N.Y. Acad. Sci. (Evaluation of agents used in the prevention of oral disease) *153*:120–136, 1968.
Workshop conference on the physical functionality of dentifrices (abrasion-cleaning-polishing). American Dental Association (Chairman: Dr. John Hefferren), 1974.
Wilkinson, J. B., and Pugh, B. R.: Toothpastes – Cleaning and abrasion. J. Soc. Cosmetic Chemists *21*: 595–605, 1970.
Wright, K. H. R., and Stevenson, J. I.: The measurement and interpretation of dentifrice abrasiveness. J. Soc. Cosmetic Chemists *18*:387–411, 1967.

THERAPEUTIC DENTIFRICES

Accepted Dental Therapeutics, 34th Ed., 1971/1972; 36th Ed. 1975/1976; published by the American Dental Association, 211 East Chicago Avenue, Chicago, Illinois, 60611.
American Dental Association, Clinical testing of dental caries preventatives – Report of a conference to develop uniform standards and procedures in clinical studies of dental caries. Published by the American Dental Association, 1955.
American Dental Association, Conference on clinical trials of drugs used in dentistry. Published by the American Dental Association, 1960.
American Dental Association, Proceedings of the conference on the clinical testing of cariostatic agents, published by the American Dental Association, 1968.
Backer-Dirks, O., Baume, L. J., Davies, G. N., and Slack, G. L.: Principal requirements for controlled clinical trials. Int. Dent. J. *17*:93–103, 1967.

Bartelstone, H. J., Mandel, I. D. and Chilton, N. W.: Critical evaluation of clinical studies with stannous fluoride dentifrices. N.Y. State Dent. J. *28*:147–156, 1962.

Bibby, B. G.: Caries: Preventive effects of topical fluoride applications: A review of recent clinical trials in North America. Bull. Acad. Med. N.J. *14*:210–226, 1968.

Caries Symposium Zürich: The present status of caries prevention by fluoride-containing dentifrices. (H. R. Mühlemann and K. G. König, Eds.) Hans Huber Publishers, Berne, Switzerland, 1961.

Duckworth, R.: Fluoride dentifrices, A review of clinical trials in the United Kingdom. Br. Dent. J. *124*: 505–509, 1968.

Duckworth, R.: Review of recent clinical trials outside North America. Bull. Acad. Med. N.J. *14*:226–239, 1968.

Evaluation of agents used in the prevention of oral disease. Ann. N.Y. Acad. Sci. (Ward Pigman, Consulting Ed.) *153*:1–388, Dec. 23, 1968.

Fluorides in the control of caries, A symposium on recent clinical advances in the use of fluorides for controlling caries. Bull. Acad. Med. N.J. *14*:201–265, Dec., 1968.

Gish, C. W., and Mercer, V. H.: "Doctor, which toothpaste do you recommend?" Consumer Bull., pp. 12–16, May, 1968.

Grøn, P., and Brudevold, F.: The effectiveness of NaF dentifrices. J. Dent. Child. *34*:122–127, 1967.

Hartles, R. L.: Toothpaste as anticaries agents. Am. Perfumer. *77*:53–55, 1962.

Heifetz, S. B., and Horowitz, H. S.: An appraisal of therapeutic dentifrices. J. Public Health Dent. *30*:206–211, 1970.

Hill, T. J.: Fluoride dentifrices. J. Am. Dent. Assoc. *59*:1121–1127, 1959.

Horowitz, H. S.: Clinical trials of preventives for dental caries. J. Pub. Health Dent. *32*:229–233, 1972.

Mandel, I. D., and Cagan, R. S.: Pharmaceutical agents for preventing caries—A review. Part I—Dentifrices. J. Oral Therap. Pharm. *1*:218–227, 1964.

Muhler, J. C.: Fifty-two pearls and their environment. Chapter 12—Dentifrices and Oral Hygiene. Bloomington: Indiana University Press, pp. 124–143, 1965.

Pader, N.: Dentifrices: Problems of growth. Drug and Cosmetic Industry *108*: Part I (from p. 36) June, 1971; *109*: Part II (from p. 36) July, 1971.

Peterson, J. K.: The current status of therapeutic dentifrices. Ann. N.Y. Acad. Sci. (Evaluation of agents used in the prevention of oral disease) *153*:334–349, Dec. 23, 1968.

Radike, A. W.: Current status of research on the use of a stannous fluoride dentifrice. J. Indiana Dent. Assoc. *39*:82–92, 1960.

Rapoport, S.: Toothpaste—Should it whiten and brighten? Can it give you the breath of springtime? Consumer Bull., pp. 7–9, Aug., 1971.

United States Code of Federal Regulations, Title 21, Part 130.

Volpe, A. R.: Summary of clinical findings with a monofluorophosphate dentifrice. Bull. Acad. Med. N.J. *14*:256–260, 1968.

Wallace, D. A.: Therapeutic dentifrices. A review of the literature on clinical investigations. Dent. Prog. *2*:242–248, 1962.

Ware, A. L.: A review of dentifrices as therapeutic agents. Aust. Dent. J. 9:203–208, 1964.

MOUTH RINSES

Darlington, R. C.: O-T-C topical oral antiseptics and mouthwashes. J. Am. Pharm. Assoc. *NS8*:484–496, 1968.

Gjermo, P.: Some aspects of drug dynamics related to oral soft tissues. Presented at Sixth International Conference on Oral Biology, Toronto, 1974. J. Dent. Res. *54*:B44–B56, 1975.

Gucklhorn, I. R.: Antimicrobials in cosmetics, Toilet Goods Assoc. Cosmetic J. *1*:15–32, Fall, 1969.

Horowitz, H. S.: The prevention of dental caries by mouth rinsing with solutions of neutral sodium fluoride. Int. Dent. J. *23*:585–590, 1973.

International workshop on fluorides and dental caries reductions, University of Maryland School of Dentistry (Chairman: Dr. Donald Forrester), 1974.

McCormick, J.: A critical review of the literature on mouthwashes. Ann. N.Y. Acad. Sci. (Evaluation of agents used in the prevention of oral disease) *153*: 374–385, Dec. 23, 1968.

Parsons, J. C.: Chemotherapy of dental plaque—A review. J. Periodont. *45*:177–186, 1974.

Rosenthal, M. W.: Mouthwashes (Chapter 16), Cosmetics-Science and Technology. (E. Sagarin, Ed.) Interscience Publishers, Inc., New York, pp. 361–379, 1957.

Rosenthal, M. W.: Mouthwashes, Cosmetics-Science and Technology. (M. Balsam and E. Sagarin, Eds.) Vol. 1, 2nd Ed. New York: John Wiley and Sons, pp. 533–563, 1972.

Torell, P., and Ericsson, Y.: The potential benefits to be derived from fluoride mouth rinses. International workshop on fluorides and dental caries reductions, University of Maryland School of Dentistry, 1974.

Volpe, A. R.: Indices for the measurement of hard deposits in clinical studies of oral hygiene and periodontal disease. J. Periodont. Res. 9:31–60, 1974.

Wedderburn, D. L.: The use of antiseptics and germicides in toilet preparations (Chap. XXI), Handbook of Cosmetic Science. (H. W. Hibbott, Ed.) Oxford University Press, Fairlawn, New Jersey, pp. 445–472, 1963.

chapter 13

ORAL HYGIENE TECHNICS AND HOME CARE

by

WALLACE V. MANN, JR., D.M.D.

INTRODUCTION

The term "oral hygiene" often has a different meaning for different people. Nevertheless, almost everyone agrees that the phrase implies oral cleanliness. Some use it to designate the condition or state of cleanliness which is present at a given point in time, while others use it to designate the procedures or practices which are used to establish the state of cleanliness. By definition, however, hygiene includes all of the measures which are necessary to establish and maintain health. Consequently, oral hygiene could include any or all of the procedures that contribute to a state of oral health. Under these circumstances the definition could be limitless. For the purposes of this chapter, the term oral hygiene will include those procedures which cleanse the teeth, periodontal tissues and mouth and thus contribute to a state of cleanliness in the oral cavity.

THE RELATIONSHIP OF ORAL HYGIENE TO CARIES AND PERIODONTAL DISEASE

Other sections of this text have stressed the importance of bacteria in the etiology of caries and periodontal disease. In addition, many investigators have established the fact that proper oral hygiene is extremely important in the prevention of both the occurrence and recurrence of caries and periodontal disease.[14, 22, 39, 50]

After an extensive review of the literature on the relation of caries to oral hygiene, Davies[18] concluded that it is more important to clean the teeth when the forces which attack the teeth are intense. These intense conditions would be found in more highly civilized societies. Conversely, cleansing the teeth would not be as important when the intensity of the forces attacking the teeth is low. Such conditions would be found in more primitive societies. Also, he concluded that cleaning the teeth will reduce caries only if carried out immediately after eating. This supported the earlier observations of Fosdick,[22] who examined approximately 700 young adults over a period of two years. He showed that the experimental group (which brushed within ten minutes after food ingestion) had 41 per cent fewer cavities when these patients were examined and contrasted with the control group.

Mansbridge[38] examined 426 children between the ages of 12 and 14 and rated the oral hygiene in each child "good" or "neglected." He concluded that there was a significantly lower prevalence of caries in those individuals with good oral hygiene. These and other studies suggest a cause and effect relationship between caries and oral hygiene. However, there are conflicting reports on this question. Some studies have shown that there is no difference in caries activity among individuals with good and poor hygiene. In fact there may be a higher rate of caries activity in those with good oral hygiene. In other words, a higher standard of oral cleanliness may result in more, and not less, caries.[28, 39] Davies[18] has commented on these conflicting reports and has suggested that the measurement of the oral hygiene at a given point in time might be misleading, since the caries which is present reflects an accumulation over a time period. Thus, the state of oral hygiene at this given point may not represent the true condition of cleanliness over the period it took to develop the caries.

Greene[25] has published a thorough review of the literature on oral hygiene as it relates to periodontal disease. In the summary of this review he has written: "The one consistent factor associated with the prevalence and severity of periodontal disease is the status of oral cleanliness." Many epidemiologic and clinical studies support this statement. It has also been shown that there is a direct relation between the amount of oral debris and the severity of the disease. Arno et al.[7] have determined that the prevalence and severity of gingivitis in 1346 factory employees in Oslo were significantly higher in the non-administrative personnel. They attributed this to the lower level of oral hygiene in this group than that found in the administrative staff. Brandtzaeg[14] also showed that the amount of periodontal disease is a linear function of the amount of debris on the teeth. In this same study it was shown that instruction in cleansing the teeth resulted in a 45 per cent improvement in periodontal health and a 40 per cent improvement in oral hygiene. Other studies have clearly established a relationship between brushing frequency and periodontal disease severity. In the past few years a number of well-controlled clinical studies have shown that the amount of gingival inflammation is related to the level of oral hygiene.[34, 47, 51] Perhaps the most significant studies have been done by a group of investigators in Denmark.[35, 36, 49] They have reported a series of experiments which are based on the development of experimental gingivitis in man. In addition to other findings not listed here, these individuals have established the following facts about the relationship of oral hygiene to gingivitis:

1. The withdrawal of toothbrushing in healthy persons with excellent oral hygiene and normal gingiva led to a rapid accumulation of bacterial plaque.
2. A gingivitis developed in these subjects in 10 to 21 days.
3. When oral hygiene was reinstated, the plaque was reduced and the gingiva returned to a healthy state.
4. Cessation of oral hygiene led to a characteristic bacteriologic change in the plaque as the gingivitis progressed. However, when good oral hygiene was resumed the bacterial flora changed to the types of organisms that existed prior to the withdrawal of oral hygiene.

Similar studies[3] have been done in laboratory animals. These also confirm the epidemiologic and clinical studies in humans that oral hygiene is directly related to the development of periodontal disease.

One may conclude from these different approaches to the problem that oral hygiene is a major factor, if not the most important factor, in caries and periodontal disease. Although this relationship has been established with fairly convincing evidence, the evidence put forth on the *methods* to achieve good oral hygiene have largely been based on opinion and empiricism. There are a limited number of well-designed and well-controlled studies which seem to indicate the best approach to the problem of mechanically removing bacteria from the teeth and from the gingiva. However, the best that can be said at present is that conclusive evidence is not yet available. The proof of the superiority of one technic or one device (or even a series of technics or devices) has not as yet been established. There is a wide variety of opinion, and we must also consider the number of different factors associated with the problem. Such variables as the physical capacity of the patient to perform proper oral hygiene, the age and level of understanding of the patient and the condition of a patient's mouth are just a few examples of the factors which affect the performance of adequate oral hygiene.

The problem is also complicated by conflicting opinion on the technics and materials to use. Nevertheless, the most practical way at present to prevent oral disease is to develop a procedure for each patient which will result in the best possible oral hygiene for that particular patient. This means the maintenance of cleanliness primarily by the mechanical dispersion and removal of adherent microorganisms from the oral cavity.

This view is expressed by Löe[37] who has written a succinct review of the methods by which plaque may be prevented and controlled. He discussed three major categories. These were natural, mechanical and chemical cleansing. Listed under the chemical category were such things as enzymes, antibiotics and agents which would change the physical properties of the surface to which the plaque is attached. Löe concluded the following:

> Available data from dental research seem to justify the clinical hypothesis that bacterial plaque is the direct cause of marginal periodontal disease and that caries will not develop in the absence of plaque. Consequently, the control of plaque represents the essential measure in the prevention of the two main dental diseases.
>
> Since natural cleansing of the dento-gingival areas is inadequate, plaque control can only be achieved through its active removal at regular intervals. The addition of various enzymes, theoretically capable of interfering with plaque development, to dentifrices, chewing gums, etc. has not as yet been promising. Prevention of plaque adhesion by changing the surface charge of the teeth is also at the experimental stage. Tests of various antibiotic substances have confirmed that complete prevention of plaque is possible. However, the problems inherent to continuous use of antibiotics suggest that they will not be acceptable for the lifelong control of plaque. Experiments with antibacterial agents other than antibiotics have demonstrated that bacterial colonisation on the teeth can be inhibited by suppressing the oral flora. More knowledge of the effect of such ecological shifts and possible side effects is needed before antibacterial substances can be introduced for clinical use.

It is with this in mind that the following portion of this chapter will present the equipment necessary for the mechanical removal of plaque and a discussion of the various methods by which this equipment can be used.

EQUIPMENT

Kimery and Stallard[32] have written a thorough review of the procedures that are currently used in oral hygiene. One of the items mentioned by them for its historical interest was the chewstick. It is also of current interest as illustrated in Figures 13–1 and 13–2. The patient carried this with him and used it after meals and throughout the day after eating. It would have been hard to improve on this patient's oral hygiene, and it emphasizes the point that motivation and a habitual pattern of using a device are the important factors. The device itself is not critical as long as it does not injure the patient and is effective in removing plaque. In addition to the chewstick, tooth picks of wood or ivory were early mechanical devices to clean the teeth. Subsequently, the tooth brush was introduced in the early part of the nineteenth century. In addition to the brush, there has been a proliferation of many different types of devices to aid in plaque removal. Some examples of these

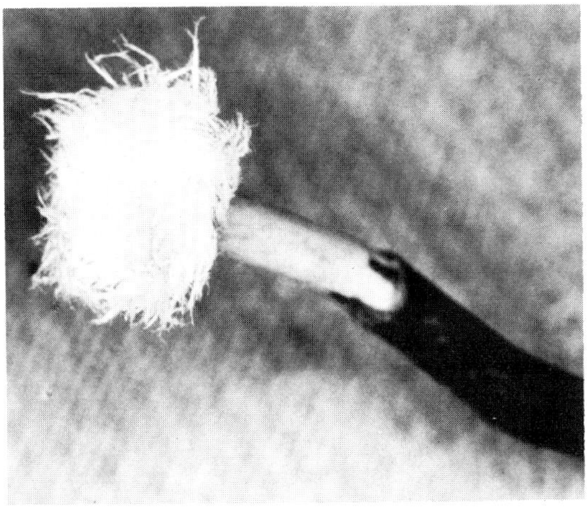

Figure 13–1 A twig from a black gum tree found in the southeastern United States. The bark is removed and the end chewed until it is frayed. (Courtesy of Dr. T. Weatherford, University of Alabama.)

will be discussed but primary emphasis will be on three items. These include the disclosing tablet, brush and dental floss. These may be considered the essential components of a plaque control program for the majority of child and adult patients. With these an effective method can be established which eliminates plaque from the areas of the teeth and periodontal tissues where plaque accumulates most readily and is removed with most difficulty, that is, the interproximal areas and the subgingival space.

The original ideas concerning this approach to plaque removal and control were developed primarily by Bass and Arnim. Much credit should be given these men. They have directed the attention of many clinicians from primary emphasis on restorative care to preventive care. Their work has been summarized and the rationale for this program has been presented in an article by Arnim.[4] Also, this article lists almost all of the pertinent references to the origin and development of this concept.

The accumulation of plaque in the interproximal areas and close to the free margin of the gingiva is shown in Figure 13–3. This demonstrates the accumulation of plaque along the gingival margin and on the tooth surfaces which form the lateral borders of the interproximal space. Notice also the oval depression on the labial surface of the central incisor. Plaque has formed here since this area was somewhat protected from the movement of the lips or tongue. The formation of plaque is shown more dramatically in Figure 13–4. The top half of the illustration shows the patient

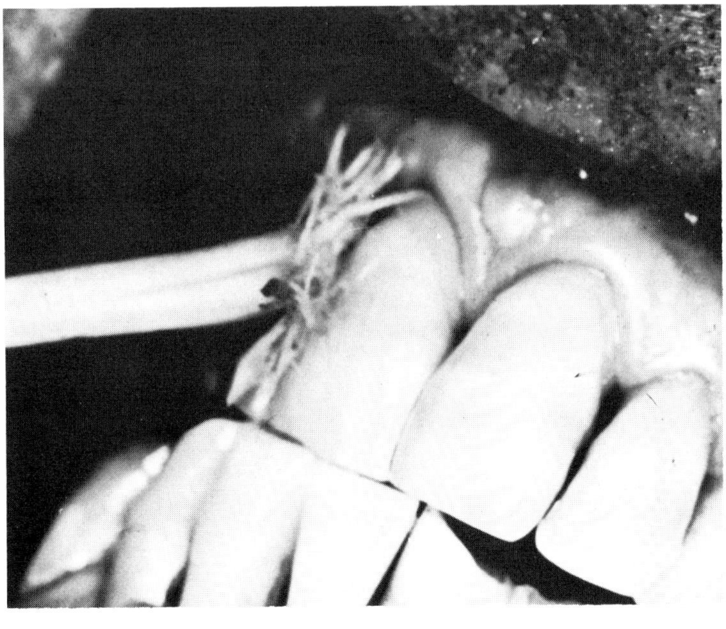

Figure 13–2 The chew stick as it is used by the patient. There are minimal caries and the periodontal tissues are healthy. (Courtesy of Dr. T. Weatherford, University of Alabama.)

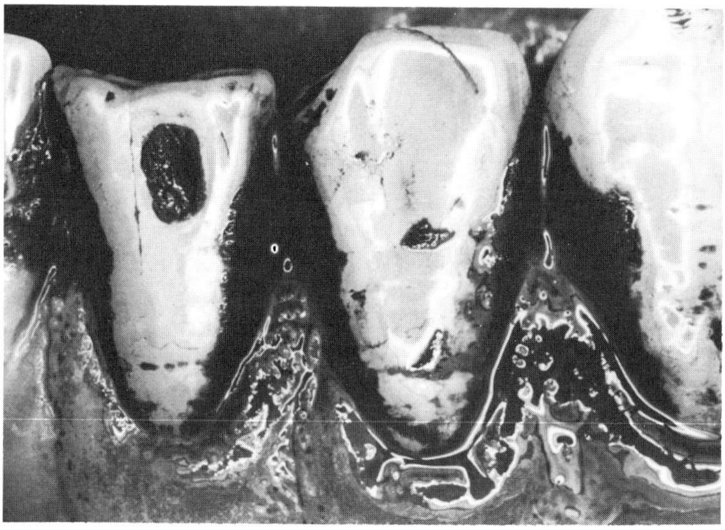

Figure 13–3 Plaque accumulation pattern in a patient who has not brushed for 24 hours.

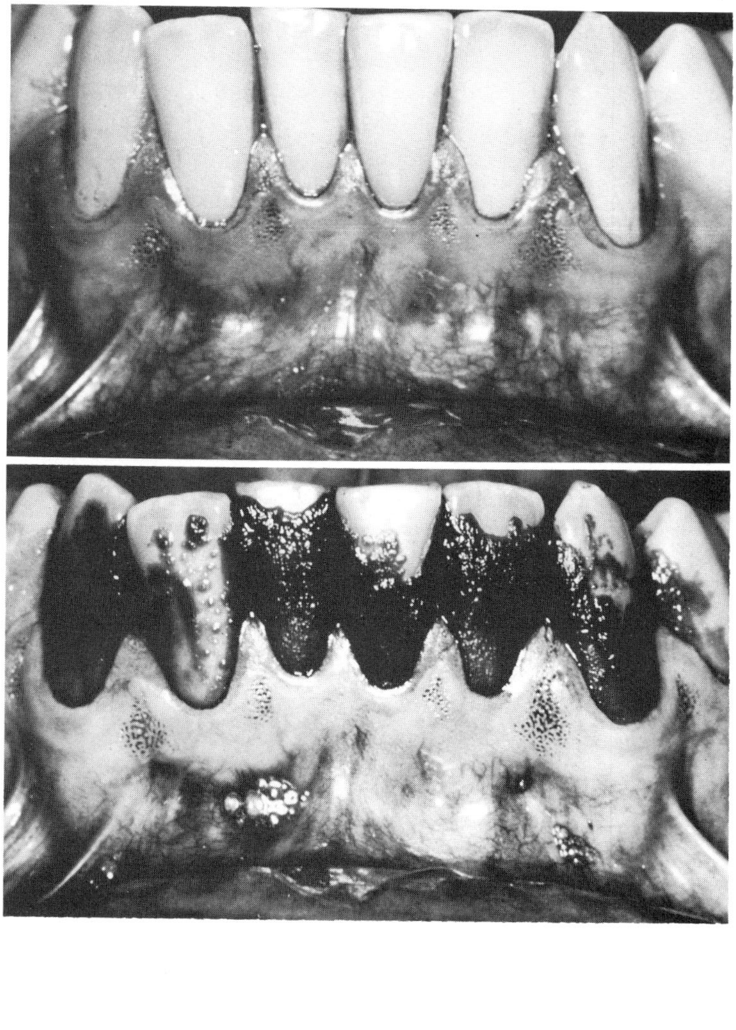

Figure 13–4 Top: Staining immediately after prophylaxis. Bottom: Plaque accumulation pattern in a patient who has not brushed for six days.

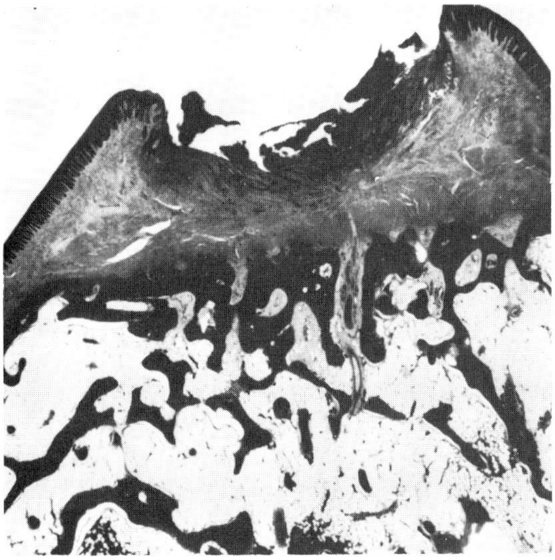

Figure 13–5 Interdental gingiva with plaque in close proximity to ulcerated epithelium. There is a characteristic chronic inflammatory reaction in this area. (Courtesy of Dr. S. Hazen, University of Connecticut.)

after a cleaning and polishing by a hygienist. The lower half shows this patient after six days during which he rinsed with an experimental mouth rinse three times daily but did not brush. This suggests that bacterial colonization over all the tooth surfaces can take place at a fairly rapid rate in the absence of brushing. The histopathologic features of the lesion are shown in Figure 13–5. This is not interdental tissue from either of the patients in Figures 13–3 and 13–4 but represents a rather characteristic appearance of inflammation with ulceration of the epithelium lining the interdental gingiva which forms the apical border of the interproximal space. These examples illustrate the importance of cleaning the subgingival space and the interproximal area. From both the caries and periodontal disease standpoint, these two areas are primary sites for the initial lesions. It is critical to remove plaque from these areas, and Figure 13–6 offers a scheme for doing this. Disclosing wafers are used to disclose the plaque, and a disposable mirror can be used by the patient to see the areas of plaque accumulation. The brush is used to clean the teeth and subgingival area, and floss is used to clean the interproximal surfaces of the teeth. The methods of doing this will be discussed later, but the conclusion which must be drawn at this point is that the early investigations of Bass and Arnim have been verified; their findings have been accepted and put into practice by many clinicians, and the evidence is quite convincing that plaque removal can be accomplished using these mechanical devices, providing a patient is sufficiently motivated.

DISCLOSING WAFERS AND SOLUTIONS

The need for disclosing substances is shown in Figure 13–7. This is a 17-year-old

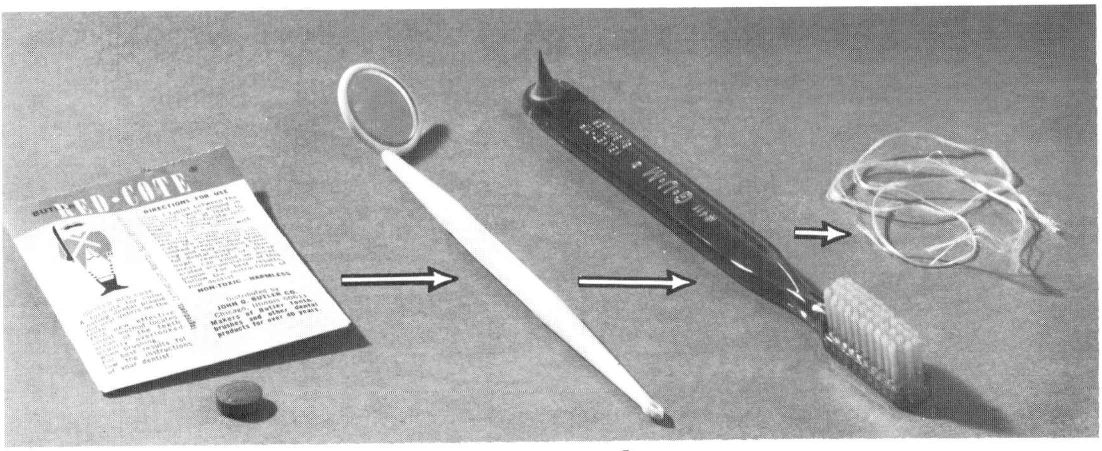

Figure 13–6 The essential equipment for plaque control. Disclosing wafers and a mirror to see the plaque, the brush and floss for plaque removal.

patient who complained of bleeding of the gingiva when he brushed in the area of the mandibular left cuspid and lateral incisor. The bacterial deposits are soft and whitish in color and are hard to distinguish from the tooth. However, the application of a dye to disclose these deposits is very helpful. It shows the patient just where these are, and the basic principle is to clean the teeth until no more stained deposit is visible.

A variety of dyes have been used in either tablet or solution form to disclose the plaque.[15, 19] Such substances as iodine, mercurochrome, neutral red, merbromin, Bismark brown and various food colorings have been used. Perhaps the two most common have been basic fuchsin and F.D.C. Red No. 3 (erythrosin). Basic fuchsin seems to stain the deposits with more contrast than erythrosin, but it must not be used over a long period of time as it might be carcinogenic. Arnim[5] has reviewed the development of disclosing agents and has said that basic fuchsin might be one of the substances which was responsible for the higher incidence of carcinoma of the bladder in workers in the aniline dye industry. Consequently, he looked for a substitute and erythrosin was suggested. He then developed the formula for a wafer. Examples of those available commercially are shown in Figure 13–8 (see also Table 13–1). Solu-

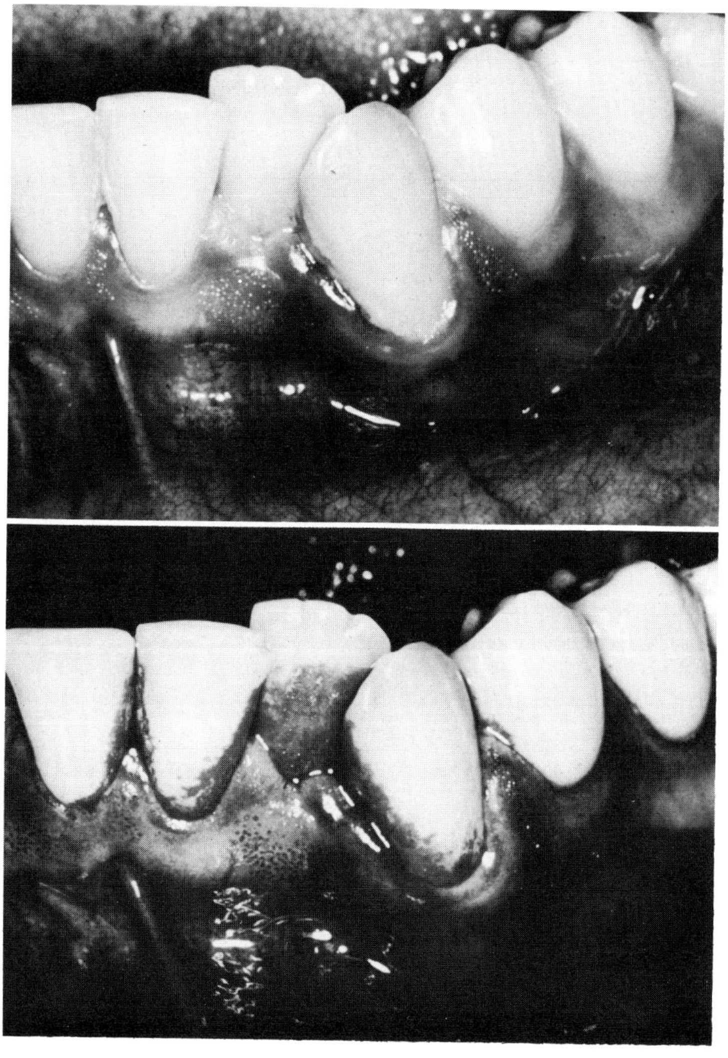

Figure 13–7 Top: Plaque which is not evident. Bottom: Plaque stained with a disclosing solution. Notice the amount of gingival inflammation in the areas of heavy plaque accumulation and minimal inflammation where there is little or no plaque.

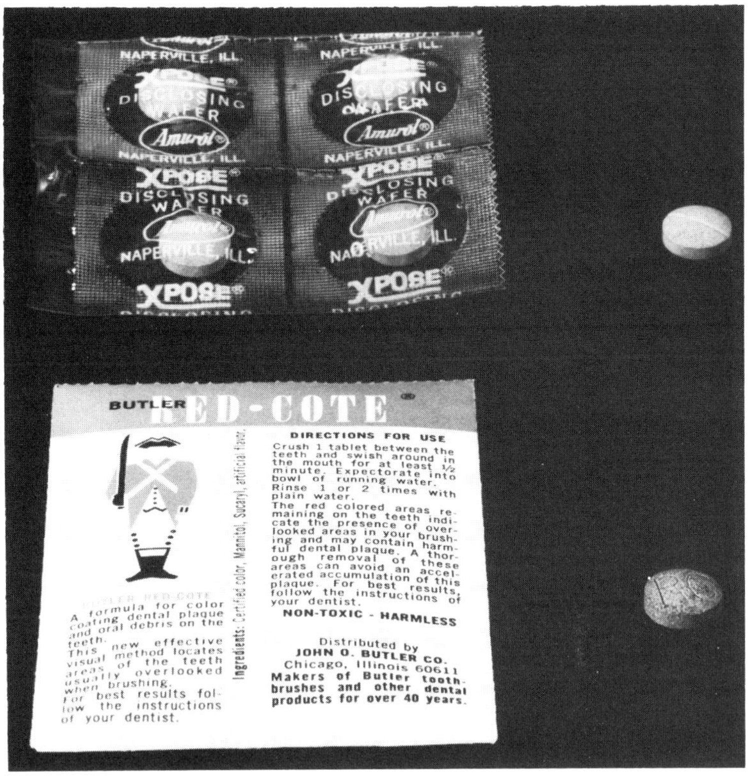

Figure 13–8 Disclosing wafers. Top is the X-pose, bottom is the Butler Red-Cote. (Names and addresses of suppliers are listed in Table 13–1.)

tions of erythrosin have also been used and the formulae for these are available.[1, 19]

A solution can also be prepared from the wafers which are purchased from commercial suppliers. The following directions can be used to make a supply of solution for office use:

30 Disclosing wafers
7 fl. oz. Warm distilled water
1 fl. oz. Alcohol (95 per cent)

Allow one-half hour for tablets to dissolve.

Generally, wafers are best for home use because such problems as spillage and excessive staining are avoided. For office use a solution of erythrosin is best. It is applied more readily and is much more convenient to use.

Little research has been done on the staining characteristics of disclosing solutions. However, the study by Downton and Castaldi[19] tested the properties of four different solutions as used under routine conditions. They concluded that erythrosin was the most suitable for office use of the four they tested (mercurochrome, erythrosin, red and green food coloring). As suggested by Bohannan,[13] the value of disclosing solutions is to allow patients to evaluate the efficiency of their program and to permit the dentist or hygienist to assess the level of care. Disclosing wafers and solutions are the first part of the program to mechanically remove plaque.

THE TOOTHBRUSH

A wide variety of brush designs is available and yet there is no evidence to support the idea that one type is better than another. The Council on Dental Therapeutics of the American Dental Association[3] clearly stated this position and Greene,[25] after an extensive review of the current knowledge of brushes, concluded at the 1966 World Workshop in Periodontics that: "The method and toothbrush of choice depend on the patient's oral health, manual dexterity,

TABLE 13-1 LIST OF PRODUCTS, MANUFACTURERS AND ADDRESSES FOR ITEMS SHOWN IN FIGURES

PRODUCT	MANUFACTURER	ADDRESS
"X-Pose" wafers	Amurol	Amurol Products Naperville, Illinois 60540
Water-Pik	AquaTec	AquaTec Corporation Denver, Colorado 80202
"Right Kind" Brush & Floss	Bass*	John O. Butler Company 540 N. Lakeshore Drive Chicago, Illinois 60611
Butler #411 "GUM Brush" "Sub Gum" brush Unwaxed floss "Red-Cote" tablets Plastic mouth mirror Proxabrush Stimulator handle with replaceable tips	John O. Butler*	John O. Butler Company 540 N. Lakeshore Drive Chicago, Illinois 60611
Flashlight type lighted hand mirror Lighted hand mirror lamp	Floxite	Floxite Company, Inc. Box 1094, Niagara Falls, N.Y. 14303
World's Fair round toothpicks for Perio-Aid	Forster	Forster Manufacturing Company Wilton, Maine 04294
Electric toothbrush	General Electric	General Electric 2126 Boston Avenue Bridgeport, Connecticut 06610
"Nupon" floss threader	Janor	Janor Company P. O. Box 1845 Grand Rapids, Michigan 49501
"ZON" dental bridge cleaners Unwaxed floss	Johnson & Johnson	Johnson & Johnson New Brunswick, New Jersey 08903
Jordan Interdental Borster	Jordan	Jordan Borste & Penselfabric Box 2023 6 RU Oslo 5, Norway

(Table continued on opposite page.)

personal preference, and his ability and desire to learn and follow prescribed procedures. No definite superiority has been shown for either natural or synthetic bristles."

Most dentists today probably recommend a soft-bristled, multitufted brush, while in the past most recommended the hard-bristled brush with two rows of tufts. The potential danger of the hard-bristled brush is shown in Figure 13–9. This patient was a 28-year-old woman who was given the brush in the illustration just one week before the photograph was taken. Notice the amount of splaying of the tufts and the short, jagged edges of the bristles. This patient was a compulsive brusher, and the amount of recession may be directly related to the toothbrush abrasion. Consequently, most people suggest a multitufted brush either identical to that recommended by Bass or somewhat similar to it. The specifications for the brush recommended by Bass[11] have been summarized by Gilson et al.:[23]

A. General form and shape
   1. Plain straight handle about six inches long and 7/16 inch wide
   2. Three rows of tufts; six tufts per row—evenly spaced
B. Filaments
   1. Made of high-quality nylon
   2. Diameter of .007 inch
   3. Length of 13/32 inch

TABLE 13–1 LIST OF PRODUCTS, MANUFACTURERS AND ADDRESSES FOR ITEMS SHOWN IN FIGURES (*Continued*)

PRODUCT	MANUFACTURER	ADDRESS
Lactona #19 Lactona #M39 nylon Tooth tip stimulator #26	Lactona	Lactona Products Division Warner Lambert Pharmaceutical Co. Morris Plains, New Jersey 07950
Perio-Aid	Marquis	Marquis Dental Manufacturing 2005 E. 17th Avenue Denver, Colorado 80206
Oral B 20 Oral B 30, 35 Oral B 40	Oral B	Oral B Company Fairfield Road Wayne, New Jersey 07470
POH Brush POH Floss "X-pose" wafers Floss caddies Oral water spray	Oral Health Products	Oral Health Products P. O. Box 4717 Tulsa, Oklahoma 74155
Pycopay Softex brush	Pycopay	Block Drug Company, Inc. 105 Academy Street Jersey City, N.J. 07302
Plastic mouth mirrors	Sherman	Sherman Specialty Merrick, New York 11566
Broxodent electric toothbrush	Squibb	E. R. Squibb & Son 745 5th Avenue New York, N.Y. 10022
Stimudents	Stimudent	Stimudent Inc. 14035 Woodrow Wilson Avenue Detroit, Michigan 48238
Dento-spray	Texell	Texell Products 3 Ashbury Place Houston, Texas 77007

*Brushes & floss according to Dr. Bass' specifications are now manufactured by the Butler Company.

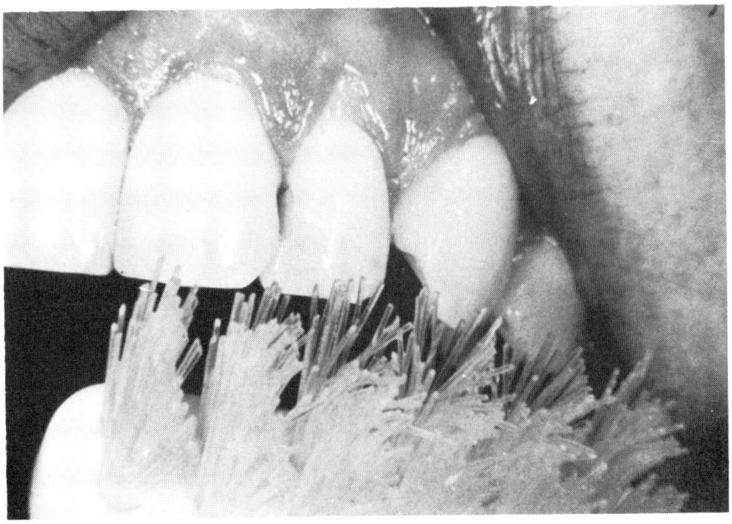

Figure 13–9 Localized moderate gingival recession associated with hard bristles and excessive brushing.

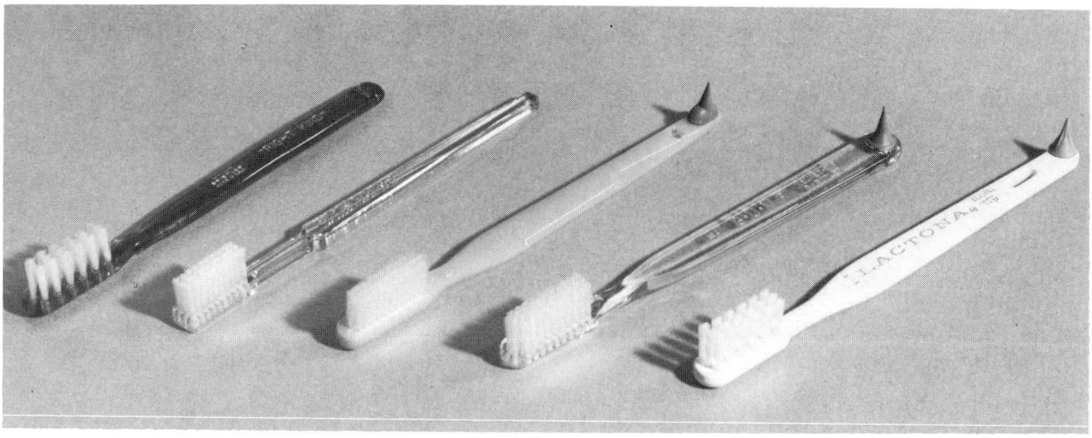

Figure 13–10 Various types of multitufted brushes with nylon bristles. From left to right: Bass' "Right Kind," Oral B-40, Pycopay Softex, Butler GUM-411, Lactona S-19.

4. Ends rounded

C. Tufts

1. 80–86 filaments per tuft

This brush is shown in Figure 13–10 on the extreme left. It is an example of the original multituft design which has been modified. Bohannan[13] stated that the modifications were made because the brush with the original design deteriorated rapidly, and another design provides more rigidity and lasts longer under normal conditions. The head of this type of brush is shown in Figure 13–11.

In addition to the overall design, the physical properties of the bristle are important considerations. An excellent report on several different brushes has been published by Gilson et al.[23] They examined the ends of the bristles of twelve different multitufted hand brushes and six brushes used in electric toothbrushes. They found a wide variation in the ends of the bristles and concluded that only one (Butler G.U.M.) had ends which were smooth and showed a "high degree of roundness." Figure 13–12 contains a magnification of the bristles of this brush. There is a slight spur on one of the bristles, but the ends appear as if they have been polished. According to Bass,[11] this can be accomplished by grinding on a wheel or abrasive belt, but the exact method by which this is done remains an industrial secret.

Another comparison of bristle ends may be seen in Figure 13–13. The bristle on the left is from a brush with the bristles polished and rounded. The bristle in the middle is from an "extra-hard" nylon brush, where the bristle end is sharp and jagged. A natural bristle is on the right and it shows the characteristic splitting at the bristle ends.

The polished, rounded bristle is pres-

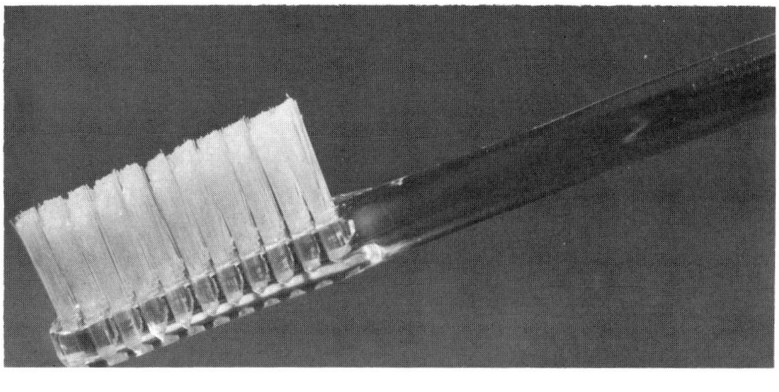

Figure 13–11 Butler GUM-411. A multitufted brush with filaments longer toward the center of the brush. There are 42 tufts, 34 bristles per tuft, .007 inch bristle diameter and bristle length of 11/32 to 14/32 inches.

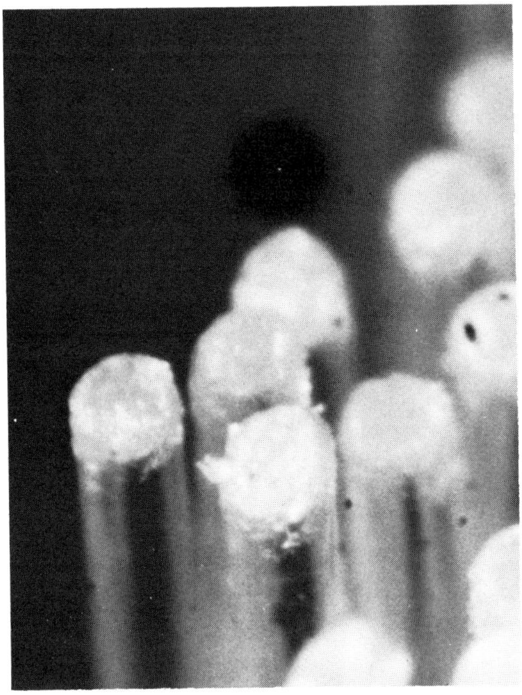

Figure 13–12 Magnification of rounded polished ends of the proper type of bristle.

ently the most widely accepted. However, there are still no objective, well-controlled studies to confirm the clinical impression that the rounded bristles are less injurious. Studies should be designed to determine the relative efficiency of cleansing and the degree of abrasion caused by different bristles. Parfitt[42] has suggested such a study and has compared the relative cleaning efficiency of hard and soft bristles in an electric brush. As yet no such studies are available for hand brushes.

Unfortunately, the brush most frequently recommended may not be the one most frequently used. A study by Fanning and Henning[20] in Australia has shown that of 51 brushes available for adults only five were acceptable in design and bristle characteristics. Of eight brushes available for children, none was acceptable. No such survey has been done in the United States. Consequently, there is little information about the quality of brushes available *for use* or the quality of those brushes *in use*. And even though the recommendation of most dentists is based on clinical experience, there is enough information available to justify the logic of using the multitufted brush with soft nylon bristles that have rounded or polished ends rather than using bristles that have sharp or jagged ends.

A question that frequently arises is the relative efficiency of the hand versus the powered brush. Parfitt[42] has discussed the various types of powered brushes and has reviewed the studies which have compared the relative efficiency of cleaning. The advantages of the hand brush are that more strokes can be applied in a shorter period of time, and it is probably used for a longer period of time as there is less fatigue. Even though Parfitt suggested that the hand brush is more versatile, he also said that in the final analysis it is the motivation of the patient that determines the degree of cleanliness that is obtained. Ash in 1964[8] and Greene in 1966[24] made very thorough reviews of the literature on this problem. Greene presented in a summary table all of the studies through 1965 which dealt with powered brushes. His review and the findings of the investigations he cited suggest that there is no essential difference in the ability of the hand and the powered brush in plaque removal. Neither one is distinctly better than the other in keeping tooth surfaces clean or in stimulating the gingiva.

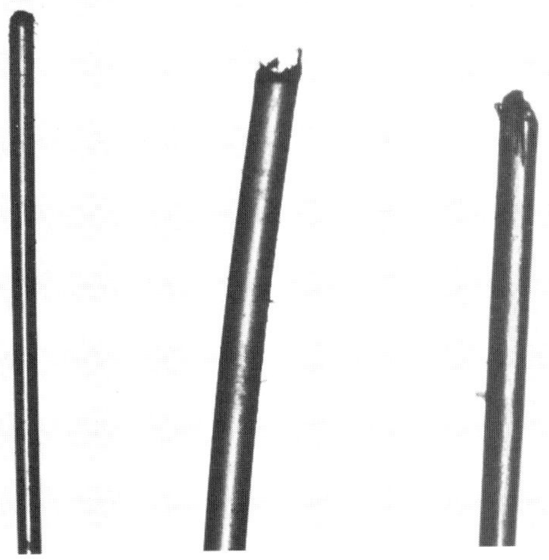

Figure 13–13 Bristle ends. From left to right: round nylon polished bristle from a multitufted brush; nylon bristle from a brush labeled "extra hard"; a bristle from a hard, natural bristled brush.

Also, one must consider the effect of the appeal of a new device which may be dropped when the newness wears off. Muhler[40] has shown that this is a demonstrable effect. He investigated 280 subjects who were given an electric brush and showed that after one year, 149 had discontinued use of the powered brush. There was an initial increase in the frequency with which this group brushed, but it steadily decreased. On the other hand, a group using the hand brush did not change their brushing frequency,

TABLE 13–2 SUMMARY OF METHODS OF BRUSHING

METHOD AND REFERENCE	BRISTLE AND PLACEMENT	MOTION	ADVANTAGES AND DISADVANTAGES
Bass[10]	apically, toward gingiva into the gingival sulcus at a 45-degree angle to the tooth surface	very short back and front vibratory, bristle ends remain in the sulcus	removes plaque from cervical area and sulcus, small area covered at one time, good gingival stimulation, easily learned
Charters[16]	coronally, with sides of bristles half on teeth and half on gingiva at a 45-degree angle to tooth surface	small circular with bristle ends remaining stationary	cleans interproximal but bristle ends do not go into sulcus, hard to learn, hard to position brush in some areas of the mouth, excellent gingival stimulation
Fones[21]	perpendicular to tooth surface	on buccal a wide circular movement to include gingiva and tooth surfaces, on lingual a back and forth horizontal motion	interproximal areas not cleaned, easy to learn, possible trauma to gingiva
"Physiologic"[44]	coronally and then along an arc over the tooth surfaces and gingiva	gentle sweeping which starts on teeth progressing over gingiva	is "physiologic," mimics the passage of food over the gingiva, does not emphasize the interproximal or sulcus areas
Roll	apically nearly parallel to the tooth surface then in an arc over tooth surfaces	on buccal and lingual slight inward pressure at first then a rolling of the head to sweep bristles over the gingiva and tooth surfaces, occlusal cleaned with horizontal stroke	does not clean sulcus area, easy to learn, requires moderate dexterity, good gingival stimulation
Stillman[46]	on buccal and lingual-apically at an oblique angle to the long axis of the tooth, ends rest on gingiva and cervical portion of tooth on occlusal – perpendicular to occlusal surface	on buccal and lingual-slight rotary with bristle ends stationary on occlusal – horizontal	excellent gingival stimulation, bristles do not enter sulcus, interproximal area is cleaned when occlusal surfaces are brushed, moderate dexterity required
Intrasulcular[16]	apically, towards gingiva into gingival sulcus at a 45-degree angle to the tooth surface or towards gingiva almost parallel to long axis of the teeth	on buccal and lingual, a very short back and forth vibratory or very small circular motion with bristle tips remaining in the sulcus then the brush head is rolled toward the occlusal surface; occlusal surfaces cleaned with horizontal stroke	good interproximal and gingival cleaning, good gingival stimulation, requires moderate dexterity

and only 39 of an original group of 254 said they had stopped using the hand brush.

In the past few years there have been fewer reports on powered brushes. At present, however, one may conclude that the powered brush is useful for patients with physical handicaps, such as paralysis or arthritis, or patients with limited manual dexterity. It probably does a better job of plaque removal in a shorter time for those patients who are not highly motivated or who spend little time in brushing. In 1968 the program of evaluating these brushes was transferred from the Council on Dental Therapeutics to the Council on Dental Materials and Devices.[26] Its publication lists the powered toothbrushes which have been classified as "acceptable." The present view of this Council is that there is no evidence to show that the powered brushes have a therapeutic potential. However, the Council has stated that manufacturers may claim effectiveness of the brushes as "an aid in the prevention of caries and some forms of periodontal disease."

METHODS OF BRUSHING

There are almost as many methods of brushing as there are types of brushes. Only the rationale and directions for one will be presented in detail here. The most common methods of brushing are listed in Table 13–2. The placement of the bristles and motion of the brush are summarized. The two basic ways a brush can be used are as a broom with the sides of the bristles in a sweeping motion or as a scrub brush by using the ends of the bristles alone.[32, 33] The requirements of any method are that it be easily learned and that it does not injure the periodontal or dental tissues. No studies have as yet determined which method meets these criteria most adequately. Kimmelman[33] has concluded that the roll technique is most easily learned and needs the least amount of instruction while the Charters'[16] method required more teaching time and more reinforcement. The roll technique has probably been most frequently recommended, and as long ago as 1932 it was the method adopted by the Hygiene Commission of the Federation Dentaire Internationale.[15] Since that time no group has had the temerity to take a similar position. However, most attention today is given the Bass technique. It involves brushing and the use of unwaxed floss. The brush is positioned as shown in Figure 13–14. The bristles are placed into the sulcus as shown in Figure 13–15. The bristle ends actually displace the marginal gingiva and the bristles are able to reach into the sulcus. Also, this angulation of the bristles is able to reach the interproximal

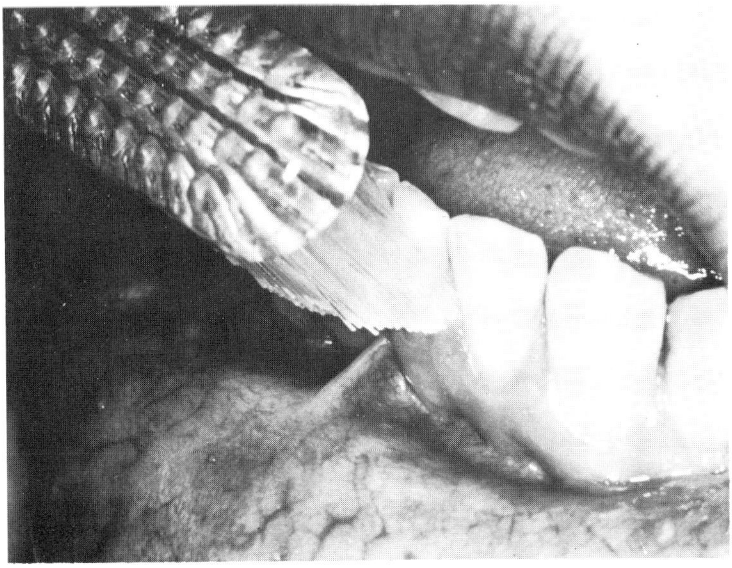

Figure 13–14 Angulation of bristles in the Bass method of brushing.

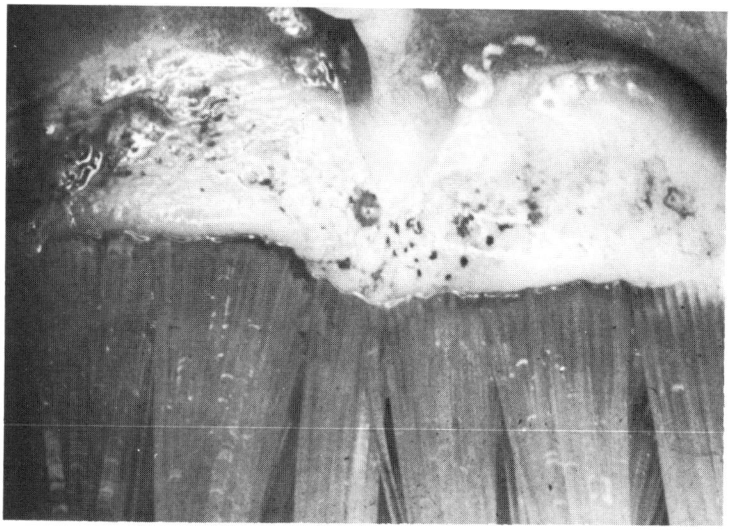

Figure 13–15 Bristles placed into the gingival sulcus. (Courtesy of Dr. G. J. Parfitt, University of British Columbia.)

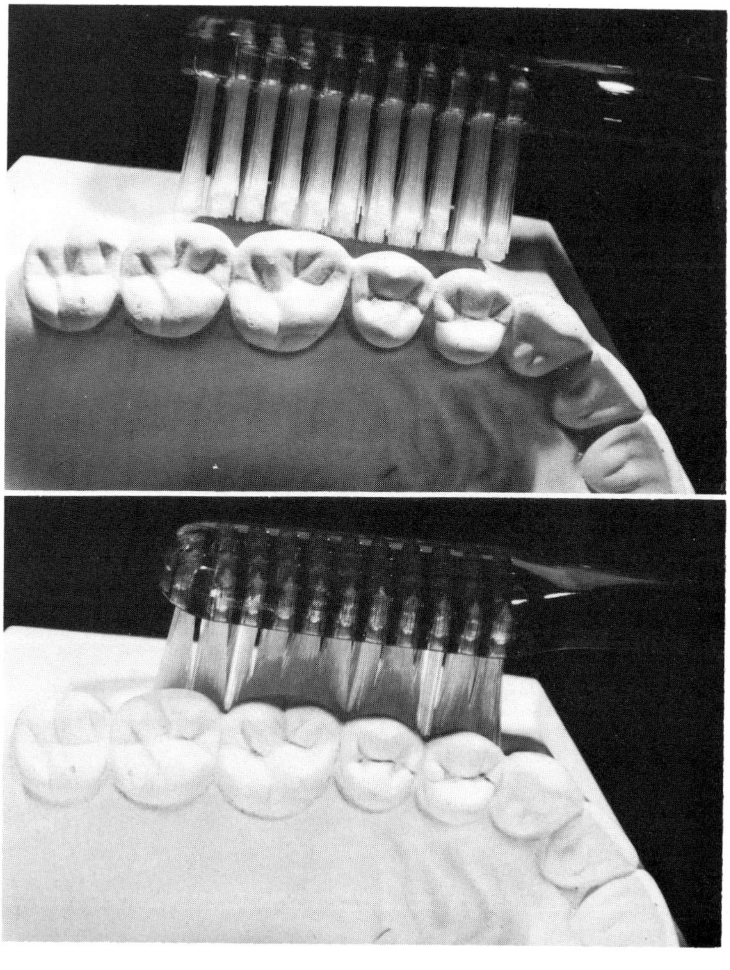

Figure 13–16 Top: Angulation of bristles at a right angle to tooth surface fails to reach interproximal. Bottom: Angulation of bristles at a 45 degree angle to tooth surface causes bristles to reach the interproximal area.

space much more efficiently. This is shown in Figure 13–16. The top half of the illustration shows the bristles placed at a right angle to the tooth surface. This angulation will clean the prominences of the tooth surface but the bristles do not reach the interproximal areas. The bottom half of the illustration shows the results of placing the bristles apically at a 45-degree angle to the tooth surface and into the sulcus. Not only is the gingival sulcus reached but the interproximal space is filled with the bristles, and the sides of these bristles can clean the cervical areas of the teeth. Even with this placement, however, the entire interproximal areas are not reached. Consequently, Bass suggested that dental floss be used to remove plaque from this area. He established the specifications for the type of floss

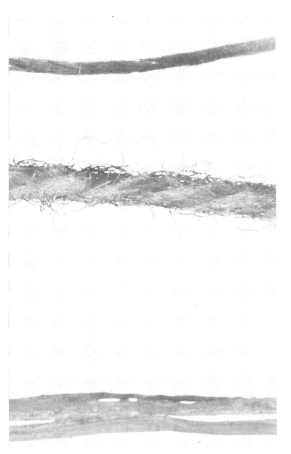

Figure 13–17 Three types of materials used for cleaning. Top: Waxed dental floss. Middle: Three-ply wool yarn. Bottom: Unwaxed dental floss.

and suggested that it should be unwaxed nylon yarn in a thin strand with approximately 35 filaments. Until this time waxed floss was very popular. However, Bass believed that unwaxed floss would cause the soft plaque to adhere more readily to the floss and become entrapped in the fine filaments. The differences in appearance of unwaxed floss, yarn and waxed floss are shown in Figure 13–17. Some individuals suggest unwaxed floss is superior, but again there are no definitive studies which compare the two types of floss. Yarn is often used when the interproximal spaces are large, particularly after periodontal surgery. Each of the materials has its advantages but the unwaxed floss is generally preferred. It must be used with care to avoid injury, and although it has a tendency to tear, it can be passed through the contact areas with less separation of the teeth. It is used as illustrated in Figure 13–18. The floss is wound around the index fingers on each hand and then placed through the contact areas by gentle pressure with the thumbs. It is placed under the gingival margin, into the sulcus and gently flattened against the tooth surface. This flattened surface is shown in Figure 13–19. The flattened floss is then moved back and forth and in a coronal direction. The tooth surface above and below the marginal gingiva is cleaned and then the floss is moved across the interproximal space to the adjacent tooth surface. This surface is cleaned and then the process is repeated for each individual interproximal area. Samples of the types of floss which are available are shown in Figure 13–20. In some cases it is not possible to place the floss through the contact area. In these situations, the floss may be used with a floss threader. Examples of these are shown in Figure 13–21.

Although one patient does not make a scientific study, an example of what can be accomplished with instruction in the Bass[10] techniques is shown in Figure 13–22. This is a twelve-year-old female with considerable plaque accumulation who was seen just after lunch one day. A disclosing solution was used (middle) and the patient was instructed in the use of a multitufted brush and floss by the methods suggested by Bass

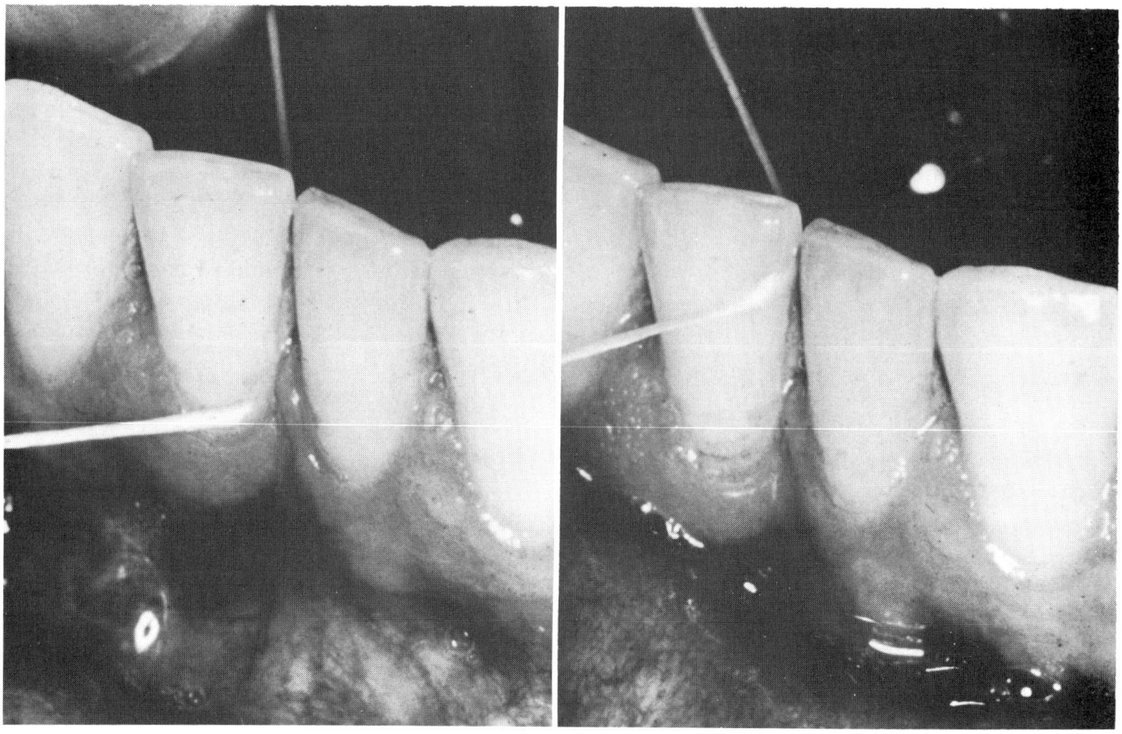

Figure 13–18 Placement of floss in the interproximal areas.

and Arnim. No other treatment was given. At the end of one week, the patient was brought back to the clinic at the same time of day and a disclosing solution was used again. The results are shown in the bottom photograph. There is some plaque in the interproximal which showed that reinforcement of the use of the floss was needed. Nevertheless, there is much less plaque than in the middle photograph taken one week earlier. A case could be made for less gingival inflammation as seen in the photographs, although this was not measured at the time.

It may be concluded that brushes and brushing methods are the subject of wide

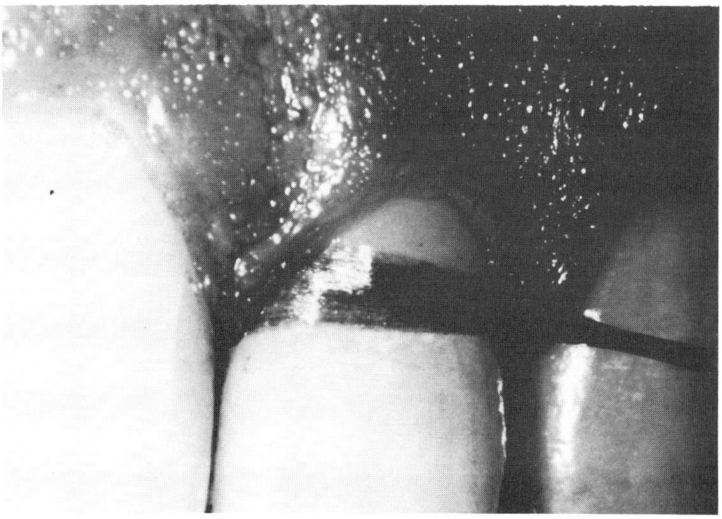

Figure 13–19 Flattening of the unwaxed floss against the surface of the tooth in the gingival sulcus. (Courtesy of Butler Brush Company and Dr. J. Seibert.)

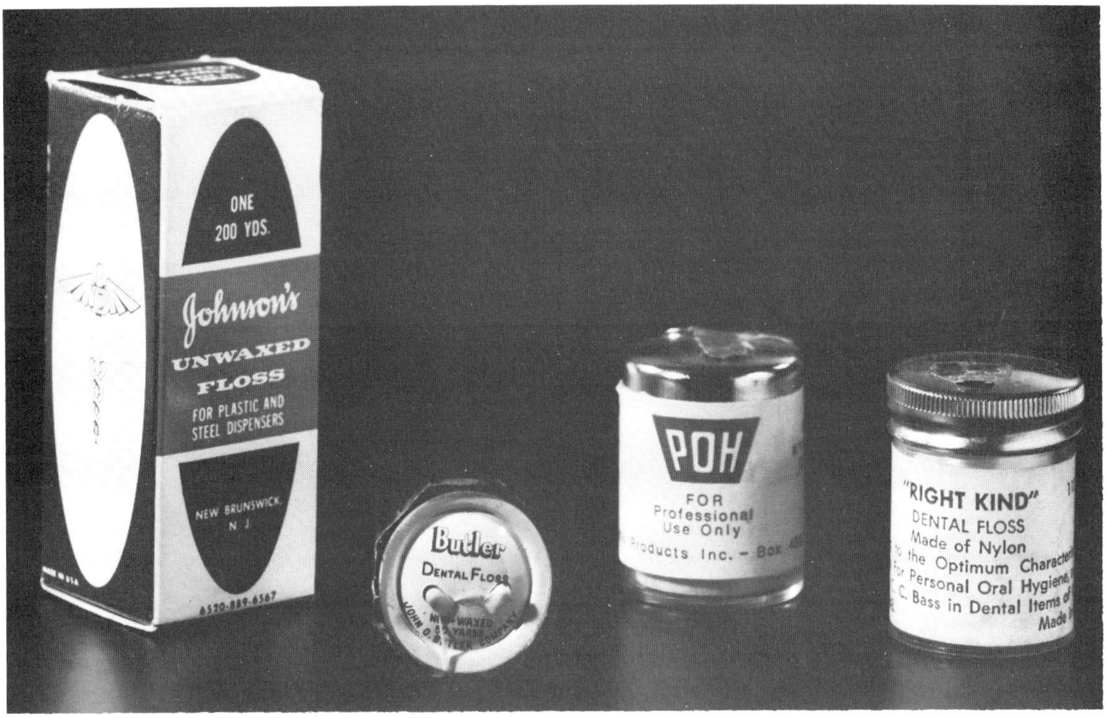

Figure 13–20 Examples of unwaxed dental floss.

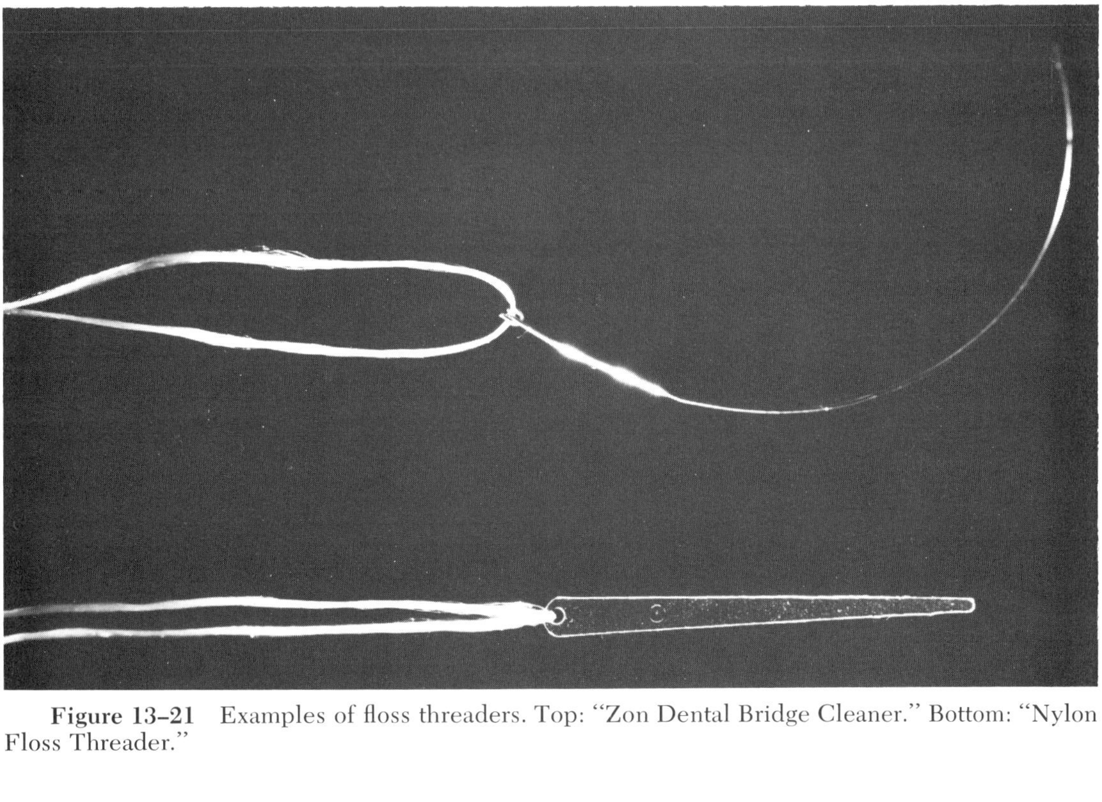

Figure 13–21 Examples of floss threaders. Top: "Zon Dental Bridge Cleaner." Bottom: "Nylon Floss Threader."

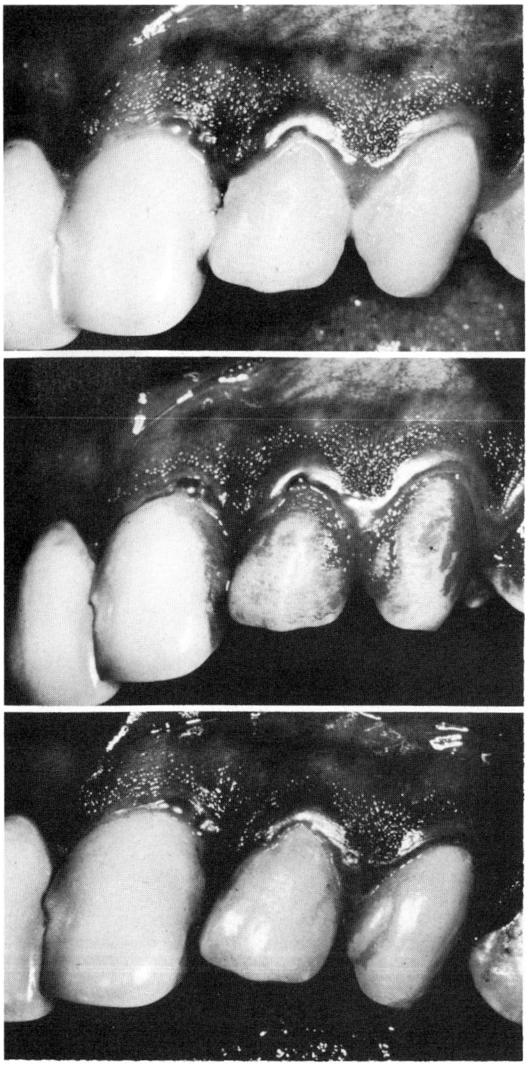

Figure 13–22 Top: Patient at initial visit with heavy plaque accumulation. Middle: Patient at initial visit with disclosing solution applied to reveal heavy plaque. Bottom: Patient seven days later with disclosing solution applied. Treatment has consisted of oral hygiene instruction with Bass technique. There is much less plaque and the gingival inflammation has been reduced.

variations. Much of the knowledge and recommendations are based on empiricism, clinical experience and personal prejudice. To be effective, however, any brushing program should be simple, easily learned, require minimal reinforcement and manual dexterity. It should remove the plaque from the critical areas where periodontal disease and caries most commonly begin, that is, the gingival sulcus and the interproximal area. For these reasons the technic suggested by Bass is the one that most closely fits these criteria and should be the one which is used. Although this recommendation is made without scientific proof, the logic for cleaning this way is valid.

Some recent investigations by Keller[30,31] and his associates do not support all of Bass' original recommendations, but they do support his idea that a brush and floss are essential items to clean the interproximal areas. These investigations are the most well-designed and carefully controlled experiments on the technics of cleansing the proximal surfaces. The experimental methods employ the use of gold crowns constructed on mandibular first molars in humans. The crowns have removable proximal inlays on the mesial surfaces. Enamel slabs from freshly extracted teeth are used interchangeably with the inlay. In this way the enamel is placed into the crown and plaque is allowed to accumulate. Different procedures for plaque removal can then be studied under a variety of experimental conditions, as the slab can be removed, the plaque stained and the area of plaque remaining can be measured. The investigators have studied the effects of various technics recommended for plaque removal and their general conclusions are as follows:

1. The best method of cleaning the proximal surfaces of posterior teeth is with a hand brush in conjunction with a dentifrice and dental floss. The brushing is followed by the use of a dental floss.
2. The second best method of cleaning is through the use of a hand brush, dentifrice and a pulsating water jet.
3. There are no apparent differences in efficiency of plaque removal between waxed and unwaxed floss.
4. There are no apparent differences between natural and synthetic bristles.
5. There are no apparent differences in plaque removal between hand and powered brushes or among the various types of movement of the brushes in the powered brushes.

6. Flossing by itself is an effective way to remove plaque.

7. Auxiliary aids, such as rubber stimulators and wooden picks, are not effective in removing plaque.

These studies should serve as a stimulus for further investigations on the most effective ways to clean teeth, especially cleaning the interproximal areas.

AUXILIARY AIDS IN ORAL HYGIENE

The previous sections have stressed the importance of the brush and floss in removing plaque according to a specific technic. There are many other types of mechanical devices which are available that have been used to help clean teeth and to provide stimulation to the tissues. Only two groups of these will be discussed here. These will be a general group of devices for interproximal cleaning and devices using forced water irrigation.

WATER IRRIGATING DEVICES

Like the powered brushes, there has been a flurry of activity in recent years on the usefulness of water irrigating devices. It is not a new idea. As far back as 1915, G. V. Black[12] suggested the use of a water-filled syringe to cleanse the subgingival space. Arnim[6] has extensively reviewed the development of water irrigators and has commented on a responsibility to advise patients about these devices. Further guidelines are available in the Guide to Dental Materials and Devices, published by the American Dental Association.[26] This also contains a list of those devices which are acceptable to the Council on Dental Materials and Devices.

There are two main types of water irrigating devices available. One is a unit which can be attached to a faucet and emits a constant stream of water with the pressure regulated by the faucet. One such device is shown in Figure 13–23, while the other is shown in Figure 13–24. This is a self-contained unit which has a motor-driven pump and supplies an intermittent stream of water at various pressures which can be regulated with a dial.

Neither of these types has been shown to be superior to the other. Also, there are conflicting reports about the relative efficiency and safety of these devices.[24] It has been fairly well established that water irri-

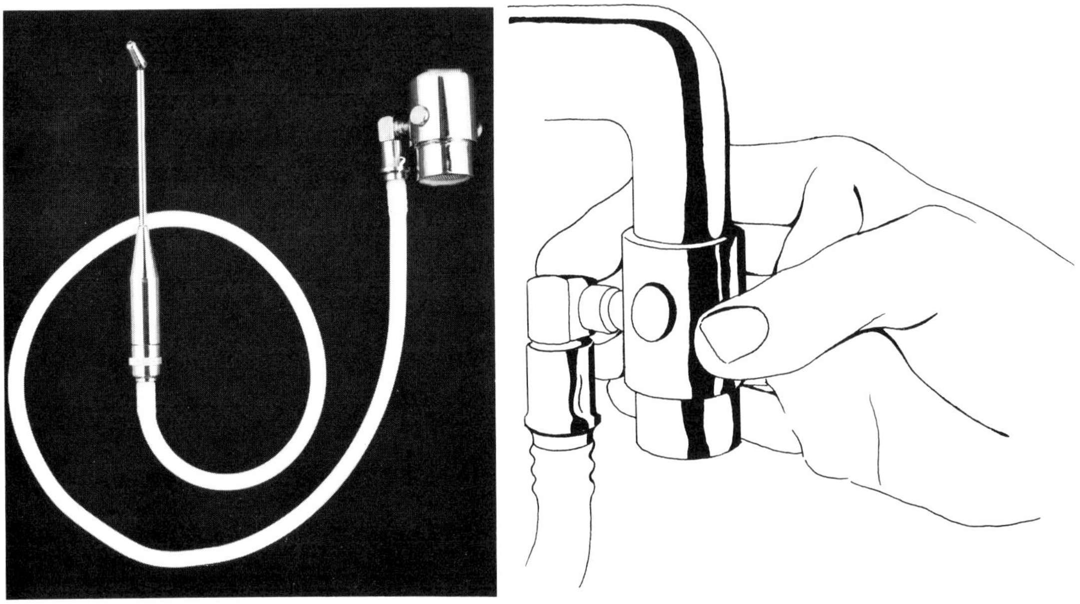

Figure 13–23 Water irrigating device which attaches to the faucet (Oral Health Products).

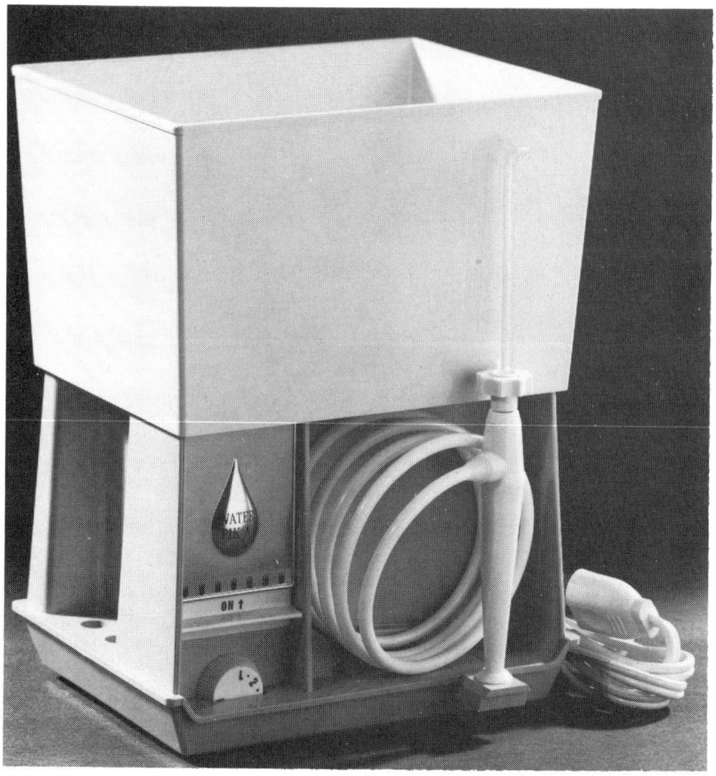

Figure 13–24 Water irrigating device which is self-contained (Water-Pik).

gation can remove loose debris from the areas around the teeth, but it is not particularly efficient in removing or preventing the accumulation of bacterial plaque. As a matter of fact, one of the definitions of plaque is that it is a bacterial deposit on teeth which cannot be removed by a stream of water. However, the magnitude of the force of the stream of water is not specified in this particular definition.

These devices might be of value in certain circumstances when used with proper guidance and adequate precaution. Patients with fixed orthodontic appliances, extensive fixed prostheses and patients with moderate periodontal disease may derive some benefit. Excessive pressure must be avoided with conditions of deep pocket formation and moderate to severe inflammation. There are some indications that fluids from oral irrigating devices might penetrate the epithelium and connective tissues lining the pockets.[6, 41] However, a recent study has shown that in a group of 30 patients with normal tissues, a gingivitis or periodontitis (10 in each group), there was no evidence of bacteremia following the use of a water irrigating device.[48]

The most important conclusion concerning water irrigation is that it cannot substitute for the brush. It is an aid to brushing under certain conditions but should not be used in place of the brush. It has yet to be shown that these devices used alone can prevent the development of caries or periodontal disease. There are some indications that they can help reduce the amount of plaque or calculus when used in conjunction with regular brushing. As with electric brushes the short-term effects may be attributed to the newness of the device and an increase in motivation on the part of the patient. The long-term effect of these devices in the prevention of the occurrence and recurrence of caries and periodontal disease has not yet been established.

MISCELLANEOUS INTERPROXIMAL CLEANING AIDS

Generally, the devices which are used to clean interproximal spaces are limited to

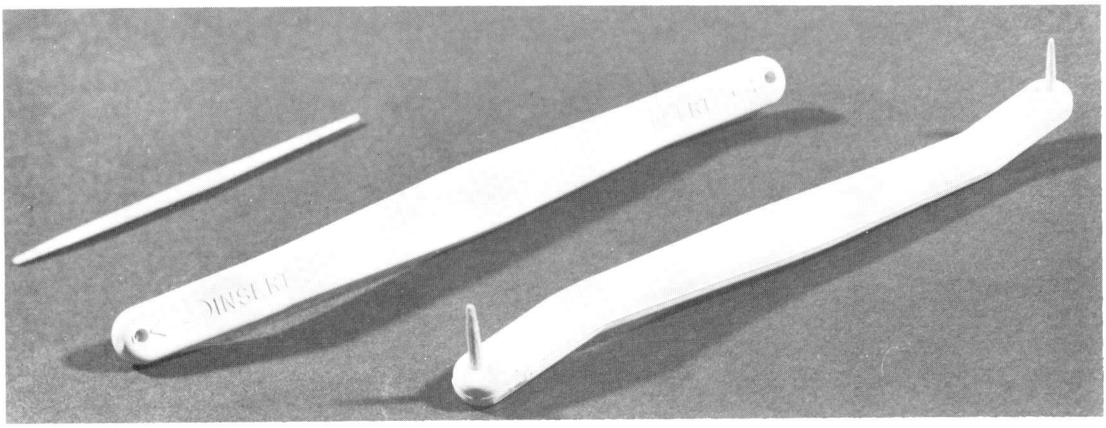

Figure 13–25 The "Perio-Aid." This plastic holder is used with a round, polished wooden tooth pick.

adult patients. In children the interdental space is filled with the papilla and there is adequate room for nothing but the tips of the bristles or floss. Some adult patients do not have room for these aids, but others who have had some recession or who have had periodontal treatment usually have adequate space. Like the water irrigators, these devices are not to be used alone but are used in conjunction with the dentifrice, brush and floss. These devices are made of various materials. They include brushes of various shapes, wooden picks (of hard or soft wood) and such things as ordinary pipe cleaners. One of the most useful of these devices is a plastic handle which holds the broken end of a round wooden tooth pick. It is shown in Figure 13–25. Like

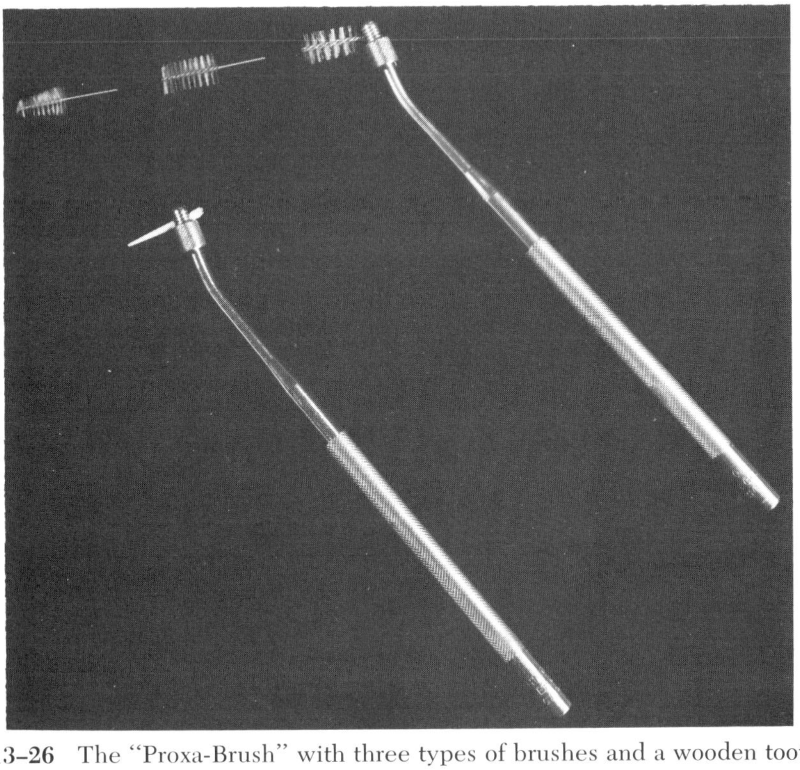

Figure 13–26 The "Proxa-Brush" with three types of brushes and a wooden tooth pick.

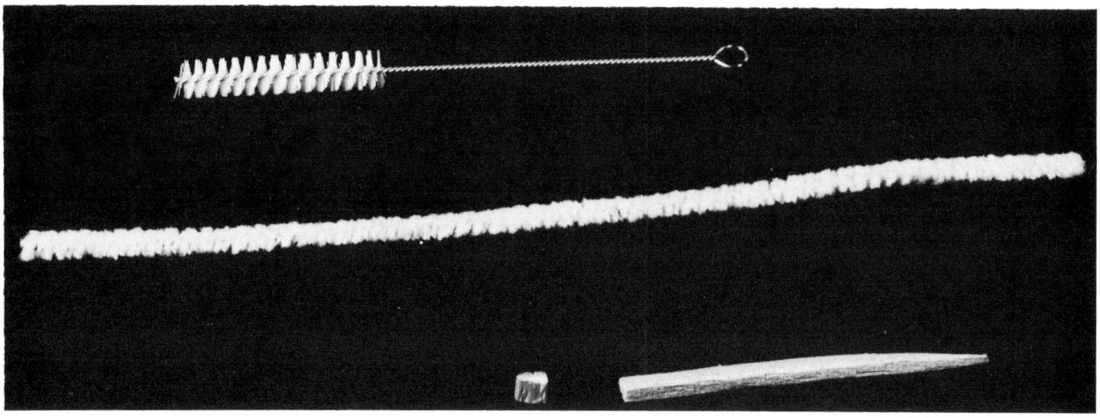

Figure 13–27 Three different devices for interproximal cleaning. Top: Jordan Interdental Borster, Middle: Pipe cleaner, Bottom: Stim-u-Dent (Balsa wood interdental stimulator).

any other device it can damage tissue if not used properly but it is particularly useful for adult patients. It is applied at right angles to the margin of the gingiva with a slight pressure to displace the gingiva and is used to polish the interproximal surfaces. It is very helpful on the distal surfaces of teeth and in areas that are impossible to floss, such as partially opened root furcations. One of the most recent devices is a brush with small conical or round brushes which attach to a handle designed to hold either a wooden tooth pick or a brush. It is shown in Figure 13–26, while other interproximal aids are shown in Figure 13–27.

SUMMARY

Many ways have been proposed to make the teeth clean. A few of these have been discussed in this chapter while others have not. Perhaps a method of reviewing some of the ways would be to look at the illustrations in Figure 13–28. This is a technique suggested by Arnim[4] to show the relative effectiveness of various agents to remove plaque. It is also an excellent teaching and learning device for students. This photograph shows a dental student who was given hard candy to eat and was told not to brush the right side of his mouth for three days. He was allowed to brush the left side. The contrast between the brushed and nonbrushed sides is evident in Figures 13–28*A* and 13–28*B*. After the plaque was stained the student was told to perform a number of procedures in the following order for a two-minute period: rinse with a commercial mouth rinse (Figure 13–28*C*), chew a carrot (Figure 13–28*D*), use a water irrigating device (Figure 13–28*E*), brush according to the Bass technique with a dentifrice (Figure 13–28*F*), and use dental floss (Figure 13–28*G*). The teeth were stained after each procedure. Slight differences can be detected depending on the procedure. However, the most obvious changes are seen when the brush is used and the final interproximal areas are cleaned with the floss. It is interesting to see the plaque retention in the carious lesion on the buccal surface of the second molar.

Until the day when chemicals or antibiotics are available, mechanical means of removing plaque remain the most effective. Toothbrushing is effective for almost all of the surfaces of the tooth, but the interproximal area must be cleaned with floss or another type of interproximal cleaning device. Any one of the devices can be used to excess and may cause damage. No one technic is clearly better than another.

The critical areas to be cleaned are the gingival sulcus and the interproximal area. Brushing according to the Bass technique, which uses a soft, multitufted brush and dental floss, is an effective way of cleaning the teeth after the plaque is stained with a disclosing solution. Additional aids are

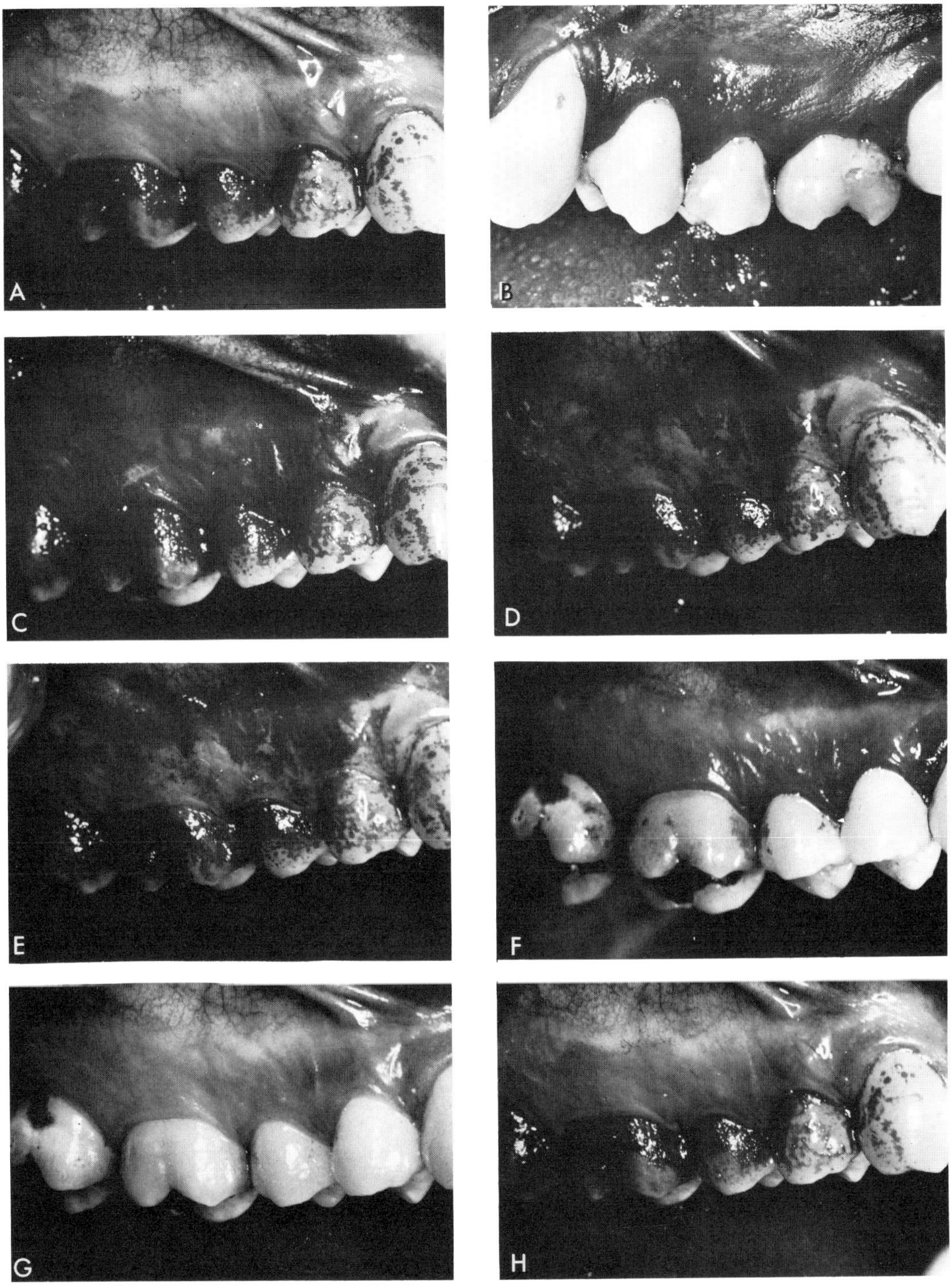

Figure 13–28 Plaque accumulation over a three-day period and a series of procedures to remove plaque. Each procedure followed in order listed: *A*, No brushing for three days on right side. *B*, Regular brushing on left side. *C*, Effect of rinsing for two minutes with a mouth rinse. *D*, Effect of chewing a carrot for two minutes. Plaque is removed primarily from the attached gingiva. *E*, Effect of two minutes' irrigation with a water irrigating device. *F*, Effect of brushing for two minutes. Bass technique with a dentifrice. *G*, Effect of using floss for two minutes and a final water rinse. Even though extensive cleaning has been done, plaque remains in the carious lesion. *H*, Contrast of cleaned versus non-cleaned tooth surface.

available but these are adjuncts and not substitutes for the brush and floss. The technics all depend on patient understanding, motivation and learning. One must consider the particular circumstances for each patient and recommend whatever devices or methods are required to get the job done, that is, to remove the plaque. This must be done with sufficient frequency and with careful attention to prevent the accumulation of the bacterial plaque, which is the single most important factor in caries and periodontal disease.

ACKNOWLEDGMENTS

The author wishes to thank Mr. Lou Audette, Mr. Ron Anderson and Miss Patricia Bohan of the Department of Biomedical Communications at the University of Connecticut Health Center for their advice and assistance with the illustrations for this chapter.

REFERENCES

1. Accepted Dental Therapeutics 1971/1972. 34th Ed. American Dental Association, Chicago, pp. 184, 265.
2. Accepted Dental Therapeutics 1971/1972. 34th Ed. American Dental Association, Chicago, p. 241.
3. Adams, R. J., and Stanmeyer, W. R. (1960): The effects of a closely supervised oral hygiene program upon oral cleanliness. J. Periodontol. *31*:242.
4. Arnim, S. S. (1967): An effective program of oral hygiene for the arrestment of dental caries and the control of periodontal disease. J. South. Calif. Dent. Assoc. *35*:264.
5. Arnim, S. S. (1963): The use of disclosing agents for measuring tooth cleanliness. J. Periodontol. *34*:277.
6. Arnim, S. S. (1967): Dental irrigators for oral hygiene, periodontal therapy and prevention of dental disease. J. Tenn. Dent. Assoc. *47*:1.
7. Arno, S., et al. (1958): Incidence of gingivitis as related to sex, occupation, tobacco consumption, toothbrushing, and age. Oral Surg. *11*:587.
8. Ash, M. M. (1964): A review of the problems and results of studies on manual and power toothbrushes. J. Periodontol. *35*:202.
9. Bass, C. C. (1948): The optimum characteristics of toothbrushes for personal oral hygiene. Dent. Items Int. *70*:967.
10. Bass, C. C. (1954): An effective method of personal hygiene (Part II). J. La. Med. Soc. *106*:100.
11. Bass, C. C. (1948): The optimum characteristics of dental floss for personal oral hygiene. Dent. Items Int. *70*:921.
12. Black, G. V. (1915): A Work on Special Dental Pathology Devoted to the Disease and Treatment of the Investing Tissues of the Teeth and the Dental Pulp. Medico-Dental Publishing Company, Chicago, pp. 108 and 433–436.
13. Bohannan, H. (1968): Oral Physiotherapy. *In* Periodontal Therapy. 4th Ed. (Goldman, H. M., and Cohen, D. W., eds.) St. Louis, C. V. Mosby Co., pp. 446–473.
14. Brandtzaeg, P. (1964): The significance of oral hygiene in the prevention of dental diseases. Odontol. Tidskr. *72*:460.
15. Bruske, J. S. (1932): Toothbrush (Abstract from Proceedings Eighth International Congress). Dent. Cosmos *74*:922.
16. Charters, W. J. (1948): Proper home care of the mouth. J. Periodontol. *19*:136.
17. Clark, J., Cheraskin, E., and Ringsdorf, M. (1969): An ecologic study of oral hygiene. J. Periodontol. *40*:476.
18. Davies, G. N. (1963): Social customs and habits and their effect on oral disease. J. Dent. Res. *42*[Suppl.]*1*:209.
19. Downton, J. M., and Castaldi, C. R. (1967): A study of four disclosing solutions. Can. Dent. Hyg., Fall 1967.
20. Fanning, E. A., and Henning, F. R. (1967): Toothbrush design and its relation to oral health. Aust. Dent. J. *12*:464.
21. Fones, A. C. (1934): Home care of the mouth. *In* Mouth Hygiene. 4th Ed. Philadelphia, Lea and Febiger, pp. 294–315.
22. Fosdick, L. S. (1950): The reduction of the incidence of dental caries. Immediate toothbrushing with a neutral dentifrice. J. Am. Dent. Assoc. *40*:133.
23. Gilson, C. M. et al. (1969): A comparison of physical properties of several soft toothbrushes. J. Mich. Dent. Assoc. *51*:347.
24. Greene, J. C. (1966): Oral health care for the prevention and control of periodontal disease. *In* World Workshop in Periodontics. Ann Arbor, University of Michigan Press, pp. 399–443.
25. Greene, J. C. (1963): Oral hygiene and periodontal disease. Am. J. Public Health *53*:913.
26. Guide to Dental Materials and Devices 1970/1971. 5th Ed. American Dental Association, Chicago.
27. Hendon, G. E., Keller, S. E., and Manson-Hing, L. R. (1969): Clearance studies of proximal tooth surfaces (Part I). Ala. J. Med. Sci. *6*:213.
28. Hewat, R., Abraham, M., and Rice, F. (1950): An experimental study on the control of dental caries. N.Z. Dent. J. *46*:78.
29. Jensen, S. B. et al. (1968): Experimental gingivitis in man IV, Vancomycin-induced changes in bacterial plaque composition as related to development of gingival inflammation. J. Periodont. Res. *3*:284.
30. Keller, S. T., and Manson-Hing, L. R. (1969): Clearance studies of proximal plaque. Part II: In vivo removal of interproximal plaque. Ala. J. Med. Sci. *6*:266.
31. Keller, S. T., and Manson-Hing, L. R. (1969): Clearance studies of proximal tooth surfaces. Parts III and IV: In vivo removal of interproximal plaque. Ala. J. Med. Sci. *6*:399.
32. Kimery, M. J., and Stallard, R. E. (1969): The evolutionary development and contemporary utilization of various oral hygiene procedures. Periodont. Abstr. *XVI*:90.

33. Kimmelman, B. B. et al. (1958): Research in toothbrush design. Pa. Dent. J. *25*:24.
34. Koch, G., and Lindhe, J. (1965): The effect of supervised oral hygiene on the gingiva of children. The effect of toothbrushing. Odontol. Review *16*:327.
35. Löe, H., Theilade, E., and Jensen, S. B. (1965): Experimental gingivitis in man. J. Periodontol. *36*:177.
36. Löe, H. et al. (1967): Experimental gingivitis in man III, The influence of antibiotics on gingival plaque development. J. Periodont. Res. *2*:282.
37. Löe, H. (1970): A review of the prevention and control of plaque. *In* Dental Plaque. (McHugh, W. D., ed.) London, E. and S. Livingstone, Ltd., pp. 259–270.
38. Mansbridge, J. N. (1960): The effects of oral hygiene and sweet consumption on the prevalence of dental caries. Br. Dent. J. *109*:343.
39. Miller, J., and Hobson, P. (1961): The relationship between malocclusion, oral cleanliness, gingival conditions and dental caries in school children. Br. Dent. J. *111*:43.
40. Muhler, J. C. (1969): Comparative frequency of use of the electric toothbrush and hand toothbrush. J. Periodontol. *40*:268.
41. O'Leary, T. J. et al. (1970): Possible penetration of crevicular tissue from oral hygiene procedures: I. Use of oral irrigating devices. J. Periodontol, *41*:3.
42. Parfitt, G. J. (1968): Therapeutic devices. Ann. N. Y. Acad. Sci. *153*:360.
43. Saxe, S. R. et al. (1967): Oral debris, calculus and periodontal disease in the beagle dog. Periodontics *5*:271.
44. Smith, T. S. (1940): Anatomic and physiologic conditions governing the use of the toothbrush. J. Am. Dent. Assoc. *27*:874.
45. Stanmeyer, W. R. (1957): A measure of tissue response to frequency of toothbrushing. J. Periodontol. *28*:17.
46. Stillman, P. R. (1932): A philosophy of the treatment of periodontal disease. Dent. Dig. *38*:315.
47. Suomi, J. D. et al. (1969): The effect of controlled oral hygiene procedures on the progression of periodontal disease in adults: Results after two years. J. Periodontol. *40*:416.
48. Tamini, H. A. et al. (1969): Bacteremia study using a water irrigating device. J. Periodontol. *40*:424.
49. Theilade, E. et al. (1966): Experimental gingivitis in man, II, A longitudinal, clinical and bacteriological investigation. J. Periodont. Res. *1*:1.
50. Waerhaug, J. (1967): Current basis for prevention of periodontal disease. Int. Dent. J. *17*:267.
51. Williford, J. W., Muhler, J. C., and Stancey, G. K. (1967): Study demonstrating improved oral health through education. J. Am. Dent. Assoc. *75*:896.

chapter 14

PREVENTION AND CONTROL OF DENTAL CARIES

by
RICHARD E. STALLARD, D.D.S., Ph.D.

Numerous methods of dental caries prevention and control are presented elsewhere in this text, and include topical and systemic fluoride, pit and fissure sealants, nutritional aspects and microbiology.

The incorporation of fluoride into the drinking-water supplies of cities has over the years had a tremendous effect on reducing the incidence of caries.[1] It is generally accepted that the beneficial effects of fluoride, whether ingested or topically applied (Fig. 14–1), is to smooth surface caries. In an ideal fluoride environment, it is estimated that pit and fissure caries are delayed one or two years, but they are certainly not prevented to the extent that smooth surface caries are.[2] Pit and fissure sealing, therefore, can have a major impact on caries incidence. The term sealant is used to describe the resin material introduced into the occlusal pits and fissures of caries-susceptible teeth, thus forming a mechanical-physical protection against the action of caries producing bacteria and substrates (Fig. 14–2).[3, 4, 5]

Two basic types of sealant material are on the market today: those that utilize an ultraviolet-sensitive catalyst requiring polymerization by exposure to ultraviolet light, and those that polymerize chemically. The main advantage of the latter is the cost savings in not having to invest in an ultraviolet light; however, with an ultraviolet light, the operator can control the setting time. The efficacy of the two systems appears, from the literature, to be equal.[3]

While nearly everyone accepts the concept that certain types of foods can be more directly related to dental caries than others, the actual quantity of sucrose in foods related to tooth decay has not been proved.[6, 7] It is also noteworthy that food additives, such as flavorings and sugar substitutes may modify the amount of acid produced by bacteria and therefore the rate of tooth decay.[8]

Food retention and between-meal eating are other major factors that influence the rate of decay.[9, 10] Since the frequency of

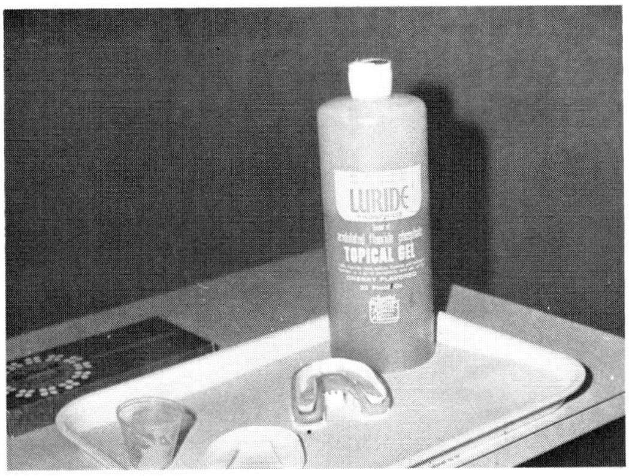

Figure 14–1 A multitude of techniques for the topical application of fluoride have appeared over the years. One of the most effective methods currently being used is the acidulated fluoride gel utilizing the ion membrane system. The need to completely remove all plaque prior to application is still being debated.

between-meal eating is directly related to tooth decay, it is interesting to compare the decay rate of several snack foods. It is obvious from Table 14–1 that factors other than sucrose are active in the development of dental caries.

A piece of hard, sugar-free candy can potentially dissolve 70 times as much tooth structure as can a ginger snap.[8] Cookies and crackers rank low on this list, for the mixture of other carbohydrates with sugar tends to neutralize the acids produced. At the same time, sorbitol (artificial sugar) enhances the dissolving of tooth enamel.

Different flavors of the same brand of lollipops will produce different effects.

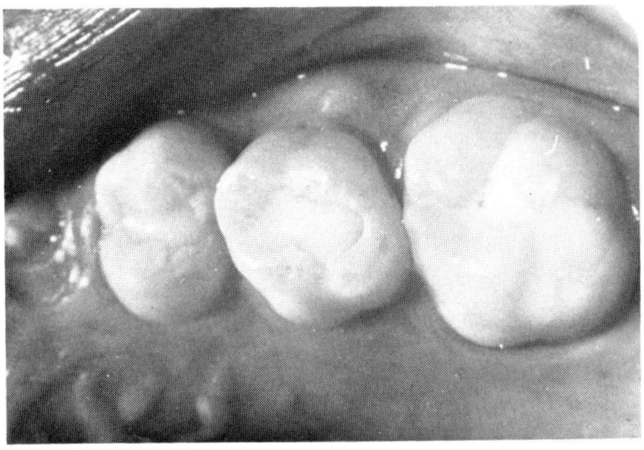

Figure 14–2 Properly applied sealant requires isolation of the teeth from any salivary contaminant during application. Both permanent and deciduous teeth can be successfully sealed, including palatal grooves.

Cherry, lemon, and grape flavors cause rapid enamel dissolution, while cinnamon, raspberry, and mint do so to a lesser degree.[8] The high concentration of acid in certain fruit-flavored candies, in some fruits, and in soft drinks has also been proved to cause erosion of tooth enamel.

One additional factor influencing the decay rate is retention of food by the teeth, coupled with frequency of between-meal snacks. Although bread has a relatively low sugar content, the starch content increases its retention. In many pastries the presence of fat counteracts the retention of starch, so that pastries are not retained on the teeth for as long a time. Hard candies are almost pure sugar, and so, dissolve rapidly and do not stay on the teeth as jelly candies do. Retention is important for only the first 30 minutes after food ingestion; after that, no difference can be detected between foods.

One disorder related to food retention is seen with increasing frequency and may actually be one of the most crippling and

TABLE 14–1 DECAY PRODUCING SNACKS*

TYPE OF SNACK	HIGH RATE	LOW RATE
Candy		
Lollipops	Cherry Lemon Grape	Cinnamon Raspberry Mint
Sticky	Jelly beans	
Hard	Sugar free (sorbitol)	Sugar (boiled)
Fruit	Raisins Apples Bananas	Dates
Baked goods	Bread Cakes Puddings	Cookies Crackers
Drinks	Orange juice Colas Chocolate milk	Milk
Dry snacks	Potato chips Peanuts	Graham crackers

*As measured by amount of tooth enamel dissolved. (From Bibby, B. G., and Mundorff, S. A.: J. Dent. Res. *54*:461–470, 1975.)

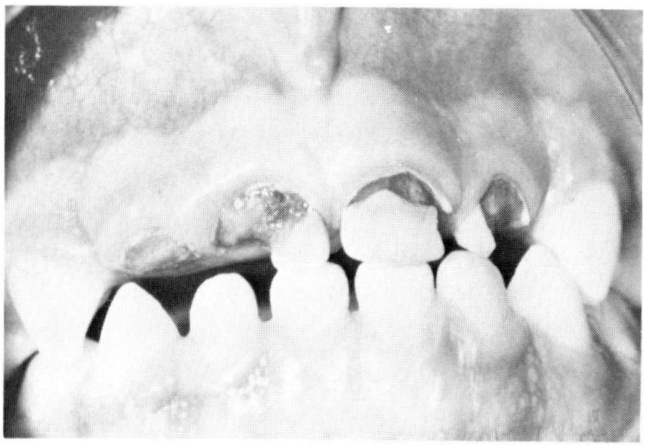

Figure 14–3 Clinical photograph of a three year old suffering from "baby bottle syndrome." The four upper anterior teeth are severely decayed, while the rest of the mouth is caries free. This child went to sleep at night with a bottle containing Kool-Aid.

damaging dental conditions of children today. This condition has many synonyms, the most common and descriptive being "baby bottle syndrome."[11] Children suffering from this disorder present themselves in the dental clinic with severe decay in the upper anterior teeth; often by the age of three the teeth have decayed off at the gum line (Fig. 14–3). The primary cause for this condition is the use of a baby bottle filled with fruit juices or other sweetened beverages which are placed in the bottle and given to the baby at night as a pacifier.

While the child is actively sucking on the bottle, the normal movement of the tongue, lips and cheeks, and the secretion of saliva will protect the teeth from the ravages of tooth decay; however, once the child falls asleep, the beverage continues to bathe the anterior teeth, where microorganisms within the dental plaque produce excess acids, resulting in a dissolving of the enamel and subsequent dental caries.[12] A similar problem has been caused, particularly in Europe, by the daytime use of pacifiers filled with fruit jellies or honey. These devices also keep a high concentration of sucrose around the upper anterior teeth.

The child who suffers from such a disorder may experience extreme pain and discomfort, caused originally by the tooth decay and secondarily by the abscess formation that often results. The persistent fever, irritability and fussiness of the child often bring the child to the pediatrician rather than the dentist. The most common treatment is removal of the severely broken-down teeth. This creates a space, which, depending on the age of the child when the teeth are lost, may allow any teeth forming posterior to them to drift forward.[13] Also, the jaw will not develop to its potential, owing to the lack of its full complement of teeth. When these two factors are combined, crowding and malaligned permanent teeth may develop, resulting in an unaesthetic situation for the child, and contributing to potential speech problems.

The cure is prevention. Unfortunately, the sweetened pacifier habit develops as a result of parental intervention, and therefore the parent must not permit the habit to start. If the child must have something to suck on, it is far better to utilize a bottle containing plain water. A baby bottle should not be used as a pacifier for children over the age of 12 to 18 months. Remember, it is far easier to prevent this problem than to subject a child to the discomfort and possible permanent deformity resulting from the diseased condition.

Dental caries is a preventable disease and one that is controllable if appropriate treatment is instituted and full cooperation is obtained from the patient and parents.

REFERENCES

1. Adler, P.: Effect of fluoride ingestion on caries experience. *In* Fluorides and Human Health. Geneva, World Health Organization, 1970, pp. 325–345.
2. Adler, P.: Effect of local fluoride treatment on caries experience. *In* Fluorides and Human Health. Geneva, World Health Organization, 1970, pp. 345–347.
3. Ripa, L. W.: The current status of occlusal sealants. J. Prevent. Dent. *3*:6–14, 1976.
4. Gwinnett, A. J.: The scientific basis of the sealant procedure. J. Prevent. Dent. *3*:15–28, 1976.
5. Handelman, S. L.: Microbiologic aspects of sealing carious lesions. J. Prevent. Dent. *3*:29–32, 1976.
6. Bibby, B. G.: The cariogenicity of snack foods and confections. J. Am. Dent. Assoc. *90*:121–132, 1975.
7. Andlaw, R. J.: The relation between acid production and enamel decalcification in salivary fermentations of carbohydrate foodstuffs. J. Dent. Res. *39*:1200–1209, 1960.
8. Bibby, B. G., and Mundorff, S. A.: Enamel demineralization by snack foods. J. Dent. Res. *54*:461–470, 1975.

9. Harris, M. R., and Stephan, R. M.: Effect of mixing water in the diet on the development of carious lesions in rats. J. Dent. Res. *32*:653, 1953.
10. Lundquist, C.: Oral sugar clearance. Odontol. Revy *3*:1–121, 1952.
11. Finn, S. B.: Dental caries in infants. Current Dental Comment, Feb. 1969, pp. 24–27.
12. James, P. M. C., Parfitt, G. J., and Falkner, F.: Study of the etiology of labial caries of the deciduous incisor teeth in small children. Br. Dent. J. *103*:37, 1957.
13. Miyamoto, W., Chung, C. S., and Yee, P. K.: Effect of premature loss of deciduous canines and molars on malocclusion of the permanent dentition. J. Dent. Res. 55:584–590, 1976.

ADDITIONAL READING

Osborn, T. W. B., Norkskin, J. N., and Staz, J.: A comparison of crude and refined sugar and cereals and their ability to produce in vitro decalcification of teeth. J. Dent. Res. *16*:165–171, 1937.

Bibby, B. G., Goldberg, H. V., and Chen, E.: Evaluation of the caries-producing potentialities of various foodstuffs. J. Am. Dent. Assoc. *42*:491–509, 1951.

Lundstrom, A.: The significance of early loss of deciduous teeth in the etiology of malocclusion. Am. J. Orthodont. *41*:819–826, 1955.

Posen, A. L.: The effect of premature loss of deciduous molars on premolar eruption. Angle Orthod. *35*:249–252, 1965.

Kroll, R. G., and Stone, J. H.: Nocturnal bottle-feeding as a contributory cause of rampant dental caries in the infant and young child. J. Dent. Child. XXXIV: 454–459, 1967.

Winter, G. B., Hamilton, M. C., and James, P. M. C.: Role of the comforter as an aetiological factor in rampant caries of the deciduous dentition. Arch. Dis. Child. *41*:207, 1966.

Horowitz, H. S., Heifetz, S. B., and Poulsen, S.: Adhesive sealant clinical trial: An overview of results after four years in Kalispell, Montana. J. Prevent. Dent. *3*:38–49, 1976.

Whitehurst, V., and Soni, N. N.: Adhesive sealant clinical trial: Results eighteen months after one application. J. Prevent. Dent. *3*:20–22, 1976.

Council on Dental Materials and Devices: Pit and fissure sealants. J. Am. Dent. Assoc. *88*:390, 1974.

Cueto, E. I., and Buonocore, M. G.: Sealing of pits and fissures with an adhesive resin. Its use in caries prevention. J. Am. Dent. Assoc. *75*:121–128, 1967.

chapter 15

PERIODONTAL DISEASE: PREVENTION AND CONTROL

by
LEONARD SHAPIRO, D.M.D., M.S.

The practice of dentistry is changing from one of treatment and repair of previous damage to one of prevention of disease. The patient's role is being altered from that of a passive bystander to one of an active participant in disease prevention. The dental office is also changing from a repair oriented facility and is assuming a teaching role in the prevention of pathology. A need will always exist for excellence in restorative therapy, but dentistry can no longer be practiced without patient education and motivation for prevention of these lesions.

Motivation, on the part of both the teacher and the student, is the key factor for the success of a plaque control program. Chronic lesions, such as those associated with the inflammatory periodontal lesion, are not usually sufficient to bring a patient to the office seeking care. One of the main motivating factors in dental disease—pain—is absent. Past experience of relief from noxious stimuli, rather than the prevention and elimination of future painful experiences, may be the only reference the patient has for seeking dental care.

The behavior of the patient must be modified to seek early preventive care rather than relief from pain. The drive to seek dental care must come from within the patient, and then usually only after he has been exposed to the benefits of preventive rather than reparative care. The patient is not motivated by an adequate zone of attached gingiva or knife-edged papillae, but rather by selfish drives, e.g., improving his appearance, improving social acceptability, and finally, the maintenance of his dentition. These needs or drives will lead to action on the part of the patient to achieve the goal of oral health (Table 15–1).

It may well be that the patient who presents in the dental office is sufficiently motivated, but this may not be sufficient to make him accept preventive therapy. It is then necessary to establish an educational rapport with the patient to make him aware of oral disease and the means by which the disease and repair cycle can be stopped. Once rapport has been established, communication between the patient and dentist is easy, provided that the common language

TABLE 15-1*

		Pretreatment					One Year Posttreatment		
		OHI-S	*Expect to Retain Their Teeth*	*Brush to Improve Gum Health*			*OHI-S*	*Expect to Retain Their Teeth*	*Brush to Improve Gum Health*
30–39	Male	1.83	59%	15%	30–39	Male	1.45	66%	50%
	Female	1.55	61%	36%		Female	1.30	58%	66%
40–49	Male	2.17	35%	12%	40–49	Male	2.70	40%	60%
	Female	1.78	58%	40%		Female	1.82	62%	75%
50–59	Male	1.92	30%	21%	50–59	Male	1.81	25%	100%
	Female	1.30	63%	38%		Female	1.10	75%	83%
60 + over	Male	1.72	42%	25%	60 + over	Male	1.32	62%	75%
	Female	1.32	74%	51%		Female	1.55	80%	66%
Means	Male	1.91	42%	18%	Means	Male	1.82	48%	71%
	Female	1.48	64%	41%		Female	1.44	69%	67%
	Overall	1.70	53%	30%		Overall	1.63	59%	69%
Total N = 100					Total N = 89				

*From Awwa, I., and Stallard, R. E.: Periodontal prognosis: Educational and psychological implications. J. Periodont. *41*: 55–57, 1970.

is commensurate with the patient's ability to understand. Failure to achieve this common language will negate the previously established rapport and make communication as well as motivation impossible.

PLAQUE CONTROL PROGRAMS

Once the rapport has been established, mechanisms must be instituted to carry out an adequate plaque control program. Office procedures for preventive dentistry vary from office to office. A dentist, control therapist, or hygienist may be the teacher. Regardless of who the teacher is, however, the motivation which brought the patient to seek preventive care must be carried over to this phase of the learning experience. Before the patient can accept preventive therapy, he must be taught the rationale for this phase of treatment and more important, the cause of this problem. If the patient is taught the cause of his disease, he can better appreciate practicing the techniques necessary for its prevention. It is not necessary to delve into the esoteric aspects of the controversy whether sulcular fluid is an exudate or a transudate, but rather the teacher should go into the development of dental plaque and the effects of bacterial products on the hard and soft tissues of the oral cavity.

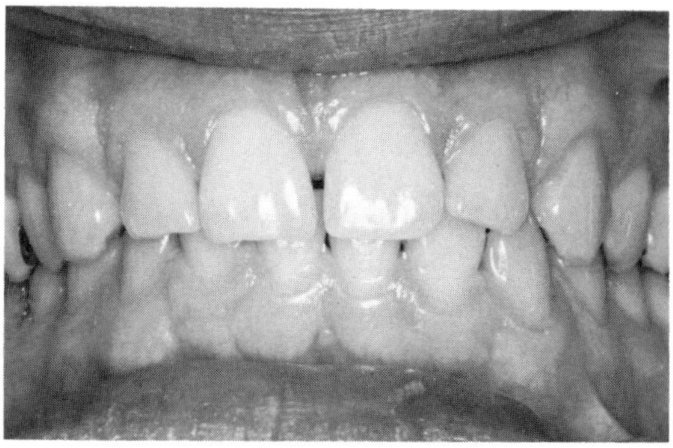

Figure 15–1 The primary objective of complete elimination of dental plaque from all surfaces of teeth can be seen in this clinical photograph. The patient is free of dental plaque and accompanying gingival disease.

The primary objective of oral hygiene procedures is the elimination of dental plaque from all tooth surfaces (Figs. 15–1 and 15–2). In the past, patients have been presented with a myriad of items which required an inordinate amount of time and a degree of dexterity which many patients lacked. In addition, little or no instruction was given concerning the etiology of the lesion.

ARMAMENTARIUM

The basic armamentarium for effective plaque control should consist of a disclosing

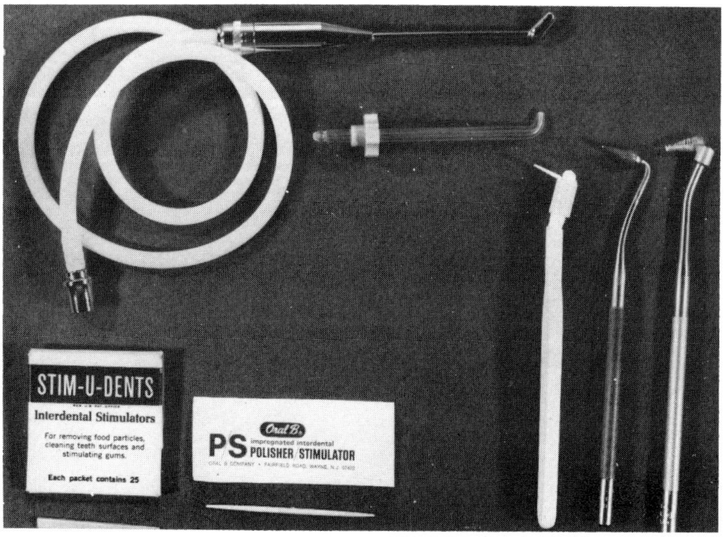

Figure 15–2 The market is flooded with numerous devices claiming to be superior in the elimination of dental plaque. A few such devices can be seen in this illustration. To date none of these has been shown to be superior to routine tooth brushing, flossing, or other interproximal cleaning.

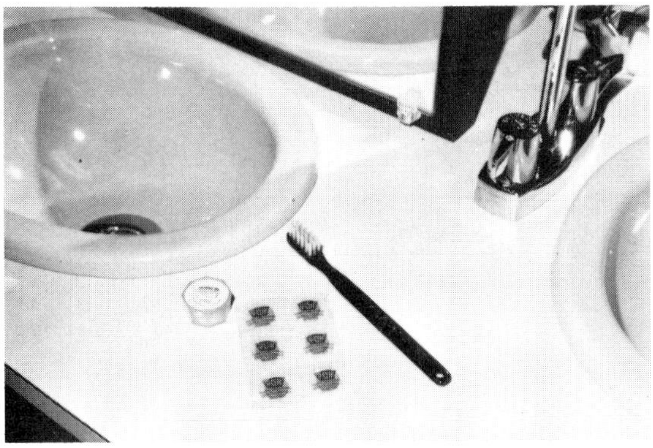

Figure 15–3 The basic armamentarium for a preventive and control program in periodontal disease consists of the tooth brush, disclosing tablets and dental floss.

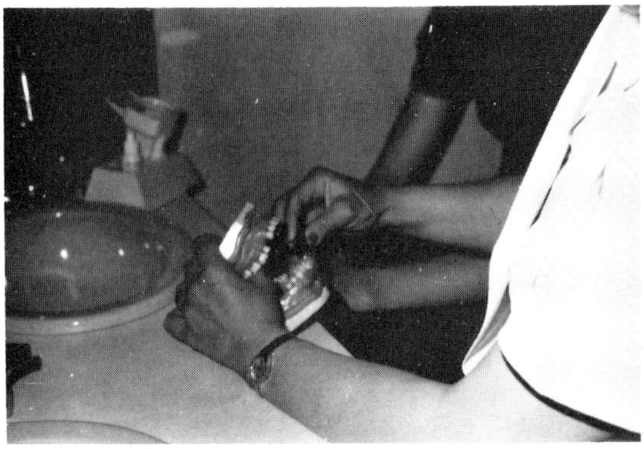

Figure 15–5 For the patient's first exposure to presentation of oral hygiene procedures, demonstration on a model has proved to be the most effective teaching method.

agent, toothbrush, and a method for interproximal cleaning (Fig. 15–3).

Disclosing Agents. Disclosing agents are used so that the patient can better visualize the dental plaque, the cause of his problem. Basically, three types of disclosing solutions are available—a red dye (FDC #3) in either a tablet or liquid which colors the plaque relatively uniformly, a fluorescein dye which must be activated by a fluorescent light and has the advantage of being relatively invisible when the light is not used, and a temporal agent which selectively stains plaque by its age rather than by amount. With the temporal dye, newer plaque is red while older plaque is blue (Fig. 15–4). It has the advantage of allowing the patient to visualize more easily the problem areas of his dentition which he may have had difficulty in cleaning.

In addition to being a guide to areas to be cleaned, the disclosing solution also acts as an efficient method for evaluating plaque control once all the procedures have been performed.

Toothbrush. Once the presence of plaque has been shown on the teeth, it must be removed. Plaque is removed by mechanical methods. The toothbrush is an aid in the removal of soft accumulated debris which has collected on the tooth. The method to be used is demonstrated first on a model (Fig. 15–5), next in the patient's mouth, and third by the patient himself

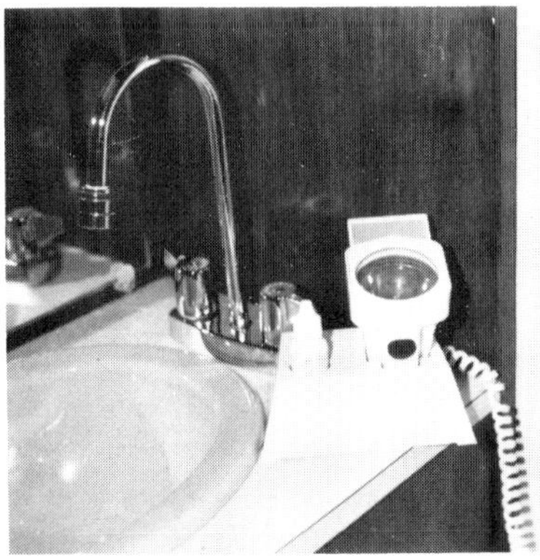

Figure 15–4 The Plak-Lite, utilizing a fluorescent dye and an ultraviolet light, offers an innovative method of disclosing the presence of dental plaque. One of its principal advantages is with the adult patient who looks somewhat askance at leaving the dental office with a red mouth.

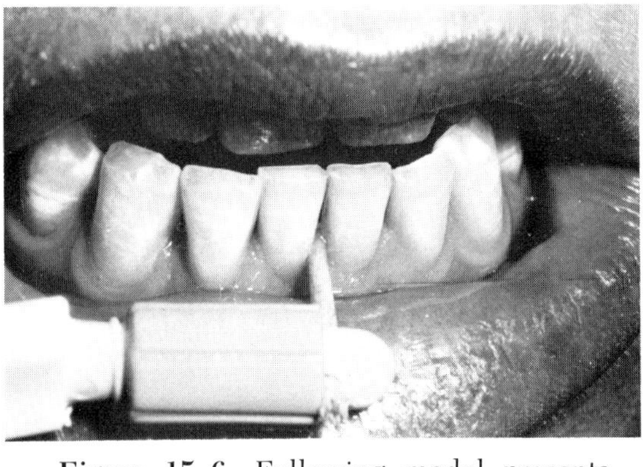

Figure 15–6 Following model presentation, demonstration in the patient's own mouth followed by utilization of the toothbrush or other device by the patient is essential.

(Fig. 15–6). Recent studies have indicated that a modification of the Bass technique, the use of a soft multituft nylon brush with the bristles inclined into the gingival sulcus, is the most efficient technique for removal of plaque from the sulcular area. The brush is moved from one area of the dentition to the adjacent area until the facial and lingual surfaces of all teeth have been cleaned. Unfortunately, a single technique cannot be used by all patients, and modifications of a basic technique are necessary to adapt to the individual situation. Most important, however, is not the technique taught, but rather the thoroughness with which it is performed.

The toothbrush has the disadvantage of being unable to cleanse the proximal surfaces of the teeth. Even after the most thorough brushing, plaque remains interproximally (Fig. 15–7). Various modalities have been developed for interproximal plaque control, ranging from dental floss to plastic stimulators. The most efficient method of interproximal plaque control appears to be dental floss. The floss is gently eased through the contact area and rubbed along the proximal surfaces until they are plaque free (Fig. 15–8). As was the case with the toothbrush, however, modifications must be made to compensate for dexterity, fixed splinting and anatomic variations. To this end other modalities such as soft balsa wood and rounded tooth picks, as well as interproximal brushes, have been developed to reach areas which the patient is unable to reach with the dental floss.

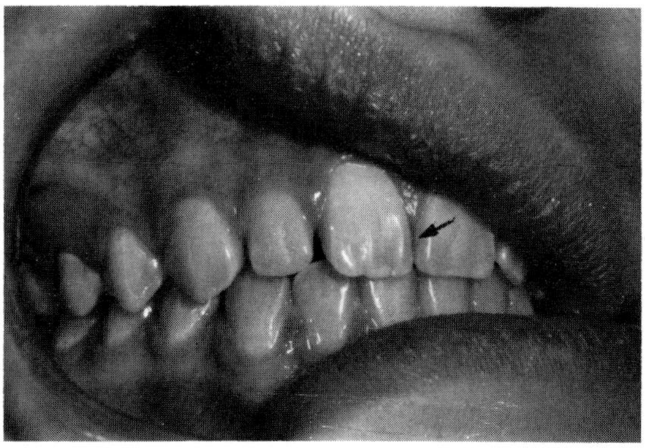

Figure 15–7 Note the plaque remaining in interproximal areas after thorough brushing. This can only be removed by the use of an interproximal cleaning aid such as dental floss.

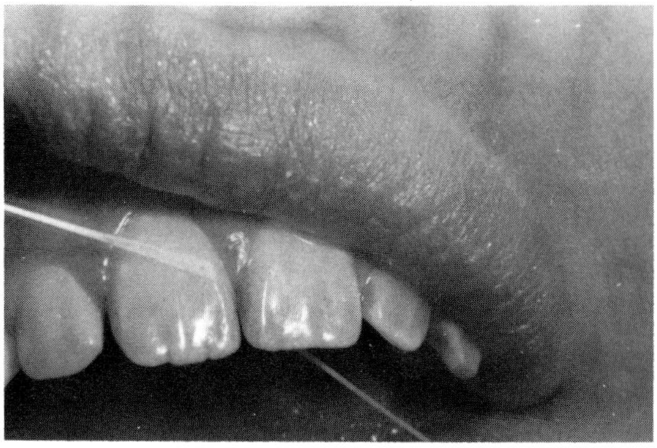

Figure 15–8 The dental floss is drawn taut across the surface of the tooth so that it can rub gently on the tooth surface, eliminating dental plaque both supra- and subgingivally.

Other instruments such as the electric toothbrush and water pressure devices have been introduced into the plaque control armamentarium. There is no available data to indicate that a powered toothbrush is any more efficient in plaque removal than the manual brush. Initial success with the electric brush may be due more to a novelty effect rather than to increased efficiency. Water pressure devices have been advocated for removal of sulcular debris. Again, there is no available data to indicate they have any efficiency in plaque removal.

CHEMICAL PLAQUE CONTROL

From past experience it is apparent that mechanical means alone are not sufficient to prevent dental disease. Recent investigations have dealt with chemical control of disease, thereby eliminating the dexterity now necessary to practice adequate plaque control. The chlorhexidine group of compounds has shown promise as a means of preventing plaque formation without eliminating entirely the resident bacterial population of the oral cavity. Much more investigation along this line is needed, however, to develop a substance which is both nontoxic to the host, yet capable of preventing new plaque formation.

PATIENT RECALL

Once the patient has been instructed in the methods of disease control in his mouth, he must be sufficiently motivated to carry on these procedures in his home. It is not sufficient that he demonstrate a complete understanding in the office. The instruction must also be integrated into a daily habit pattern in order to prevent a recurrence of disease. Closely integrated with good home care is a carefully planned recall sequence.

All patients are not compulsive personality types; therefore, they do not exhibit perfect plaque control, and it is probably also true that most patients are incapable of maintaining a satisfactory level of plaque control over a long period of time without some assistance. The recall visit presents an opportunity to reorient and re-educate the patient in the rationale and methods of plaque control.

Without this continuous reinforcement to remain highly motivated, patients may relapse into old comfortable habits.

The prevention of periodontal disease requires a sufficiently motivated patient practicing adequate plaque control. With an understanding of the disease process the patient can better appreciate the methods used to control disease in his mouth. At present only mechanical methods are available for disease control, but current research has shown promise for a chemical means of individual plaque control.

REFERENCES

1. Anderson, J.: Integration of plaque control into the practice of dentistry. Dent. Clin. North Am. *16*:621, 1972.
2. Arnim, S. S.: The use of disclosing agents for measuring tooth cleanliness. J. Periodontol. *34*:227, 1963.
3. Awwa, I., and Stallard, R. E.: Periodontal prognosis: Education and psychological implications. J. Periodontol. *41*:55–57, 1970.
4. Bass, C. C.: An effective method of personal oral hygiene. J. La. State Med. Soc. *106*:100, 1954.
5. Bass, C. C.: The optimum characteristics of tooth brushes for personal oral hygiene. Dental Items of Interest *70*:697, 1948.
6. Cohen, D. W., Stoller, N. H., Chace, R., and Laster, L.: A comparison of bacterial plaque disclosants in periodontal disease. J. Periodontol. *43*:333, 1972.
7. Hill, H. C., Levi, P. P., and Glickman, I.: The effects of waxed and unwaxed dental floss on interdental plaque accumulation and interdental gingival health. J. Periodontol. *44*:411, 1973.
8. Less, W.: Mechanics of teaching plaque control. Dent. Clin. North Am. *16*:647, 1972.
9. Lifer, L.: Motivation of the patient by the dentist. Dent. Clin. North Am. *16*:609, 1972.
10. Loe, H., Theilade, E., and Jensen, S. B.: Gingivitis in man. J. Periodontol. *36*:177, 1965.
11. Radentz, W. G., Barnes, G., Carter, H., Ailor, J., and Johnson, R.: An evaluation of two techniques for teaching proper dental flossing procedures. J. Periodontol. *44*:177, 1973.
12. Van de Voorde, H. E.: A movie versus chairside instruction to present preliminary oral hygiene information. J. Periodontol. *43*:277, 1972.

chapter 16

PREVENTIVE DENTAL RADIOLOGY

by
ARTHUR H. WUEHRMANN, D.M.D

INTRODUCTION

Concepts of prevention related to dental radiology take at least two forms. The appropriate use of radiologic procedures can assist in preventing advanced dental disease through the early recognition and treatment of various pathological entities. Alternatively, preventive radiology can, through the implementation of good radiological health principles, reduce somatic and genetic alterations which could result from using ionizing radiation.* Preventive dental radiology encompasses both concepts, and this chapter will touch on salient features related to both.

Of maximum importance in understanding the concepts of preventive radiology is an appreciation of the term *diagnostic yield.* Regardless of its type, human exposure to ionizing radiation has a deleterious effect. From a purely biologic standpoint, it would be best if humans were not subjected to man-made ionizing radiation. This statement is true until the balance between risk and gain is examined. Man's longevity has increased materially in civilized countries during the 20th century because of the many advances in health care. Among these advances must be included the diagnostic use of x-radiation. Thus, the undesirable effects of x-radiation exposure are offset but not eliminated by health benefits. Since use of x-radiation is potentially harmful, each exposure should result in the greatest amount of diagnostic information possible per unit of x-radiation used. Diagnostic yield can be defined as the amount of diagnostic information made available per unit of x-radiation absorbed by the patient.

It becomes immediately obvious that diagnostic yield is related directly to three aspects of x-radiation use: 1) radiation reduction methods employed by the dentist, 2) adequacy of chairside radiographic techniques, and 3) competency to interpret diagnostic information available on radio-

*Ionizing radiation is any particulate or electromagnetic energy that causes atoms or molecules to ionize. Except in research endeavors, the dental profession uses, with few exceptions, only x-radiation. Therefore, the use of the terms ionizing radiation and x-radiation (and x-rays) is synonymous.

graphic films. Weakness in one or more of these three facets of the science lowers the diagnostic yield either by causing the patient to receive more radiation than is necessary in order to attain the desired diagnostic end product or by causing the patient to be exposed unnecessarily because of the non-use of available diagnostic information.

A complete discussion of the abovementioned three factors that interrelate in producing diagnostic yield would require a textbook on dental radiology rather than a chapter in a preventive dentistry text. Accordingly, the material to follow will not be complete, and the reader is encouraged to study in considerably greater detail all matters which relate to dental radiology. Although interpretation and chairside radiographic techniques will be mentioned, emphasis will be given to radiation reduction methods in the dental office. Prior to such discussion, attention will be given to certain general considerations for the purpose of clarifying issues to follow.

GENERAL CONSIDERATIONS

It must be recognized by the health science professions that the use of ionizing radiation constitutes a public health problem. No facet of dental practice other than the use of x-radiation represents anything other than an interpersonal relationship between dentist and patient. Perhaps with the advent of more state and federally sponsored dental programs, government agencies will be considered a third party, but the interrelationship still will be basically between doctor and patient. An unsatisfactory denture is immediately recognizable and can be remedied or destroyed without loss except in terms of time and money. Similarly, a restoration that is dislodged or has a rough margin can be noted and corrected. Other examples are obvious. Ionizing radiation, on the other hand, can create somatic effects which are not recognizable immediately and which may not become obvious at any time during an individual's lifetime. In addition to somatic effects in the exposed individual, genetic changes can occur which may affect progeny. Much has yet to be learned by radiation biologists about the effects of low level radiation exposures on individuals and their offspring. Because the situation is so intangible, the health professions must accept professional responsibility beyond that ordinarily recognized in the course of practice.

X-radiation effects on vital tissue are fundamentally those of ionization and excitation of atoms within molecules. The result of ionization (the creation of electrical instability in an atom or molecule) is the recombination of the affected molecule with other unlike charged atoms or molecules to form incompatible substances not intended to exist in the human body. This statement, of necessity, is a gross generalization and oversimplification (textbooks have been written on the subject). It will serve for purposes of understanding certain terms that should be in the vocabulary of all practicing dentists.

X-radiation *exposure* is stated in terms of roentgens, abbreviated R. The roentgen* can be thought of as that amount of X or gamma radiation that will create a known amount of ionization in air under certain conditions. The roentgen can be considered in the same vein as other devices for measuring quantities such as the meter or the gram or the liter. The roentgen is a measure of x-radiation made in air and is used to state the amount of radiation emanating from the x-ray machine.

X-radiation *dosage* is stated in terms of rads. The rad,** which relates directly to the roentgen, is a measure of *absorbed radiation* in tissue or in any other substance. Although an understanding of radiation output (R) is important, an understanding of the amount of radiation absorbed by the body is even more so. For example, if 100 R were produced at the ra-

*The roentgen (R) is a special unit of exposure. It can be defined as that amount of X or gamma radiation which will produce in 1 cc. of air (at standard temperature and pressure) one electrostatic unit of either sign. One electrostatic unit equals 2.08×10^9 ion pairs.

**The rad is a special unit of absorbed dose equal to 100 ergs per gram of absorbing material.

diation source but the radiation were of such a character as to penetrate the human body without being absorbed, the amount of radiation would have little importance in terms of biologic effect.

Directly allied to the concept of the rad is the idea of gram-rads. It is obvious that if only one gram of tissue were to receive a given amount of radiation, the effect would be far less deleterious than if 1000 grams of tissue each received one rad. These concepts will be used in discussing radiation reduction methods, but, for purposes of understanding, it will be helpful to give a suitable example. Under certain conditions, the output of the modern dental x-ray machine at eight inches from the source of radiation (x-ray tube anode) is approximately 1 R per second. Since for x-radiation, the roentgen and the rad are approximately equivalent, each exposed gram of tissue near the skin surface will absorb approximately one rad. (This assumes an approximately eight-inch source to skin distance.) However, if one x-ray beam is well confined in comparison to another beam which has a larger diameter, the amount of tissue exposed in the first instance will be less than that of the second, and the gram-rads for the second individual will be greater than for the first. This is one reason why dentists are encouraged to use an x-ray beam collimated to just cover the film to be exposed. With these general considerations in mind, it is appropriate to think in terms of radiation reduction methods in the dental office.

RADIATION REDUCTION METHODS IN THE DENTAL OFFICE

Radiation protection methods used in the dental office should relate to two categories of individuals: patients and dental office staff. Patients may be further subdivided into those actually being exposed and those being treated in other operatories or waiting in the reception room for treatment. Similarly, the staff may be separated into persons actually operating the x-ray equipment and those working in contiguous rooms. Reference will be made later in this chapter to structural shielding; these comments will relate primarily to the protection of patients not being exposed to x-radiation and to auxiliaries other than those actually using the x-ray equipment. For the present, reference to the patient implies the patient actually being exposed and reference to the operator implies the individual operating the x-ray equipment.

PATIENT PROTECTION

Patient protection can be accomplished by suitable alterations, when necessary, in x-ray machine design, by the use of fast films of appropriate size, and by the employment of satisfactory x-ray techniques. Each of these will be discussed in detail.

X-ray Machine Alterations. Although currently produced dental x-ray equipment conforms to desirable standards, verification of conformity should be made when the machine is installed. Older machines often need modification. The changes that are more frequently needed are in x-ray beam collimation, filtration, and tube head (or tube housing) leakage.

X-RAY BEAM COLLIMATION. The x-ray beam emanates from a small area on the surface of the x-ray tube anode. For present purposes, this can be considered a point source. The beam ordinarily passes through a round aperture in the x-ray tube housing, thus giving the beam a rounded shape, the diameter of which can be determined. The remainder of the tube housing fully absorbs the radiation unless it leaks (see tube head leakage). The x-ray beam diameter used for exposure of intraoral dental films should be no more than 2.75 inches at the skin surface. If the beam is excessively large, it can be further reduced by the insertion of a suitable lead diaphragm (often called a lead washer) into the tube head housing where the x-ray beam emanates from the housing (Fig. 16–1). In addition to suitable collimation by this means, the dentist should use an open-end cylinder that is lined with a heavy metal (a lead foil

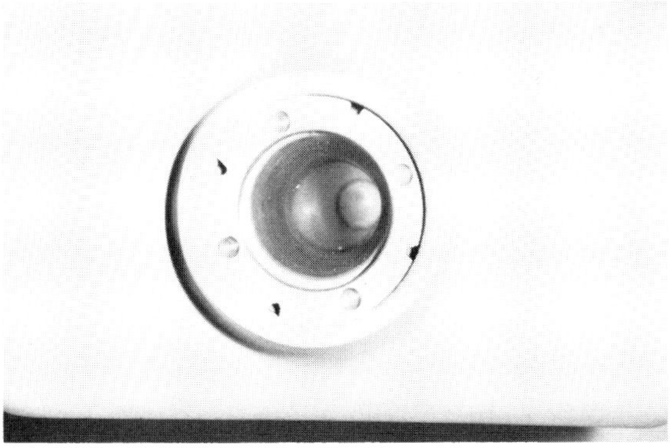

Figure 16–1 Aperture through which the x-ray beam emerges from the tube head. Cylinder with appropriate lead diaphragm, is not shown. They attach over the opening.

of approximatelyly 0.3 millimeter in thickness is usually recommended) or one that has been lead impregnated during manufacture (Fig. 16–2). The frequently used plastic pointed cone should be discarded because primary radiation striking the cone creates secondary radiation which scatters in directions other than that of the primary beam, causing exposures of the patient and the operator that do not contribute in any way to high diagnostic yield. The lining of a plastic cylinder is simple and has been described in the literature.

An x-ray beam diameter greater than 2.75 inches is frequently needed for various types of extraoral film. Consequently, different size lead collimators and different lengths of lined cylinders may be needed depending on whether the dentist makes extraoral film exposures. Extraoral films should be used frequently by the dentist in an effort to obtain a high diagnostic yield.

Filtration. Commercially pure aluminum is commonly used for the filtration of x-ray beams using kilovoltages ordinarily employed in dentistry. The purpose of the filtration is to absorb or attenuate long wavelength x-ray photons that have little likelihood of penetrating the patient's tissue and reaching the film. Such photons are absorbed in the tissue between the outside of the face and the film and cause tissue destruction but no diagnostic yield. The minimum total filtration (the inherent filtration built into the x-ray tube plus added filtration) ordinarily recommended is 0.5 millimeter aluminum for machines operating below 50 kVp, 1.5 mm Al for those operating between 50 and 70 kVp, and 2.5 mm Al for machines operating above 70 kVp. Recently manufactured machines ordinarily will conform to these recommendations, but older machines often need alteration. The dentist can easily add the needed thicknesses of chemically pure aluminum or he can have this done by qualified personnel usually available through his state health department.

The dentist frequently does not know whether the total filtration in his machine is adequate, but a very simple test is available. Preferably using a phantom,* although the use of a patient over the childbearing age is permissible, the dentist makes a conventional intraoral exposure using an exposure time he knows will produce a diagnostic film of suitable density (density is defined as the degree of blackness of a radiographic film). An additional 0.5 mm Al is then inserted in the x-ray beam by removing the cylinder, placing an aluminum disc of appropriate size in the x-ray tube head opening, and replacing the cylinder. Another exposure is made of the same phantom or patient, using exactly the same exposure technique. Both films are processed simultaneously on the same processing rack. If the original filtration was adequate, the insertion of the additional fil-

*A substance of thickness and density comparable to human tissue through which the x-ray beam is passed.

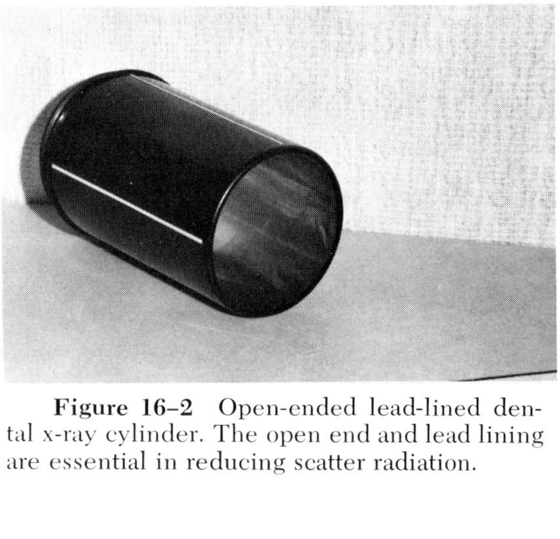

Figure 16–2 Open-ended lead-lined dental x-ray cylinder. The open end and lead lining are essential in reducing scatter radiation.

tration will produce a noticeably lighter film, and the added thickness of aluminum should be removed. If the density of the second film is not visibly reduced, additional 0.5 mm thicknesses of chemically pure aluminum should be sequentially added until the film density is definitely altered. The last thickness of aluminum that causes a reduction in density should then be removed. The rationale for this test is based on a desire to filter nonuseful radiation but not to attenuate x-ray photons that can reach the film.

Tube Head Leakage. Modern dental x-ray machines are ordinarily examined during manufacture for tube head leakage, and generally can be considered safe for dental office use. On occasion, however, new tube heads have been found to leak x-radiation, and older tube heads frequently show some degree of leakage. To determine leakage, the aperture in the x-ray tube head through which the x-ray beam emanates must be completely obliterated with an approximately 1/4 inch thickness lead disc, and the tube head surveyed while the machine is activated, using suitable monitoring equipment that ordinarily is not available in the dental office. State or city health departments often are available for this type of survey at little or no cost.

Radiation leakage sometimes occurs when the usual lead collimator (or lead washer) does not have a sufficiently large outside diameter. This leakage may not be discovered using ordinary monitoring procedures. It can be detected by using an 8 × 10 inch or larger film. The open end of the cylinder is placed in contact with the center of the film surface, and an exposure of relatively long duration is made. When processed, the exposed portion of the film should be totally black and the surrounding area should be clear. Film blackening beyond the exposed circle indicates a need for modification that can be done by the dentist or a suitable technician. The use of a pointed plastic cone instead of an open-end lined cylinder will cause film blackening beyond the exposure circle. This is not tube head leakage; it can be remedied by discarding the pointed cone.

Film Speed and Size. The sensitivity of intraoral film emulsions used in dentistry varies widely. Film speeds have been characterized by the American National Standards Institute* using alphabetical speed designations wherein A is the slowest (least sensitive) film. The fastest practical film presently available is the D speed. A speed film is no longer available on the American Market. B speed, which is available, is four times slower (hence requires four times the exposure to produce a comparable film density) than D speed film. Although not required by regulation, most American film manufacturers indicate speed of their product on the outside of the paper package containing approximately a gross of film.

The American National Standards Institute also has classified film according to size. It is suggested that the 1.00 and the 1.0 film, the very small film generally used for children, not be employed because of its small size and the lack of information that can be recorded on it. It is true that the small film is more easily inserted into the child's mouth, but the 1.1 film, a size smaller than the customarily employed 1.2 film, is ordinarily quite suitable even for small children. Tables showing the American National Standards Institute speed and size groupings for dental film are available by writing to the footnoted address.

It also is pertinent that the 2.3 bitewing film (the long, narrow film frequently used by dentists) is inadequate. It is too narrow to show both maxillary and mandibular structures adequately, and the inclusion of all posterior teeth on one side increases the likelihood of tooth overlap. For these reasons diagnostic yield decreases when 2.3 film is used.

The use of high speed film in older machines having mechanical timers often is difficult because of timer deficiencies. Most mechanical timers will not time below 1/2 second and not accurately below approximately 3/4 of a second. Electronic timers can be purchased for use with most older

*American National Standards Institute, 1430 Broadway, New York, N.Y.

machines, but there are three other alternatives that may be useful. 1) The inverse square law states that the intensity of x-radiation varies inversely with the square of the distance. Thus, if a dentist is using an 8-inch radiation source (x-ray tube anode) to film distance, a doubling of this distance to approximately 16 inches will require four times the exposure time (assuming all other exposure factors are constant) required at 8 inches. Therefore, if a dentist using a B speed film changed to a D speed, he could use the same exposure time for the D speed film as for the B speed film by doubling his source to film distance. 2) Alternatively, the milliamperage of the dental machine, which ordinarily is 10 on the older machines, could be reduced to 2½ or 3 mA by the insertion of suitable resistors in the wiring of the machine. This can be done inexpensively by a knowledgeable service man. Exposure ordinarily is the product of the mA multiplied by the number of seconds used. If a dentist employed 10 mA and used a one-second exposure for a B speed film, he could use 2.5 mA and one second for a D speed film; the exposure time can be kept constant by decreasing the mA. 3) The third alternative available to the dentist is the use of additional filtration. Added filtration hardens the beam (increases the relative proportion of short wavelength x-ray photons and decreases the proportion of usable but longer wavelength x-ray photons) and reduces the x-ray beam intensity (number of x-ray photons per unit of time). Some experimentation is necessary to determine the amount of added filtration necessary to make the mechanical timer useful with the high speed film. A combination of increased distance, decreased milliamperage, and increased filtration could be used. Film exposure determinations would have to be used and will be considered below.

Determination of Exposure Time. Suitable exposure times using exposure factors predetermined by the dentist should be made regardless of whether alterations in distance, milliamperage, and filtration have been employed to accommodate to mechanical timers. The principle involved is based on the fact that all films should be fully exposed but never overexposed. An underexposed film will always be light (appear underdeveloped) because film processing procedures can be effective only on emulsion grains that have been adequately exposed. Overexposed emulsions will be excessively dark unless darkroom procedures are modified (developing time reduced) to prevent excessive film darkening. Such procedures are contraindicated in view of previously discussed attitudes relating to diagnostic yield. Radiation exposure that is not diagnostically useful should be avoided. Failure to minimize exposure could be classified as an act of malpractice. The darkroom should be used in an entirely standardized fashion according to recommendations of solution manufacturers. The darkroom will be considered at greater length later in this chapter.

Although suitable exposure determinations are best accomplished by using a phantom, the dentist ordinarily will have to use a patient beyond the childbearing age. A series of approximately six films ordinarily are used. The dentist first determines all the exposure factors he plans to use except exposure time. These factors include kilovoltage, milliamperage, x-ray source to film distance, collimation, filtration, and film type (speed). The first exposure is made for the purpose of producing a film the dentist believes will be objectionably light but at least sufficiently dense to show an image. The remaining films are exposed so that each subsequent film exposure represents a 50 per cent increase over the exposure time used for the previous one. For example, if the first, rather light film was exposed for ½ second, the second film would be exposed for ¾ second and the third film would be exposed for 1⅛ seconds. The films are exposed sequentially and are then processed simultaneously on the same film holder using the time-temperature processing directions of the solution manufacturer. Prior to processing, the processing solutions should have been changed, the solution tanks thoroughly cleaned, and all precautions taken to ensure that the darkroom was functionally adequate (see section on darkroom). After the films have been appropriately washed and dried, they are examined, and the dentist determines the most suitable density for his use. Often the dentist will select an exposure time between two of those used for experimental purposes.

The patient employed for this type of procedure should be an adult of average structure. Exposures will have to be increased for heavy boned or obese individuals and decreased for children. The mandibular molar area is ordinarily used for this examination because it requires an average exposure in comparison to the mandibular anterior and the maxillary posterior segments of the dental arches. An exposure for the mandibular anterior area is ordinarily 1/2 that of the mandibular molar area, and exposure for the maxillary molar region utilizes about a 1/3 increase over that of the mandibular molar region. Exposure values for children and elderly persons may have to be decreased as much as 50 per cent, and for the heavy boned or obese individuals it may have to be doubled. If high kilovoltage techniques in the region of 90 to 100 kVp are employed (with a commensurate decrease in mAs), the need for material changes in exposure time is reduced both for exposure area in the same individual and for people of varying bodily structures.

Technique. Excellence in the performance of all mechanical dental radiological procedures is essential if high quality films are desired. Patient protection can be accomplished by avoiding repetitious exposure due to poor technique and by increasing the diagnostic yield through the availability of optimum quality films.

Radiographic technique is ordinarily divided into chairside and darkroom procedures, and the former is subdivided into intra- and extraoral methods. Space does not permit adequate discussion. Extraoral technique will not be mentioned, and only a few salient features of intraoral and darkroom methods will be discussed. The reader should recognize his responsibilities and take adequate steps to ensure the delivery of highly diagnostic radiographic film.

INTRAORAL TECHNIQUE. Intraoral techniques ordinarily used in dentistry include the bisecting angle technique and the right angle-paralleling technique. The former ordinarily employs the use of an eight inch source to film distance while the latter requires an extended distance of 16 inches minimum. The techniques themselves will not be discussed in this chapter. It is pertinent that the right angle or paralleling technique (the film and the object are placed parallel with each other and the x-ray beam is directed at right angles to both the film and the object) will produce a superior intraoral radiograph to one produced using the bisecting procedure. However, both techniques are capable of producing acceptable film, particularly when bite-wing films are used in conjunction with a complete radiographic series made using the bisecting angle procedure. Of considerably greater importance than a discussion of the pros and cons of one technique versus another is the essentiality of using the selected technique with care to produce the best possible intraoral film without the need for re-exposing the patient or being satisfied with less than satisfactory films. Although the use of an increased radiation source to film distance as well as the use of higher kilovoltages (90 or 100 kVp as compared to from 50 to 70 kVp) does result in some decreased patient radiation exposure, the difference between absorbed x-radiation using long versus short distances and/or high versus low kilovoltages is too small to recommend technique changes entirely on this basis. However, increased radiation source to object distance does improve the film definition and reduces film distortion, and kilovoltage alterations do change the contrast of the radiographic film. The dentist may also wish to alter distance and kilovoltage for purposes other than patient protection.

DARKROOM. As was mentioned earlier, the darkroom should be used for standardized processing of radiographic film

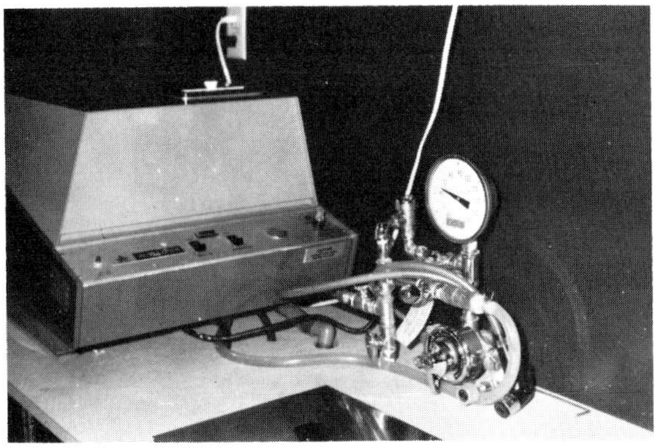

Figure 16–3 Cleanliness and the utilization of proper techniques are essential in the darkroom to achieve the greatest diagnostic yield from the image recorded on the x-ray film.

using a strict time-temperature method according to the manufacturer's directions. Adequate technique requires a clean darkroom (Fig. 16–3) and the careful scrubbing of solution tanks with bland soap and a non-abrasive cloth or sponge prior to solution replacement. After the use of soap all tanks should be carefully rinsed with water. Flushing the fixing tank with dilute acetic acid to insure the complete removal of all alkali before replacing the fixing solution is also advisable. Developing and fixing tanks and covers should not be used interchangeably. Solutions should be used within temperature ranges of 60 to 75 degrees; a developer temperature of 65 to 68 degrees is usually recommended. Maintenance of solution temperature often requires the use of refrigerated water and always requires adequate plumbing, the details of which will not be described in this chapter.

Film fogging is often the result of inadequate facilities or poor darkroom technique. Fogging is the overall addition to the film surface of varying degrees of blackness caused by factors other than x-radiation exposure. Fogging reduces film quality and minimizes diagnostic yield. Film fogging in the darkroom is ordinarily caused by extraneous light, excessive darkroom safelighting, or contaminated or exhausted processing solutions. The darkroom should be carefully examined for extraneous light by turning off *all* lights, and standing in the darkroom for a minimum of five minutes in order to allow for eye accommodation. Chalk or other suitable marking materials should be available. Light leaks can be noted, marked, and subsequently remedied by taping, puttying or plastering. The most usual locations of light leaks are keyholes and cracks around the darkroom door but leaks are not limited to these areas.

The use of not more than a 10-watt bulb behind a Wratten 6B filter, both contained in a metal housing and placed not closer than four feet from the darkroom counter top, can be recommended for most dental office darkrooms. As with x-radiation, the intensity of visible light varies inversely as the square of the distance. Bringing the darkroom light closer to the counter top increases the intensity of the darkroom lighting and may cause film fogging.

A question often asked is, "How often should x-ray processing solutions be changed?" A very practical answer is, "As often as is necessary." Solutions that are kept covered and at the recommended temperature will last a long time. Obviously, the use of the solutions gradually exhausts the chemicals. Rather than suggest a specific time when solutions should be changed, it seems preferable to advocate placing a control radiograph on the view box ordinarily found in the darkroom (if a view box is not available in the darkroom, the control film can be put on a view box in the operatory). This control radiograph should be of optimal quality. When the subsequent radiographs do not demonstrate this quality, the dentist should investigate. Under ordinary circumstances, the reason will be exhausted processing solutions, and at this time the solutions should be changed. The replenishment of processing solutions because the level is low can be done either by adding solution replenisher or by adding ordinary developer or fixer. Replenisher is somewhat stronger but it must be purchased separately and is not generally available through dental supply houses. Because of the small quantities of solution used in dental tanks, it is customary to discard used solutions rather than to attempt to increase solution strength.

Booklets specifically describing darkroom care and utilization can be obtained from leading film and solution manufacturers. The darkroom should be an area of absolute standardization. Failure to standardize darkroom procedures results in an inability to adequately vary chairside exposure techniques in the interest of producing highly diagnostic radiographs.

Lead-Impregnated Aprons. The biologic effects of low level x-radiation are not well understood and are, for the most part, extrapolated from experiments using radiation levels far in excess of that acquired in a dental office. Experimental evidence suggests that in most instances almost no adverse effects can be anticipated from exposure to very small quantities of x-radiation. However, some x-radiation absorption effects, particularly those related to blood dyscrasias and genetic alterations, appear to be linearly related to dosage. Strictly as a preventive measure, and recognizing that the need may be minimal, it is advocated that lead-impregnated aprons (a minimum of 0.25 millimeter lead equivalent) be used when radiographing children and females through their reproductive years. There is, of course, no objection to using an apron on male patients through their reproductive years, but sperm are said to be replaced approximately every 120 days, while ova are present in the female from birth to menopause. It is a well established radiobiological fact that the more embryonic and the more metabolically active cells are most susceptible to ionizing radiation; for this reason, and others, children should be protected.

It is frequently stated that the use of the apron provokes unnecessary conversation and possibly promotes apprehension. This may be true. On the other hand, radiation is hazardous, and patients are entitled to be adequately protected. If they are apprehensive, they are deserving of assurance and of explanation as needed. Failure to use adequate preventive measures because of possibly creating obstacles which subsequently will have to be overcome is no excuse for neglect (Fig. 16–4).

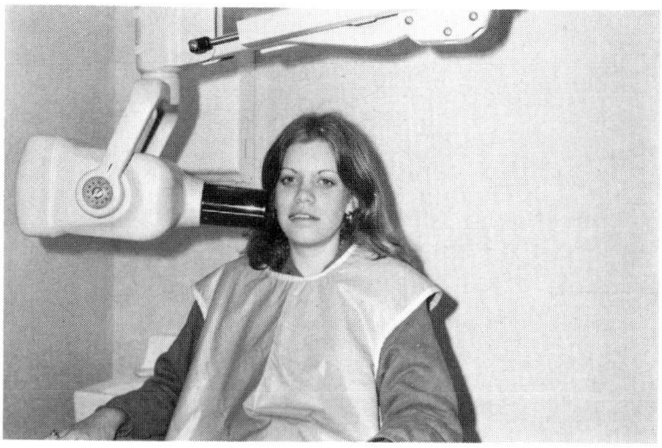

Figure 16–4 Protection against primary and secondary radiation is provided to the patient by both safety factors built into the equipment and the use of a lead apron.

Structural Shielding. Suitable radiation barriers of a structural nature (permanently fixed) should be incorporated in any new structure and should be added to present structures. However the amount of barrier material designed to protect people, both patients and employees, in rooms adjoining the radiation exposure area will depend greatly on the workload,* the occupancy factor,** and the use factor.† Lead is usually the structural shielding material of choice, but other materials such as ceramic tile, stainless steel, and certain types of plaster, in addition to the distance between the radiation source and the individual who might be exposed, can be suitable barriers depending on a variety of considerations (Fig. 16–5). These matters will not be discussed in detail; rather, the reader is referred to the report of the National Council on Radiation Protection and Measurements No. 35, entitled "Dental X-Ray Protection," which can be secured at a cost of $1.50 each from NCRP Publications, P. O. Box 4867, Washington DC 20008. This report as it relates to structural shielding design is excellent; however, the report as it relates to *General Considerations* and to

*Workload is expressed in milliampere seconds per week.

**Occupancy factor is the factor by which the workload should be multiplied to correct for the degree of occupancy of the area in question while the x-ray machine is "ON."

†Use factor (or beam direction factor) is the fraction of the workload during which the useful x-ray beam is directed at the barrier under consideration.

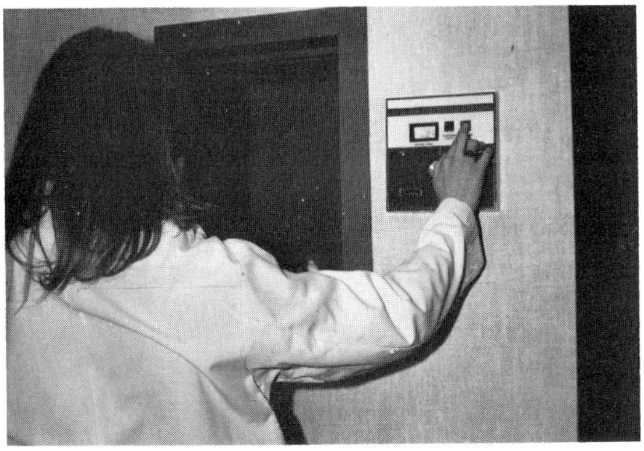

Figure 16–5 The operator is protected from radiation by structural shielding. Federal standards have been set to protect against both primary and secondary radiation. Here the operator is standing behind a lead-lined wall with a lead-glass window.

X-ray Equipment is excessively permissive and in the opinion of this author is not in the best interests of the public. Similarly, certain portions of the section entitled *Operating Procedures* are weak. Appendix A, which includes definitions of radiological terms, is excellent. The shortcomings as well as the strong points of this report are mentioned for reader guidance.

OPERATOR PROTECTION

The operator, unless he stands directly in the path of the primary radiation beam (the useful beam as it emanates from the x-ray tube head), is exposed primarily to secondary or scattered radiation from the patient. Accordingly, everything that the operator does to minimize the radiation received by the patient in turn reduces the amount of radiation received by him (unless he is standing behind a barrier designed specifically for his protection).

The use of barriers in the dental office is advocated but may not be necessary unless x-radiation is used frequently. For example, it is essential to have a barrier for operator protection in a clinic where radiographs are being taken almost constantly as part of the clinic's diagnostic procedure. Conversely, the need for a barrier simply does not exist in an office where very minimal usage is made of x-radiation. Thus, in the average dental office barriers probably should be placed in the "nice to have" category. Barriers for operator protection should not be confused with structural shielding for non-occupationally exposed individuals.

Of considerably greater importance than barriers in the average situation is distance and position. These factors will be discussed in some detail.

Distance. As has been mentioned several times earlier, the intensity of x-radiation varies inversely with the square of the distance. If a dentist foolishly standing one foot from the patient during exposure receives "x" amount of scattered radiation, he will receive ¼ of that amount if he moves two feet away from the patient. It is ordinarily recommended that the dentist stand a minimum of five feet from the patient and from the x-ray tube head and that he definitely not stand in the primary x-ray beam. If the operatory situation makes this impossible, the need for a suitable x-ray barrier must be considered; in all probability the need for a barrier will no longer be in the "nice to have" category, it will be needed. However, other factors, particularly the workload, enter into these deliberations. Naturally, the existence of any leakage radiation (which definitely should not exist) is an important consideration.

Operator Position. When exposing the anterior part of the face, the operator should stand on either side of the patient, toward the back of the patient's head, in a position between 90 and 135 degrees to the x-ray beam. Secondary and scattered radiation produced at the anterior part of the face is well filtered by the head, and little of it emanates from the side of the head near the occipital region. When an exposure is made of the side of the face, the operator is advised to stand in a position from 90 to 135 degrees to the x-ray beam in back of the patient's head. The advantages of this position are identical with those above. It is preferable that the operator not stand 90 to 135 degrees to the x-ray beam in front of the patient's face because more secondary and scattered radiation can emanate out of the soft tissues of the patient's face than through the denser portions of the patient's skull.

Maximum Permissible Dose. Radiation protection standards permit users of x-radiation, namely the operator, to absorb 10 times more whole body exposure than that allowed the average individual in the population. This is not because the operator has or acquires more resistance to the radiation. The percentage of individuals in the population who are using radiation is extremely small in comparison with those who are exposed to x-radiation for diagnostic purposes, and, from a genetic standpoint, the accumulation of genetic alterations in the entire population (the genetic mutation pool) is affected very minimally by x-radiation users.

While the concept of a maximum permissible dose (MPD) for operators generally is not publicized because it tends to produce a false sense of security, a formula does exist which states that radiation workers may receive an accumulated dose to critical organs (hence whole body radiation) of $(N-18) \times 5$ rem (roentgen equivalent man). For dental purposes, the rem can be thought of as equivalent to the roentgen or rad. The N in this formula is the present age of the patient. The product of this formula indicates the amount of whole body radiation that a radiation worker can accumulate through any given age, with the important stipulation that the radiation dose in any 13 consecutive weeks must not exceed 3 rem. An analysis of this formula indicates that individuals 18 years of age and younger should not be using x-radiation. It is also important to emphasize that a weekly accumulation in excess of 25 milliroentgens of whole body radiation (approximately 1/4 of the average weekly permissible accumulation using the above formula) should be considered maximum, and means should be taken to greatly reduce total exposure. The MPD for users has no direct relationship to the exposure of users for diagnostic purposes. There is no maximum permissible dose for non-users.

DIAGNOSTIC YIELD IN RELATION TO TECHNIQUE AND INTERPRETATION

It was emphasized in the opening paragraphs of this chapter that "diagnostic yield" is a measurement of the effectiveness with which x-radiation is used. It was pointed out that diagnostic yield is heavily interrelated with radiation protection methods, chairside technique, and radiographic interpretation. Radiation protection methods in the dental office have been discussed and certain aspects of chairside and darkroom technique have been incorporated into radiation reduction methods. Space did not permit more detailed discussion. The reader is encouraged to use appropriate dental radiology texts to become more informed.

It is equally impossible to discuss radiographic interpretation adequately within the space permitted. However, a chapter of this nature must include certain pertinent matters related to interpretation if the concepts of preventive dentistry as related to radiology are to be even reasonably complete. Discussion will be limited to a description of 1) what constitutes an adequate single film or complete mouth radiographic survey, and 2) what are the most frequently made radiographic interpretive errors related to preventive dentistry.

CRITERIA OF AN ADEQUATE INTRAORAL RADIOGRAPHIC SURVEY

Radiographs should be taken for specific purposes (Fig. 16–6). Single films or complete radiographic surveys ordinarily are taken to examine crowns, periodontal structures, and periapical regions of the dentition. Accordingly, the apices of all teeth should be observed at least once in a complete survey. Ths does not mean that all radiographic films of a region must demonstrate the apical portion of the tooth adequately in all films, but the apex of each tooth root must be clearly observable at least one time in the survey. This criterion is necessary in order to detect apical pathology. Additionally, the interproximal

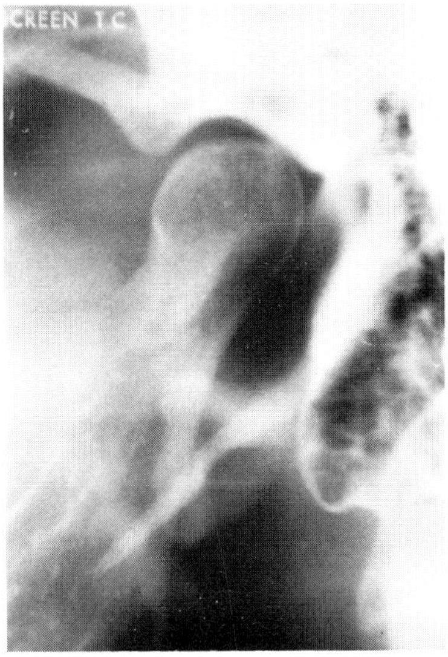

Figure 16–6 Example of a radiograph taken with an S. S. White Panorex unit utilizing appropriate techniques for visualization of the temporomandibular joint and surrounding structures.

contacting surfaces of abutting teeth must be observable at least once without any overlapping of contiguous teeth and, in the case of the posterior teeth, with the buccal cusps superimposed on the lingual or palatal cusps. The detection of incipient caries and incipient periodontal bone changes definitely requires a lack of interproximal surface superimposition and an angulation technique that will neither distort the height of the periodontal bone level nor hide small carious lesions in the bulk of remaining enamel in the contact point region. To fulfill these criteria, it becomes absolutely necessary to utilize the principles of the right angle-paralleling technique, either through employing the technique itself or through the use of bite-wing films. If bite-wing films are used, it is strongly advocated that two 2.2 films be used in each quadrant (or alternatively two 1.2 films can be used if the dentist chooses to place his own bite-wing tabs) rather than a 2.3 bite-wing film (through age approximately 12 years only one film per side is necessary). American National Standards Institute classification of intraoral film and the reasons for the above recommendations were stated earlier in this chapter.

FREQUENT INTERPRETIVE ERRORS RELATED TO PREVENTIVE DENTISTRY

Radiographic interpretation of hard tissue abnormalities is an essential aspect of oral diagnosis. Detection of a diseased state usually prevents progress of pathologic conditions; within this concept all radiographic interpretation is a part of preventive dentistry. There are, however, a few interpretive errors related to caries, periodontal disease, and apical pathology that are very commonly made. Because of space limitations, only these will be discussed.

Interpretive Errors Related to Dental Caries. Among numerous errors in the interpretation of dental caries made frequently are two that must be mentioned in this chapter. It is essential to emphasize that a dental caries lesion observed radiographically *always* appears smaller than the carious lesion actually is when observed either clinically or microscopically. Consequently, there is no such thing as a radiographically "small" lesion. The statement: "That carious area is small. Let's leave it and watch it," if made with respect to children and young adults, is synonymous with neglect unless there are other extenuating circumstances which suggest need for delaying treatment. The location of these "small" lesions is usually interproximal, just below the contact area, but it may be occlusal, at the dentoenamel junction. The latter, however, is usually detected clinically. In a patient over approximately 30 years of age, a small-appearing lesion is probably arrested caries and often will not need treatment.

The second frequently made error is in the interpretation of pulp exposure based on observing a large carious lesion and its *apparent* continuity into the pulp chamber. The position of the lesion in relation to the pulp or angulation of the x-ray beam can easily superimpose a carious lesion onto the pulp chamber and create an erroneous interpretation. The radiograph is very useful in demonstrating the presence of the carious lesion, and it gives some idea of the lesion's extent, but clinical methods should be used to determine the actual depth of the carious lesion. Less reliance on the radiographic film may prevent tooth loss in such instances.

Interpretive Errors Related to Periodontal Disease. Probably the most neglected field of dental practice is periodontology. Similarly, one of the more important diagnostic shortcomings of dental practitioners is a failure to recognize radiographic incipient signs of periodontal disease. These incipient manifestations include triangulation, lack of continuity, and hence irregularity, of the crestal alveolar bone surface between abutting teeth, and a tendency to produce excessive bone condensation, particularly near the crest of the interproximal alveolar bone.

The other frequent error relates directly to the x-ray beam angulation used to produce the radiograph. Intraoral films taken for periodontal purposes are most useful when the film and the tooth are parallel to each other and the x-ray beam is directed at a right angle to both. The right angle-paralleling technique or a well taken bite-wing film accomplishes this purpose. Failure to follow these directions distorts the anatomic relationship of tooth and supportive bone, causing the buccal bone shadow to be cast closer to the tooth crown than it actually is. An impression is gained that more supportive bone exists than is actually the case.

Interpretive Errors Related to Apical Pathology. The periapical radiograph serves the important objective of demonstrating the existence of apical pathology when it exists in a chronic state unaccompanied by subjective patient symptoms. In doing so, it is extremely valuable. The radiograph cannot be used to differentiate between the abscess, the granuloma, and the cyst, and treatment should not be based on the dentist's efforts to do the impossible. Accordingly, endodontic and oral surgery decisions relative to the treatment of apical lesions should not be based on radiographic information. One exception seems to exist: a lesion that appears "typically" cystic is likely to be cystic. (Cysts are described radiographically as a *distinctly* radiolucent area clearly delineated by a peripheral opaque lamina that may or may not be continuous with the lamina dura of the involved tooth.) Conversely, a lesion can appear to be "typically" an abscess or granuloma (Fig. 16–7) (typical in terms of descriptions found in many textbooks and criteria used generally by the profession) and yet contain epithelial cells in lumen formation, the usual histologic criterion for a cyst. While the need for enucleating cysts is not a radiographic problem (Fig. 16–8), it is pertinent to mention that apical lesions measuring not more than approximately a

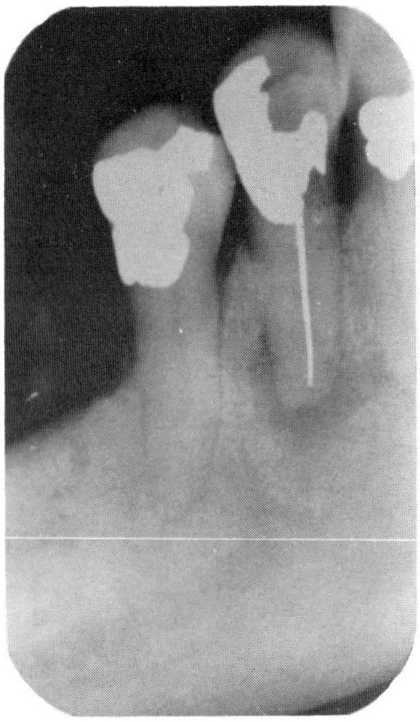

Figure 16–7 X-ray demonstrating periapical lesion. Diagnosis of a periapical granuloma was made histologically on retreatment.

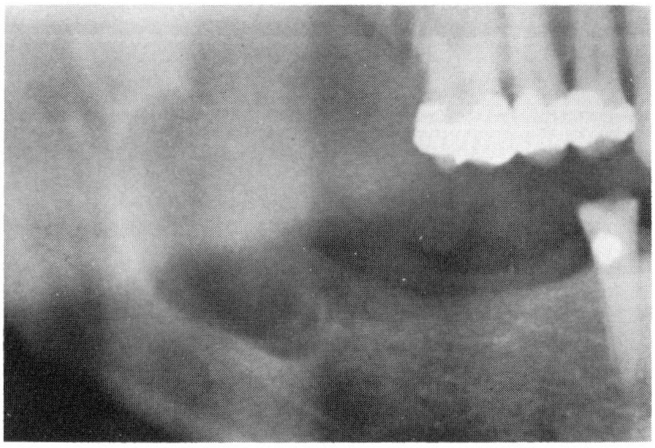

Figure 16–8 Radiograph of a residual dental cyst resulting from the incomplete removal of a third molar. The lesion was treated surgically and diagnosis confirmed histologically.

centimeter in diameter, regardless of their radiographic appearance (thus regardless of whether they are abscesses, granulomas or cysts), ordinarily will be replaced by normal bone without surgical interference if the agent causing the lesion is eliminated.

SUMMARY

This chapter has interrelated dental radiology with preventive dentistry and has emphasized the justification of x-radiation usage by the dental profession on the basis of *diagnostic yield.* It has intimated that dentists whose diagnostic yield is consistently low probably should be denied the use of x-radiation. In the interest of present and future generations, technical and interpretive competency should be determined. The adequacy of equipment should be certified by local or state agencies. Everything possible should be done to increase the balance between risk and gain in the use of x-radiation in dentistry by heavily outweighing gain as opposed to risk. This is preventive dentistry.

It now remains, not as a summary of previous material but as an additional statement of fact, to relate patient whole body (hence genetic organ) exposure to background radiation received from the cosmos and from surrounding environmental situations. Such background radiation has been in existence since man evolved and has probably contributed substantially to his evolution. A complete mouth survey of 17 periapical films and four bite-wing films can be taken using less than 5 R of exposure at skin. For each R of exposure at skin, it is estimated that the gonadal exposure is approximately 1/10,000 of an R or 0.5 mR for the full mouth survey. This amount of radiation is approximately equivalent to the background radiation received by the patient each day of his normal life if he resides at or near sea level. People in higher altitudes receive more background exposure. Thus, it can be fairly stated that the whole body exposure received from a complete mouth radiographic film survey is roughly the equivalent of "a day in the sun." Such minimal exposure can be justified. However, the above stated 5 R total exposure is based on the optimal use of x-radiation by the dentist. Dental practice habits commonly in vogue frequently result in a total exposure from 25 to 60 R instead of the 5 R, and grossly poor technique no doubt could increase the total exposure to 300 R, or 60 times that needed. Obviously the diagnostic yield would be materially decreased under such circumstances. These data relate entirely to x-ray machine adequacy and to technical excellence. They cannot be related to interpretive ability, but unless this ability is high, even the additional exposure equivalent to "a day in the sun" cannot be justified. It is hoped that the remarks in this chapter will encourage the reader to become more radiographically conscious and to utilize to an appropriate extent the services of dental radiology specialists when such a specialty status becomes recognized by the American Dental Association.

---

*Illustrations for this chapter furnished by Richard E. Stallard, Group Health Medical Center, Bloomington, Minnesota.

ADDITIONAL READING

American Dental Association: Radiation hygiene and practice in dentistry. I to V. J. Am. Dent. Assoc. *74*:1032, 1967; *75*: 1197, 1967; *76*:115, 363, 602, 1968.

American Dental Association: Radiation hygiene and practice in dentistry: state regulation of dental x-rays. J. Am. Dent. Assoc. *76*:107, 1968.

American Dental Association, and Alcox, R. W.: Diagnostic radiation exposures and doses in dentistry. J. Am. Dent. Assoc. *76*:1066, 1968.

Berkman, M. D.: Pedodontic radiographic interpretation. Dent. Radiogr. Photogr. *44*:27, 1971.

Cheraskin, E.: Roentgenographic manifestations of osseous changes in the jaws. Oral Surg. *12*:442, 1959.

Clark, D. E.: Association of irradiation with cancer of the thyroid in children and adolescents. J. Am. Dent. Assoc. *159*:1007, 1955.

Curby, W. A., and Wuehrmann, A. H.: Utilization of constant exposure factors for intraoral roentgenographic studies. J. Dent. Res. *32*: 790, 1953.

Duffy, B. J., Jr., and Fitzgerald, P. J.: Cancer of the thyroid in children: a report on 28 cases. J. Clin. Endocr. *10*:1296, 1950.

Dummett, C. O.: Review of the clinical and roentgenologic manifestations of incipient periodontal disease. Ann. Dent. *4*:47, 1945.

Ennis, L. M., Berry, H. M., and Phillips, J. E.: Dental Roentgenology, 6th ed., Philadelphia, Lea & Febiger, 1967.
Fitzgerald, G. M.: Dental roentgenography. I. An investigation in adumbration, or the factors that control geometric unsharpness. J. Am. Dent. Assoc. *34*:1, 1947.
Goepp, R., et al.: The reduction of unnecessary x-ray exposure during intraoral examinations. Oral Surg. *16*:39, 1963.
Manson-Hing, L. R.: On the evaluation of radiographic techniques. Oral Surg. *27*:631–634, 1969.
Manson-Hing, L. R.: Kilovolt peak and the visibility of lamina dura breaks. Oral Surg. *31*:268–273, 1971.
Manson-Hing, L. R.: The fundamental biologic effects of x-rays in dentistry. Oral Surg. *12*:562, 1959.
Manson-Hing, L. R.: Vision and oral roentgenology. Oral Surg. *15*:173, 1962.
Menezer, L. F.: The open-ended metal column for the dental x-ray machine. J. Am. Dent. Assoc. *73*:1083, 1966.
National Council on Radiation Protection and Measurements: Dental x-ray protection, NCRP report no. 35, Washington, D.C., 1970, NCRP Publications.
Parfitt, G. J.: An investigation of the normal variations in alveolar bone trabeculation. Oral Surg. *15*:1453, 1962.
Prichard, J.: The role of the roentgenogram in the diagnosis and prognosis of periodontal disease. Oral Surg. *14*:182, 1961.
Priebe, W. A., et al.: The value of the roentgenographic film in the differential diagnosis of periapical lesions. Oral Surg. 7:979, 1954.
Report of the Radiation Protection Committee, American Academy of Oral Roentgenology: The effective use of x-radiation in dentistry. Oral Surg. *16*:294, 1963.
Richards, A. G.: Roentgen-ray doses in dental roentgenography. J. Am. Dent. Assoc. *56*:351, 1958.
Richards, A. G., et al.: X-ray protection in the dental office. J. Am. Dent. Assoc. *56*:514, 1958.
Richards, A. G.: New concepts in dental x-ray machines. J. Am. Dent. Assoc. *73*:69, 1966.
Richards, A. G.: Sources of x-radiation in the dental office. Dent. Radiogr. Photogr. *27*:51, 1964.
Richards, A. G.: Radiation barriers. Oral Surg. *25*:701, 1968.
Shafer, W. G., Hine, M. K., and Levy, B. M.: A Textbook of Oral Pathology. 2nd ed., Philadelphia, W. B. Saunders Co., 1963.
Shira, R. B.: Roentgenographic interpretation as an aid in oral surgical procedures. J. Am. Dent. Assoc. *65*:449, 1962.
Stafne, E. C.: Oral roentgenographic diagnosis, Philadelphia, W. B. Saunders Co., 1958.
Trout, E. D., et al: Conventional building materials as protective barriers in dental roentgenographic installations. Oral Surg. *15*:1211, 1962.
Worth, H. M.: Principles and Practice of Oral Radiologic Interpretation. Chicago, Year Book Medical Publishers, Inc., 1963.
Wuehrmann, A. H.: Radiation Protection and Dentistry, St. Louis, The C. V. Mosby Co., 1960.
Wuehrmann, A. H.: Procedure for lining open-end dental x-ray cylinders with lead foil. Oral Surg. *30*:64–65, July 1970.
Wuehrmann, A. H.: The long cone technic. P.D.M., pp. 1–30, July, 1957.
Wuehrmann, A. H.: Roentgenographic interpretation of dental caries. P.D.M. pp. 3–46, Sept. 1959.
Wuehrmann, A. H., and Manson-Hing, L. R.: Dental Radiology. 4th ed., St. Louis, The C. V. Mosby Co., 1977.

chapter 17

THE PREVENTION AND DETECTION OF ORAL CANCER

by
THEODORE E. BOLDEN, D.D.S., PH.D.

At present, total prevention of cancer *before* its occurrence is difficult, if not impossible; however, cancer can be prevented from causing rapid destruction of tissues and death to the patient by early detection and treatment. In other words, cancer can be cured and prevented from causing sequelae and complications prior to the appearance of the classical symptoms and signs of the disease. Therefore, in thinking in terms of prevention in its truest sense, early detection and the use of control methods can prevent mutilation of tissues and metastasis of the disease, providing the greatest chance of survival and complete cure for the patient.

THE "FACE" OF ORAL CANCER

VARIABILITY

The *first* step toward the prevention and detection of oral cancer for the individual patient is for the health professional to develop an awareness for the high degree of variability in the appearance, in the "face," of oral cancer.

TISSUES AND AREAS INVOLVED

The *second* step is for the health professional to develop an appreciation for the fact that oral cancer may involve any of the basic tissues of the oral cavity as the "primary" site and conversely that any of the tissues of the oral cavity may be involved as the "secondary" site for malignant processes primary to other parts of the body.

We define the basic tissues as epithelium, connective tissue, muscle, nerve and blood. What the dentist "sees" when he examines the oral tissues is primarily epithelium, the mucous membrane which lines the oral cavity. For convenience, we divide the oral cavity into anatomical areas designated as: (1) lips, (2) gingiva, (3) jaws, (4) floor of the mouth, (5) tongue, (6) buccal

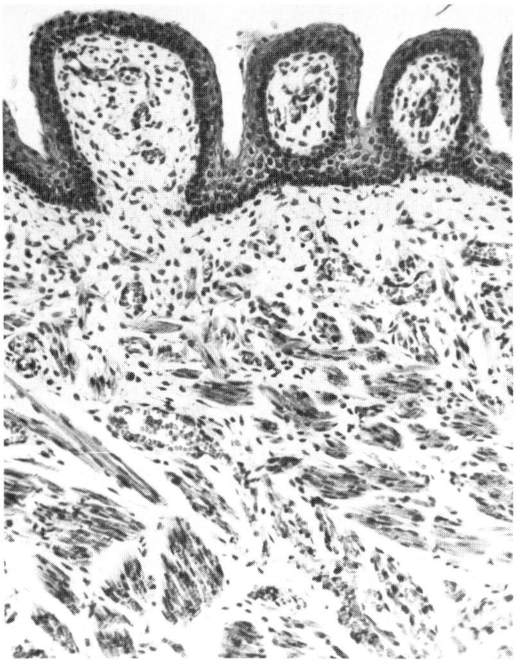

Fig. 17–1

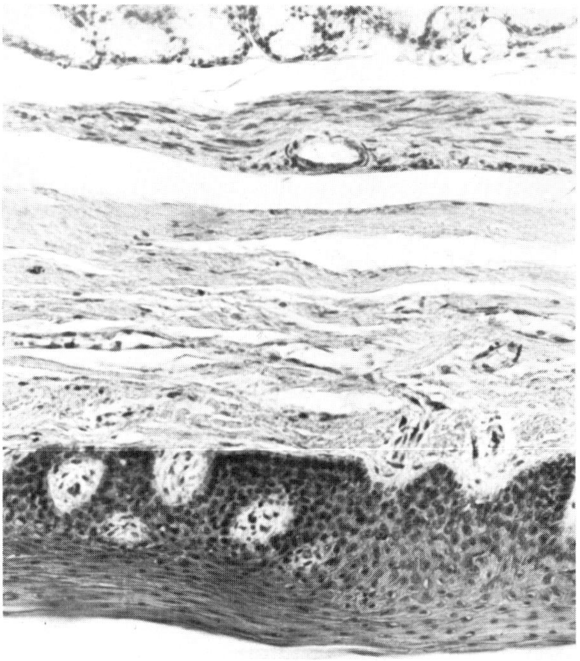

Fig. 17–2

Figure 17–1 Photomicrograph of a normal human tongue demonstrating the stratified squamous epithelium on the surface with an underlying layer of connective tissue. Note the thick muscular layer beneath. (×120)

Figure 17–2 Compare this photomicrograph of human palate with Figure 17–1. Note the absence of muscular tissue in the section. (×120)

mucosa, (7) palate, (8) pulp, and (9) para-oral tissues. These areas are readily accessible for direct observation, palpation and inspection. A section through each one would be composed of a representative of each of the five basic tissues. Only the proportion of these would differ. For example, a section of tongue would show a preponderance of muscle while a section through the palate would show little muscle (Figs. 17–1 and 17–2).

The Lips. The lips, with the cheeks, form the outer boundary of the vestibular portion of the oral cavity. The inner boundary is formed by the alveolar ridges and the teeth. The lips are covered externally by a keratinized stratified squamous epithelium, the skin, and internally by a non-keratinized mucous membrane. The vermilion border, or red area, connects the two as a transitional zone. Sebaceous glands, hair follicles and sweat glands are present in the skin surface. The transitional zone has few sebaceous glands. Numerous labial glands are present in the submucosa.[99]

The Gingiva. The gingiva are composed of dense fibrous tissue, closely connected to the periosteum of the alveolar process and surrounding the necks of the teeth. They are covered by a smooth and vascular mucous membrane whose outer layer is stratified squamous epithelium. The gingiva can be subdivided into free and attached types. The free gingiva includes the papillary and marginal gingiva. Its inner surface lines the gingival sulcus and is attached to the tooth as the epithelial attachment. The attached gingiva has a rough or stippled appearance (orange peel). The stippling is produced by the dense connective tissue which binds (attaches) the gingiva to the alveolar bone.

The Jaws. Alveolar bone is a special bone produced in response to the growth and development of the teeth—teeth are found in both jaws, maxilla and mandible.

The mandible is the longest and strongest bone of the face and forms the lower jaw. It consists of a curved horizontal portion, the body, and two perpendicular portions, the *rami,* which are nearly at right angles with the ends of the body. The body is curved somewhat like a horseshoe and has two surfaces, lateral and medial, and two borders, superior or alveolar and inferior. The lateral and medial surfaces serve as sites of origin or insertion of muscles; the superior border is hollowed into cavities for the reception of teeth.

Floor of the Mouth. The mucous membrane of the lingual surface of the tongue continues at the sublingual sulcus as the sublingual mucosa and the alveolar mucosa. The lingual gingiva is a distinct line, the mucogingival line. The mucous membrane of the floor of the mouth is loosely attached to the underlying structures and permits the free mobility of the tongue. The epithelium is nonkeratinized. The submucosa contains adipose tissue and the sublingual glands.

The Tongue. The tongue is a specialized muscular organ which occupies the greatest portion of the floor of the mouth. It has two surfaces, dorsal and ventral, a tip and two lateral borders. It is curved somewhat like a horseshoe, corresponding to the curvature of the lower jaw. The tip, lateral borders and ventral surface are smooth, the dorsal surface is roughened due to the presence of projections, the lingual papillae. Taste buds are present on the sides of the large papillae in the posterior third of the tongue. The entire surface is covered by stratified squamous epithelium. In the wall of the pharynx and in the posterior part of the tongue are found solitary follicles of adenoid tissue. These lie in the tunica propria and invade the epithelium. These follicles, the lingual tonsils, form one-third of the lymphatic pharyngeal ring. The other two masses form the palatine tonsil and the pharyngeal tonsil. The palatine tonsil lies between the pillars of the fauces and is associated with the palate. The pharyngeal tonsil is located on the posterior wall of the pharynx above the level of the palate. All three have crypts lined either by stratified squamous epithelium or ciliated epithelium (pharyngeal).[120]

The Buccal Mucosa. The buccal mucosa forms the inner lining of the cheek and its outer lining is skin. The two meet in the midface where they serve as lining of the lips. Between the two linings, buccal mucosa and skin, are buccal glands, nerves, vessels, areolar tissue, a muscular stroma and large quantities of adipose tissue—the buccal fat pad.

The mucous membrane is reflected above and below upon the gingiva and is continuous posteriorly with the mucous membrane lining the soft palate. The mucous membrane, like the integument, is stratified squamous epithelium.

The Palate. The superior portion of the oral cavity is formed by the palate. The palate is divided into a hard palate anteriorly and a soft palate posteriorly. The hard palate forms the roof of the mouth and separates the oral and nasal cavities. It is bound anteriorly and laterally by the maxillary alveolar arches and gingiva. Posteriorly it is continuous with the soft palate. It is lined by a mucous membrane whose outermost layer is stratified squamous epithelium. The palatal mucosa is furnished with numerous palatal salivary glands and is intimately adherent to the palatine process of the maxilla and the horizontal plate of the palatine bone.

The soft palate is a movable fold suspended from the posterior border of the hard palate. It consists of a fold of mucous membrane enclosing muscle fibers, an aponeurosis, blood vessels, nerves, lymphoid tissue and mucous glands. The upper border is attached to the posterior margin of the hard palate. Its sides are blended with the pharynx. Its lower border is free. Hanging from the middle of its lower border is a small, conical, pendulous process, the palatine uvula. Arching laterally and downward from the base of the uvula on either side are two curved folds of mucous membrane, containing muscular fibers, called the arches or pillars of the fauces.

The Dental Pulp. The dental pulp is the connective tissue occupying the cavity in the center of the dentin of the tooth. It is composed of odontoblasts, connective tissue cells, intercellular substance, blood vessels, lymphatic vessels and nerves. The pulp also serves a sensory and defensive function. Among changes that occur within the pulp is a gradual narrowing of the canal with age.

The pulp differs from connective tissue in that it is encased in rigid walls, the dentin. This means that the viability of the pulp is severely impaired by processes having an inflammatory component. Why is this so? This is true because the blood supply to the pulp enters the diminishing root canal at the apex of the tooth. Inflammation is characterized by increase in diameter of blood vessels and loss of fluid into the surrounding tissue spaces with subsequent edema. The rigid walls prohibit and severely limit the degree of expansion of loose connective tissue. Consequently, the more severe the pulpitis, the more severe the edema and the greater chance for strangulation of the flow of blood. Strangulation leads to the death of the pulp.

The dental pulp is subject not only to local diseases, but also to pathologic states of a systemic nature. It is extremely vascular, and the blood vessels are terminal in type with an absence of a collateral circulation.

The dental pulp contains cells and definitive structures comparable to connective tissues elsewhere in the body. It is reasonable to assume that these may undergo malignant change or that these may be involved in a malignant process because of the pulp's vascularity.

Para-oral Tissues. The para-oral tissues are those tissues which lie contiguous to, bound or surround the oral cavity. They include the face, head and neck. As the patient sits, one can observe changes in the appearance of the eyes, ears, nose, chin, neck and scalp. Pre- and post-auricular, nasal, labial, and other sinuses can be readily observed. Thyroglossal duct cysts in the midline of the neck present as fluctuant bulges to be distinguished from lateral cysts of the neck. Asymmetry accompanying cherubism, unilateral condylar hyperplasia, jaw tumors and growth defects are rather obvious. Evidence of pigmentary changes, hypo-, hyper-, de- and re-pigmentation,[48] is readily detectable by looking at the paraoral tissues. The oral cavity may become the site of malignant change following direct extension or spread from the para-oral tissues.

CANCER OF THE LIP

A 20-year survey, 1940–1959, showed 4,357 cancers of the lip. Ninety-four per cent involved the lower lip and more were observed in males than females. Most labial cancers are squamous cell carcinomas. Localization showed no sex predilection (Table 17–1).

Basal cell carcinoma presents with equal frequency on the upper and lower lip (Table 17–2). Lip cancer is associated with the use of tobacco, most frequently as a cigarette (Table 17–3).[72]

Carcinoma of the lip has also been attributed to such factors as smoking of short hot pipes, leukoplakia and chronic inflammatory fissuring of the lip. The consumption of alcohol does not appear to be significant in the production of lip cancer. This is more often a disease of men with the average age 66 years. The incidence of lip cancers increases with increase in age (Table 17–4). Metastasis to the submental and submandibular lymph nodes occurs in about 25 per cent of patients, often appears late and is predominantly from the lower lip. The five-year survival rate is remarkably high, rang-

TABLE 17–1 ORAL CANCER*

SITE	NO. PATIENTS	SEX RATIO	PERCENTAGE LOCALIZED	
			Male	*Female*
Lip	4,357	13:1	85	86
Tongue	3,335	4:1	39	54

*Adapted from Latourette, H. B., and Myers, M. H.: End-results of treatment of oral and laryngopharyngeal cancer. Fifth National Cancer Conference Proceedings. Philadelphia, J. B. Lippincott Co., 1964.

TABLE 17-2 CELLULAR TYPES OF LIP CARCINOMAS BY ANATOMICAL SITES AMONG NEGRO AND WHITE MALES*

	ANATOMICAL SITES							
	LOWER LIPS		UPPER LIPS		BOTH LIPS		TOTAL	
CARCINOMAS	*No.*	*Per Cent*	*No.*	*Per Cent*	*No.*	*Per Cent*	*No.*	*Per Cent*
Squamous cell	279	88.8	12	3.8	3	1.0	294	93.6
Basal cell	6	1.9	9	2.9	1	0.3	16	5.1
Both 1 and 2			1	0.3	3	1.0	4	1.3
Total	285	90.7	22	7.0	7	2.3	314	100.0

*From Keller, A. Z.: Cellular types, survival, race, nativity, occupations, habits and associated diseases in the pathogenesis of lip cancers. Am. J. Epidemiol. *91*(5):486–499, 1970.

ing from approximately 70 per cent (Table 17–5)[72] to 85 per cent, but is lower in females than in males.[74]

CANCER OF THE GINGIVA

The highest incidence of gingival cancer occurs in South India where it constitutes roughly nine per cent of all cancer cases seen. Twenty-five per cent of all oral cancers in South India, and 16 per cent and 12 per cent of all oral cancers seen in Georgia and at Memorial Hospital respectively were epidermoid cancers of the gingiva.[25] The distribution by sex of 606 patients with epidermoid cancer of the gum (1942–1961) was 77 per cent men (465) and 23 per cent women (141). In 79 per cent of all females and 88 per cent of all males, the cancer occurred between 50 and 80 years of age. Symptoms consist of ulceration or pain or both in nearly every case. An occasional patient complained primarily of inability to

TABLE 17-3 TYPE OF TOBACCO SMOKED BY CASES OF LIP CANCERS AND THEIR CONTROLS (WHITE MALES ONLY)*

	CASES OF LIP CANCER		CONTROLS			
			CANCER†		GENERAL‡	
CLASSIFICATION	*No.*	*Per Cent*	*No.*	*Per Cent*	*No.*	*Per Cent*
Non-smokers	22	7.3[b]	16	5.3[a]	44	16.6[a,b]
Ex-smokers	7	2.3[d]	2	0.7[d]	3	1.1
Cigarettes only	181	60.2	194	64.5	140	52.8
Cigars only	7	2.3	10	3.3	10	3.8
Pipes only	18	6.0	14	4.6	9	3.4
Cigarettes and cigars	4	1.3	1	0.3	0	0.0
Cigarettes and pipes	13	4.3[c]	6	2.0	0	0.0[c]
Cigars and pipes	4	1.3	10	3.3[c]	0	0.0[c]
Cigarettes, cigars and pipes	2	0.7	2	0.7	1	0.4
Not stated	43	14.3	46	15.3	58	21.9
Total	301	100.0	301	100.0	265	100.0

*From Keller, *ibid.*
†Males with squamous cell carcinomas of the intra-oral cavity and pharynx.
‡Males from all diagnostic categories of medical and surgical patients.
[a]: $p < 0.00001$.
[b]: $p < 0.001$.
[c]: $p < 0.01$.
[d]: $p < 0.05$.

TABLE 17–4 MINIMUM ANNUAL RATES OF CASE INCIDENCE AND THE TOTAL DISTRIBUTION BY AGE FOR WHITE MALES WITH LIP CANCERS*

	TOTAL CASES		ANNUAL INCIDENCE	
AGE IN YEARS	*No.*	*Per Cent*	*No.*†	*Rate*‡
25–29	2	0.6	2	0.07
30–34	3	1.0	2	0.06
35–39	23	7.4	22	0.53
40–44	26	8.4	23	0.74
45–49	24	7.7	21	1.20
50–54	24	7.7	21	1.95
55–59	15	4.8	12	1.89
60–64	45	14.5	41	3.55
65–69	94	30.2	86	9.07
70+	55	17.7	53	9.73
Total	311	100.0	283	1.43

*From Keller, *ibid.*
†Newly diagnosed cases of lip cancer from 1958 through 1962.
‡Number of cases per 100,000 living veterans.

TABLE 17–5 FIVE-YEAR RATES OF SURVIVAL FOR MALES WITH LIP CANCERS BY STAGE, SITE AND CELLULAR TYPE OF THE DISEASE AND BY RACE*

CLASSIFICATION	NO.	RATE†	STANDARD ERROR‡
Total			
Cases	314	95.23	1.20
U. S. males[a]	314	86.44	0.61
Race			
Negroes[b]	3	98.69	0.00
Whites	311	95.20	1.20
Stage of disease			
Localized	283	96.61	1.12
Metastasized	31	82.34	4.58
Site of disease			
Lower lip	285	94.74	1.35
Upper lip[b]	22	100.00	0.00
Both lips[b]	7	96.99	0.00
Cellular type of disease			
Squamous cell	294	94.84	1.32
Basal cell	16	100.00	0.00
Both cell types[b]	4	97.80	0.00
Cases with skin cancers of head, face and neck			
Present	38	91.98	3.96
Absent	276	95.65	1.19

*From Keller, *ibid.*
†Each rate and standard error is adjusted to the age distribution of the total cases.
‡One standard error of the rate.
[a]United States males of the case's age and race.
[b]Among each of these, there were no deaths; thus each unadjusted survival rate is 100 per cent and standard error of the rate is zero.

TABLE 17–6 SIZE OF PRESENTING LESION*

SIZE	NO. OF CASES	PER CENT
Less than 2 cm.	134	22
2–3 cm.	176	29
3–5 cm.	193	32
Greater than 5 cm.	72	12
Unknown	21	

*From Cady, B., and Catlin, D.: Epidermoid carcinoma of the gum. A 20-year survey. Cancer *23*: 551–564, March 1969.

wear previously well-fitting dentures or of bleeding. When pain was cited as the primary symptom, 51 per cent of the patients had symptoms for less than three months, while with the complaint of relatively painless ulceration, 42 per cent sought care within this period.

An accurate history of smoking was obtained in 452 of the 606 cases. Thirty-four per cent of male patients were either *cigar* or *pipe* smokers.[25] The majority of gingival lesions averaged between three and five centimeters when first observed by the dentist (Table 17–6).

In radiologic examination of 216 of the 606 cases, 81 per cent (97 of 113 cases) proved to have histologic evidence of bone invasion, if no roentgenographic evidence of bone distribution was seen. Pathologic examination of the surgical specimen removed indicated that the epidermoid cancer extended to medial soft tissues, such as the floor of the mouth and tongue, or to lateral soft tissues, such as the gingivobuccal gutter, cheek, lip and retromolar space, in a high proportion of patients. The use of snuff in the gingivobuccal sulcus is considered causative for gingival carcinoma.[109]

Spontaneous gingival hemorrhage and/or gingival hypertrophy may be the first clinical evidence of leukemia, the most frequent cancer in children. More adults are struck by leukemia than children, but approximately one-half of the cancer cases of children in America is due to leukemia. It was predicted that 1973 would produce 19,000 new cases of, and 15,000 deaths from, leukemia.

TABLE 17-7 NUMBER OF PATIENTS AND PER CENT AGE DISTRIBUTION BY SEX CANCER OF FLOOR OF MOUTH IN CONNECTICUT, 1935-1959*

	TOTAL		MALE		FEMALE	
AGE	*No.*	*Per Cent*	*No.*	*Per Cent*	*No.*	*Per Cent*
0-49	56	11.8	49	11.3	7	16.7
50-59	129	27.1	116	26.7	13	31.0
60-69	196	30.7	137	31.6	9	21.4
70-79	106	22.3	97	22.4	9	21.4
80+	39	8.2	35	8.1	4	9.5
All Ages	476	100.0	434	100.0	42	100.0
Median Age	63		64		61	

*From Shedd, D. P., Von Essen, C. F., Ferraro, R. H., Connelly, R. R., and Eisenberg, H.: Cancer of the floor of the mouth in Connecticut, 1935-1959. Cancer *21*:97-101, January 1968.

CANCER OF THE FLOOR OF THE MOUTH

Epidermoid carcinoma is the most frequent malignant lesion of the floor of the mouth and it is seen more often in males.[127] Other malignancies which are encountered in the floor of the mouth are adenocarcinoma, transitional cell carcinoma, basal cell carcinoma, myxosarcoma and unspecified sarcoma. The incidence in males increases with increase in age (Table 17-7). The lowest incidence for males is experienced in Sweden, and the highest figure for male and female was reported from Puerto Rico (Table 17-8). The most frequent sites of oral cancer in Puerto Rico are the tongue and the floor of the mouth. The highest incidence in males is seen in the fifth decade and in females in the sixth decade.[41] The disease is usually localized at the time of original diagnosis and responds well to surgery (Table 17-9). Women tend to survive better than men (Tables 17-10 and 17-11), with localized lesions offering the best five year survival rate.[127] As the disease progresses, the tongue and mandible are invaded and the cervical lymph nodes become permeated with cancer.

CANCER OF THE TONGUE

Comparative data show that squamous cell carcinoma is the most frequent malignant lesion of the tongue (Table 17-12) and involves men more frequently than women, except in Sweden (Table 17-13).

In Britain, cancer of the tongue is most

TABLE 17-8 ANNUAL INCIDENCE OF CANCER OF FLOOR OF MOUTH BY SEX AND GEOGRAPHIC AREA*

		ANNUAL INCIDENCE RATES (per 100,000)					
		NO. OF PATIENTS		CRUDE		AGE-ADJUSTED†	
GEOGRAPHIC AREA	PERIOD	*Male*	*Female*	*Male*	*Female*	*Male*	*Female*
10 U.S. Cities	1947	89	19	1.4	0.3	–	–
Sweden	1958-61	25	11	0.2	0.1	0.1	0.1
Norway	1953-61	107	61	0.7	0.4	0.6	0.3
New York‡	1958-60	160	45	1.2	0.3	1.2	0.3
Puerto Rico	1950-61	194	66	1.4	0.5	2.4	0.8
Connecticut	1935-59	434	42	1.7	0.2	1.8	0.1

*From Shedd, et al., *ibid.*
†The total population of the continental United States (1950) was used as the standard.
‡Exclusive of New York City.

TABLE 17–9 NUMBER OF PATIENTS AND PER CENT STAGE DISTRIBUTION BY TYPE OF TREATMENT – CANCER OF FLOOR OF MOUTH IN CONNECTICUT, 1935–1959*

STAGE OF DISEASE	SURGERY ALONE		RADIATION ALONE		SURGERY PLUS RADIATION		NO TREATMENT	
	No.	*Per Cent*	*No.*	*Per Cent*	*No.*	*Per Cent*	*No.*	*Per Cent*
Localized	62	56.4	114	47.1	25	37.9	10	31.3
Regional	33	30.0	101	41.7	34	51.5	16	50.0
Distant	3	2.7	10	4.1	3	4.5	4	12.5
Unknown	12	10.9	17	7.0	4	6.1	2	6.2
All Stages	110	100.0	242	100.0	66	100.0	32	100.0

*Live diagnoses only. Excludes cases reported only by autopsy and death certificate. (From Shedd, et al., *ibid.*)

TABLE 17–10 NUMBER OF PATIENTS AND RELATIVE SURVIVAL RATES BY TIME PERIOD OF DIAGNOSIS – CANCER OF FLOOR OF MOUTH IN CONNECTICUT, 1935–1959*

PERIOD	NO.	RELATIVE SURVIVAL RATES (%)		
		1-year	*3-year*	*5-year*
1935–49	216	60.2	33.0	27.5
1950–59	234	70.9	48.3	42.3
All Cases	450	65.8	40.9	35.2

*Live diagnoses only. Excludes cases reported only by autopsy or death certificate. (From Shedd, et al., *ibid.*)

TABLE 17–11 FIVE-YEAR RELATIVE SURVIVAL RATES BY TYPE OF TREATMENT AND STAGE OF DISEASE – CANCER OF FLOOR OF MOUTH IN CONNECTICUT, 1935–1959*

TYPE OF TREATMENT	FIVE-YEAR RELATIVE SURVIVAL RATES (%)		
	Total all Stages	*Localized*	*Regional*
Surgery alone	58.2	72.7	31.3
Surgery plus radiation	32.3	57.0	17.7
Radiation alone	28.5	40.1	17.8
No treatment	9.4	0.0	8.0
Treated and Not Treated	35.2	50.3	19.3

*Based on live diagnoses only. For number of cases, see Table 18–18. (From Shedd, et al., *ibid.*)

TABLE 17–12 NUMBER OF PATIENTS AND PER CENT HISTOLOGIC TYPE DISTRIBUTION BY SEX*

HISTOLOGIC TYPE	TOTAL		MALE		FEMALE	
	No.	*Per Cent*	*No.*	*Per Cent*	*No.*	*Per Cent*
Squamous cell carcinoma	722	74.2	590	73.1	132	79.5
Carcinoma, NOS	104	10.7	85	10.5	19	11.4
Other specified types	22	2.3	18	2.2	4	2.4
Unspecified types	125	12.8	114	14.1	11	6.6
All Types	973	100.0	807	100.0	166	100.0

*From Shedd, et al., *ibid.*

TABLE 17–13 CRUDE AND AGE-ADJUSTED RATES FOR INCIDENCE OF CANCER OF TONGUE PER 100,000 POPULATION BY SEX AND GEOGRAPHIC AREA*

		INCIDENCE RATES PER 100,000			
		CRUDE		AGE-ADJUSTED†	
GEOGRAPHIC AREA	PERIOD	*Male*	*Female*	*Male*	*Female*
10 U.S. Cities[11]	1947	4.1	1.2	4.2	0.8
Finland[5]	1953–62	0.8	0.6	1.0	0.6
Sweden[8]	1958–61	0.8	0.9	0.6	0.6
Norway[6]	1953–61	1.0	0.7	0.9	0.5
New York[8+14] ‡	1958–60	2.6	0.8	2.4	0.7
Puerto Rico[7]	1950–61	3.9	1.3	6.6	2.2
Denmark[9]	1943–57	0.8	0.7	0.8	0.6
S. E. England[23]	1960–62	1.9	1.0	1.4	0.6
Connecticut	1935–59	3.3	0.7	3.3	0.6

*From Shedd, et al., *ibid.*
†The total population of the continental United States (1950) was used as the standard.
‡Exclusive of New York City.

often seen in men in the lower income bracket, and the mean age at diagnosis is 62 years. Etiological factors are trauma from adjacent teeth, dental sepsis, tobacco and alcohol. Approximately one-half of the patients seen at diagnosis have a primary neoplasm still confined to the tongue; two-fifths of these are two centimeters in size or smaller. Nodal metastasis occurs in about 40 to 50 per cent of patients at first and is likely to develop 20 per cent further.[122]

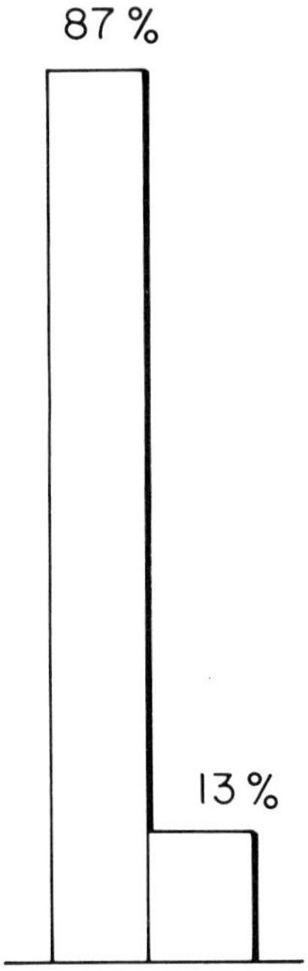

Figure 17–3 Sex ratio. Eighty-seven per cent of the patients were men and 13 per cent were women. The ratio of male to female patients was 6.7. (From Flamant, et al.: Cancer of the tongue: A study of 904 cases. Cancer *17*(3): 377–385, March 1964.)

Out of the 904 cases of cancer of the tongue studied between 1943 and 1959 inclusive by Flamant et al., 87 per cent were male and 13 per cent were female (Fig. 17–3).[53] The average age was 59 years. The largest per cent of patients were in the 55-year age group.[53]

Patients could be placed in three groups according to the site of origin of the cancer as follows:

Group I	mobile portion of the tongue	513 patients
Group II	base of the tongue	368 patients
Group III	origin not determined because of poor anatomic description	23 cases

In group I, 396 cases had the site of origin in the lateral border of the tongue, anterior to insertion of the anterior pillars; 37 cases had the origin in the dorsal surface, anterior to the circumvallate papillae; 16 cases in the tip of the tongue; 64 cases on the ventral surface, excluding the borders.

In group II, 274 cases had the cancer origin in the posterior portions, posterior to the circumvallate papillae. In 94 cases there were instances of massive or total involve-

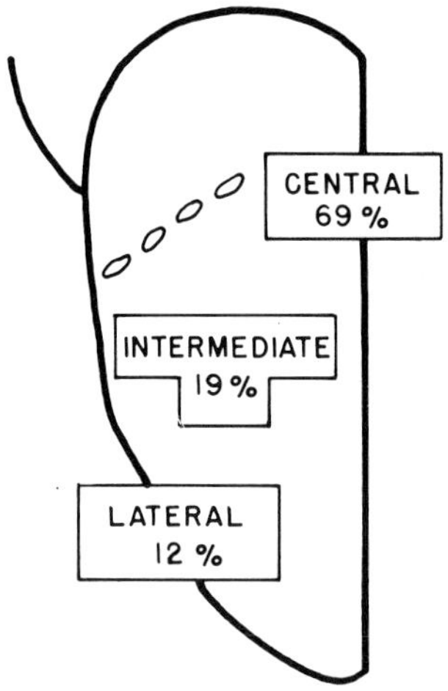

Figure 17–4 The site of origin of the primary tumors along the transverse axis. Sixty-nine per cent were centrally located. (From Flamant, et al., *ibid.*)

ment of the base of the tongue. The primary tumor tended to favor the left side rather than the right. However, the majority (69 per cent) were in the central area, while 19 per cent were in the intermediate area and only 12 per cent were situated laterally. The primary was larger at the base of the tongue and smaller at the tip (Fig. 17–4).[53]

In another population, carcinoma of the tongue showed a sex ratio of 3:1, males to females, for the anterior two-thirds and 6:1 for the base of the tongue. The five-year survival rate varied from 31 per cent to 54 per cent for cancer of the anterior two-thirds to 22 per cent to 43 per cent for cancer of the base of the tongue (Table 17–14).[74]

In Connecticut, cancer of the tongue is more often found on the anterior two-thirds of the tongue without inclusion of the base (Table 17–15). Based on a classification of localized regional spread and distant or remote spread, females have a more favorable stage distribution (Table 17–16). The tumor is localized at the time of diagnosis in 60 per cent of the female patients as compared to five per cent of the male patients.

Survival patterns differ greatly, depending upon the stage of the disease at the time of diagnosis (Table 17–17), the location of the lesion (Table 17–18), and the mode of therapy (Table 17–19). Treatment varies from surgery alone, surgery plus radiation, radiation alone and no therapy (Table 17–20).[127] The shortest five-year survival is experienced by patients with distant metastases (0 per cent) and the longest by those with localized tumors (45 per cent) (Table

TABLE 17–14 CANCER OF THE TONGUE*

SITE OF ORIGIN (Where Specified)	NO. CASES	SEX RATIO	PER CENT LOCALIZED	5-YEAR RELATIVE SURVIVAL RATES (Male Cases Diagnosed 1940–1954)	
				All Stages	*Localized*
Anterior 2/3 of tongue	549	3:1	49:65	31	54
Base of tongue	498	6:1	32:47	22	43

*From Latourette and Myers, *op cit.*

TABLE 17–15 NUMBER OF PATIENTS AND PER CENT SUBSITE DISTRIBUTION BY SEX*

SUBSITE	TOTAL		MALE		FEMALE	
	No.	*Per Cent*	*No.*	*Per Cent*	*No.*	*Per Cent*
Base plus other locations	151	15.5	124	15.4	27	16.3
Base only	203	20.9	172	21.3	31	18.7
Other than base	398	30.9	323	40.0	75	45.2
Tongue, NOS	221	22.7	188	23.3	33	19.9
All Locations	973	100.0	807	100.0	166	100.0

*From Shedd, et al., *op. cit.*

TABLE 17-16 NUMBER OF PATIENTS AND PER CENT STAGE DISTRIBUTION BY SEX*

	TOTAL		MALE		FEMALE	
STAGES OF DISEASE	*No.*	*Per Cent*	*No.*	*Per Cent*	*No.*	*Per Cent*
Localized	399	47.4	306	44.5	93	60.4
Regional	313	37.2	273	39.7	40	26.0
Distant	47	5.6	39	5.7	8	5.2
Other and unknown	82	9.7	69	10.0	13	8.4
All Stages	841	100.0	687	100.0	154	100.0

*From Shedd, et al., *ibid.*

TABLE 17-17 NUMBER OF PATIENTS AND PER CENT TREATMENT DISTRIBUTION BY SEX*

	TOTAL		MALE		FEMALE	
TYPE OF TREATMENT	*No.*	*Per Cent*	*No.*	*Per Cent*	*No.*	*Per Cent*
Surgery alone†	242	28.8	180	26.2	62	40.3
Radical	100		80		20	
Limited	130		91		39	
Surgery plus radiation†	101	12.0	86	12.5	15	9.7
Radical	56		48		8	
Limited	42		35		7	
Radiation alone	423	50.3	360	52.4	63	40.9
No treatment	75	8.9	61	8.9	14	9.1
All Types of Treatment	841	100.0	687	100.0	154	100.0

*Live diagnosis only. Excludes cases reported by autopsy and death certificate only. (From Shedd, et al., *ibid.*)
†Includes cases with unspecified extent of surgery.

TABLE 17-18 FIVE-YEAR OBSERVED SURVIVAL RATES BY ANATOMICAL LOCATION OF THE TUMOR–TONGUE CANCER IN CONNECTICUT, 1935-1959, AND OTHER SELECTED SERIES*

		5-YEAR OBSERVED SURVIVAL RATES (%)		
			LOCATION OF TUMOR	
AUTHOR	PERIOD	ALL PATIENTS	*Base*	*Anterior Two-thirds*
Cade and Lee[2]	1925-55	27	11	35
Frazell and Lucas[18]	1939-53	35	21	42
Fletcher et al.[17]	1948-59	44	32	51
Latourette and Myers[20]	1940-59	21	17	24
Poppe[24]	1932-58	22	13	25
Shedd et al.	1935-59	23	13	29

*From Shedd, et al., *ibid.*

TABLE 17–19 NUMBER OF PATIENTS AND FIVE-YEAR OBSERVED, EXPECTED AND RELATIVE SURVIVAL RATES BY STAGE OF DISEASE AND SEX*

		5-YEAR SURVIVAL RATES (%)		
STAGE OF DISEASE AND SEX	NO.	*Observed*	*Expected*	*Relative*
Localized	399	35.8	78.9	45.4
Males	306	33.0	77.8	42.5
Females	93	45.0	82.4	54.6
Regional	313	11.1	78.0	14.2
Males	273	9.8	77.3	12.7
Females	40	19.7	82.9	23.8
Distant	47	0.0	†	0.0
Males	39	0.0	†	0.0
Females	8	0.0	†	0.0
Other and unknown	82	16.4	78.9	20.8
Males	69	10.4	77.5	13.4
Females	13	46.2	86.8	53.2
All Stages	841	22.8	78.7	28.9
Males	687	19.8	77.6	25.4
Females	154	36.2	83.4	43.4

*Live diagnosis only. Excludes cases reported by autopsy and death certificate only. (From Shedd, et al., *ibid.*)
†Expected rates not computed.

17–17). Five-year survival is greater for patients with lesions involving the anterior two-thirds only (Table 17–18). Surgery alone offers the best prognosis and five-year survival rate (Table 17–19). Survival over a ten-year period when plotted logarithmically shows an excess mortality (Fig. 17–5).[127]

Oral Cancer Mortality

The case incidence rate of cancer of the tongue in California is twice that of cancer of the floor of the mouth. Mean annual deaths from cancer of the tongue are more than two times that of cancer of the floor of the mouth (Table 17–21).[152]

TABLE 17–20 NUMBER OF PATIENTS AND FIVE-YEAR OBSERVED, EXPECTED AND RELATIVE SURVIVAL RATES BY TYPE OF TREATMENT AND SEX*

		5-YEAR SURVIVAL RATES (%)		
TYPE OF TREATMENT AND SEX	NO.	*Observed*	*Expected*	*Relative*
Surgery alone	242	46.0	81.5	56.4
Males	180	44.0	80.7	54.5
Females	62	51.8	84.0	61.6
Surgery plus radiation	101	18.6	84.1	22.1
Males	86	17.3	84.5	20.4
Females	15	26.7	82.2	32.4
Radiation alone	423	14.4	76.8	18.8
Males	360	11.7	75.6	15.5
Females	63	29.9	83.3	35.9
No treatment	75	1.3	73.1	1.8
Males	61	0.0	†	0.0
Females	14	7.1	82.1	8.7
All Types	841	22.8	78.7	28.9
Males	687	19.8	77.6	25.4
Females	154	36.2	83.4	43.4

*Live diagnoses only. Excludes cases reported by autopsy and death certificate only. (From Shedd, et al., *ibid.*)
†Expected rates not computed.

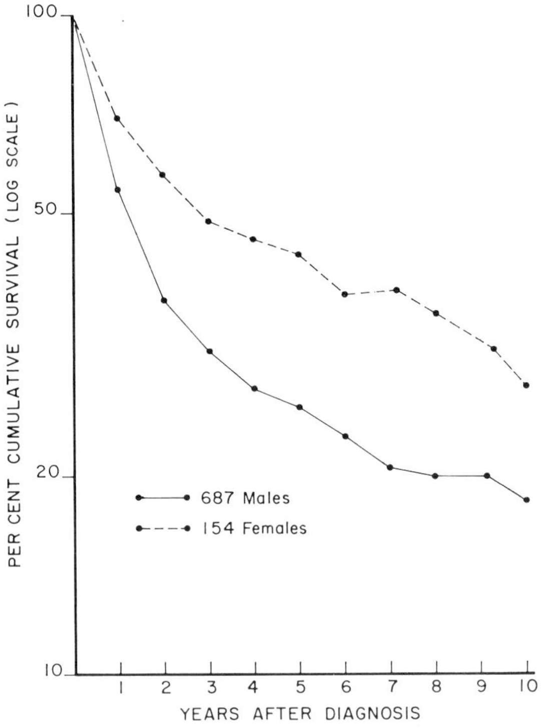

Figure 17–5 Relative survival rates during 10 years for men and women diagnosed while alive with cancer of the tongue in Connecticut, 1935–1959. (From Shedd, et al.: Cancer of the tongue in Connecticut, 1935–1959. Cancer *21*: 89–96, January 1968.)

CANCER OF THE BUCCAL MUCOSA

Cancer of the buccal mucosa is less common than the other oral cancers and is nearly as common in females as males. Of 819 patients with cancer of the buccal mucosa, palate or gingiva, 74 per cent were male, all patients were in the fifth to eighth decades of life, and the majority of the lesions were localized epidermoid carcinoma. The incidence rate for cancer of the cheek, palate and gingiva increases with age. The highest incidence is found in Puerto Rico. Causative agents are tobacco chewing, snuff dipping and heavy pipe smoking.

Carcinoma of the buccal mucosa tends to be a flat plaque-like lesion often associated with long-standing leukoplakic changes.[62] The histology is divided between squamous carcinoma and adenocarcinoma with tumors of the salivary origin providing a third alternative. Tumors may be localized, have regional involvement, or distant metastases at the time of diagnosis.[128]

Localization is higher in women than in men. Women have a higher survival rate than men. The response is better to surgery alone when the lesion is localized. The five-year relative survival pattern is improved when the lesion is localized and is just under 40 per cent.

CANCER OF THE PALATE

Squamous cell carcinoma is the most frequent cancer of the *palatine arch* (mouth, the soft palate, the tonsil and its bed and the tonsillar pillar) and the palate and is pri-

TABLE 17–21 ORAL CANCER MORTALITY AND MORBIDITY BY SPECIFIC SITES*

ORAL CANCER SITE *(ICD Code)*	MEAN NO. OF ANNUAL DEATHS, CALIFORNIA *(1960–1962)*†	AGE-ADJUSTED AVERAGE ANNUAL CASE INCIDENCE RATES/100,000 POPULATION *(Alameda County, California)*‡
Lip (140)	10.33	4.7
Tongue (141)	106.33	3.6
Salivary (142)	26.67	0.9
Floor (143)	42.33	1.6
Other mouth (144)	50.33	1.5
Mesopharynx (145)	47.00	1.7
Nasopharynx (146)	33.00	0.7
Hypopharynx (147)	25.67	1.2
Unspecified pharynx (148)	67.00	0.7
Total (140–148)	408.66	16.6

*From Weir, J. M., Dunn, J. E., Jr., and Buell, P. E.: Smoking and oral cancer: epidemiological data, educational responses. Am. J. Public Health 59(7):959–966, June 1969.

†Sum of site-specific deaths for California in 1960, 1961 and 1962, divided by 3.

‡Incidence for males, from "Incidence of Cancer in Alameda County, California 1960–1964." (Table 18–15) State of California, Department of Public Health.

TABLE 17–22 DISTRIBUTION BY AGE AND SEX*

AGE	MALES (%)	FEMALES (%)	TOTAL
20	0	0	0
20–30	2	0	2
30–40	1	1	2
40–50	19–65	10–35	29
50–60	62–80	14–20	76
60–70	87–90	13–10	100
70–80	68–90	5–10	73
80+	19	4	23
Total	258–85	47–15	305

*From Schulz, M. D., Lintner, D. M., and Sweeney, L.: Carcinoma of the palatine arch. Am. J. Roentgenol. Radium Ther. Nuclear Med. 89(3):541–548, March 1963.

marily a disease of elderly males (Table 17–22). Other cancers include transitional cell carcinoma, lympho-epithelioma and malignant lymphoma. Sore throat, pain on swallowing, pain in ear, lump or ulcer in throat, lump in neck, or bleeding may be the primary symptom and may be present up to one year before the patient seeks relief.

The tumor varies greatly in appearance. It may be soft and fluctuant, hard and indurated, cauliflower-like or present as an oro-antral fistula.

Reverse smoking frequently produces or is directly associated with cancers of the palate.[107]

CANCER OF THE SALIVARY GLANDS

Carcinoma of the salivary glands is predominantly adenoid cystic, acinic cell, adenocarcinoma, mucoepidermoid or undifferentiated (Table 17–23).

The majority of salivary cancers arise from the parotid gland and present in the male.

The majority appear to have a predilection for the Caucasian since the highest incidence for both male and female is reported from the United Kingdom, Sweden, and the German Democratic Republic; for males, the United Kingdom, Connecticut and Finland; and for females, Hawaii (Caucasian), Nevada, Canada and Newfoundland. In each location cited above, the annual average incidence of cancer of the salivary glands per 100,000 by age is 85.[46]

The survival pattern for cancer of the salivary glands is high. Nearly 53 per cent of patients with malignant tumors of the parotid gland were alive and free of the disease five or more years after therapy (Table 17–24).

CANCER OF THE PULP

Cancer has been reported in pulps of molar and cuspid teeth of Caucasians as sec-

TABLE 17–23 CYTOLOGIC FEATURES OF SALIVARY-GLAND CARCINOMA*

CARCINOMA	CYTOLOGY *Nuclei*	*Cytoplasm*	*Other*
Adenoid Cystic	Round	Little	Globules of mucus
Acinic Cell	Central	Foam abundant	No ductal epithelium
			No cellular atypia
			Solid plugs of acinic cells
Other Adenocarcinomas			Plugs of overlapping cells
			Sheets of cells regularly arranged
Mucus producing		Abundant	Occasionally globules of mucus-like material-red in MGG stained smears
Muco-epidermoid			
Low malignancy			Monomorphic cells-resembled oncocytes
High malignancy			Polymorphic
Undifferentiated			Decrease in cytoplasmic/nuclear ratio

*From Zajicek and Eneroth: Cytological diagnosis of salivary-gland carcinomata from aspiration biopsy smears. Acta. Otolaryng. *263*:183–185, 1970.

TABLE 17-24 RESULTS AFTER FIVE YEARS OR LONGER IN 111 PATIENTS WITH MALIGNANT TUMORS OF PAROTID GLAND*

TYPE OF TUMOR	NO. OF PATIENTS	NO EVIDENCE OF DISEASE	DIED OF DISEASE	DIED OF OTHER CAUSES
Malignant mixed	34	15	12	7
Mucoepidermoid	32	23	6	3
Squamous	8		6	2
Adenoid cystic	13	6	4	3
Acinic cell	8	8		
Adenocarcinoma	16	6	8	2
Total	111	58	36	17

*From Bardwill, J. M.: Tumors of the parotid gland. Am. J. Surg. *114*:498–502, October 1967.

ondary lesions only. Pulp cancer occurs predominantly in teeth on the right side. The greatest incidence occurs in male subjects who range from three to seventy years of age.[18] Primary sites include the mandible, antrum, lower lip and the oral mucous membrane (Table 17–25). Roentgenologic examination of the affected jaw shows a general loss of lamina dura and bone architecture around the involved teeth, areas of radiolucency and multiple lytic lesions. The principal clinical symptoms are pain and/or swelling and loosening of the affected teeth. Histologically, the affected pulp shows invasion by tumor cells (Fig. 17–6).

TABLE 17-25 SITE OF PRIMARY TUMORS IN PATIENTS WHOSE TEETH WERE EXAMINED FOR PULP INVOLVEMENT*

NUMBER OF CASES	SITE OF ORIGIN	PERCENTAGE OF TOTAL
12	Mandible	30.8
8	Antrum	20.5
8	Lower Lip	20.5
3	Floor of Mouth	7.7
3	Tongue	7.7
2	Gingiva of Mandibular Alveolus	5.1
1	Upper Lip	2.3
1	Maxilla	2.3
1	Tibia	2.3

*Modified after Stewart and Stafine, 1955. (From Bridgewater, V. R. C., and Bolden, T. E.: Cancer of the pulp–A review of the literature–1904–1967. The Meharri-Dent. *28*(2), March 1969).

ADVANCED ORAL CANCER

Clinical "Face"

Cancer may involve any one of the basic tissues, or their derivatives. Cancer may present at any one of the anatomical sites enumerated. The "face" of advanced cancer is quite variable. The high death rate from oral cancer is directly related to the late diagnosis of the disease. The initial diagnosis of oral cancer at the advanced stage of the disease may be related to the insidious, silent and grotesque changes in the clinical "face" of cancer (Fig. 17–7*A*–*AA*).[14]

Appearance

Clinically, cancer may present as an ulcer, a swelling, a fungating mass, an osteolytic radiolucency, a pathologic fracture, facial asymmetry, a white indurated zone, an area of hyperpigmentation, an oro-antral fistula, an oro-facial fistula, a fluctuant mass, zones of erythema, or extraction sites which do not heal.[14]

Presenting Symptoms

Even the advanced oral cancer may be painless until late in the disease or until there is impingement upon the growth during mastication. Halitosis, bleeding or hemorrhage, ulceration, rapid growth, rapid change in color, trismus, "my face looks different, my tongue is sore," difficulty on swallowing and difficulty eating are some of

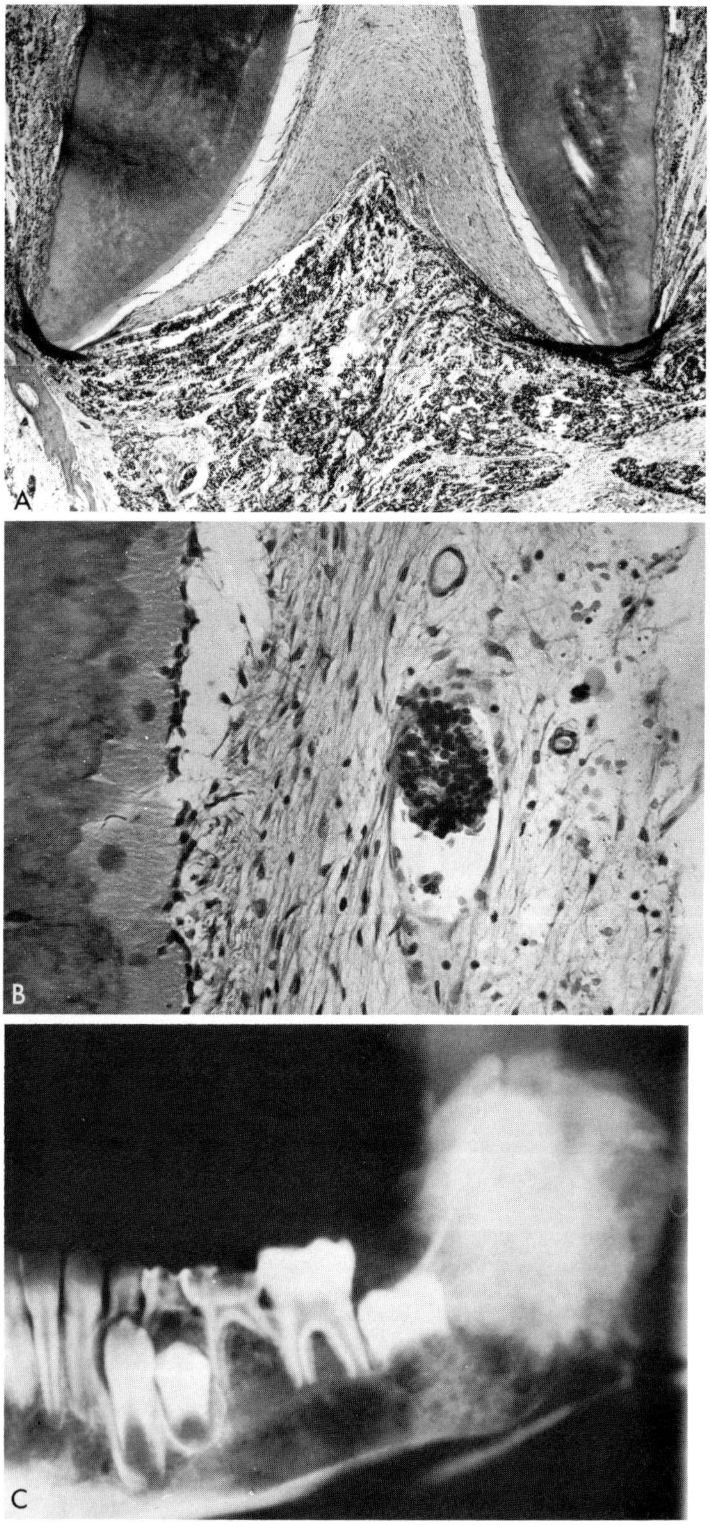

Figure 17–6 *A*, Indentation and compression of the apical pulpal tissue of the permanent first molar. (Hematoxylin and eosin stain. Original magnification, × 40). *B*, Nest of tumor cells within a pulpal blood vessel in the deciduous second molar. Compare the morphology of these tumor cells to those seen in other areas of the jaw. (Hematoxylin and eosin stain. Original magnification, × 200). *C*, Panoramic radiographic appearance of the involved portion of the jaw. Note the bulk of tumor overlying the ramus, with destruction of the condyle and coronoid process. There are also osteolytic changes in the body of the mandible. (From Snyder, M. B., and Cawson, R. A.: Jaw and pulpal metastasis of an adrenal neuroblastoma. Oral Surg. *40*(6): 775–784, Dec. 1975).

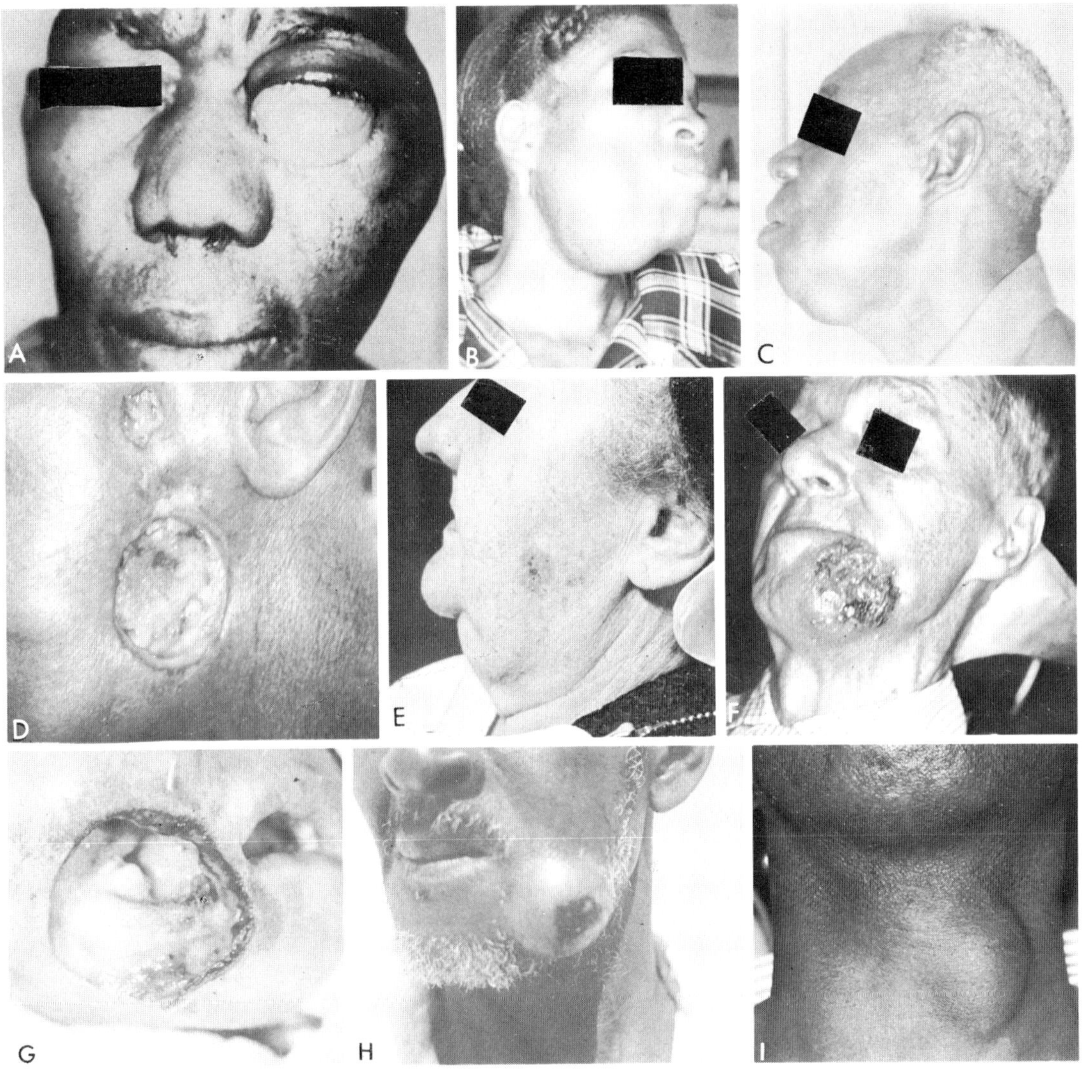

Figure 17–7 The clinical and histologic "face" of oral cancer.

Clinical "face": *A*, Eye, facial asymmetry, squamous cell carcinoma; *B* and *C*, submaxillary gland, facial asymmetry, benign mixed tumor; *D* and *E*, cheek, facial asymmetry, ulceration, pigmentation, basal cell carcinoma; *F*, chin, facial asymmetry, squamous cell carcinoma; *G*, cheek, facial asymmetry, ulceration, noma; *H*, mandible, facial asymmetry, ulceration, fibrosarcoma; *I*, thyroid gland, asymmetry.

Oral cavity: *J* and *K*, Lip, squamous cell carcinoma; *L*, gingiva-mandible, squamous cell carcinoma; *M*, gingiva-maxilla, squamous cell carcinoma; *N*, gingiva-mandible, pigmented papilloma; *O*, floor of the mouth, squamous cell carcinoma; *P* and *Q*, alveolar ridge, squamous cell carcinoma; *R*, tongue, papilloma; *S*, tongue, squamous cell carcinoma; *T*, tongue, squamous cell carcinoma; *U*, palate, papillary carcinoma; *V* and *W*, palate, squamous cell carcinoma; *X*, palate, adenocarcinoma; *Y* and *Z*, palate, squamous cell carcinoma;

Illustration continued on the following page.

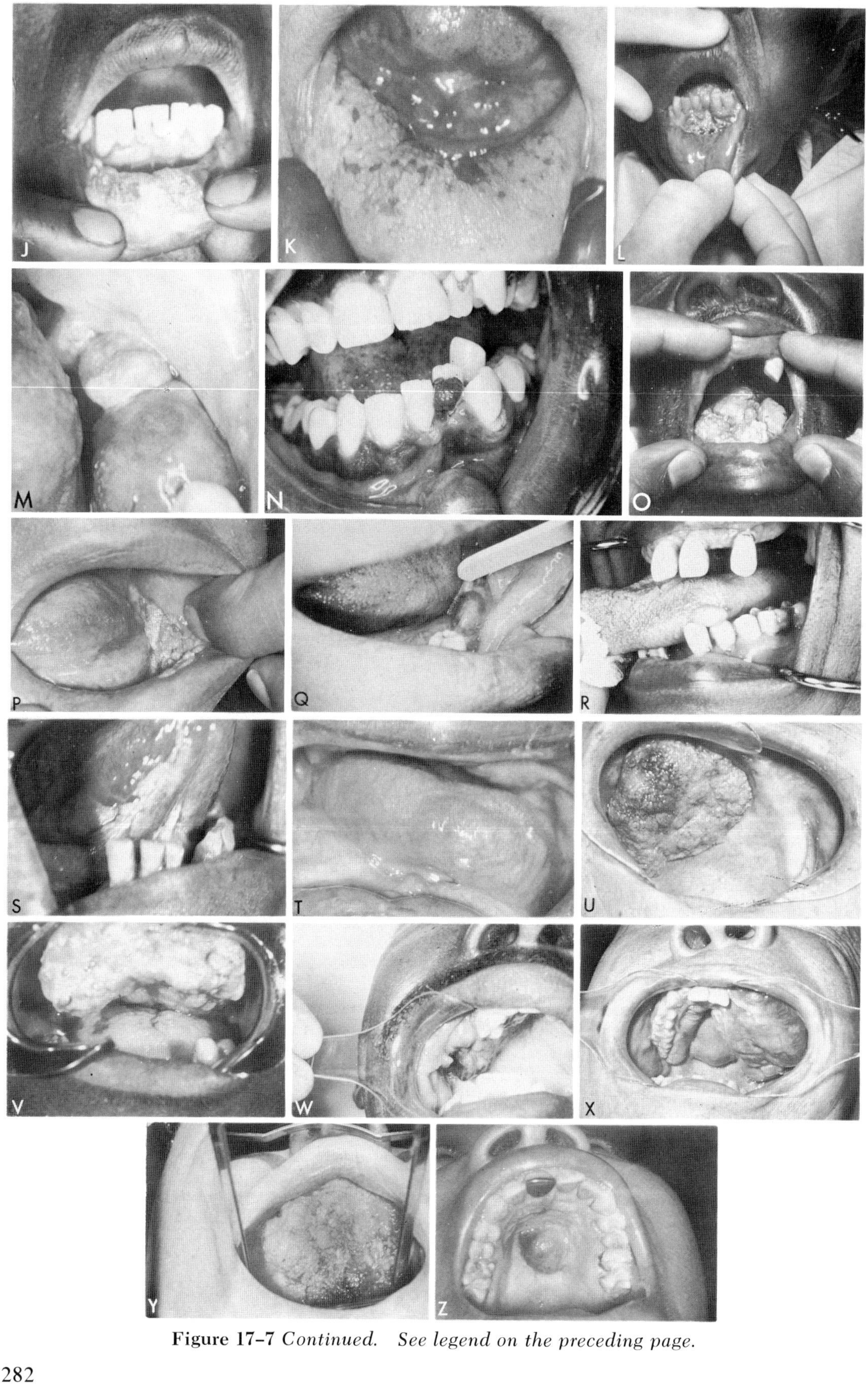

Figure 17–7 *Continued. See legend on the preceding page.*

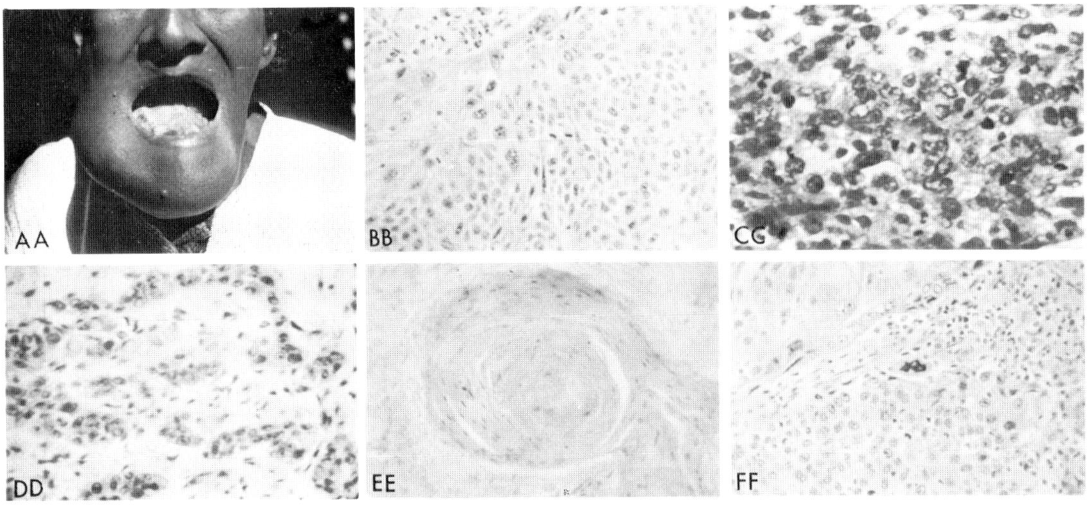

Figure 17-7 *Continued Histologic "face"*: *AA*, mandible, ameloblastoma; *BB*, abnormal mitosis and pleomorphism, H and E, ×120; *CC*, mitotic figure, H and E, ×120; *DD*, invasion, H and E, ×120; *EE*, horn pearl, H and E, ×120; *FF*, hyperchromatism, H and E, ×120.

the more prevalent signs and symptoms of the advanced oral cancer.

Histologic "Face"

Histologically, the advanced cancer will show several features depending upon the tissue source and the biology of the tumor. Among these are invasion, pleomorphism, hyperchromatism, increased mitotic activity, abnormal mitotic figures, gigantism, dyskeratosis, intracellular keratinization, increased deposition of melanin, destruction of basement membranes and central necrosis (Figs. 17-7*BB-FF* and 17-8).[14]

The "face" of cancer may histologically be almost indistinguishable from the adjacent normal mature tissue or may resemble the most embryonic tissue. This face depends upon the degree of differentiation of the cancer. The more differentiated the cancer growth, the greater its resemblance to its tissue of origin. The less differentiated the tumor, the more difficult it is to determine its tissue of origin—the more embryonic. In general, the less differentiated the greater is its malignancy.

Cytological "Face"

The cytology of oral malignant lesions varies according to the tumor. A typical scraping from a well-differentiated squamous cell carcinoma would show sheets of cells or single cells (Fig. 17-9*A*, *C*, *E*, *F*). They would vary widely in shape and size. Characteristic shapes are polygonal, spindle, tadpole and cells with horn pearl formation. Typical nuclei are pyknotic or vesicular, occasionally binucleate or multinucleate. The chromatin may show clumping. The nuclear membrane may be indented, irregular and thick. A prominent nucleolus may be present. Cytoplasm is thick and varies in

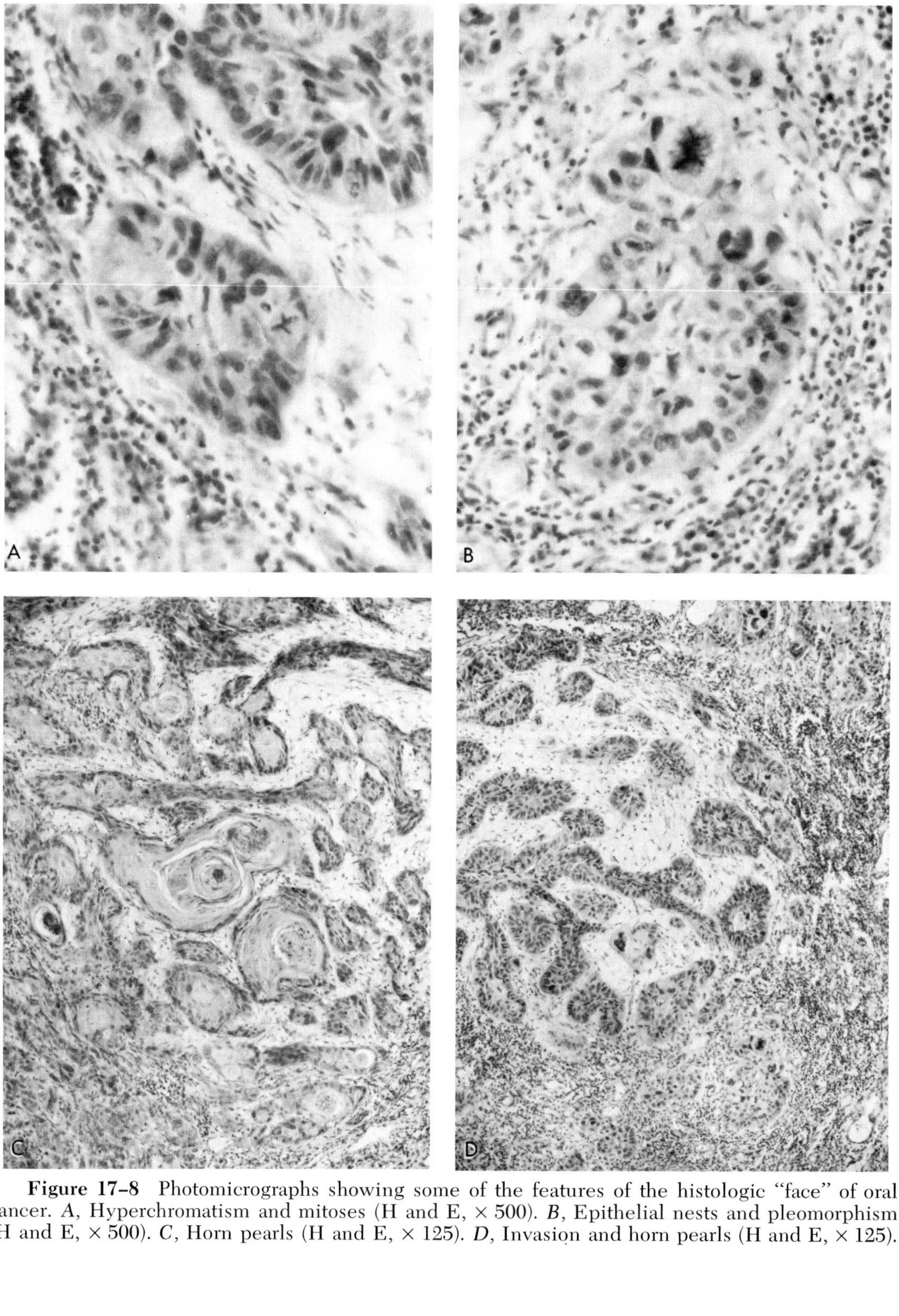

Figure 17–8 Photomicrographs showing some of the features of the histologic "face" of oral cancer. *A*, Hyperchromatism and mitoses (H and E, × 500). *B*, Epithelial nests and pleomorphism (H and E, × 500). *C*, Horn pearls (H and E, × 125). *D*, Invasion and horn pearls (H and E, × 125).

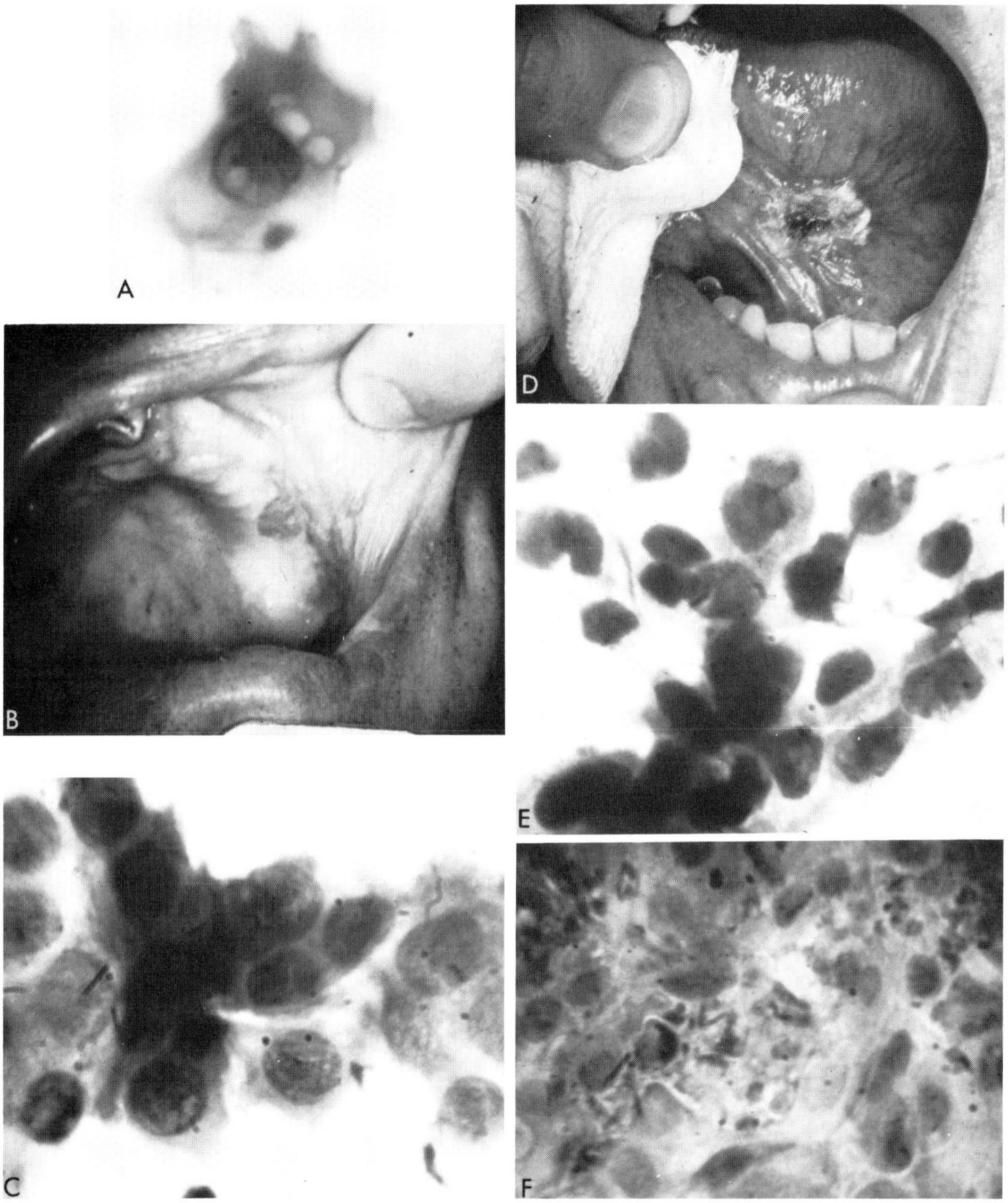

Figure 17-9 Squamous cell carcinoma. *A*, Malignant cell. *B* and *C*, Early lesion. *D* and *E*, Advanced lesion. *F*, 1° breast, 2° metastatic to mandible. (Courtesy of Dr. Maston Nelson, Meharry Medical College, School of Dentistry.)

size. The fundamental change is in the nuclear-cytoplasmic ratio and this helps to differentiate scrappings from malignant lesions and benign lesions.[97]

CHARACTERISTICS OF SPECIFIC ADVANCED ORAL CANCERS

SQUAMOUS CELL CARCINOMA

Epidermoid Carcinoma

The clinical *face* of advanced squamous cell carcinoma presents little challenge to identify since it is well known. A highly variable face, it may be exophytic or endophytic, ulcerated or non-ulcerated, papillary, smooth or rough, white, red or black, foul-smelling, purulent or hemorrhagic, painful or silent. The advanced epidermoid carcinoma may be recognized by changes in size, color, texture, continuity and/or consistency of the oral and/or para-oral tissues (Fig. 17–9, *B* and *D*). The distinction is made between epidermoid cancer and squamous carcinoma. Epidermoid cancer has keratinization or pearl formation while squamous carcinoma is the type which has no pearl formation and usually has a necrotic mass in central foci.[71]

Squamous cell cancer from the oral cavity histochemically shows alkaline phosphatase and aminopeptidase activity in the stroma, acid phosphatase in the epithelium, esterase in parakeratotic and necrotic cells, and succinic dehydrogenease in the peripheral cell layer. Lactic acid, malic acid, glycerophosphate, glucose-6-phosphate and isocitrate dehydrogenase localize in the peripheral layer to the subhornified layer of the squamous-cell cancer.[71]

Verrucous Carcinoma

Verrucous carcinoma is a variant of epidermoid carcinoma with predilection for the buccal mucosa and the mandibular gingiva (Table 17–26). It rarely metastasizes. It appears as a warty fungating elevated ulcerated mass. It varies in size from 0 to 10.0 cm. (Table 17–27). The tumor tends to erode the mandible with a sharp margin without infiltrating into the marrow spaces (Fig. 17–10).[73] Secondarily the tongue, floor of the mouth, hard palate and paranasal sinuses become involved.

The tumor starts as a blister or sore, grows slowly for years then suddenly grows more rapidly. The majority of patients are in the fifth to eighth decades of life (Table 17–28).

The tumor appears more often in men than women, in Caucasians more often than Negroes, and seems to be related to the use of chewing tobacco and snuff. The initial symptoms vary greatly but the predominant one seems to be the presence of a mass (Table 17–29). The tumor is radioresistant and may undergo anaplasia following radiation.[73]

TABLE 17–26 LOCATION OF VERRUCOUS CARCINOMA*

LOCATION		NO. PATIENTS
Oral cavity		77
Buccal mucosa	50	
Gingiva	21	
Tongue	3	
Anterior tonsillar pillar	1	
Hard palate	2	
Larynx		12
Nasal Fossa		4
Genitalia		12
Penis (glans)	8	
Vagina	1	
Vulva	1	
Scrotum	1	
Perineum	1	
Total		105

*From Kraus, F. T., and Perez-Mesa, C.: Verrucous carcinoma: clinical and pathologic study of 105 cases involving oral cavity, larynx and genitalia. Cancer *19*:26–38, January 1966.

TABLE 17–27 SIZE (LARGEST DIAMETER) OF ORAL CAVITY LESIONS*

SIZE	NO. PATIENTS
1.0–1.9 cm	19
2.0–4.9 cm	36
5.0–10.0 cm	15
Not recorded	7

*From Kraus and Perez-Mesa, *ibid.*

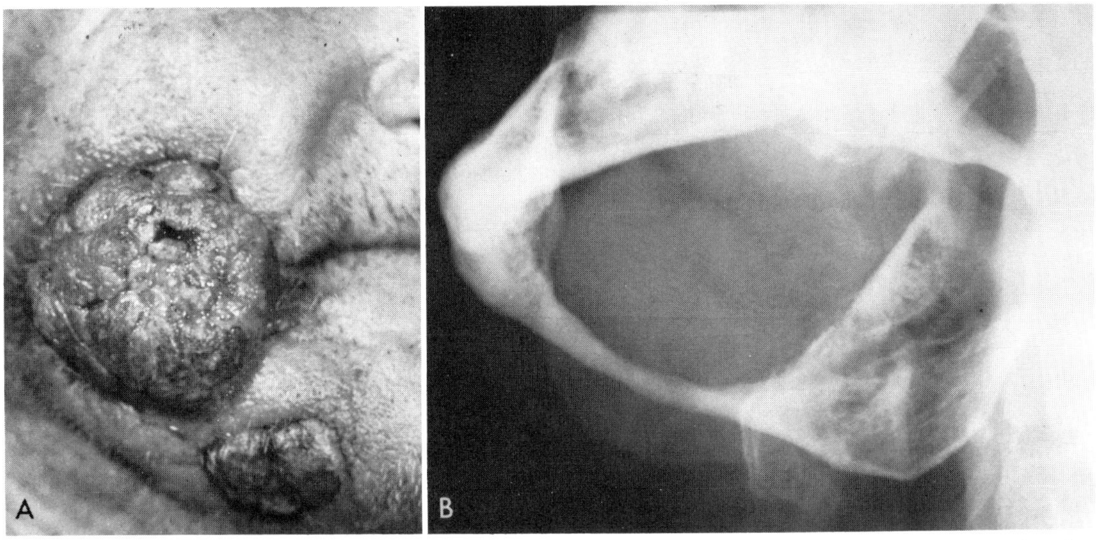

Figure 17–10 *A*, Verrucous carcinoma of the buccal mucosa that has invaded through the skin of the cheek and floor of the mouth. *B*, The mandible has been invaded and eroded extensively as shown by x-ray examination. (From Kraus, F. T., and Perez-Mesa, C.: Verrucous carcinoma: Clinical and pathologic study of 105 cases involving the oral cavity, larynx and genitalia. Cancer *19*:26–38, January 1966.)

Ameloblastoma

The incidence of ameloblastoma varies from one to 13 to 40 per cent among all cysts and tumors of the jaws. These tumors usually involve the mandible and are usually treated by partial mandibulectomy or maxillectomy. When first seen they are usually extremely large, cystic or fungating masses which may fill the mouth and may interfere with mastication.[38] The tumor predominates in the male. The injection of sclerosing agents into the tumor has proved to be an effective method for causing regression of the tumor (Fig. 17–11.[148] See also Fig. 17–7AA).[14]

Primary tumors of the bony and odontogenic tissues of the jaw accounted for 0.8 per cent of all malignancies in Uganda (Table 17–30).[45] Ameloblastomas, ossifying fibromas and antral carcinomas were the most common tumors in 92 tumors of jaws of Ugandans.

The frequency of ameloblastomas among dental tumors, malignancies and epithelial tumors varies among African, Korean and American populations (Table 17–31).

Malignant Ameloblastoma. Ameloblastomas rarely become malignant.[136] Of 22 cases of malignant ameloblastomas reported during the interim 1953–1966, five were

TABLE 17–28 AGE INCIDENCE OF VERRUCOUS CARCINOMA OF THE ORAL CAVITY*

AGE SPAN†	DECADE	NO. OF PATIENTS
30–39	4	1
40–49	5	4
50–59	6	13
60–69	7	26
70–79	8	26
80–89	9	7

*From Kraus and Perez-Mesa, *ibid.*
†Range: 34–85 years.

TABLE 17–29 SYMPTOMS OF ORAL VERRUCOUS CARCINOMA*

SYMPTOM	NO. PATIENTS
Presence of mass	31
Presence of "sore" or ulcer	29
Pain or tenderness	19
Blister	5
Hard white patch	4
Fistula	5
Bleeding	3
Loose teeth	1

*From Kraus and Perez-Mesa, *ibid.*

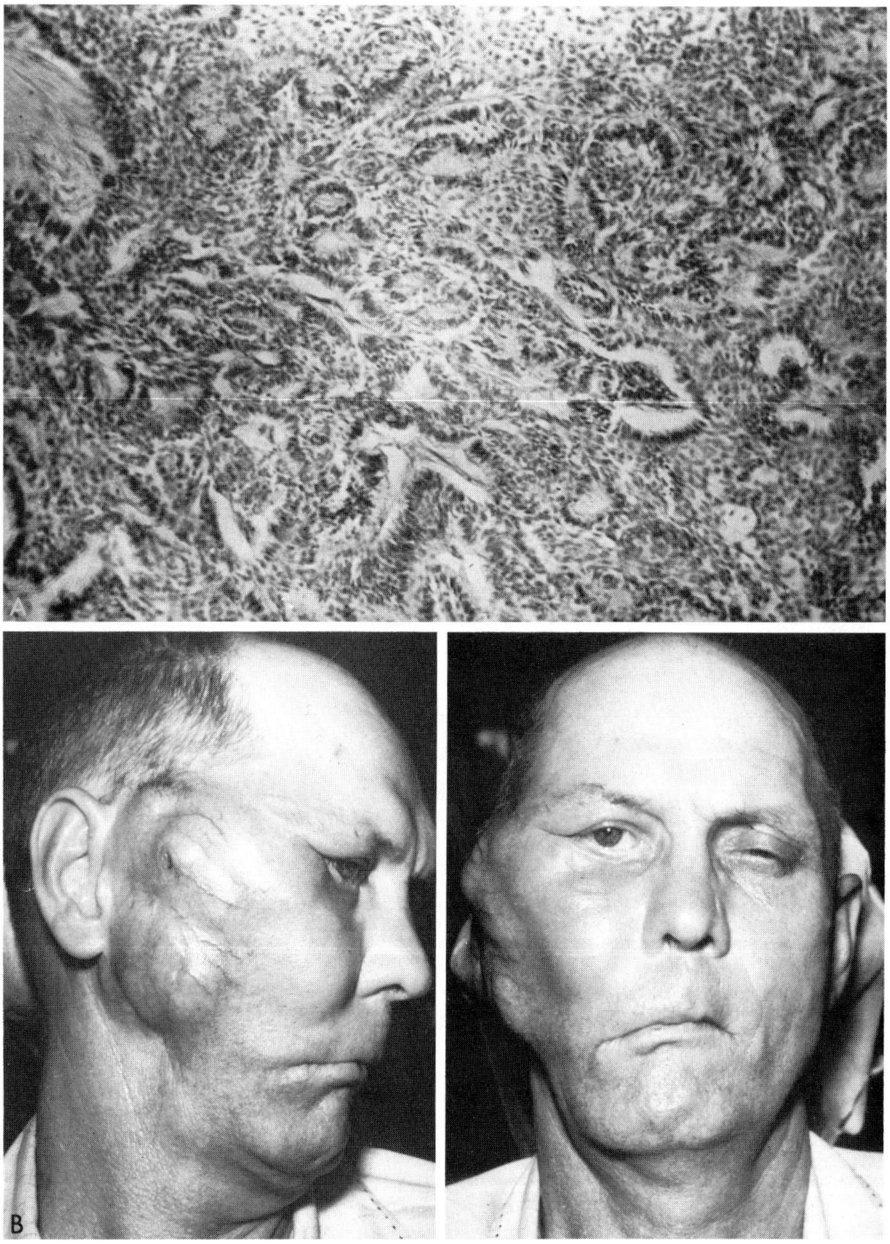

Figure 17–11 *A*, Photomicrograph showing typical appearance of ameloblastoma. *B*, Lateral and frontal views of the patient showing recurrent ameloblastoma involving the maxillofacial structures during the past 22 years. He has had "multiple" surgical procedures. The patient now presents an inoperable condition (December 1958). *C*, The sclerosing agent Sylnasol was injected into the tumor mass. After eight weeks a biopsy specimen was taken, the microscopic findings showing dense fibrous connective tissue with some fragmentation of collagen fibers and chronic inflammation. No evidence of ameloblastic cells was noted in the biopsy material. Repeated biopsies showed the same microscopic findings. *D*, Clinical appearance of the patient (April 1962) shows marked "regression" of the tumor mass. He had received eight injection treatments; each dose was 10 to 15 cc. injected over a 12-month period. (From Vazirani, S. J., and Schultz, L. W.: Sclerosing agent in treatment of ameloblastoma: 15 years follow-up. Oral Surgery Transactions of the Fourth International Conference, Amsterdam, Edinburgh, E. & S. Livingstone, May 1971.)

Illustration continued on the opposite page.

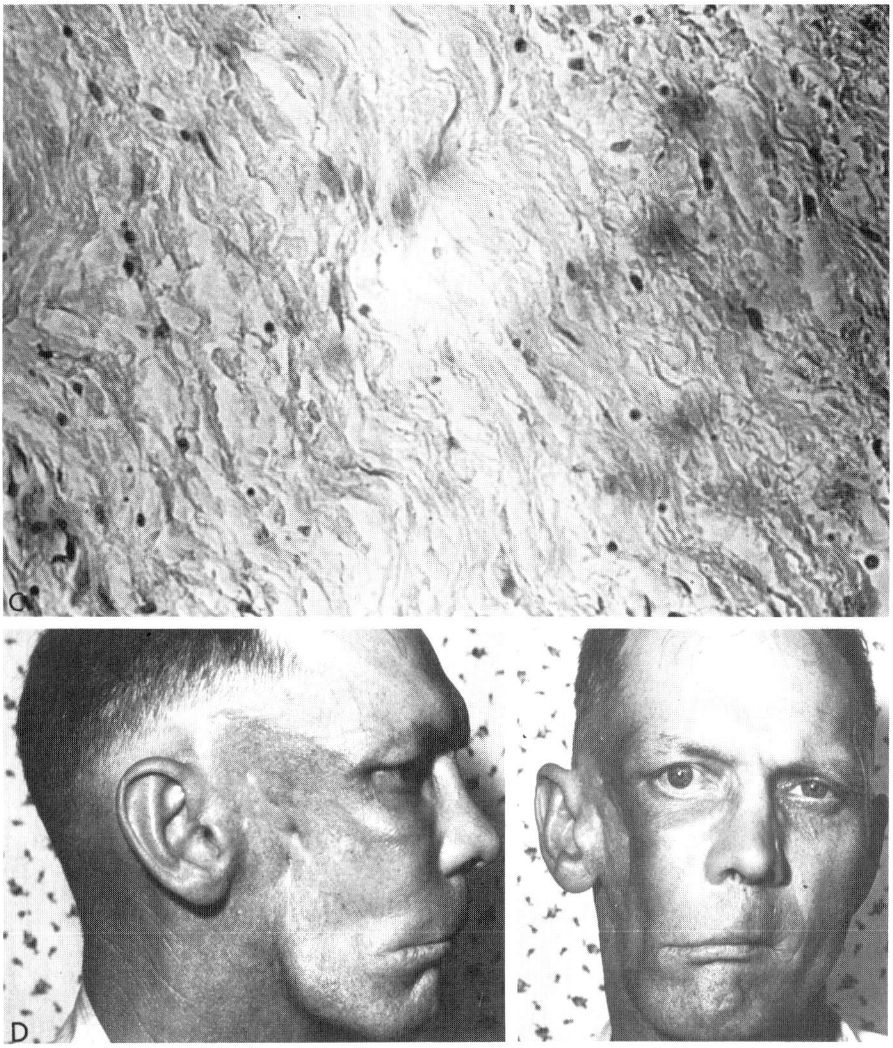

Figure 17–11 *Continued.*

evaluated as proved examples of malignancy, 12 as possible and four as doubtful. The proved metastatic lesions showed atypical keratinization, acanthotic or granular-cell variation.[28] The sites of metastasis are to the deep cervical lymph nodes, the lungs and the breast.

BASAL CELL CARCINOMA

Intraoral basal cell carcinomas are usually associated with the lip, though they may occur in the left lower molar region or on the buccal gingiva in the lower third molar region as slow growing, soft-tissue masses (see Fig. 17–7).[14] Both oxidative and hydrolytic enzymes may be detected in the tissues from these tumors,[94] especially alkaline and acid phosphatase, esterase β-glucuronidase, aminopeptidase, succinate dehydrogenase and NAD- and NADP-dependent dehydrogenases.[94]

NEVOID BASAL CELL CARCINOMA

The nevoid basal cell carcinoma syndrome is a rare disorder which has been recognized as early as two years,[66] but usually manifests about puberty or before the twenty-fifth year.[11, 59]

TABLE 17–30 HISTOLOGIC CLASSIFICATION OF TUMORS INVOLVING THE JAWS IN UGANDA AFRICANS (Burkitt Lymphomas Excluded)

Odontogenic tumors		26
Ameloblastoma	24	
Ameloblastic fibroma	2	
Ossifying fibroma		14
Osteogenic sarcoma		4
Carcinomas involving jaws		35
Antral carcinoma	31	
Buccal carcinoma	3	
? origin	1	
Malignant melanoma of buccal cavity		3
Granular-cell congenital epulis		2
Pigmented congenital epulis		2
Salivary tumors		2
Malignant lymphoma		2
Neurofibrosarcoma		2
Total histologically confirmed tumors		92
Histologically non-neoplastic lesions		7
Clinical malignancy; no histologic examination		18
Total		117

*From Dodge, O. G.: Tumors of the jaw, odontogenic tissues and maxillary antrum (excluding Burkitt lymphoma) in Uganda Africans. Cancer *18*(2):205–215, February 1965.

TABLE 17–31 FREQUENCY OF AMELOBLASTOMAS

Sudan	17 of 1337 (1.3%) epithelial tumors recorded
Transvaal	0.6% 1.6 cancers
Johannesburg	0.8% 0.4 cancers
Kenya	0.6% 0.4 cancers
Kampala Cancer Registry	0.3% of all tumors
U. S. A.	0.07% of all malignant tumors 1.0% of all dental tumors
Uganda	0.8% of all malignancies
Korea	12.7% of all 157 tumors of the jaws (59–65)

*Compiled from Dodge, *ibid.* and Chung, D. H., Kiunman, J. E. G., Lee, B. C., and Lee, Y. T.: Tumors of the jaws in Korea. Oral Sug. *27*(6):716–728, June 1969.

The signs, "face," and symptoms include multiple basal cell tumors of the skin (Fig. 17–12),[84a] cysts of the jaws, rib anomalies, vertebrae anomalies, brachymetacarpalism, mandibular and maxillary cysts, and sexual, ophthalmologic, and neurologic abnormalities. The jaw cysts in the basal cell nevus syndrome are of particular importance.[59] They are believed to be odontogenic cysts representing developmental disturbances during tooth development and they are lined by thin, flattened keratinizing squamous epithelium. They may vary from microcysts to several centimeters in size and may present in the maxilla and mandible.[65]

The syndrome is inherited as an autosomal-dominant polymorphic trait with good penetrance but with variable expressivity (Table 17–32 and Fig. 17–12).[85]

SALIVARY GLAND TUMORS

The behavior of primary tumors of the salivary glands is such that benign tumors are seldom fatal and that the majority of malignant tumors can be controlled by surgical intervention.[8] Malignant tumors of the parotid gland may exhibit lymphogenous spread to regional lymph nodes, and hematogenous spread to the lungs, long bones, abdominal viscera, soft tissue, spine and scapula.[8]

Adenoid Cystic Carcinoma

Adenoid cystic carcinomas or cylindromas constitute approximately 16 to 20 per cent of all salivary gland tumors.[1] The tumor is found most frequently in the fifth to sixth decades and exists for one year or less. However, cases have been reported in which the tumor existed for up to 35 years.[36] Adenoid cystic carcinoma is more common in women than in men. It is distinguishable from the benign adenoma by a slow-spreading ulceration. The site of this tumor is the hard and soft palates.

The five-year cure rate of palatal cancer is just under 40 per cent. Chemotherapeutic agents are being increasingly used in the management of uncontrolled malignant disease.[122]

Acinic Cell Carcinoma

Acinic cell carcinoma is a tumor of the salivary glands constituting from 2.3 to 7.7 per cent of major salivary gland tumors, and 12 per cent of all malignant tumors of the

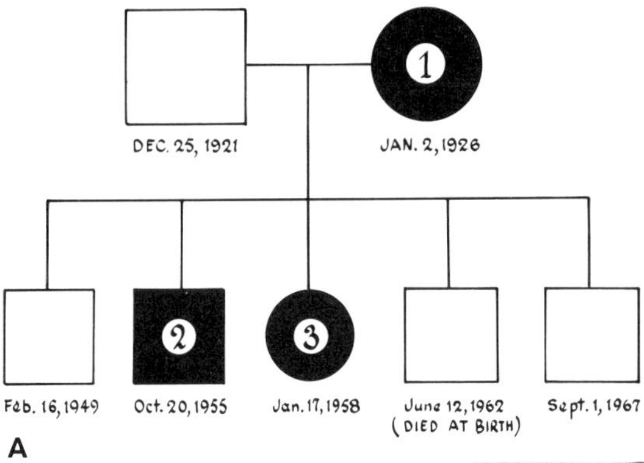

A

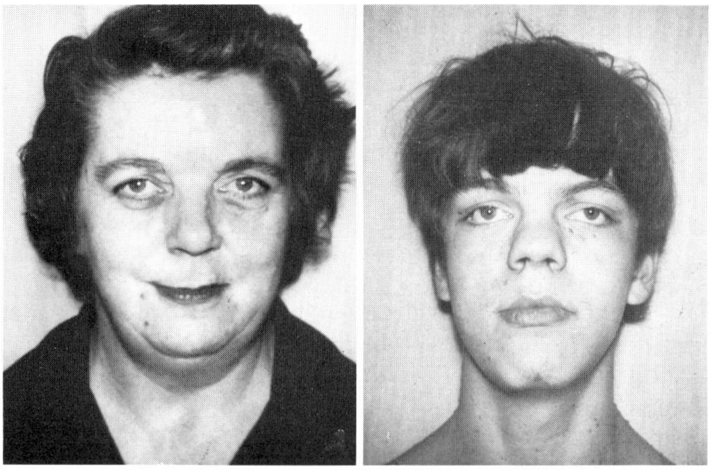

B

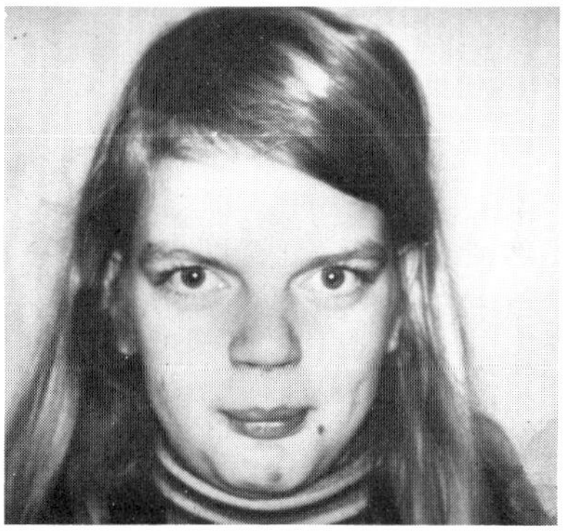

Figure 17–12 *A*, Pedigree of an affected family. *B*, Affected family members. Mother, age 46 (A). Son, age 16 (B). Daughter, age 14 (C). Forehead bossing and hypertelorism are apparent.

Illustration continued on the following page.

major salivary glands. It appears to arise from the serous acinic portion of the glands, but one author considers the primary source to be the ductal epithelium which is pluripotent rather than acinic cells. Acinic cell carcinoma of the sublingual gland was the final diagnosis of a 45-year-old white male who developed a lump under the tongue. The final growth size of the tumor was about five centimeters in diameter. The entire sublingual gland and cyst were removed.

Upon microscopic observation, the cytoplasm in the tumor cells contained fine granules which were mucin positive. The observations in this case appear to support the hypothesis of acinic cell origin of this tumor rather than the hypothesis of duct cell origin.[143]

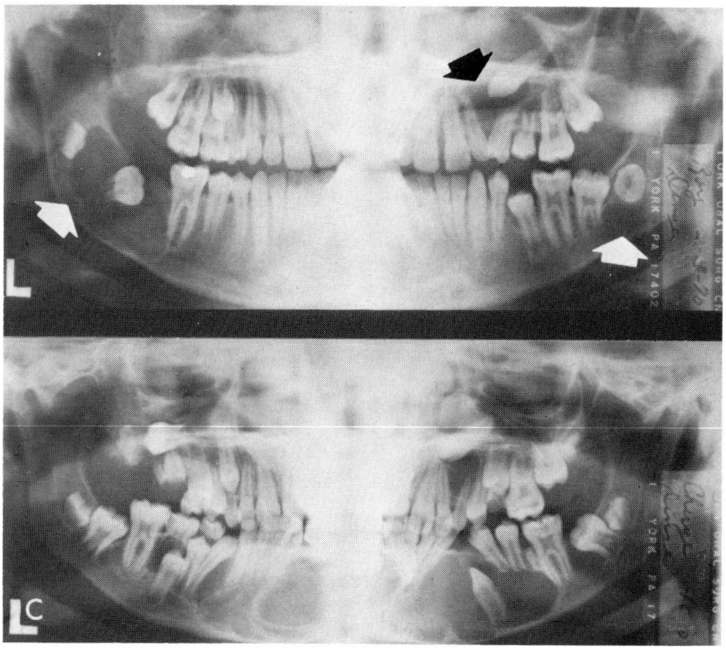

Figure 17–12 *Continued* *C*, Panographic radiographs of son (top) and daughter (bottom). Jaw cysts in the affected boy are indicated by arrows. (From Miller, A. S., et al. Nevoid basal-cell carcinoma syndrome. Oral Surg. *36*(*4*):533–543, October 1973.)

Mucoepidermoid Carcinoma

The parotid gland and the palatal glands are the frequent sites for mucoepidermoid carcinoma. The tumor is seen predominantly in males (55 per cent) and comprises approximately six to eight per cent of all tumors of the salivary glands. Nearly one-half of the tumors present in patients in the third to fifth decade. Nearly 850 mucoepidermoid carcinomas have been reported.[52]

Mucoepidermoid carcinoma, adenoid cystic carcinomas and adenocarcinomas are included in aberrant salivary gland tumors which are primary within lingual salivary gland depressions or within the jaw bones.[84]

Sebaceous Cell Tumors

Lesions involving sebaceous cells in the parotid region are considered very rare. An asymptomatic mass in the superior portion of the right or left parotid gland which enlarges slowly over a period of two years may be a sebaceous lymphadenoma or a low-grade carcinoma. Sebaceous cells are apparently the dominant part of most tumors in this region. In comparison, a lymphoid background is a prominent part of the lesion called sebaceous lymphadenoma.[37]

The first report of malignant sebaceous cell carcinoma of the parotid region not related to another tumor was presented in 1966. Histologic examination indicated that the tumor was composed of sebaceous-like cells and ruled out skin appendages as a site of origin (Fig. 17–13).[134]

ORAL MALIGNANT MELANOMA

Oral malignant melanomas are rare. They may appear on the mucous membrane as a painless black discoloration or swelling or raised mass which may grow slowly for long periods, six to eight years, before they become friable, hemorrhagic, ulcerated and infected or may terminate early with widespread metastases. From 0.4 to 1.3 per cent of melanomas occur in the oral cavity and about 80 per cent of these are found in the maxilla.[35]

Oral malignant melanoma represented 1.7 per cent of all cases of melanoma reported from Sao Paulo, Brazil, 1953–1965. The most common site was the palate (Table 17–33).

TABLE 17-32 CHARACTERISTICS OF THE BASAL CELL NEVUS SYNDROME*

	DEFECT	FREQUENCY
Age of occurrence		Early childhood, puberty, before 25 years
Dental anomalies	Mandibular cysts	Almost constant
	Maxillary cysts	Occasional
Skeletal anomalies	Bifid ribs	
Rib	Anterior flattening	
	Synostoses	
	Partial agenesis	
	Rudimentary cervical ribs	
Vertebral	Scoliosis	
	Cervical fusion	Significant when present
	Thoracic fusion	
Metacarpals	Spina bifida occulta	20% of patients
Brachymetacarpalism	Shortening of fourth metacarpal	Occasionally pronounced Usually not marked
Defective Dentition	Caries	Marked
	Misshapen	Permanent
Cutaneous Anomalies	Basal cell epitheliomas	2–25 years Multiple – several hundred
	Benign cysts and tumors	One or two present usually; sometimes many present
	Milia	
	Epithelial cysts	
	Lipomas	
	Fibromas	Red
	Dyskeratosis of palms and soles	Areas 1 to 1 mm. in diameter with marked decrease in production of melanin
Neurological Anomalies	Mental retardation and aberration	Infrequent individual occurrence
	Electroencephalographic changes	Defects of the system frequently noted
	Calcification of the dura	
	Agenesis of the corpus callosum	
	Medulloblastomas	
Ophthalmologic	Hypertelorism	Fairly common
Abnormalities	Dystropia canthorum	Fairly common
	Internal strabismus	
	Congenital blindness	Questionable significance
Sexual Abnormalities		
Hypogonadism	Absent or undescended testes	
	Infantile external genitalia	Increased frequency recorded
	Female pubic hair pattern	
	Scanty facial hair	
	Ovarian fibromas (non-interference with reproductive ability)	Constant feature
Miscellaneous Abnormalities	Inheritance pattern	Inherited
	Hyporesponsiveness to parathormone	Autosomal dominant polymorphic trait with good penetrance but with variable expressivity; occurs equally in males and females
	Lymphatic cysts	

*Compiled from Berlin, N. I., Van Scott, E. J., Clendenning, W. E., Archard, H. O., Block, J. B., Witkop, C. J., and Haynes, A.: Basal cell nevus syndrome. Ann. Int. Med. *64*:403–421, February 1966.

Lesions were most frequent in Caucasian males over 30 years of age (Table 17–34).

Five-year survival was obtained in only one case of the lip.[12] Most patients died of intense dissemination of the melanoma. Three cases of oro-nasal malignant melanoma had an unusual survival rate varying from 4 to 30 years.[87]

Six cases of primary malignant melanoma of the oral cavity were seen at Mulago Hospital, Kampala, between 1960 and 1965 (Table 17–35).[19] Eighty-three per cent occurred in females. The incidence of male

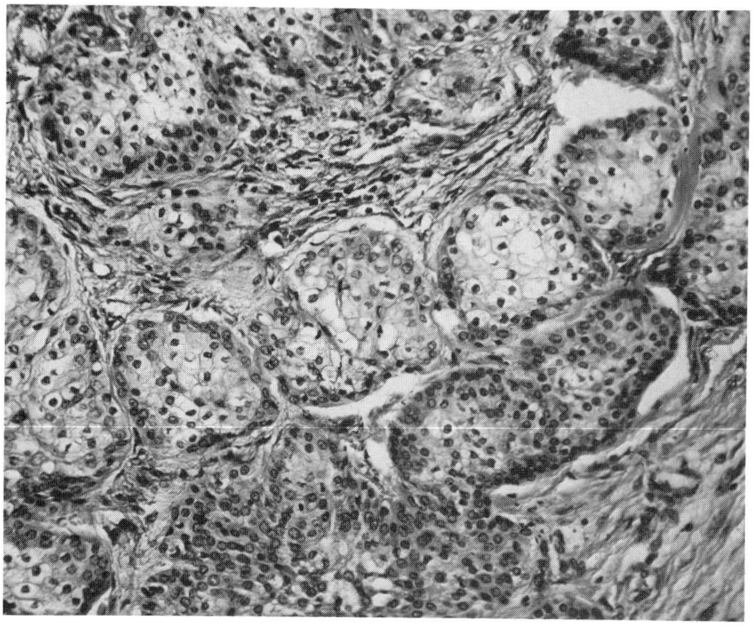

Figure 17–13 Clusters of malignant sebaceous glands. (× 240) (From Silver, H., and Goldstein, M. A.: Sebaceous cell carcinoma of the parotid region. Cancer *19*:1773–1779, 1966.)

to female was 1:5. Most were clinically silent, grew slowly, and involved the maxilla and/or palate. The incidence of oral melanomata varies from 2 to 21 per cent among all cases of malignant melanoma (Table 17–36).[19]

By 1967, less than 10 cases of malignant melanoma had been reported in albinos and only one of these gave the maxillary gingiva as the primary site.[57] The lesion presented as an epulis-like mass on the buccal gingiva anterior to the maxillary left first molar in a 45-year-old Caucasian. Of 24 cases reported, 1964–1971, the majority (33 per cent) occurred in the eighth decade. Most (33 per cent) involved the palate.

TABLE 17–33 SPECIFIC ANATOMICAL INCIDENCE OF ORAL MALIGNANT MELANOMA (Sao Paulo, Brazil, 1953–1965)*

SITE	TOTAL MALIGNANT TUMORS	MELANOMA
Palate	242	4
Lower Lip	928	1
Buccal Mucosa	105	1
Upper Gum	98	1

*From Bertelli, A.: Malignant melanoma of the mouth. Arch. Otolaryngol. 87:68–71, January 1968.

Culture of cells from cases proved by biopsy to be malignant melanoma have been maintained for periods up to four months. Four cell types have been identified with the electron microscope.[20] The cells were primarily oligodendritic on primary culture and bi-polar tyrosinase-positive melanocytes on subculture.

Premelanosomes have been detected.[86] These observations are in keeping with those of other investigators made on explants of malignant melanoma from other sites.[39]

Under the electron microscope malignant cells were polydendritic, with large indented nuclei and prominent nucleoli. The cytoplasm contained individual "melano-

TABLE 17–34 GENERAL INCIDENCE OF ORAL MALIGNANT MELANOMA (Sao Paulo, Brazil, 1953–1965)*

SEX	RACE	AGE	
4 = Male	4 = White	31–40	1
3 = Female	3 = Negro	41–50	2
		51–60	2
		61–70	2

*From Bertelli, *ibid.*

TABLE 17-35 PRIMARY MALIGNANT MELANOMA (Uganda, 1960–1965)*

	AGE	SEX	LOCATION	SIZE/BIOLOGY	LYMPHADENOPATHY
Case 1	55	Female	Rt. side mandible, 2 mo., painless swelling	5 cm. long; ulcerated, friable	Rt. smg lymphadenopathy
Case 2	27	Female	Lt. mandible, 2 yr., slowly growing	5 cm. long; black mass, alveolar margin, left maxilla and roof of mouth	Lt. smg and cervical lymphadenopathy
Case 3	60	Female	Lt. mandible, 3 mos., swelling following tooth extraction	3 × 2 cm.; black mass, superior alveolus, left mandible firm, painless, non-ulcerated	No palpable lymphnodes
Case 4	42	Female	Palate, 9 mo., painless swelling	Raised pigmented, ululcerated, friable mass	No palpable lymphnodes
Case 5	35	Female	Lt. mandible, 6 mo., painless swelling	Bluish-black mass, hard palate bilaterally—left buccal sulcus for about 6 cms.	
Case 6	60	Male	Lt. mandible	Black mass; rt. buccal sulcus extends from lower incisors to the fauces maxilla and palate	Metastases to lungs, pancreas, adrenals, stomach, gall bladder, urinary bladder

*From Broomhall, C., and Lewis, M. G.: Malignant melanoma of the oral cavity in Ugandan Africans. Brit. J. Surg. *54*(7):581–584, July 1967.

somes" and clumps of melanin cell surfaces and many microvillous projections.[86]

PLEOMORPHIC RHABDOMYOSARCOMA

Extraoral swelling of the mandible coupled with a hard, elastic mass intraorally on the gingiva which rapidly enlarges and is accompanied by pain, hemorrhage and impaired chewing should alert one to the possibility of a rare malignant tumor of muscle.[70]

Rhabdomyosarcoma is a malignant tumor of mesenchymal origin and striated muscle. It may present on the gingiva or be located in the tongue as a painless, fleshy, red hard mass.[70] Males are affected twice as often as females. The tumor usually occurs in the fifth decade of life. Rhabdomyosarcomas show local recurrences or distal metastases. The time of appearance of local recurrences and distal metastases varies from two weeks to 24 months.

Survival from the time of diagnosis varies from 22 months[44] to 17 months[141] to 10

TABLE 17-36 DATA IN REVIEW OF MALIGNANT MELANOMA*

AUTHOR	YEAR	NO. OF CASES OF MELANOMA	NO. OF CASES IN ORAL CAVITY	RACE
Baxter	1949	170	2 (1–2 per cent)	Colored (mostly Negroes)
Morris and Horn	1951	287	7 (2–4 per cent)	Negroes
Pack, Gerber and Scharnagel	1952	1190	21. (1–8 per cent)	All races
Moore and Martin	1955	1557	12 (0–8 per cent)	All races
Broomhall and Lewis	1967	125	10 (8–0 per cent)	Negroes

*From Broomhall and Lewis, *ibid.*

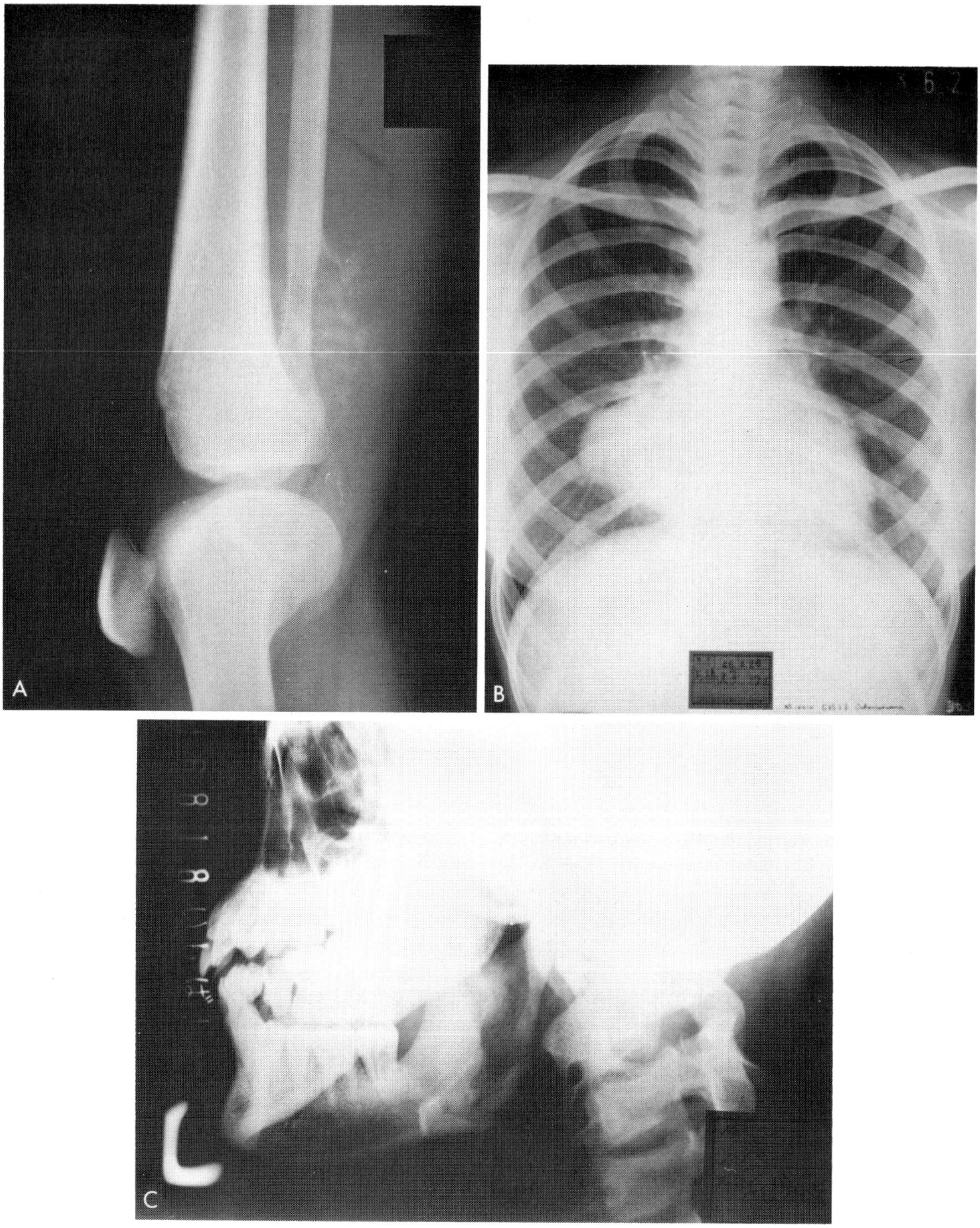

Figure 17–14 *A*, Lateral radiograph of the knee and proximal leg. There is destruction of the cortex in the left proximal fibula with amorphous calcification in the soft tissue. Codman's triangle is noted. These changes are suggestive of malignant bone tumor. *B*, Frontal chest radiograph showing a large mass in the right lower lung medially that obscures the right cardiac border. The tumor has a slightly lobulated appearance. *C*, Lateral oblique radiograph of the mandible showing ill-defined mandibular bone destruction just posterior to the third molar socket. (From Ohba, T., Katayama, H., Nakagawa, E. and Takeda, N.: Mandibular metastasis of osteogenic sarcoma. Oral Surg. *39*(5):821–825, May 1975.)

months.[93] Rhabdomyosarcoma constituted less than one per cent of all tumors of the jaws seen in Koreans during the period 1939 through 1965.[38]

OSTEOGENIC SARCOMA

A sun-ray roentgenographic appearance should alert one to the possibility of osteogenic sarcoma. Wide resection is apparently curative for osteogenic sarcoma of the mandible due to the tendency of the tumor to spread late and to grow slowly. The presenting symptoms may be as vague as a "sensation of tightness" of the maxilla[78] and a slowly increasing swelling of the soft tissue or pain, trismus or hemorrhage from the mandible.[34] Osteogenic sarcoma of the mandible is frequently found in individuals averaging from 30 to 40 years of age and causes death by extensive local recurrence.

Early diagnosis is directly related to early roentgenologic survey showing an osteolytic lesion with occasional destruction of the alveolar plate. High-intensity radiation followed by wide excision of the mandible and adjacent soft tissue provides the best cure rate (Fig. 7–14).[100a]

Ewing's Sarcoma

As late as 1968 only 36 cases of Ewing's sarcoma of the mandible and maxilla had been reported in the scientific literature. The patient may be as young as three years of age. The lesion may present on the gingiva as an exophytic radiosensitive tumor mass accompanied by pain and swelling and extensive areas of necrosis.[108]

CHONDROSARCOMA

Chondrosarcoma of the mandibular symphysis occurs in approximately 19 per cent of cases of the disease that are primary to the mandible. Less than 70 cases of chondrosarcoma of the jaws have been reported. The first symptom may be loosening of the incisor teeth, associated with a radiolucent bony defect. The local destruction may be extensive.

Distant metastases occur to the lungs and bone and usually terminate the disease. The tumor is responsive to local excision.[55]

Chondrosarcoma must be differentiated from chondromas, exostoses, hyperplastic deformities and other malignant tumors of the condyle which may produce facial asymmetry. Marked facial asymmetry with prognathism with unilateral deviation of the chin, cross bite and increased height of the ramus is characteristic of hyperplasia and exostosis of the mandibular condyle.

FIBROSARCOMA

Oral fibrosarcoma is relatively rare. The tumor is solid, single and well encapsulated. Growth is along lines of least resistance. Mesenchymal elements predominate.

The presence of a slowly or rapidly growing mass in the maxilla, producing mobility of the teeth, swelling of the alveolar process, ulceration of the gingival mucosa, unilateral nasal obstruction, mucopurulent or serosanguineous discharge, headaches and ocular disturbances is the typical clinical feature of oral fibrosarcoma. X-ray may show extensive destruction of the hard palate and antrum and cloudiness of the antrum. The tumor is most common in the second and third decades (Fig. 17–7*H*).[14, 147]

Fibrosarcoma of the head and neck is treated by surgical removal only. The malignancy shows no sex predilection and presents between 21 and 50 years of age. Metastases are predominantly hematogenous. Undifferentiated fibrosarcoma has aggressive local recurrence and widespread metastasis. Differentiated fibrosarcomas (fibromatosis) rarely metastasize but do recur locally.[40]

LYMPHOSARCOMA

Enlargement of the cervical lymph nodes, a painless swelling in the floor of the

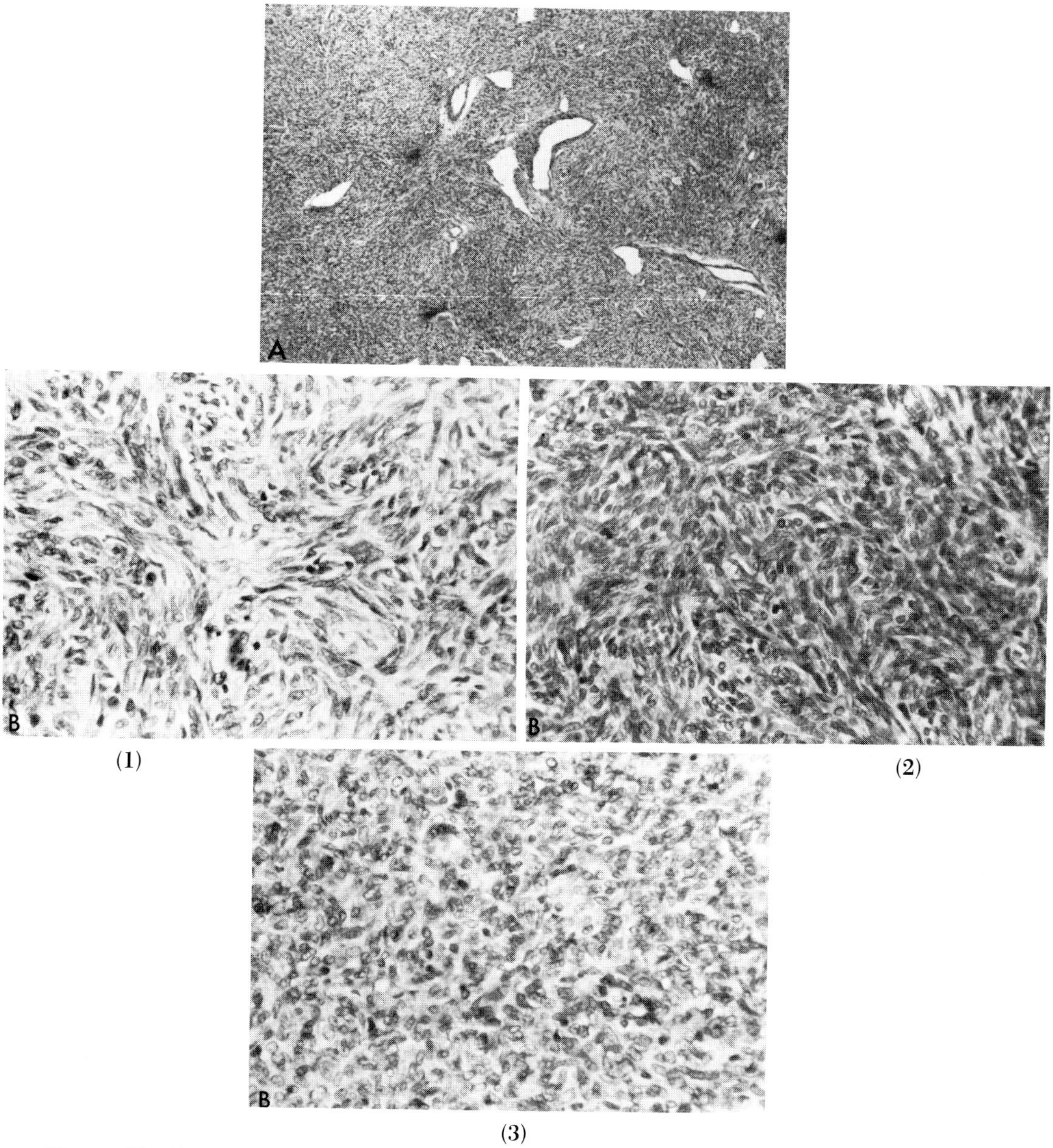

Figure 17–15 *A*, Low-power view showing vascular spaces of different sizes and shape. Lesion is predominantly cellular. Blood vessels are absent in regions of densely packed cells. *B*, Medium-high-power view showing (1) loosely packed elongated cells, (2) dense elongated cells, and (3) rounded cells. *C*, High-power view of region showing mitotic figure (arrow). Mostly cells are elongated and nuclei are vesicular. *D*, High-power view of silver stain showing no tumor on inside of sheath around blood vessels. (From Das, A. K., and Gans, B. J.: Hemangiopericytoma of oral cavity: Review of literature and report of case. J. Oral Surg. Anesth. Hosp. D. Serv. *23*:456–460, July 1965.)

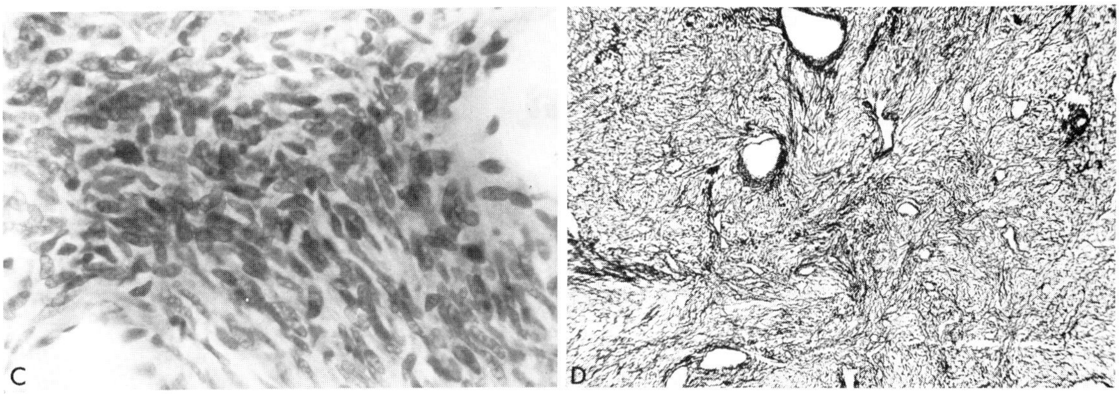

Figure 17-15 *Continued.*

mouth, on the gingiva, in the cheek or on the palate, is frequently the first clinical evidence of the presence of a malignant tumor of lymphoid tissue, the lymphosarcoma. The disease has been shown to arise from or to involve any of the oral tissues, including the salivary glands. The disease may present without pain, difficulty in swallowing or elevation of temperature. The only presenting symptom may be facial asymmetry. The predominant cell may be lymphoblastic or lymphocytic.[146]

RETICULUM CELL SARCOMA

Reticulum cell sarcoma is usually fatal after an acute course and is predominantly observed in young adults and children, approximately 70 per cent under 40 and 35 per cent under 20 years of age.[145] It may be metastatic or primary to the jaws.[4] The tumor is characterized by rapid osteolytic changes of a diffuse nature, widespread metastasis and death. Jaw lesions show radiosensitivity.[4]

Nearly one-half of the sarcomas seen in Korea from 1959 through 1965 were reticulum-cell sarcomas (12 of 25).[38] Eight cases of primary reticulum-cell sarcoma of the mandible reviewed in 1955 showed swelling and bony destruction constantly. Most were asymptomatic.[58] The mandibular lesion may present as a "firm, non-tender, smooth mass in the right side of the neck from the mastoid process to the clavicle and from the sternocleidomastoid muscle anteriorly to the posterior cervical triangle." The periodontal spaces may be widened, especially in the molar region. Biopsy may show large polygonal cells with large vesicular nuclei, or cuboidal cells with poorly defined borders, marked nuclear pleomorphism and prominent nuclei surrounded by fibrous tissue.

ANGIOSARCOMA

Angiosarcoma is a rare malignant tumor of blood vessel origin and may occur anywhere there are blood vessels, muscle, deep tissues or periosteum.[26] It is especially rare in the oral cavity.

In the soft tissues of the oral cavity, the lesion appears as a rapidly enlarging tumor mass on a sessile base which may be tender and fluctuant. Only seven instances of angiosarcoma in the mouth have been reported (Table 17-37).

TABLE 17-37 ORAL ANGIOSARCOMA CASES*

LOCATION	NUMBER	PRIMARY	METASTATIC
Mandible	3	2	1
Maxilla	1	1	
Tongue	1		1
Floor of Mouth	1	1	
Gingiva	1	1	

*From Albright, C. R., Shelton, D. W., Vatral, J. J., and Hobin, F. C.: Angiosarcoma of the gingiva: A case report. J. Oral Surg. *28*:913-917, December 1970.

The first case occurring in the gingiva and the first case in the oral cavity of a Negro, a 34-year-old male, was reported in 1970. The lesion appeared pathologically as a malignant neoplasm producing abnormal vascular spaces containing blood.[3] The etiologic factors are unknown and the frequency of occurrence has apparently not been established.

There appears to be a predilection in the Jewish population (14 out of 20 patients or 70 per cent), with both sexes about equally affected (55 per cent male, 45 per cent female).

HEMANGIOPERICYTOMA

Hemangiopericytoma has been reported in the tongue, salivary glands and pharynx[43] as rare benign tumors (Fig. 17–15).[43] The tumor arises from pericytes around capillary walls. Most demonstrate aggressive behavior and frequently recur after local excision.

The malignant hemangiopericytoma occurs in approximately 22 per cent of the tumors. They metastasize to the peritoneum, lung, bone, liver, lymph nodes and subcutaneous tissue. One case of oral malignant hemangiopericytoma presented in the cheek and mandible of a 16-year-old boy in an area where an ameloblastoma had been removed four years previously[114] without signs of recurrence of the ameloblastoma.

LEUKEMIA

The most frequent cancer in children is leukemia. The gingivae are distended by leukemic infiltrates but frank hemorrhage, as observed in adults, seldom occurs.[112] Leukemia is a neoplastic disease originating in the blood-forming tissues of the body. Its "face" presents as an abnormal and uncontrolled proliferation of mature and immature leukocytes in the peripheral blood and the infiltration of these cells into the various tissues of the body. Leukemias are usually fatal whether acute, chronic or subacute, monocytic, lymphocytic, granulocytic or myelocytic. The acute leukemias are seen predominantly in children, while the chronic leukemias occur more often in adults beyond 40 years of age.

The presenting oral lesions include ecchymoses, ulcerations, infections and bleeding. Spontaneous gingival bleeding and/or gingival hypertrophy, petechial and submucosal hemorrhage may be the initial presenting oral finding (Fig. 17–16). There may be an associated anemia, hepatosplenomegaly and generalized lymphadenopathy. Mucosal ulcers, cervical or submandibular lymphadenopathy, atrophy of the lingual papillae, pain, pallor of the oral tissues and mucosal ulcers may also be observed.[118]

The white cell count may be less than 5,000. Hypofibrinogenemia, thrombocytopenia and clot degeneration may be seen, especially in acute promyelocytic leukemia.[5] The chief complete figure includes weakness, fever, chills, shortness of breath, nosebleeds and abdominal, back or leg pain.[118]

BURKITT'S LYMPHOMA

Multicentric lymphoma of childhood[23] presents as isolated cases among the South African Bantu,[98] but accounts for approxi-

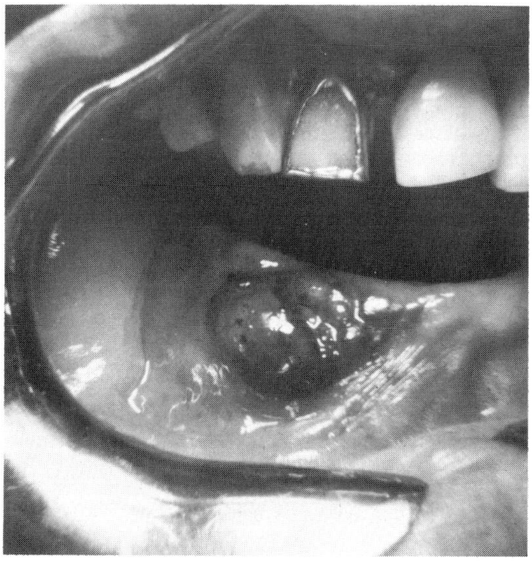

Figure 17–16 Intraoral photograph showing wall demarcated nodular, bulbous, hemorrhagic lesion on alveolar ridge of 38 year old black female. Chronic myelogenous leukemia.

TABLE 17–38 CLINICAL DISTRIBUTION OF BURKITT'S TUMOR IN JAWS OF 285 PATIENTS IN UGANDA*

Unilateral maxilla	113
Unilateral mandible	57
Four quadrants	45
Ipsilateral maxilla and mandible	31
Bilateral maxilla	10
Three quadrants	9
Incisor region	3
Opposite quadrants	1
No details	16
	285

*From Adatia, A. K.: Dental tissues and Burkitt's tumor. Oral Surg. 25(2):221–234, February 1968.

mately 50 per cent of all cancers in children in Uganda.[23, 24] This tumor is also reported to be common in New Guinea.[63]

Cases of Burkitt's lymphoma have been found in South America.[10] Of 21 cases of malignant lymphoma observed between 1954 and 1964 in Cali, Colombia, in patients 15 years or younger, 10 had a histologic picture similar to that of Burkitt's tumor, nine had clinical features resembling those described in Africa, and seven presented the same clinical form but not the histologic pattern.[9]

No area of the jaws of the oral cavity has been omitted. The clinical and radiologic distribution of Burkitt's tumor is shown in the following two tables (Tables 17–38 and 17–39).

Lymphoma cells from patients with Burkitt's lymphoma have been grown *in vitro* in suspension cultures,[51] and a line of lymphoreticular cells (AL-J-G) which adhere to glass surfaces has been derived from similar cultures.[104] Tissue from a jaw tumor produced floating clumps of round lymphoid cells after 59 days of culture, and from these clumps the suspension line AL-1 was determined. AL-1-G cells were round or oval cells which became adherent to the glass surface. With hematoxylin-eosin stain these cells had features of a malignant lymphoma, histiocytic type. On the coverslip, they were elongated and polygonal with pleomorphic lobulated nuclei and small to moderate amounts of pale basophilic cytoplasm. Under the electron microscope they were large (15–20 μ in diameter) and usually ovoid or elongated. Nuclei were large, often lobulated and indented, with one or more large nucleoli and massed projections. Many cells contained multiple areas of Golgi complex and smaller smooth or coated vesicles. Cytogenetically, the percentage of polyploid cells increased over a three-year period from 39 to 100 per cent (Table 17–40). Marker chromosomes included: (1) a long acrocentric chromosome the size of No. 2; (2) a long submedium chromosome the size of No. 4 but with a much longer arm; and (3) a long acrocentric chromosome the size of No. 10. The AL-1 suspension contained from 45 to 49 chromosomes with only 24 per cent of the cells polyploid (over 90 chromosomes per cell): 100 per cent of AL-1-G cells in the third year of culture had more than 90 chromosomes.[104] No herpes-virus or viral particle was found in the AL-1-G cultures.

TABLE 17–39 DISTRIBUTION OF BURKITT'S TUMOR IN JAWS ON RADIOLOGIC EXAMINATION OF SEVENTY-TWO PATIENTS IN UGANDA*

Four quadrants	30
Ipsilateral maxilla and mandible	13
Bilateral mandible	9
Unilateral maxilla	8
Bilateral maxilla	4
Unilateral mandible	4
Three quadrants	4
	72

*From Adatia, *ibid.*

TABLE 17–40 OVERALL PERCENTAGES OF POLYPLOIDY AND MARKERS SEEN IN AL-1 AND AL-1-G CELL LINES*

	AL-1		AL-1-G	
	POLYPLOID	(MARKER)	POLYPLOID	(MARKER)
1967	12%	(80%)	39%	(100%)
1968	20%	(80%)	100%	(100%)
1969	24%	(100%)	100%	(100%)

*From Rabson, A. S., Chu, E. W., Berezesky, I. K., Legallais, F. Y., and Grinley, P. M.: Morphologic and cytogenetic studies in vitro of surface-adherent lymphoreticular cells derived from Burkitt lymphoma tissue. Int. J. Cancer 5:217–223, March 1970.

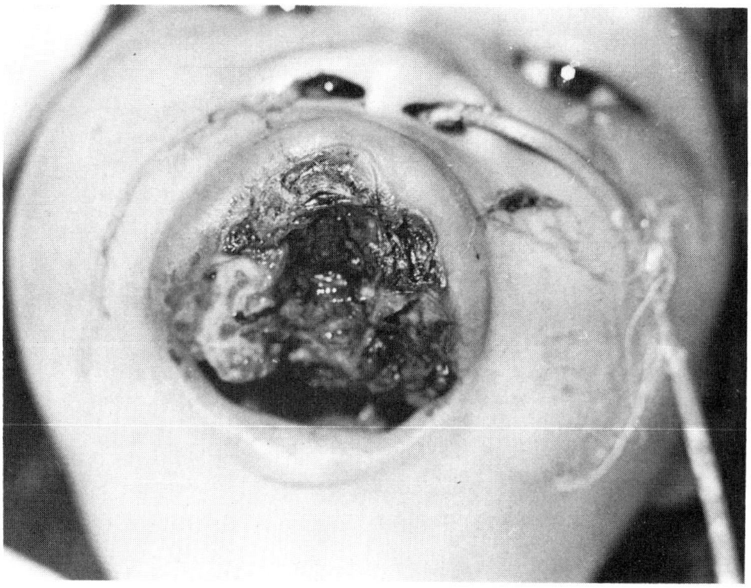

A

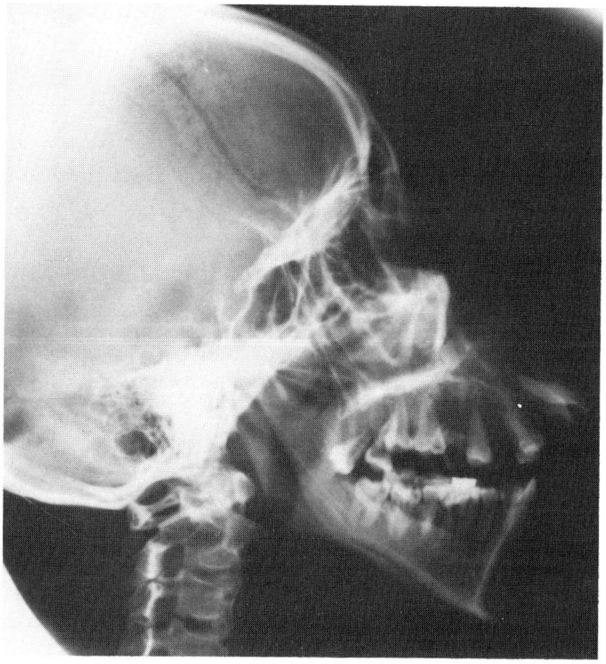

B

Figure 17–17 *A*, Patient at time of admission. *B*, Roentgenogram showing most of anterior part of maxillary bone destroyed and teeth displaced. (From Ramanathan, et al.: Metastatic choriocarcinoma involving the maxilla. Oral Surg. *26*(5):688–693, November 1968.)

METASTASES TO THE ORAL CAVITY

Metastatic tumors to the oral cavity have been estimated to represent approximately one per cent of all oral malignancies.[106] Choriocarcinoma is a malignant tumor of the fetus which grows and metastasizes in the mother, producing chorionic gonadotropin. Metastases are common to the lung, vagina, brain, liver, and kidney, but rare to the oral cavity.[106] It may, however, metastasize to the maxilla, causing destruction of the jaw and displacement of teeth (Fig. 17–17), and present as a fungating mass involving the gingiva without lymphadenopathy.

A painless, raised area resembling fibrous hyperplasia of the gingiva, such as is observed following prolonged use of an ill-fitting denture, may represent metastatic lesions from the stomach,[76, 115] lung,[131] kidney[99a] or uterus.[50a]

The chief complaint may be inability to wear the artificial appliance. Biopsy of the lesion would usually show replacement or infiltration of submucosa by tumor cells (Fig. 17–18).[76]

Renal carcinoma may involve the mandibular gingiva.[42] Distant metastases to the oral tissues have been reported as primary in the breast,[13] bronchus and lung,[69, 149] prostate,[7, 29] testes,[27] colon,[67] ovary, kidney and rectum,[21, 140] pancreas[22] and retina.[83]

Hepatocellular carcinoma with metastasis to the oral cavity is considered rare. When it does occur, metastatic lesions most often involve the bones of the jaws and, with less frequency, soft tissues. The lesion may present as an innocuous, small gingival swelling causing little pain or bleeding. Frequently it is mistaken for a pyogenic granuloma.[15, 105]

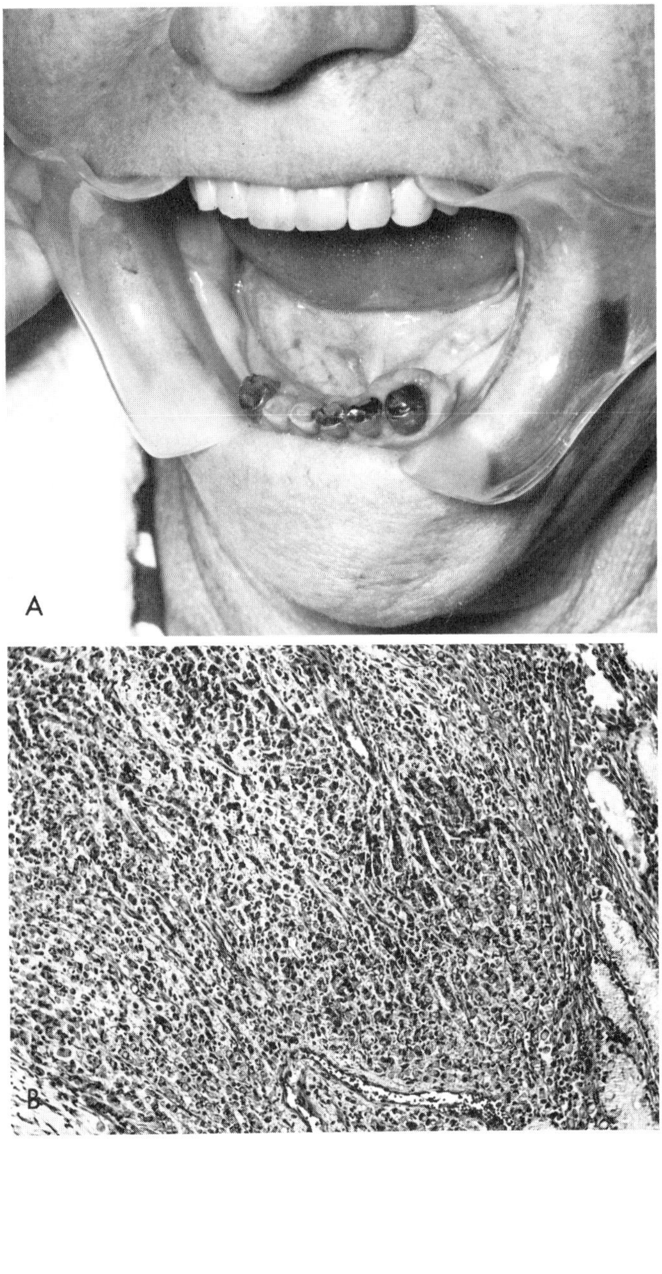

Figure 17–18 *A*, Appearance prior to biopsy procedure. Clinically, tissue surrounding lingual aspect of mandibular left cuspid was normal in color, with no surface ulceration. *B*, Section of primary lesion identified as adenocarcinoma of stomach. (× 85) (From Lund, et al.: Metastasis of gastric adenocarcinoma to oral mucosa. Oral Surg. *26*(6):805–809, June 1968.)

Primary hepatocellular carcinoma of the liver is rare in whites (.01 to 2 per cent) but fairly prevalent in natives of South China. The tumor spreads through the hepatic and portal veins as well as the regional lymphatic vessels.[77] Metastases to the jaws may accompany Wilm's tumor.[47, 96]

Metastasis is more frequently found in the mandible than in the maxilla. The common site in the mandible is the molar-premolar region. This may be explained by the rich deposit of hematopoietic tissue in this region. Metastatic tumors to the jaws usually occur late in the course of malignant disease.

The most common primary sites of mandibular metastases are the breast, thyroid and lung.[21, 124]

Less than 10 per cent of cases of osteogenic sarcoma are primary to the maxilla and/or mandible. This may have wide significance since osteogenic sarcoma is the most malignant tumor of bone and is observed in patients primarily in the first three decades of life. Whereas metastases occur via blood channels and chiefly to the lungs, when they do involve bones, those bones are usually the vertebral column, skull and pelvis – not the jaws.[31, 137]

Firm, tender and egg-sized "lumps" in the tongue should be suspect, especially beyond the fourth and fifth decades of life. Though rare, malignant melanoma, esophageal sarcoma, and carcinomas of the lung, breast, kidney, uterus, prostate and pharynx[153] metastasize to the tongue.

Neuroblastoma

The neuroblastoma is generally a malignancy of early childhood. It is an extremely malignant tumor which has origin from the developing sympathetic ganglion or the undifferentiated proliferating neural tissue of the adrenal medulla. Nine cases of metastasis of neuroblastoma to the oral tissues have been recorded.[136] The angle of the mandible is the most frequent site in children ranging in age from two to eight years. The oral involvement may be noted before, simultaneous with, or following recognition of the primary source.

The oral lesion may resemble a gum boil, with expansion of the lingual aspect of the mandible, enlarged lymph nodes, loosening and separation of the teeth, and displacement of tooth germs. The patient usually experiences weight loss and abdominal discomfort. Radiographic survey may show well marked radiolucencies with irregular margins and numerous small peripheral radiolucencies,[17] or a large radiopaque soft-tissue mass enveloping the mandibular ramus with destruction of the condyle and coronoid process (see Fig. 17–6).[137]

METASTASES FROM THE FLOOR OF THE MOUTH

Generally, carcinoma of the floor of the mouth is associated with only regional lymph node metastases. Distant metastases have been reported at 11.5, 3.8 and 6.8 per cent respectively and may include the mandible, myocardium, lungs, liver, clavicular and hilar lymph nodes. Hypercalcemia is not generally associated with this disease, but may lead to calcification of the lungs and kidneys in the presence of phosphate therapy.

Lymphoma and carcinoma of the kidney, lung and breast are the neoplasms most often associated with hypercalcemia. Of 430 patients with hypercalcemia and cancer, 3.2 per cent (14) had head and neck tumors. Three of the 14 head and neck tumors involved the tongue, and two involved the floor of the mouth (Table 17–41).

Hypercalcemia is directly related to phosphate therapy. Only 36 cases have

TABLE 17–41 CASES OF HEAD AND NECK TUMORS IN A SERIES*

SITE OF TUMOR	NO. OF CASES
Floor of the Mouth	2
Larynx	4
Tonsil	3
Tongue	3
Nasopharynx	2

*From Sheiman, R. A., and Wayne, K. S.: Oral carcinoma and hypercalcemia. Arch. Otolaryngol. 92:198–200, August 1970.

been reported of metastasis to the phalanges from a primary oral squamous cell carcinoma. Terminal phalanges are more often involved than the proximal phalanges by a ratio of 2:1.[30] Late pain in the phalanx accompanied by destructive bony radiographic lesions associated with tenderness, gradually increasing edema and ulceration of the tip of the tongue may be the presenting "face" of distant metastasis.[30]

A 65-year-old Caucasian male was seen in 1958 for pain in his tongue and floor of the mouth which was of six weeks' duration. Oral examination showed four teeth on the left side, an advanced ulcerated lesion (4 × 6 cm.) involving the floor of the mouth, inferior surface of the tongue and the lateral border of the tongue on the left side, and a palpable node (1 × 2 cm.) in the left subdigastric region. The biopsy was reported as squamous cell epidermoid carcinoma (intermediate type). Aspiration biopsy of the left subdigastric region showed the same type of carcinoma. (Occasional involvement of the left and right aspects of the neck occurs from time to time.) Ultimately, in June 1959, the patient complained of pain in the left thumb. Examination revealed swelling and tenderness in the left thumb. Radiograph revealed destruction of bony distal phalanx of the left thumb.

The diagnosis based on histopathologic findings, after disarticulation of the distal phalanx of the left thumb, was squamous cell epidermoid carcinoma. On autopsy there was (1) extensive infiltration of adipose tissue and blood vessels of the tongue by squamous cell epidermoid carcinoma; (2) excessive metastasis of the carcinoma in the heart; (3) squamous cell carcinoma metastasis to lung, spleen, thyroid gland, kidneys and liver; and (4) metastatic infiltration of the lymph nodes, skin and large blood vessels.

METASTASES FROM THE SALIVARY GLANDS

Malignant tumors of the major salivary glands metastasize to the cervical lymph nodes, the lungs, the skin and less frequently, the bones (Table 17–42).[87a]

Metastases originate from adenoid cystic carcinoma, mucoepidermoid carcinoma, anaplastic carcinoma and poorly differentiated carcinoma (Table 17–43).

The average onset of metastasizing disease of the salivary glands is 40 years with an average 14-year span between onset of the disease and diagnosis of the malignancy (Table 17–44).

INCIPIENT ORAL CANCER

Today there seems to be an increasing demand for prevention of dental diseases. During the past decade there has been a great emergence and awakening of the philosophy of prevention of dental diseases in modern dental practice. This present trend in the philosophy of preventive dentistry focuses on all aspects of clinical dental practice. Bearing this concept in mind, one of the major aspects of the preventive dentistry philosophy involves the prevention of

TABLE 17–42 NUMBER OF CASES IN THE HISTOLOGIC-CLINICAL STUDY OF SALIVARY-GLAND TUMORS FROM PATIENTS TREATED AT THE DEPARTMENT OF OTOLARYNGOLOGY AND RADIUMHEMMET, KAROLINSKA SJUKHUSET, STOCKHOLM, 1921–1964

SITE	TOTAL NO. OF TUMORS	MIXED TUMORS *Benign*	*Malignant*	*Total*
Parotid gland	2020	1510	31	1541
Submandibular gland	181	89	3	92
Total	2211	1599	34	1633

*From Moberger, J. G., and Eneroth, C. M.: Malignant mixed tumors of the major salivary glands. Cancer *21*(6):1198–1211, June 1968.

TABLE 17–43 CLINICAL AND HISTOLOGIC FEATURES OF MALIGNANT MIXED TUMORS OF THE MAJOR SALIVARY GLANDS IN NINE CASES WITH METASTASES*

CASE	PRIMARY TUMOR *Gland*	PRIMARY TUMOR *Recurrence*	SITE *Lymph node Neck*	SITE *Lungs*	SITE *Skin*	SITE *Bone*	TYPE OF TUMOR
4	Parotid	X	X		X		Adenoid cystic carcinoma
6	Parotid		X	X			Adenoid cystic carcinoma
8	Parotid	X			X		Adenoid cystic carcinoma
7	Parotid	X	X	X		X	Mucoepidermoid carcinoma
11	Submandibular		X				Mucoepidermoid carcinoma
1	Parotid	X	X	X	X		Poorly differentiated carcinoma
2	Parotid	X		X	X		Anaplastic carcinoma
9	Parotid		X			X	Anaplastic carcinoma
10	Submandibular	X	X	X		X	Anaplastic carcinoma

*From Moberger and Eneroth, *ibid.*

oral cancer because of its seriousness. Moreover, lack of knowledge of definite etiology and primary preventive measures to preclude the initiation of the disease necessitates the orientation of the dentist, the dental profession and the public toward secondary preventive measures; namely, early diagnosis and treatment of incipient oral cancer.

Since the dental office is the first place where recognition of an abnormality in the oral cavity usually occurs, the dentist's responsibility is that of recognition and the identification of any oral lesion which has the potential to become cancerous, as well as referral to specialists if cancer is suspected. Therefore, in order to accept his responsibility as a member of the health team for prevention of oral cancer, the dentist should have a knowledge of the natural history of oral cancer which includes the following:

1. Description of the disease or what it looks like and what it is
2. Ways of diagnosing or detecting the disease
3. How to differentiate oral cancer from other diseases
4. The most frequent locations of oral cancer
5. What happens clinically or identifiable clinical features

As a part of the health team that is involved in the management of oral cancer, it is primarily important that the dentist be informed and motivated so that he will be able to recognize the occurrence of oral cancer and assume the responsibility for

TABLE 17–44 CLINICAL COURSE IN NINE CASES OF METASTASIZING MALIGNANT MIXED TUMORS OF THE MAJOR SALIVARY GLANDS*

CASE	AGE AT ONSET	TIME INTERVAL FROM ONSET TO DIAGNOSIS OF MALIGNANCY (*yr.*)	FIVE-YEAR SURVIVAL	TIME FROM DIAGNOSIS OF MALIGNANCY TO DEATH (*yr.*)
4	54	5		4
6	22	10		2
8	40	20		4
7	27	40		2
11	56	5	X	
1	36	5		2
2	22	34		10
9	51	1		1
10	54	2		1

*From Moberger and Eneroth, *ibid.*

forestalling the ravages of this disease in the incipient stage.

The purpose of early detection of oral cancer is to improve the survival rate, the five- and ten-year survival rate, of the patient. These rates can be enhanced greatly the earlier the appropriate therapy is started. That therapy may be surgery, irradiation, chemotherapy[39] or any combination of these.

Incipient oral cancer is extremely difficult to recognize clinically because the accompanying changes may be so subtle as to produce only minor alterations in function, color, texture, continuity or consistency of the affected tissues.[14]

In regard to the relatively high incidence of oral cancer, the practicing dentist, through the performance of a thorough oral examination, has a very important role to play in the prevention of oral cancer or the early detection of cancerous lesions. Careful attention should be paid to certain critical areas that are known to be common sites of oral cancer.

There are several clinical procedures which the dentist may employ for the early detection and prevention of oral cancer. He can (1) listen, (2) look, (3) examine, (4) x-ray, (5) perform simple diagnostic tests, (6) scrape, (7) aspirate, (8) order clinical tests, (9) biopsy and (10) educate. The ultimate weapon is the biopsy. Let us examine the various possibilities for prevention and detection of oral cancer in terms of their application and *degree of reliability.*

Listen. Listen to the patient! The patient probably thinks that the role of the dentist or other health professionals is to ferret out what is wrong with him. The dentist becomes an agent 007, a professional Killmaster. This frequently means that the patient will not *volunteer* information. The dentist has to drag it out of him. Frequently, too, the patient will not *know* what kind of information is important and pertinent, and hence may respond with only a "yes" or "no" to a battery of questions. The patient frequently fails to remember bits of information until *after* the visit. However, the patient *will* talk and it behooves the astute diagnostician to listen. The dentist is also obliged to conduct the interview in such a manner that the following information may be learned: a complete history of the present complaint, previous dental complaints, previous medical complaints, previous dental and medical history and therapy, life style and personal habits, oral habits, medical and dental phobias and fears, nutritional and religious background, family history, socio-economic status, family size and occupational pursuits. The patient talks, the dentist listens—clues are obtained upon which the dentist can draw logical conclusions. The patient knows his case better than any other person!

Look. Look at the patient! The structures of primary interest to the dentist are usually in full view, though occasionally obscured by a cosmetic veneer. But even though the lips may be red, the eyelashes long and black, the eyelids shadowed white and the cheeks a sunburst brown, it still may be possible to see the edematous ankles, the heightened respiration, the pallor to the nail bed, the vitiliginous or hyperpigmented zones, the facial asymmetry, the open bite, the cervical lymphadenopathy, the keratotic zones, or the butterfly lesions. These signs may be the first evidence of abnormality. They may already represent the advanced "face" of disease. They may, however, be the first "face," the early face of cancer. One can learn a great deal about the health of the patient and the potential for the development of oral or para-oral cancer by astute observation of the patient. *The look* when added to *the listen* may result in the early diagnosis of cancer.

Examine. Examine the patient! Every patient deserves complete examination of the oral and paraoral tissues. Techniques may differ from examiner to examiner, but the basic principles remain the same. The tissues should be examined so as to locate and to describe deviations from the normal. Consequently, when examining the external face and the oral cavity, one should look for changes in color in three basic areas—white, red and black. White patches, erythematous zones, petechiae and zones of hypo- and hyperpigmentation should be noted—as well as the duration of such color changes. Four other features need to be evaluated:

1. Consistency—is the tissue flaccid, fluctuant, hard, firm or nodular?
2. Contour—is the surface rough, asymmetric, ulcerated or pitted; is a sinus or fistula present?
3. Temperature—is the tissue cold, flushed, hot, dry or moist?
4. Function—can the patient open his mouth fully; can he eat, talk and breathe normally?

The troika—look-listen-examine—increases the possibility for detection of an abnormality and improves the diagnostic acumen of the dentist.

X-ray. Take an x-ray! Routine bitewing and periapical x-ray examinations of the teeth and jaws frequently reveal the presence of osteolytic and osteosclerotic changes in the bones of the face as unexpected findings. The complete x-ray evaluation may necessitate the taking of appropriate occlusal film, anteroposterior and lateral views of the skull and face.

The x-ray is a fairly reliable tool for the detection of changes in bone contour, bone profile and patterns of bone growth. The x-ray points the way as a reliable indicator of changes in bone metabolism and of the presence of forces which act beyond physiologic limits or which augment its deposition.

Simple Diagnostic Tests. Perform a test! Perhaps the two oral diagnostic tests which hold the most promise in terms of early detection of oral cancer are the sialograph and the toluidine blue test.

The sialograph permits a roentgenographic evaluation of the parotid or submaxillary gland following its instillation with a radiopaque material such as Ethiodol. The technic requires the cannulation of Stenson's or Wharton's duct with polyethylene tubing. Using a Leur-Lok syringe and constant pressure, 1 cc. of Ethiodol is slowly introduced into the duct system. X-rays are taken while the gland is full and at appropriate intervals—one hour, two hours, three hours, four hours, eight hours and 12 hours—to measure the emptying capacity of the gland.

Parenchymal changes in the gland associated with cancer produce specific changes in the sialograph.

Intrinsic lesions produce a filling defect outlined by a displaced duct system. Malignant lesions are generally infiltrative and result in the pooling of radiopaque material on filling. Retention of the contrast medium and its permeation of the surrounding parenchyma upon stimulation of the gland is also characteristic of the malignant process.[113]

The toluidine blue test permits a topographic evaluation. Toluidine blue, an acidophilic metachromatic nuclear stain, has affinity for areas of carcinoma-in-situ and invasive carcinoma but not for normal mucosa. Consequently it affords the dentist a painless method for obtaining information quickly without evoking *de novo* or enhancing a pre-existing fear of cancer in the patient.

Whereas initial observations were limited to the stainability of areas of epidermoid carcinoma,[125, 126, 142] recent evidence indicates that lymphosarcoma, fibrosarcoma and melanoma also yield positive staining.[95]

TECHNIQUE OF USE. Patients with suspected lesions are instructed to rinse the mouth with water and to swallow some water. Excess saliva is removed by suction. A mucolytic agent, one per cent acetic acid, is applied to the mucosa with a cotton applicator. Toluidine blue (one per cent) is then applied with a cotton applicator. The dye should cover the entire lesion and clinically normal margins. Excess toluidine blue is removed by rinsing with water. Lesions which retain the dye stain blue and are classified as positive. Negative lesions do not retain the dye. A mucolytic agent is used so that the dye will come into direct contact with the surface of the lesion.

Lesions which stain should be biopsied. Negative lesions should be followed clinically for variable periods and restained. False positives have not been reported by this technique.[95]

The toluidine test holds great promise for (1) differential diagnosis of dysplastic or hyperkeratotic lesions, traumatic ulcers, and inflammatory ulcers; (2) determination of resection margins; (3) multicentric malignancies; (4) recurrences and (5) differentiation of benign from malignant lesions.

Scrape (acquire a surface sample). It is estimated that 80 per cent of the deaths from oral cancer could be prevented by early detection and prompt adequate therapy.[103]

Cyto-detection, exfoliative oral cytology and oral smears provide the dentist with a third diagnostic weapon which may lead to the early detection of oral malignancy. It too is painless and produces no fear of cancer in the patient.

Oral cytology or oral exfoliative cytology is the study of normal and abnormal desquamated cells of the oral cavity. Cells may be induced to desquamate artificially, by scraping, or may accumulate in the natural fluids of the body and be recovered by aspiration.

The normal oral living cell goes through its life cycle and drops from the surface mucosa to become part of the saliva. Those changes associated with age, i.e., pyknosis of nuclei, loss of nuclei, loss of granules, parakeratosis and keratosis, can be observed in the regular hematoxylin and eosin preparation. Individual cells are desquamated.

The surface biopsy, surface scraping, usually produces sheets of cells in various stages of maturation. Depending upon the vigor of the clinician, they may be *all* surface – seldom are basal cells included.

The cytologic picture of normal human oral mucosa collected by this method demonstrates three predominant cell types representing various stages of keratinization of the squamous epithelial cell. These were blue cells, red cells and yellow cells when treated according to the method of Papanicolaou. The size and stainability of the cells are shown in Table 17–45.[90]

When these cells are grouped according to the predominant types, blue, red and yellow, certain significant cytological patterns emerge (Table 17–46). Blue cells predominated on the soft palate, cheek and vestibular area. The tongue showed a predominance of red cells. The gingiva had a high incidence of yellow cells.[90]

No relationship between age and sex and the distribution of cell types in the oral cavity is shown. Cells may also be collected by using a moist wooden tongue blade. Scrapings taken in this manner from the dorsal and ventral aspects of the tongue and the buccal mucosa of 50 male students, aged 20 to 30, show two cell types – one large, red staining with irregular outline and pyknotic nucleus and one blue staining with more regular outline and longer granular nucleus.

The gingiva released a third cell type – yellow with indefinite outline and no nuclear detail. The degree of cornification was greatest in descending order on the gingiva, dorsum of the tongue, the cheek and ventral surface of the tongue.[85] These cytologic findings agree with histologic and clinical observations.

Smears from oral leukoplakia from six areas of the oral cavity revealed no typical "leukoplakia cell" nor any abnormality in the nucleus or nucleolus. Yellow staining cells without nuclei are found in increased number.[91]

Smears from the center of oral carcinoma are more valuable than those taken

TABLE 17–45 CHARACTERISTICS OF EPITHELIAL CELLS OF THE ORAL MUCOSA*

DENOMINATION	NUCLEUS *(Size)*	CYTOPLASM *(Amount)*	CYTOPLASM *(Color)*
Small blue	Large	Small	Blue
Large blue	Small	Large	Blue
Large mixed	Small	Large	Blue-red
Large red	Small	Large	Red
Red-yellow	Small	Small	Red-yellow
Yellow	Absent	Small	Yellow

*From Montgomery, P. W.: A study of exfoliative cytology of normal human oral mucosa. J. Dent. Res. *30*(1): 12–18, February 1951.

TABLE 17-46 PERCENTAGE DISTRIBUTION OF CELLS

REGION	CELL TYPE	MEAN PERCENTAGE	STANDARD DEVIATION	CONFIDENCE INTERVALS
Soft palate	Blue	50.8	28.8	35.96–77.69
	Red	41.7	27.2	19.82–54.70
	Yellow	7.5	12.9	0.31–20.81
Cheek	Blue	51.5	26.6	37.81–62.48
	Red	43.8	23.8	25.89–60.29
	Yellow	4.7	12.3	0.0 - 9.54
Vestibule	Blue	45.0	28.9	25.29–64.74
	Red	42.9	26.8	28.77–64.01
	Yellow	12.1	21.7	0.50–30.11
Tongue (anterior)	Blue	19.7	16.7	6.93–31.74
	Red	47.3	20.7	33.01–58.33
	Yellow	33.7	21.4	19.32–47.24
Tongue (posterior)	Blue	30.9	16.8	17.77–45.34
	Red	35.5	15.9	25.20–47.19
	Yellow	33.5	15.4	23.27–42.09
Gingiva	Blue	7.3	9.1	0.0 -13.41
	Red	17.8	18.1	4.51–33.30
	Yellow	75.0	21.5	56.98–83.65

TABLE 17-47 CHARACTERISTICS OF ISOLATED MALIGNANT CELLS AND TUMOR TYPE

Hornifying epidermoid carcinoma (21 cases)	Marked pleomorphism	
	Chromatin – salt and pepper, thread-like or in heavy opaque masses	
	Nuclear membrane – thickened, irregular or indented	
	Nuclei – angular or cigar-shaped or round, multinucleated and/or binucleated	
	Excessive cornification, epithelial pearls	
Well differentiated Epidermoid Carcinoma with Minimal Hornification (2 cases)	Nuclei – round or oval; nucleoli large	
	Chromatin – granular	
	Cytoplasm – pink or orange	
	Tadpole or snake cells – few	
Anaplastic Carcinoma (10 cases)	(1) Uniform in Size and Shape	(2) Round or oval
	Cytoplasm – scant	Scant or no blue
	Nuclei – hyperchromatic	Vesicular
	Chromatin – net-like and coarse	Irregularly placed
	Arrangement – clumps	Single/scattered
Transitional Cell Carcinoma (1 case)	Nuclei – large, elongated, vesicular; lobulated	
	Nucleoli – multiple and prominent	
	Cytoplasm – pale, scanty, indistinct borders	
Verrucous Carcinoma (1 case)	Papillary clusters of small round squamous cells	
	Nuclei – round or oval	
	Cytoplasm – scant clear blue or colorless	
	Some keratinized	
Carcinoma in situ (15 cases)	Nuclei large, regular, hyperchromatic	
	Chromatin – granular	
	Cytoplasm (parabasal) – blue, pink or orange with sharp cytoplasmic borders	
Melanoma	Tumor cells – little or no cytoplasm and indistinct borders	
	Cytoplasm – vacuolated stained blue, pink or orange	
	Nuclei – hyperchromatic; pleomorphic	
	Nuclear membrane – delicate	
	Chromatin – small clumps, evenly distributed	
	Nucleoli – large irregular internal vacuoles; central densities; anastomosing filaments	
	Granules – melanin – inside and outside the cell sometimes fused into round aggregates up to 100 μ; sometimes evenly dispersed throughout cytoplasm; orange, black or brown	

*From Medak, H., McGrew, E. A., Burlakow, P., and Tiecke, R. W.: Correlation of cell populations in smears from the oral cavity. Acta Cytol. (Balt.) *11*:279–288, July–August 1967.

from the periphery or margin of the lesion.[92] The most frequent abnormality found in a series of 15 cases of oral carcinoma was an abnormally large nucleus with a definitely altered nuclear-cytoplasmic ratio and with a typical nucleolus.

Smears and biopsies from the same oral mucosal site were evaluated, by different observers in 50 selected patients with carcinoma. Five types of carcinoma were identified in the material and classified as follows:

Type I	21 cases	Hornifying epidermoid carcinoma
Type II	2 cases	Well-differentiated epidermoid carcinoma with minimal hornification
Type III	10 cases	Anaplastic carcinoma
Type IVa	1 case	Transitional cell carcinoma
Type IVb	1 case	Verrucous carcinoma
Type V	15 cases	Carcinoma *in situ*

The cytologic characteristics of each carcinoma type and of malignant melanoma were distinctive enough to permit definitive identification of the tumor mass of the primary tumor (Table 17–47).

Disproportionate enlargement of the nucleus, marked nucleoli and increase in nucleoli, scant cytoplasm and slight anisokaryosis are features of the various types of maxillo-oral sarcoma.[150]

USEFULNESS. Smear of clinically evident abnormalities yielded 45 positive smears from 1,297 smears submitted—a two per cent incidence of cancer. Three patients with existing cancer had their cancer undetected by oral smear.[139]

Over 3,600 smears taken over a three-year period yielded 37 oral malignancies in a Canadian population,[68] 34 of which were confirmed by biopsy. Twenty of these were not clinically diagnosed as cancer and thus the cytological smear provided the early detection of the disease.[68]

Cytologic examination of 1,561 cases (56–67) revealed 312 malignant neoplasms. The correct diagnosis of carcinoma and sarcoma was made in 80.4 per cent (185/230) and 78.5 per cent (22/28) of them.[151]

MULTIPHASIC SCREENING. Automated multiphasic health screening of 14,749 apparently healthy patients 35 years of age and older included exfoliative cytology of all lesions of abnormalities. One intraoral malignancy was found. Ten per cent or 1,468 examinees had an intraoral lesion or abnormality for which a cytology smear was taken. All except six of these lesions clinically appeared innocuous and all except 34 of the cytology reports were returned Class I (no abnormal cells). Of the six lesions which clinically appeared malignant, none was so confirmed on biopsy. One lesion which clinically appeared innocuous, a 0.3 cm. "keratosis" on the lateral border of the tongue of a 56-year-old female, was returned as Class IV (suggestive of cancer) and on biopsy was confirmed as squamous cell carcinoma—one malignancy in under 15,000 patients.[110]

RELIABILITY. The reliability of oral cytology as a prognosticator of oral malignancy varies according to the experience of the user. One series yielded a 98 per cent reliability,[116] another 85.4 per cent[131] (Table 17–48).[131]

The false negatives reported in those series where cytology and biopsy are performed on the same lesion vary from 0 per cent[81] to 26.15 per cent.[111]

False negative percentages fall as one gains experience. The decrease relates directly to multiple examinations, careful collecting technique or adoption of a different collecting technique. Fifty-two false negatives out of 237 cases of carcinoma and sarcoma (21.9 per cent) was reduced to 20 out of 175 (12.0 per cent) and subsequently to 24 out of 268 (9.0 per cent) during the period 1956 to 1965.[151]

Correlative cytology and biopsy of 75 patients with visible oral lesions revealed 34 (45.3 per cent) malignant and 41 (54.7 per cent) non-malignant lesions. All malignant lesions were squamous cell carcinoma. Cytologically, 10 (13.3 per cent) of the lesions diagnosed as malignant by biopsy, were classified as Class I or Class II (false-negative), and one (1.3 per cent) benign lesion was classified as Class III (false-positive).[56]

Twenty-seven per cent of 22 oral malignant tumors were cytologically negative for cancer.[123] In another study of 1,500 oral biopsies and smears, from 10 to 15 per

TABLE 17-48 FALSE NEGATIVES REPORTED WITH ORAL CYTOLOGY*

	NO. OF ORAL LESIONS	HISTOLOGICALLY PROVED	NEGATIVE CYTOLOGY	FALSE NEGATIVE INCIDENCE (%)
Rowe, 1967	372	Carcinomas (65)	17	26.15
Sklar, Meyer, Cataldo, Taylor, 1968	2,052 Biopsy + Cytology	Carcinomas (82)	12	14.6 Reliability 85.4
Dizner et al., 1967	500	Carcinoma epidermoid (39)	4	10.3
		Reticulosarcoma (1)		
		Cylindroma (1)	1	100
Dargent et al. 1968	65	Well differentiated Carcinoma Malpighie (1)	1	7–8
Masson, Faucon	28			7–8
Sandler, 1966	2,758 (592 biopsies)	Malignant (315 of 592 biopsies)	7	2 Reliability 98

*From Shklar, G., Meyer, I., Cataldo, E., and Taylor, R.: Correlated study of oral cytology and histopathology. Oral Surg. 23(1):61–69, January 1968.

cent of oral carcinomas gave negative cytology.[32]

Radiation Changes

If the predictability of the radiosensitivity of oral carcinoma could be determined by the percentage of exfoliated epithelial cells showing radiation effects, thus good radiation response (RR) and good clinical result or survival rates, one could also predict survival rates.[82]

Twenty-two biopsy-proved cases of oral carcinoma receiving radiation therapy were followed by oral smear taken from the tumor and from the surrounding normal tissue, (1) prior to therapy, (2) at intervals of four to seven days during therapy, (3) on completion of therapy and (4) at follow-up visits. The criterion for good clinical result was regression of the primary growth.[82]

The effects of radiation on benign epithelial cells included cell enlargement, cytoplasmic vacuoles, multinucleation, nuclear enlargement, chromatin clumping, chromatolysis, karyorrhexis, pyknosis and nuclear vacuoles.[82]

No correlation could be found between radiation responses and the clinical outcome. There was poor correlation between the cytology at the end of radiation and the clinical outcome up to the end of one year. There appeared to be a correlation between the pre-treatment size of the tumor and the clinical outcome at the end of the follow-up period.

These results were different from those found for predictability of radiosensitivity of carcinoma of the cervix uteri during radiation therapy, where a significant association between good RR and good clinical result and between poor RR and poor clinical result was found.[60, 61]

ULTRASTRUCTURE. Ultrastructural changes of cells exposed to radiation included nuclear and cytoplasmic damage occasionally as independent phenomena. Increases in cytoplasmic fibrils, vacuoles and lysosomes, altered mitochondria and endoplasmic reticula, disruption of nuclear DNA and rupture of membranes were the characteristic alterations.

Malignant cells differed from normal cells by numerous multivesicular bodies, increases in Golgi complexes and endoplasmic reticula and a marked diminution of cytoplasmic fibrils.[135]

Aspiration Biopsy Smears. Aspiration biopsy of salivary gland lesions yields a high degree of reliability in those cases with histologically verified tumors.[49]

In 33 of 413 primary benign tumors of the salivary glands (1953–1965), no tumor cells were identified cytologically—a false negative of approximately eight per cent. The papillary cystadenoma proved to be the most difficult to identify.[49]

Eight of 89 malignant salivary-gland tumors (nine per cent) were denoted as cysts. In 81 malignant salivary gland tumors in which tumor cells were found, only 44 to 54 per cent were evaluated cytologically as malignant or of suspected malignancy.[49] Cytologic and histologic findings were compared in 632 cases where surgery was performed *after* aspiration biopsy of suspected salivary gland tumor. In 31 of 377 cases of benign tumor, no tumor cells were found at cytologic examination—false negative of 8.4 per cent; reliability of 92 per cent.

In 105 histologically verified malignant tumors, 53 were identified as carcinomas and eight as suspected malignant epithelial tumors; 52 cases presented with no malignant tumor cells on cytologic examination—false negative of 49 per cent.[50]

Adenoid cystic carcinoma aspirates were characterized by cells with round or oval nuclei surrounded by a thin rim of cytoplasm. Cells were usually tightly packed in clusters, with "cylinders" of homogeneous mucoid material—spherical bodies surrounded by carcinoma cells.[50,156]

DEEP SUCTION ABRASION. The Waldemar cytoaspirator (CA) is an instrument designed to improve oral tissue sample collection and to reduce the incidence of false negatives. The cytoaspirator produced more than twice the number of parabasal cells as did the tongue blade method (Fig. 17–19).[119]

Clinical Tests. Assay visceral function!

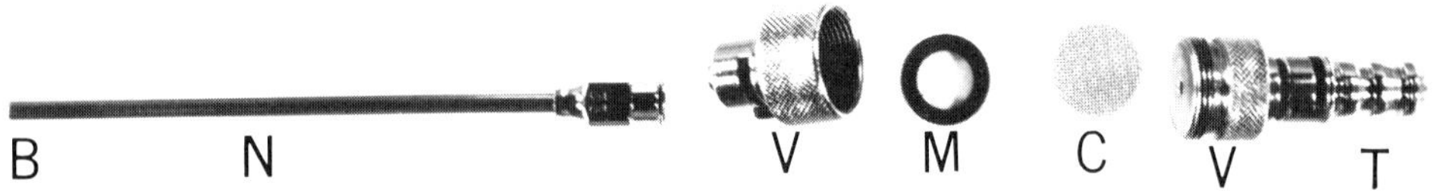

A

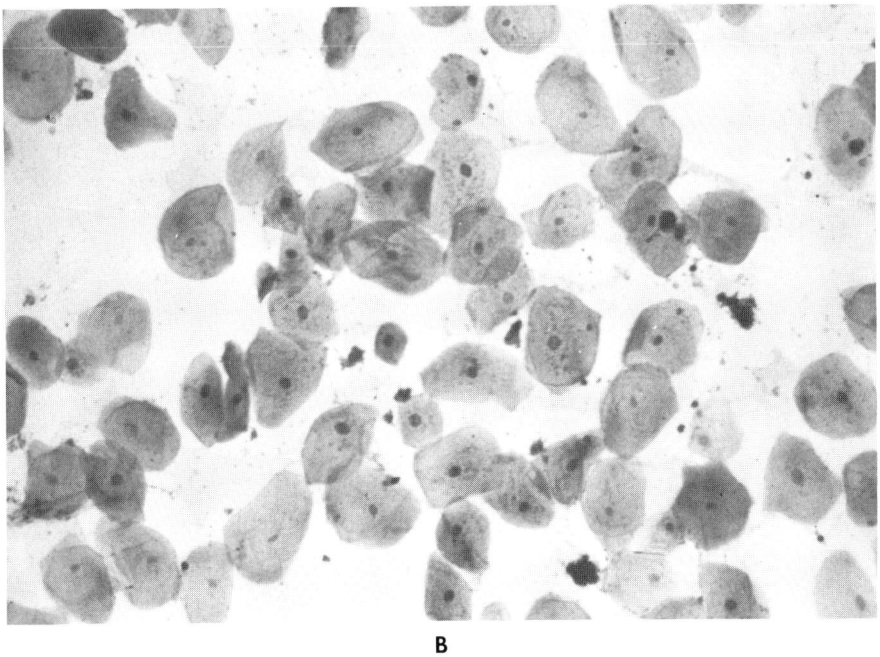

B

Figure 17–19 *A*, The cytoaspirator disassembled: B, abrasive, beveled end; N, 12 gauge needle; V, Ventura chamber to prevent distortion of cells; M, magnetic rubber washer; C, cell screen; V, other half of vacuum chamber; T, suction hose adapter.

B, Specimen, typical field. (Magnification, ×100; reduced 2/5.)

The clinical laboratory is or should be a close friend of the patient suspected of having cancer—advanced or incipient. Analysis of blood, urine and bone marrow will reveal much about the blood cells, their immaturity, composition and hematopoietic properties, hormone output (17-ketosteroids and estrogen levels), liver function and kidney function. These may help to rule out leukemia, diabetes, hepatoma and prostatic carcinoma as causative for oral symptomatology.

Consultation with obstetricians and gynecologists, proctologists and specialists in internal medicine can help to rule out cervical, breast and prostatic cancer as the primary site for oral tumorogeneses. The frequency with which visceral lesions metastasize to the oral tissues and the graphic changes in the maturity of hematopoietic cell type would tend to impart a high level of reliability to these clinical tests, thus providing good diagnostic evidence to support the clinical impression.

Biopsy. When in doubt, take it out! The biopsy is the most important and reliable test to provide the definitive diagnosis for the suspicious oral lesion. The technique requires that a portion of the lesion plus a wide margin of normal tissue be removed for histologic preparation and examination.

The biopsy may be incisional or excisional. The incisional biopsy takes a part of the lesion and is especially useful when the lesion is large. The excisional biopsy provides the opportunity to take the entire lesion and is especially useful when the lesion is small.

In either case, a wedge of tissue is removed, under local or general anesthesia, to sufficient depth as to provide a good opportunity for the oral pathologist to gauge the degree of invasion or extension of the malignancy. What happens to the biopsy specimen? It is placed immediately into an appropriate fixative (10 per cent formalin, Helly's fluid or formalin-alcohol-calcium acetate) and sent to the oral pathology laboratory along with a complete history, x-rays and clinical photographs of the lesion and a clinical impression. After fixation the specimen is processed routinely in paraffin, sectioned at six microns, stained with hematoxylin and eosin, and read under the microscope. The final report is forwarded to the submitting health professional.

Ten per cent formalin is the most widely used fixative and has the advantage that tissues can remain in it for long periods of time without harm or deterioration. Helly's fluid contains potassium dichromate and bichloride of mercury. It provides good cytologic preservation. Formalin, alcohol and calcium acetate (FAC) is a specific fixative for the identification of mast cells in the tissue section.

Educate. Inform the laity! The battle to protect and save lives from intercurrent oral malignancy in the final analysis depends upon the existence of an alert, non-apathetic patient. The necessity for patient education cannot be overemphasized.[75] Patient education starts as a one-to-one relation between the patient and the dentist. To be effective, the dentist has to know how to relate, how to communicate and how to motivate the patient to get him to change his behavior and his attitudes toward his own oral health. Patient

TABLE 17-49 WHAT THE DENTIST CAN DO TO DETECT CANCER

1. Listen to the patient talk
2. Observe the patient grossly
3. Examine the oral and paraoral tissues
4. Use exfoliative cytology on suspected lesions
5. Biopsy suspected lesions
6. Employ diagnostic tests routinely, i.e., x-ray, toluidine blue, sialography
7. Use the clinical laboratory for screening
8. Aspirate when convenient
9. Refer to colleagues for visceral evaluation
10. Correct oral habits and inadequacies

TABLE 17–50 SIGNALS WHICH SHOULD ALERT THE PATIENT AND THE DENTIST TO THE POSSIBILITY FOR INCIPIENT OR ADVANCED ORAL CANCER

1. A persistent, scaly, white patch
2. A pigmented spot which suddenly increases in size
3. An ulcer which does not heal
4. Puffy bleeding gums in the absence of medication
5. Progressive facial asymmetry
6. Teeth which loosen suddenly, without a history of trauma or a blow to the jaw
7. Paresthesia, anesthesia and oral numbness
8. Trismus and pain upon movement of the jaw
9. A lump in the neck, on the face, or in the oral tissues
10. An extraction wound which does not heal
11. Altered taste

education continues as a dentist-community relation. The dentist must not only provide education about oral cancer to the individual patient who comes to his office for services, but he must also educate the wider community.

One mechanism for doing this is through case-finding projects.[88] In these a two- or three-man team (dentist, dental assistant, dental hygienist) visits nursing homes, prisons, low-rent housing projects, high schools, civic organizations, churches, colleges, industrial plants and professional health organizations.

The *approach* is to:

1. Shock the attendees with the grotesqueness of advanced oral cancer
2. Show how debilitating the disease is
3. Provide assurances that the disease can be corrected, if detected early
4. Demonstrate techniques which the dentist and the patient can use which may lead to early detection and diagnosis (Table 17–49)
5. Provide a list of danger signals which the patient can look for (Table 17–50)
6. Provide a list of things the patient can do to prevent cancer (Table 17–51)
7. Perform on-the-spot screening examinations and oral smears of those in attendance

The public health nurse, as part of her home visitation program to shut-ins, can instruct members of the family in terms of good oral health (Fig. 17–20). Film strips, rear projection screens, automatic projectors, hand-outs, throw-aways, animated film, 8 and 16 mm. movies and closed-circuit T.V. may be used to help the dentist meet this responsibility. The effectiveness of this approach hinges upon the ability of the dentist to "tell it like it is," to talk about the "face" of cancer in the language of the population with which he is dealing. Shock, sympathy, rapport and empathy must be established and felt!

In summary, besides the role of the dentist to recognize and identify suspicious oral lesions, another important role is that of educating his patients and the public so that they may be aware of lesions that may predispose to oral cancer and understand that cancer is preventable, although difficult. Finally, it is the responsibility of the dentist to

TABLE 17–51 WHAT THE PATIENT CAN DO TO PREVENT CANCER

1. Don't use snuff, nasally or in the mucobuccal fold
2. Use alcohol moderately
3. Maintain balanced, adequate, nutritious diet
4. Have dental deficiencies corrected
5. Avoid excessive direct exposure to sunlight
6. Use tobacco sparingly
7. Don't pick, lance or burn bumps or pimples
8. Keep the lighted end of the cigar or cigarette outside the mouth
9. Don't use lime and tobacco as a chew
10. See your dentist twice yearly

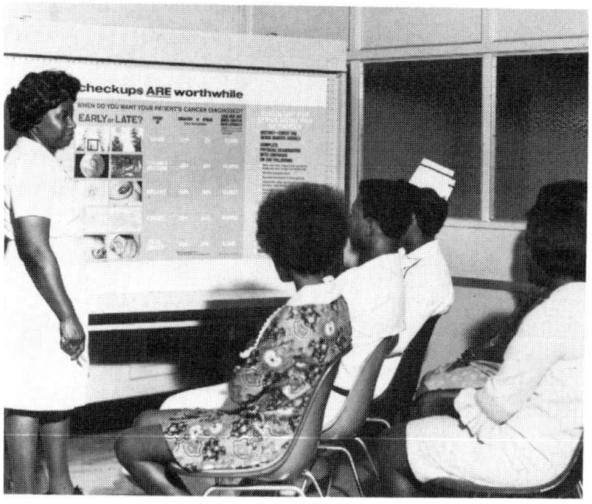

LAY EDUCATION

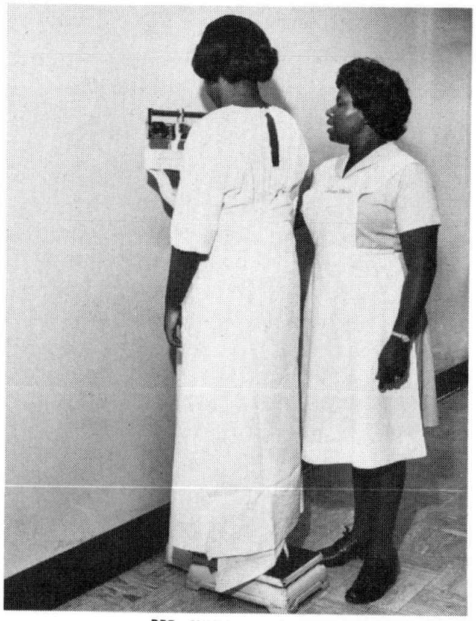

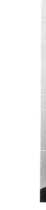

PRE- CLINIC EVALUATION

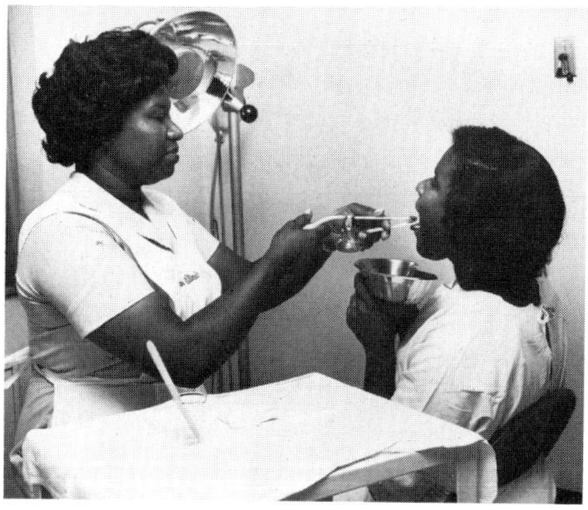

ORAL SPRAY

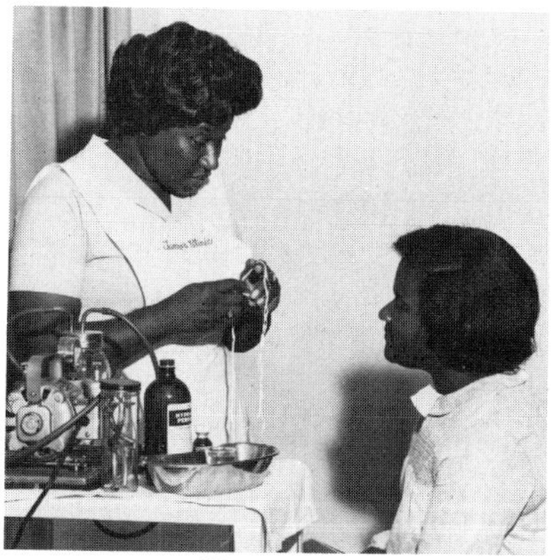

CLINICAL NURSING

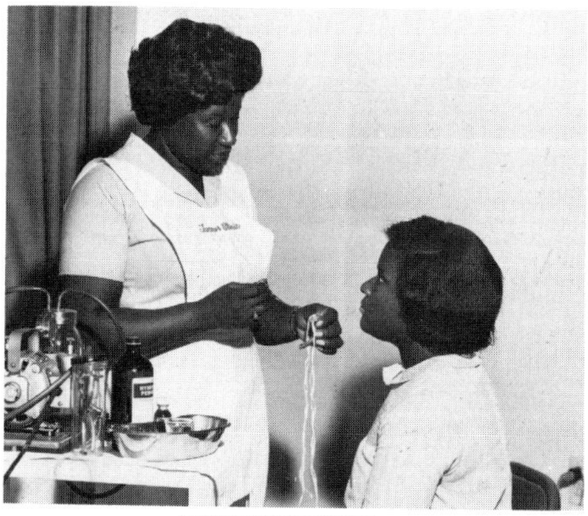

POST-TRACHEOSTOMY CARE

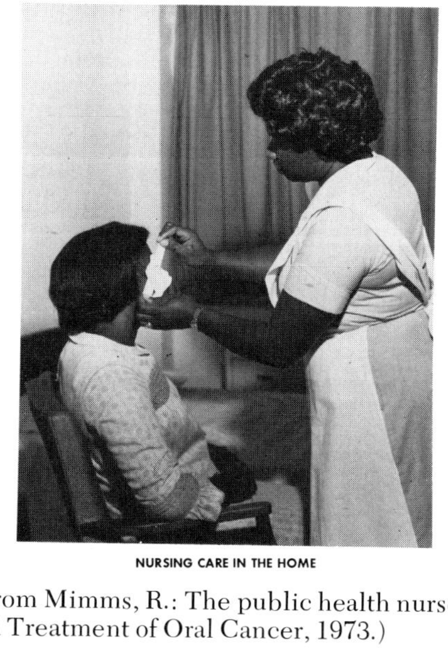

NURSING CARE IN THE HOME

Figure 17–20 The public health nurse in oral cancer. (From Mimms, R.: The public health nurse in oral cancer. In Bolden: A Symposium on the Diagnosis and Treatment of Oral Cancer, 1973.)

refer any patient suspected of having cancer to specialists who are experts in the management and treatment of oral cancer.

DIFFERENTIAL DIAGNOSIS

The prevention and early detection of oral cancer requires that the dentist be able to differentiate between the "face" of oral cancer and several of the *look-alikes* which appear on the oral mucosa. These include (1) leukoedema (2) lichen planus (3) leukoplakia (4) moniliasis and (5) syphilis.

LEUKOEDEMA

Leukoedema affects the buccal mucosa (Fig. 17–21).[79] It presents as a whitish-gray lesion which either persists or disappears when the tissue is stretched. It may involve any age group but tends to predominate in individuals around 40 years of age. In one study, the youngest subject was 14 and the oldest 89.[79] The incidence varies among population groups. It has been reported as high as 90 per cent and as low as 68 per cent in the Negro, 43 per cent in American Caucasians,[117] and from 2.4 to 16.9 per cent in Papuans and New Guineans.[101] The entity is asymptomatic. Biopsy reveals an irregular surface without keratinization, intracellular edema, acanthosis, elongated and irregular epithelial ridges.

LICHEN PLANUS

Lichen planus is a subacute or chronic dermatitis which is usually extremely pruritic and tends to be generalized but may be localized. It is characterized by small flat-topped, violaceous papules, oftentimes with minimal scaling. The lesions vary in size from two to nine millimeters or more. The disease appears in three principal forms: (1) lichen planus, (2) lichen planus hypertrophicus and (3) lichen planus atrophicus.

Lichen planus may occur on the cheek as white lacy lines producing a white lesion or as a red, ulcerated lesion in its erosive form. It may involve the gingiva, palate or tongue. On the latter, white plaques with little or no evidence of linear pattern may be produced. Areas of oral mucosa affected by lichen planus become more pronounced upon stretching. The cause of lichen planus is unknown. The typical history of exacerbations and remissions of dermal and mucosal lesions preceding moments of stress tends to highlight psychogenic factors as causative.[80]

Lichen planus in a 29-year-old freshman dental student presented during periods of examination. Lesions on the buccal mucosa tended to follow the line of occlusion (Fig. 17–22). Lesions on the dorsal surface of the left hand were scaly and dry. The dorsal surface of the right foot contained approximately 16 flat to elevated violaceous, dry, scaly lesions varying in size from two to nine millimeters.[80]

LEUKOPLAKIA

Leukoplakia, a precancerous lesion, may present as a developmental defect, be associated with syphilis, be invaded by candida,[33] be associated with the use of various forms of tobacco,[16, 89] or result from chronic irritation or friction. An incidence of leukoplakia as high as 32 per cent[99a, 155] may rise to 90 per cent in the presence of reverse smoking. The lesion presents as a white patch or plaque on the oral mucosa.

The developmental leukoplakia may be a widespread edematous thickening of the surface epithelium in an irregular fashion or may present as a non-inflammatory, soft, well-defined, butterfly-like lesion on the ventral surface of the tongue.[33] The lesions are generally not seen until middle age.

Leukoplakia associated with the chronic friction afforded the oral mucosa by abraded teeth or smoking will usually reverse itself if the irritant is removed.

Papuans and New Guineans

The prevalence of oral cancer among Papuans and New Guineans had been reported to represent 23.0 per cent and 10.8 per cent of all types of cancer in males and

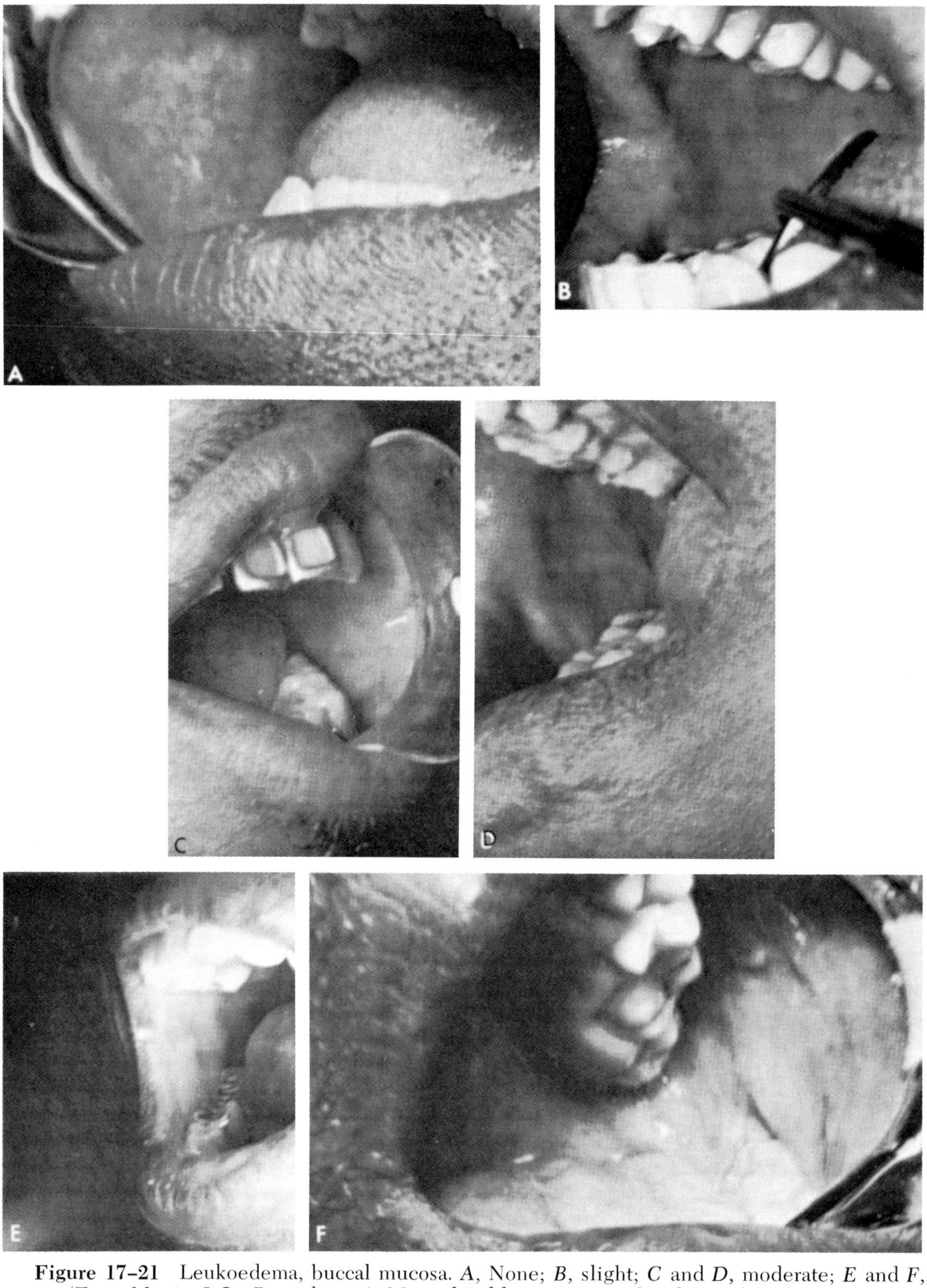

Figure 17–21 Leukoedema, buccal mucosa. *A*, None; *B*, slight; *C* and *D*, moderate; *E* and *F*, severe. (From Martin, J. L., Buenahora, A. M., and Bolden, T. E.: Leukoedema of the buccal mucosa. Meharri-Dent. *24*(3):7–9, June 1970.)

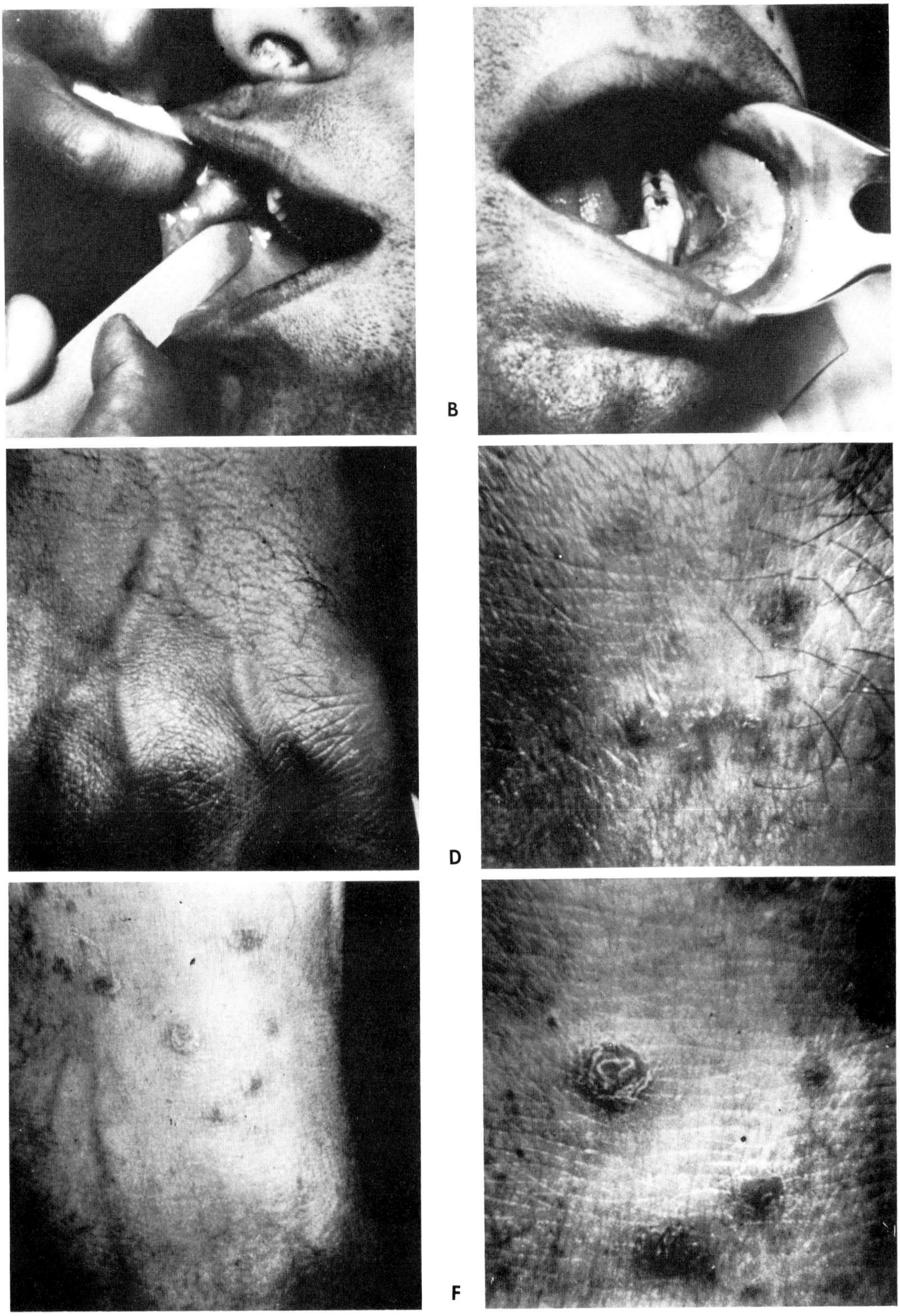

Figure 17–22 Lichen planus. *A*, Buccal mucosa; *B*, mandibular mucobuccal fold; *C*, left hand, dorsal surface; *D*, left hand, closer view; *E*, right foot, dorsal surface; *F*, right foot, closer view. (From Massey, R. M., and Bolden, T. E.: Chronic lichen planus: A case report. The Meharri-Dent. *28*(2): 12–13, March 1969.)

females respectively. Leukoplakia ranged from 11.0 to 13.8 per cent with the highest prevalence among the betel-nut-chewing population.[6] An equally high prevalence of leukoplakia was reported among betel-nut-chewing coastal New Guineans.[54] Recent studies found preleukoplakia in 10.6 to 13.4 per cent and leukoplakia in 3.1 to 6.2 per cent of Papuans and New Guineans. The highest percentages were apparently associated with smoking and betel-nut chewing.[101]

Britain

More than 1,850 cases of oral cancer occur in Britain per year and the incidence rises sharply with age. The mortality is close to 50 per cent. The incidence of cancer in leukoplakia is estimated at 50 to 100 times greater than in the normal mouth.[33] The majority of these leukoplakias are benign. However, the drainage areas of the oral cavity are the most frequent site of oral cancer, and leukoplakias within this area should be expected to develop into cancer more frequently.[33]

MONILIASIS

Moniliasis produces a white patch and is usually observed in the very young and the aged without teeth. The lesion of moniliasis is a surface phenomenon caused by the mycelia of the fungus *Candida albicans.* When the lesion is scraped, the fungi are removed, leaving a raw bleeding surface. There is evidence that the Candida invades the tissue, causing hyperplasia of the epithelium. It is suggested that infective diseases, such as syphilis and severe candidiasis, may be more carcinogenic than tobacco.[33]

SYPHILIS

Syphilis, infection by *Treponema pallidum,* is the great mimic. One must always be alert to the possibility of this marauder. In addition to the mucous patches and fistula of the palate, seen in tertiary syphilis, one should be aware of ulcerations, especially of the dorsum of the tongue. The lesion may resemble the typical leukoplakia. That oral syphilitic leukoplakias may develop into cancer is seen in the evidence presented by Weisburger.[152a] He reported that 100 per cent of patients with serological evidence of syphilis and leukoplakia developed carcinoma in the areas of the leukoplakias.

REFERENCES

1. Abazal, N. A., El-Khanhab, M. M., and Fahim, M. S.: Adenoid cystic carcinoma (cylindroma) of the palate. Oral Surg. *22*:429–440, October 1966.
2. Adatia, A. K.: Dental tissues and Burkitt's tumor. Oral Surg. *25*(2):221–234, February 1968.
3. Albright, C. R., Shelton, D. W., Vatral, J. J., and Hobin, F. C.: Angiosarcoma of the gingiva: A case report. J. Oral Surg. *28*:913–917, December 1970.
4. Appel, P. W.: Reticulum cell sarcoma of the jaws: Report of two cases. Oral Surg. *26*(1):92–95, July 1968.
5. Arthur, A. L., and Salman, S. A.: Leukemia—Report of two cases. Oral Surg. *27*(4):460–466, April 1969.
6. Atkinson, L., Chester, I. C., Smyth, F. G., and ten Seldam, R. E. J.: Oral cancer in New Guinea—A study in demography and etiology. Cancer *17*:1289–1298, 1964.
7. Banerjee, S. C.: Metastasis to the mandible. Oral Surg. *23*:71–77, January 1967.
8. Bardwill, J. M.: Tumors of the parotid gland. Am. J. Surg. *114*: 498–502, October 1967.
9. Beltran, G.: Childhood lymphoma in Colombia, South America. Cancer *19*:1124–1130, August 1966.
10. Beltran, G., Baez, A., and Correa, P.: Burkitt's lymphoma in Colombia. Am. J. Med. *40*:211–216, 1966.
11. Berlin, N. I., Van Scott, E. J., Clendening, W. E., Archard, H. O., Block, J. B., Wiltrop, C. J., and Haynes, A.: Basal cell nevus syndrome. Ann. Int. Med. *64*:403–421, February, 1966.
12. Bertelli, A.: Malignant melanoma of the mouth. Arch. Otolaryngol. *87*:68–71, January 1968.
13. Blake, H., and Blake, F. S.: Breast carcinoma metastatic to maxilla. Oral Surg. *13*:1099–1102, September 1960.
14. Bolden, T. E.: The "face" of oral cancer. the Meharri-Dent. *29*(3):11–16, June 1970.
15. Bolden, T. E., and Smith, R. E.: Hepatoma metastatic to the oral cavity. Quart. Nat. Dent. Assoc. *22*:53–55, January 1964.
16. Borota, A.: Tobacco and the oral mucosa. J. Am. Geriat. Soc. 9: 774, 1961.
17. Bradley, P. F., and Rowe, N. L.: Mandibular metastasis of the neuroblastoma: Report of a case. J. Oral Surg. *28*(10):781–784, October 1970.

18. Bridgewater, V. R. C., and Bolden, T. E.: Cancer of the pulp—A review of the literature—1904-1967. the Meharri-Dent. *28*(2) March 1969.
19. Broomhall, C., and Lewis, M. G.: Malignant melanoma of the oral cavity in Ugandan Africans. Brit. J. Surg. *54*(7):581-584, July 1967.
20. Brown, M. M. L., Borland, R., and Milton, G. W.: Human oral malignant melanoma in cell culture. Cancer *19*:648-656, May 1966.
21. Buchner, A., and Raymon, Y.: Distant metastasis to the jaws: Report of four cases. J. Oral Surg. *25*:246-250, May 1967.
22. Burch, R. J.: Metastasis of neuroblastoma to the mandible. J. Oral Surg. *10*:160-162, April 1952.
23. Burkitt, D. P.: A sarcoma involving the jaws in African children. Brit. J. Surg. *46*:218-223, 1958.
24. Burkitt, D. P., and Connor, G. T.: Malignant lymphoma in African children I. A clinical syndrome. Cancer *14*:258-269, 1961.
25. Cady, B., and Catlin, D.: Epidermoid carcinoma of the gum. A 20-year survey. Cancer *23*:551-564, March 1969.
26. Calhoun, J. J.: Malignant hemangioendothelioma (angiosarcoma). Oral Surg. *27*(2):156-160, February 1969.
27. Cameron, J. R., and Stetzer, J. J., Jr.: Metastatic carcinoma of the mandible: Report of a case. J. Oral Surg. 5:227-229, July 1947.
28. Carr, R. F., and Halperin, V.: Malignant ameloblastomas from 1953 to 1966: Review of the literature and report of a case. Oral Surg. *26*(4):514-522, October 1968.
29. Cash, C. D., Royer, R. Q., and Dahlin, D. C.: Metastatic tumors of the jaws. Oral Surg. *14*:897-905, August 1961.
30. Castigliano, S. G.: Metastasis to the distal phalanx from primary malignancy of the oral cavity: Report of case. J. Oral Surg. *24*:467-469, September 1966.
31. Castigliano, S. G., and Rominger, J.: Metastatic malignancy of the jaws. Am. J. Surg. *87*:496-507, 1954.
32. Cataldo, E.: Comments, J. Oral Surg. *25*:464, September 1967.
33. Cawson, R. A.: Leukoplakia and oral cancer. Proc. Roy. Soc. Med. *62*(6):610-615, June 1969.
34. Chambers, R. G., and Mahoney, W. D.: Osteogenic sarcoma of the mandible: Current management. Am. Surgeon. *36*(8):463-471, August 1970.
35. Chaudry, A. P., Burke, R. J., and Gorlin, R. J.: Malignant melanoma of the oral cavity: A review of 105 cases. Cancer *11*:923-928, 1958.
36. Chaudry, A. P., Vickers, R. A., and Gorlin, R. J.: Intraoral minor salivary gland tumors: An analysis of 1,414 cases. Oral Surg. *14*:1194-1226, 1961.
37. Cheek, R., and Pitcock, J. A.: Sebaceous lesions of the parotid. Arch. Path. *82*:147-150, August 1966.
38. Chung, D. H., Kiunman, J. E. G., Lee, B. C., and Lee, Y. T.: Tumors of the jaws in Korea. Oral Surg. *27*(6):716-728, June 1969.
39. Cobb, J. P., and Kupfer, A.: Environmental influences of the growth of Cloudman S-91 mouse melanoma in organ culture. *In*: Bolden, T. E.: Proceedings of an Oral Research Seminar, School of Dentistry, Meharry Medical College *3*, 1971.
40. Conley, J., Stout, A. P., and Healey, W. V.: Clinicopathologic analysis of eighty-four patients with an original diagnosis of fibrosarcoma of the head and neck. Am. J. Surg. *114*:564-569, October 1967.
41. Correa, J. N., Bosch, A., and Marcial, V. A.: Carcinoma of the floor of the mouth: Review of clinical factors and results of treatment. Am. J. Roentgenol. Rad. Therap. Nuclear Med. *99*(2):302-312, February 1967.
42. Cranin, A. N., Berman, S., and Tucker, N.: Renal cell carcinoma of the mandibular periodontium. Oral Surg. *21*(5):626-631, May 1966.
43. Das, A. K., and Gans, B. J.: Hemangiopericytoma of oral cavity: Review of literature and report of case. J. Oral Surg. Anesth. Hosp. D. Serv. *23*:456-460, 1965.
44. Dito, W. R., and Batsakis, J. G.: Intraoral pharyngeal and nasopharyngeal rhabdomyosarcoma. Arch. Otolaryngol. *77*:123-128, 1963.
45. Dodge, O. G.: Tumors of the jaw, odontogenic tissues and maxillary antrum (excluding Burkitt lymphoma) in Uganda Africans. Cancer *18*(2):205-215, February 1965.
46. Doll, R., Muir, C. S., and Waterhouse, J. A. H.: Cancer incidence in five continents II. Union Internationale Contre le Cancer, Geneva, 1970.
47. Doykos, J. D.: Wilm's tumor metastatic to mandible and oral mucosa. Oral Surg. *27*(2):220-224, February 1969.
48. Dummett, C. O.: Oral pigmentation. J. Periodontol. *31*:356-360, October 1961.
49. Eneroth, C. M., Franzen, S., and Zajicek, J.: Cytologic diagnosis on aspirate from 1000 salivary gland tumors. Acta. Otolaryng. [Suppl.]*224*: 168-172, 1966.
50. Eneroth, C. M., Franzen, S., and Zajicek, J.: Aspiration biopsy of salivary gland tumors: A critical review of 910 biopsies. Acta Cytol.(Balt.) *11*(6):470-472, November-December 1967.
50a. Englert, R. J., and Pasqual, H. N.: Metastatic chorionepithelioma of gingival tissue: Report of a case. Oral Surg. *10*:813-818, 1957.
51. Epstein, M. A., and Barr, Y. M.: Characteristics and mode of growth of a tissue culture strain (EBI) of human lymphoblasts from Burkitt's lymphoma. J. Nat. Cancer Inst. *34*:231-240, 1965.
52. Eversole, L. R.: Mucoepidermoid carcinoma: Review of 815 reported cases. J. Oral Surg. *28*(7):490-494, July 1970.
53. Flamant, R., Hayes, M., Lazar, P., and Denoix, P.: Cancer of the tongue: A study of 904 cases. Cancer *17*(3):377-385, March 1964.
54. Forlen, H. P., Howstein, O., and Stuttgen, G.: Betelkaven und Leukoplakie. Arch. Klin. Exper. Dermat. *221*:463-480, 1965.
55. Fronstein, M. H., Hutcheson, J. B., and Sanders, H. L.: Chondrosarcoma of the mandibular symphysis. Oral Surg. *25*(5):665-669, May 1968.
56. Gaither, W. D.: Comparison of exfoliative cytodiagnosis and histodiagnosis of oral lesions:

Review of the literature and report of 75 cases. J. Oral Surg. *25*:446–453, September 1967.
57. Garrington, G. E., Scofield, H. H., Coryn, K., and Lacy, G. R., Jr.: Intraoral malignant melanoma in a human albino. Oral Surg. *24*(2): 224–230, August 1967.
58. Gerry, R. G., and Williams, S. F.: Primary reticulum cell sarcoma of the mandible. Oral Surg. *8*:568, 1955.
59. Graham, J. K., McJimsey, B. A., and Hardin, J. C., Jr.: Nevoid basal cell carcinoma syndrome. Arch. Otolaryngol. *87*:72–77, 1968.
60. Graham, R. M.: The effects of radiation on vaginal cells in cervical carcinoma: I. Description of cellular changes. II. Prognostic significance. Surg. Gynec. Obstet. *84*:153–173, 1947.
61. Graham, R. M., and Graham, J. B.: Cytologic prognosis in cancer of uterine cervix treated radiologically. Cancer *8*:59–70, 1955.
62. Hendrick, J. W.: Malignancy of buccal mucous membrane, gingiva, soft and hard palate. Ann. Otol. *61*:1094–1113, 1952.
63. Higginson, J.: Environment and cancer. The Practitioner *198*:621–630, 1967.
64. Holland, S., and Bolden, T. E.: Malignant melanoma of the oral cavity. In press.
65. Howell, J. B., Byrd, D. L., McClendon, J. L., and Anderson, D. E.: Identification and treatment of jaw cysts in the nevoid basal cell carcinoma syndrome. J. Oral Surg. *25*:129–138, 1967.
66. Howell, J. B., and Caro, M. R.: The basal cell nevus; Its relationship to multiple cutaneous cancers and associated anomalies of development. Arch. Derm. Syph. (Chicago) *79*:67–80, 1959.
67. Humphrey, A. A., and Amos, N. H.: Metastatic gingival adenocarcinoma from a primary lesion of the colon. Am. J. Cancer *28*:128–130, 1936.
68. Hunter, H. A.: Three year experience with an oral cytology service for the Ontario Dental Profession. Laval Med. *39*:8–10, January 1968.
69. James, P. L.: Metastasis in upper jaw from a carcinoma of the bronchus. Brit. Dent. J. *107*: 308–309, November 1959.
70. Kaloyannides, T. M.: Pleomorphic rhabdomyosarcoma of the gingiva. Oral Surg. *27*(2): 150–155, February 1969.
71. Kawakatsu, K., and Mori, M.: Histochemical evaluation of enzymatic activities in human squamous cell cancer. Cancer Res. *23*:539–545, May 1963.
72. Keller, A. Z.: Cellular types, survival, race, nativity, occupations, habits and associated diseases in the pathogenesis of lip cancers. Am. J. Epidemiol. *91*(5):486–499, 1970.
73. Kraus, F. T., and Perez-Mesa, C.: Verrucous carcinoma: Clinical and pathologic study of 105 cases involving oral cavity, larynx and genitalia. Cancer *19*:26–38, January 1966.
74. Latourette, H. B., and Meyers, M. H.: End results of treatment of oral and laryngopharyngeal cancer. Fifth National Cancer Conference Proceedings. Philadelphia, J. B. Lippincott Co., 1964, p. 281.
75. Lemeh, D.: Personal communication.
76. Lund, B. A., Moertel, C. G., and Gilbilisco, J. A.: Metastasis of gastric adenocarcinoma to oral mucosa. Oral Surg. *25*(6):805–809, June 1968.
77. Lund, B. A., Soule, E. H., and Moertel, C. G.: Hepatocellular carcinoma with metastasis to gingival mucosa: Report of case. J. Oral Surg. *38*:604–607, August 1970.
78. McDonald, R. C., and Fredricks, W. H.: Osteogenic sarcoma of the maxilla: Report of a case. Oral Surg. *26*(5):736–741, November 1968.
79. Martin, J. L., Buenahora, A. M., and Bolden, T. E.: Leukoedema of the buccal mucosa. The Meharri-Dent *29*(3):7–9, June 1970.
80. Massey, K. M., and Bolden, T. E.: Chronic lichen planus—A case report. The Meharri-Dent *28*(2):12–13, March 1969.
81. Medak, H., McGrew, E. A., Burlakow, P., and Tiecke, R. W.: Correlation of cell populations in smear from the oral cavity. Acta Cytol. (Balt.) *11*:279–288, July-August 1967.
82. Memon, M. H., and Jafarey, N. A.: Cytologic study of radiation changes in carcinoma of the oral cavity: Prognostic value of various observations. Acta Cytol. (Balt.) *14*(1):22–24, January 1970.
83. Merrill, R. G., and Westheimer, F. W.: Metastatic retinoblastoma of the mandible: Report of a case. J. Oral Surg. *22*:341–345, July 1964.
84. Miller, A. A., and Winnick, M.: Salivary gland inclusion in the anterior mandible. Oral Surg. *31*(6):790–797, June 1971.
84a. Miller, A. S., Leifer, C., Apllon, P. L., and Bowser, M. W.: Nevoid basal-cell carcinoma syndrome. Report of a pedigree with electron microscopy of skin lesions. Oral Surg. *36*(4): 533–543, October 1973.
85. Miller, S. C., Soberman, A., and Stahl, S. S.: A study of the cornification of the oral mucosa of young male adults. J. Dent. Res. *30*(1):4–11, February 1951.
86. Milton, G. W., and Brown, M. M. L.: Malignant melanoma of the nose and mouth. Brit. J. Surg. *52*(7):484–493, July 1965.
87. Moberger, J. G., and Eneroth, C. M.: Electron microscopic studies of human leukemia and lymphoma. Cancer *20*:760–777, May 1967.
87a. Moberger, J. G., and Eneroth, C. M.: Malignant mixed tumors of the major salivary glands. Cancer *21*(6):1198–1211, June 1968.
88. Mobley, E. L.: Oral Cancer Detection Program. Unpublished data.
89. Moertal, C., and Foss, E.: Multicentric carcinomas of the oral cavity. Surg. Gynec. Obstet. *106*:652–654, 1958.
90. Montgomery, P. W.: A study of exfoliative cytology of normal human oral mucosa. J. Dent. Res. *30*(1):12–18, February 1951.
91. Montgomery, P. W., and Von Hamm, E.: A study of the exfoliative cytology of oral leukoplakia. J. Dent. Res. *30*(1):260–264, April 1951.
92. Montgomery, P. W., and Von Hamm, E.: A study of the exfoliative cytology in patients with carcinoma of the oral mucosa. J. Dent. Res. *30*(1):308–313, June 1951.
93. Moore, O., and Grossi, C.: Embryonal rhabdomyosarcoma of the head and neck. Cancer *12*:69–73, 1959.
94. Mori, M., Morimoto, Y., Yoshimura, Y., and Kawamura, H.: Enzymatic histochemical demon-

stration of basal cell carcinoma in the oral cavity. Oral Surg. *25*(5):746–755, May 1968.
95. Myers, E. N.: The toluidine blue test in lesions of the oral cavity. Ca-A Cancer Journal for Clinicians *20*(3):135–138, May-June 1970.
96. Meyers, W. L.: Metastatic nephroblastoma of the mandible. Oral Surg. *23*:375–378, March 1967.
97. Naib, Z. M.: Exfoliative Cytopathology. Boston, Little, Brown & Co., 1970.
98. Oettle, A. G.: Cancer in Africa, especially in regions south of the Sahara. J. Nat. Cancer Inst. *33*:383–436, 1964.
98a. Ohba, T., Katayama, H., Nakagawa, E., and Takeda, N.: Mandibular metastasis of osteogenic sarcoma. Oral Surg. *39*(5):821–825, May 1975.
99. Orban, B. J.: Oral Histology and Embryology, 4th Ed. St. Louis, C. V. Mosby Co., 1957.
99a. Paymaster, J. C.: Oral and pharyngeal cancer in India. *In* Cancer of the Head and Neck. International Workshop on Cancer of the Head and Neck, New York, May 10–14, 1965, pp. 308–316.
99b. Persson, P. A., and Wallenius, K.: Metastatic renal carcinoma (hypernephroma) in the gingiva of the lower jaw. Acta Odontol. Scandinav. *19*:289–296, 1961.
100. Pindborg, J. J.: Oral cancer from an international point of view. J. Canad. Dent. Assoc. *31*:219–226, April 1965.
101. Pindborg, J. J., Barnes, O., and Roed-Petersen, B.: Epidemiology and histology of oral leukoplakia and leukoedema among Papuans and New Guineans. Cancer *22*:379–384, August 1968.
102. Pindborg, J. J., Mehta, F. S., and Daftary, D. K.: Occurrence of epithelial atypia in 51 Indian villagers with oral submucous fibrosis. Brit. J. Cancer *24*:253–257, June 1970.
103. Putnam, W. J.: The early detection of oral cancer through the application of exfoliative cytology. Hemispheric Conference for Better Oral Health for the Americas, 35–36, September 1966.
104. Rabson, A. S., Chu, E. W., Berezesky, I. K., Legallais, F. Y., and Grinley, P. M.: Morphologic and cytogenetic studies in vitro of surface-adherent lymphoreticular cells derived from Burkitt lymphoma tissue. Int. J. Cancer *5*:217–223, March 1970.
105. Radden, B. G., and Reade, P. C.: Gingival metastasis from a hepatoma. Oral Surg. *21*(5):621–625, May 1966.
106. Ramanathan, K., Eravelly, J., and Ken, T. P.: Metastatic choriocarcinoma involving the maxilla. Oral Surg. *26*(5):688–693, November 1968.
107. Reddy, D. G., and Rao, V. K.: Cancer of the palate in coastal Andhra due to smoking cigars with the burning end inside the mouth. Indian J. Med. Sci. *11*(10):791–797, October 1957.
108. Roca, A. N., Smith, J. L., MacComb, W. S., and Jing, Bao-Shan: Ewing's sarcoma of the maxilla and mandible. Oral Surg. *25*(2):194–203, February 1968.
109. Rosenfeld, L., and Calloway, J.: Snuff dipper's cancer. Am. J. Surg. *106*:840–844, 1963.
110. Ross, N. M., and Gross, E.: Oral findings based on an automated multiphasic health screening program. J. Oral Med. *26*(1):21–26, January-March 1971.
111. Rovin, S.: An assessment of the negative oral cytologic diagnosis. J. Am. Dent. Assoc. *74*:759–762, 1967.
112. Rowe, N. H., and Kwapis, B. W.: Oral and perioral cancer detection. Dent. Clin. N. Amer. 189–201, March 1968.
113. Rubin, P., and Hoot, J. F.: Secretory sialography in diseases of the major salivary glands. Am. J. Roentgenol. Rad. Therap. Nuclear Med. *77*(4):575–598, April 1957.
114. Sage, H. H., and Salman, F.: Malignant hemangiopericytoma in the area of a previous ameloblastoma of the mandible. Oral Surg. *26*(3):275–283, September 1968.
115. Salman, I., and Darlington, C. G.: Rare (unusual) malignant tumors of the jaws. Am. J. Orthodont. *30*:725–739, December 1944.
116. Sandler, N. C.: Errors of oral cytodiagnosis. Report of follow-up of 1,801 patients. J. Am. Dent. Assoc. *72*:874–888, 1966.
117. Sandstead, H., and Lowe, J. W.: Leukoedema and keratosis in relation to leukoplakia of the buccal mucosa in man. J. Nat. Cancer Inst. *14*:423–433, October 1953.
118. Sarnquist, J. L.: Oral manifestations of leukemia. J. Am. Dent. Hygienist Assoc. *43*(3):145–150, 1969.
119. Schemen, P., Lumerman, H., and Altchuler, S: Improved oral cytologic sampling by means of deep suction abrasion. Oral Surg. *26*(4):505–513, October 1968.
120. Schour, I: Oral Histology and Embryology, 8th Ed. Philadelphia, Lea & Febiger, 1960.
121. Schulz, M. D., Lintner, D. M., and Sweeney, L.: Carcinoma of the palatine arch. Am. J. Roentgenol. Rad. Therap. Nuclear Med. *89*(3):541–548, March 1963.
122. Shaheen, O. H.: Malignant disease of the mouth. The Practitioner *203*:23–29, July 1969.
123. Shapiro, B. L., and Gorlin, R. J.: An analysis of oral cytodiagnosis. Cancer *17*:1477–1479, November 1964.
124. Sharp, G. S., Bullock, W. K., and Hazlet, J. W.: Oral cancer and tumors of the jaw. New York, McGraw-Hill Book Co., 1956.
125. Shedd, D. P., Hukitt, T. B., and Bahn, S.: In vivo staining properities of oral cancer. Am. J. Surg. *110*:631–634, 1965.
126. Shedd, D. P.: Further appraisal of in vivo staining properties of oral cancer. Arch. Surg. (Chicago) *95*:16–22, 1967.
127. Shedd, D. P., Von Essen, C. F., Ferraro, R. H., Connelly, R. R., and Eisenberg, H.: Cancer of the floor of the mouth in Connecticut, 1935–1959. Cancer *21*:97–101, January 1968.
128. Shedd, D. P., Von Essen, C. F., Connelly, R. R., and Eisenberg, H.: Cancer of the buccal mucosa, palate, and gingiva in Connecticut, 1935–59. Cancer *21*:440–446, March 1968.
129. Shedd, D. P., Von Essen, C. F., Ferraro, R. H., Connelly, R. R., and Eisenberg, H.: Cancer of the tongue in Connecticut, 1935–59. Cancer *21*(1):89–96, January 1968.
130. Sheiman, R. A., and Wayne, K. S.: Oral carcinoma and hypercalcemia. Arch. Otolaryngol. *92*:189–200, August 1970.

131. Shklar, G., and Taylor, R.: Metastasis of pulmonary carcinoma to oral mucosa: Report of case. J. Oral Surg. Anesth. Hosp. D. Serv. *23*:549–552, 1965.
132. Shklar, G., Meyer, I., Cataldo, E. and Taylor, R.: Correlated study of oral cytology and histopathology. Oral Surg. *23*(1):61–69, January 1968.
133. Shultz, L. W., Vazirani, S. J., and Bolden, T. E.: Unilateral hyperplasia and exostosis of the mandibular condyle. Oral Surg. *13*(4):387–395, April 1960.
134. Silver, H., and Goldstein, M. A.: Sebaceous cell carcinoma of the parotid region. Cancer *19*:1773–1779, 1966.
135. Silverman, S.: Ultrastructure observations of radiation response in oral exfoliative cytology. Acta Cytol. (Balt.) *13*(5):292–301, May 1969.
136. Snyder, M. B., and Cawson, R. A.: Jaw and pulpal metastasis of an adrenal neuroblastoma. Oral Surg. *40*(6):775–784, December 1975.
136a. Small, I. A., and Waldron, C. A.: Ameloblastoma of jaws. Oral Surg. *8*:281–296, 1955.
137. Snyder, S. L., and Marks, I.: Osteogenic sarcoma metastatic to the mandible. Oral Surg. *25*(2):216–220, February 1968.
138. Statistics on Cancer. New York, American Cancer Society, 1967, p. 5.
139. Stahl, S. S., Koes, L. B., Brown, R. C., and Murray, D.: Oral cytology screening in a large metropolitan area. J. Am. Dent. Assoc. 1385–1388, December 1967.
140. Straith, F. E.: Metastatic adenocarcinoma of the mandible. Oral Surg. *24*(1):1–5, July 1967.
141. Strobbe, G. D., and Dargeon, H. W.: Embryonal rhabdomyosarcoma of head and neck in children and adolescents. Cancer *3*:826–836, 1960.
142. Strong, M. S., Vaughn, C. W., and Incze, J. S.: Toluidine blue in the management of carcinoma of the oral cavity. Acta Otolaryngol. (Chicago) *87*:527–531, 1968.
143. Suzuki, H., and Henderson, R.: Acinic cell carcinoma of the sublingual gland. Arch. Otolaryngol. *87*:146–149, February 1968.
144. Schultz, L. W., and Vazirani, S. J.: Use of sclerosing agent in treatment of ameloblastoma. Preliminary report. Oral Surg. *13*:150, 1960.
145. Taylor, C. G., Alexander, L. E., and Kramer, H. S., Jr.: Primary reticulum cell sarcoma of the mandible. Report of case. J. Oral Surg. *28*:281–321, March 1970.
146. Vazirani, S. J., and Bolden, T. E.: Lymphoblastoma of the submaxillary gland: A case report. Bull. Nat. Dent. Assoc. *15*:81–87, 1957.
147. Vazirani, S. J., and Bolden, T. E.: Oral fibromyxosarcoma of the maxilla. Oral Surg. *11*(3):227–234, March 1958.
148. Vazirani, S. J., and Schultz, L. W.: Sclerosing agent in treatment of ameloblastoma. Fifteen-year follow-up Oral Surg. Transactions of the Fourth International Conference on Oral Surgery, Amsterdam, May 1971.
149. Vrebos, J. E., Masson, J. K., and Harrison, E. G., Jr.: Metastatic carcinoma of the mandible with primary tumor in the lung. Am. J. Surg. *102*: 52–57, July 1961.
150. Watanabe, Y.: Exfoliative cytology of maxillo-oral sarcoma. Twelfth Annual Meeting, American Society of Cytologists, Pittsburgh, November 1964.
151. Watanabe, Y.: Methods for the early diagnosis of oral tumors. Int. Dent. J. *18*(4):708–723, 1968.
152. Weir, J. M., Dunn, J. E., Jr., and Buell, P. E.: Smoking and oral cancer: epidemiological data, educational responses. Am. J. Public Health *59*(7):959–966, June 1969.
152a. Weisburger, D.: Precancerous lesions. J. Am. Dent. Assoc. *54*:507–513, 1957.
153. Weitzner, S., and Hentel, W.: Metastatic carcinoma in the tongue: Report of a case. Oral Surg. *25*(2):278–281, February 1968.
154. Wright, D. H., and Roberts, M.: The geographical distribution of other types of malignant lymphoma in Uganda. Brit. J. Cancer *20*:469–474, 1966.
155. Yashar, J. S., Guralnick, E., and McHuby, R. L.: Multiple malignant tumors of the oral cavity, respiratory system and upper digestive system. Experience at the Pondville State Hospital from 1949–1959. Am. J. Surg. *112*:70, 1966.
156. Zajicek, J., and Eneroth, C. M.: Cytological diagnosis of salivary gland carcinomata from aspiration biopsy smears. Acta Otolaryngol. *263*:183–185, 1970.
157. Ziegler, J. L., Morrow, R. H., Jr., Templeton, C., Bluming, A. Z., Fass, L., and Kyalwazi, S. K.: Clinical features and treatment of childhood malignant lymphoma in Unganda. Int. J. Cancer *5*:415–425, 1970.

chapter 18

ACID ETCH AS A PREVENTIVE TECHNIQUE IN DENTISTRY

by

RICHARD J. SIMONSEN, D.D.S.

One of the most far-reaching recent improvements in the practice of dentistry has been the development of the acid etch technique.

The significance of the work by Buonocore (1955), in which he reported that the bonding of acrylic restorative material to enamel could be greatly enhanced with use of an acid conditioning agent, has not even today been fully appreciated by more than a minority of dentists. Undoubtedly Buonocore's work will be recognized in the years to come as the pioneering essay into the development of one of the most widely used techniques in dentistry. Even today there are improvements in the method being made continually, as the result of new research. The technique had a long and sometimes painful birth, but it can now be said to be past its infancy stage and maturing rapidly.

Buonocore was the first to apply the industrial use of phosphoric acid to resin retention in dentistry. It took many years for others to adopt the technique, and it was not until the late 1960's and early 1970's that articles concerning various *in vivo* and *in vitro* studies were published. Today, along with its widespread use in fissure sealing for caries prevention, we see the acid etch principle widely used in both restorative and orthodontic dentistry.

Uses of the acid etch principle are as follows:

1. *Preventive Dentistry:*
   Fissure Sealants. Fissure sealing is the primary preventive use of the acid etch technique. Secondary preventive uses can also be attributed to the technique, however, inasmuch as very conservative tooth preparation is feasible. Also, secondary decay and gingivitis from the use of orthodontic bands are eliminated

when the technique is used to bond brackets directly onto teeth.

2. *Restorative Dentistry:*
   A. Restoration of fractured incisors.
   B. Restoration of carious anterior teeth.
   C. Restoration of teeth with developmental defects; for example, peg-shaped laterals, hypocalcification marks, fluorosis, and iatrogenic defects such as tetracycline stains.
   D. Splinting of teeth that have become mobile as a result of trauma or periodontal disease.
   E. Construction of temporary bridges and space maintainers. (The acid etch principle may well have a more than temporary effect on crown and bridge dentistry in the future.)
   F. Pit and fissure composite restorations. (See page 332 for a detailed description of this technique.)
3. *Orthodontics*
   A. Bonding of brackets directly onto teeth.
   B. Attachment of space maintainers.

In this chapter the important primary preventive aspect of acid etch dentistry will be discussed.

FISSURE SEALANTS

The term sealant is used to describe resin material that is introduced into the occlusal pits and fissures of caries-susceptible teeth, thus forming a mechanical physical protective layer against the action of caries-producing bacteria and substrates.

The incorporation of fluoride into the drinking water supplies of cities has over the years had a tremendous effect on reducing the incidence of caries. Studies, such as the one of Ast et al. (1956), have reported significant drops of 50 to 60 per cent in the caries rates of children of various ages. It is generally accepted that the beneficial effect of either ingested or topically applied fluoride is in prevention and control of smooth-surface caries. With ideal fluoride environment, it is suspected that pit and fissure caries is delayed one or two years, but it is certainly not prevented on the scale that smooth surface caries is. Pit and fissure sealing, therefore, can have a tremendous impact on caries incidence.

ETCHING AGENT

Buonocore (1955) initially used 85 per cent phosphoric acid for his etch of enamel. This strength was chosen apparently in deference to the industrial use of phosphoric acid in treating metal surfaces to obtain better adhesion of paint and resin coatings.

Gwinnett and Buonocore (1965) tested several etching agents and reported: "With the solutions of phosphoric acid, it was noted that with increasing concentrations progressively less change was produced on the enamel surface." The same authors in 1972 described the effect of etching on enamel as "an increase in porosity, with the prism cores being preferentially dissolved." The most recent significant work on acid strength has been done by Silverstone (1974) and by Silverstone et al. (1975). In his 1974 study, Silverstone confirmed an inverse relationship between acid strength and change in surface topography on the enamel surface when using the acid of choice, orthophosphoric acid.

Additionally, and more importantly, he found that the depth of histological change was greatest at weaker acid concentrations. This area of histologically changed enamel allows the resin to form the "tags that are the foundation for the mechanical retention of the resin within the enamel." At weaker acid solutions, however, the loss in surface contour is greatest, and the ideal acid for etching combines the least loss in surface contour with the greatest depth of histologic change. As can be seen from Table 18–1, 30 per cent H_3PO_4 produced a surface loss of 10 microns and a depth of histologic change of 20 microns, for a total depth effect of 30 microns. Silverstone's conclusion was that "unbuffered 30 per cent phosphoric acid proved to be the most satisfactory conditioning fluid . . . ." Silverstone also found the ideal etching time to be 1 minute (Table 18–2).

Silverstone's later studies (1975) confirmed his earlier results, and it has be-

TABLE 18-1 DEPTH OF ETCH AND HISTOLOGIC CHANGE IN ENAMEL (TO NEAREST μM) FOLLOWING A ONE MINUTE EXPOSURE TO VARIOUS CONCENTRATIONS OF PHOSPHORIC ACID

ONE MINUTE EXPOSURE	CONCENTRATION OF PHOSPHORIC ACID, % 20	30	40	50	50 ZnO	60	70
Depth of etch	14	10	9	7	6	2	2
Depth of histologic change	20	20	15	12	10	4	2
Total depth of enamel affected	34	30	24	19	16	6	4

(From Silverstone, L. M.: Caries Res. 8:2–26, 1974.)

TABLE 18-2 LOSS IN DEPTH OF SURFACE CONTOUR (TO NEAREST μM) AFTER EXPOSURE TO VARIOUS CONCENTRATIONS OF PHOSPHORIC ACID

EXPOSURE TIME IN MINUTES	CONCENTRATION OF PHOSPHORIC ACID, % 20	30	40	50	50 ZnO	60	70
1	14	10	9	7	6	2	2
2	17	15	14	9	7	5	2
3	40	34	27	14	11	5	2

50 ZnO = 50% phosphoric acid + 7% zinc oxide by weight

(From Silverstone, L. M.: Caries Res. 8:2–26, 1974.)

come generally accepted that etching with 30 to 40 per cent H_3PO_4 will provide the ideal surface contour for retention. Rock (1974) compared the bond strength of Silverstone's recommended 30 per cent H_3PO_4 solution with the more commonly used 50 per cent H_3PO_4 buffered with 7 per cent zinc oxide (as used in Nuva System, L. D. Caulk Company, Milford, Delaware). Rock found an increase of over 50 per cent in the tensile strength of a sealant bond when 30 per cent H_3PO_4, as compared to 50 per cent of buffered H_3PO_4, was used to etch the enamel.

Enamel is predominantly hydroxyapatite, $Ca_{10}(PO_4)_6(OH)_2$. The hydroxyapatite crystals are packed together to form prisms which, in the mature tissue, are flattened hexagons in transverse section. The prisms are oriented at right angles to the enamel

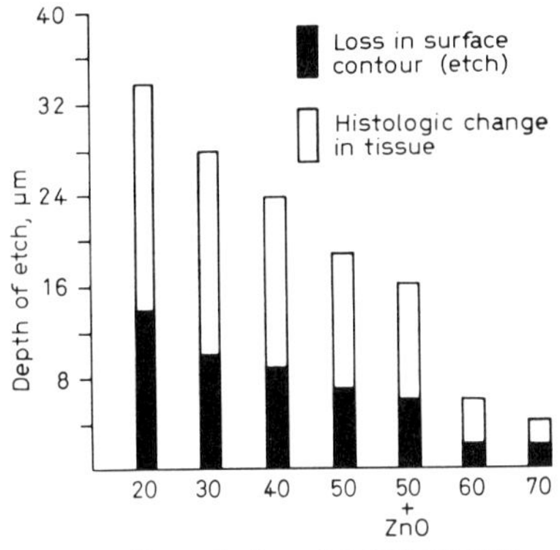

Figure 18-1 Depth of enamel affected by 1-min. exposures to various concentrations of phosphoric acid. (From Silverstone, L. M.: Caries Res. 8:2–26, 1974.)

surface, thus providing a latticework surface that when selectively etched produces an ideal base for the mechanical attachment of resins.

Silverstone et al. (1975) described three basic types of surface characteristics in etched enamel. "In the most common, called type 1 etching pattern, prism core material was preferentially removed, leaving the prism peripheres relatively intact [see Fig. 18–2]. In the second, type 2 etching pattern, the reverse pattern was observed. The peripheral regions of prisms were removed preferentially, leaving prism cores remaining relatively unaffected. In the type 3 etching pattern, there was a more random pattern, areas of which corresponded to types 1 and 2 damage together with regions in which the pattern of etching could not be related to prism morphology."

All three etching types were found in single samples of etched enamel, suggesting that "there is no one specific etching pattern produced in human dental enamel by the actions of acid solution." Gwinnett, another knowledgeable author who has done much work on the subject, reported (1973) similar findings, "Summarily the most common appearance of the conditioned enameled surface is that of rods showing a preferred loss of material from the rod cores. Less frequently, the preferred loss is from the peripheries. Such losses are not clinically predictable and preferred loss at cores and peripheries may occur at adjacent sites in the same tooth."

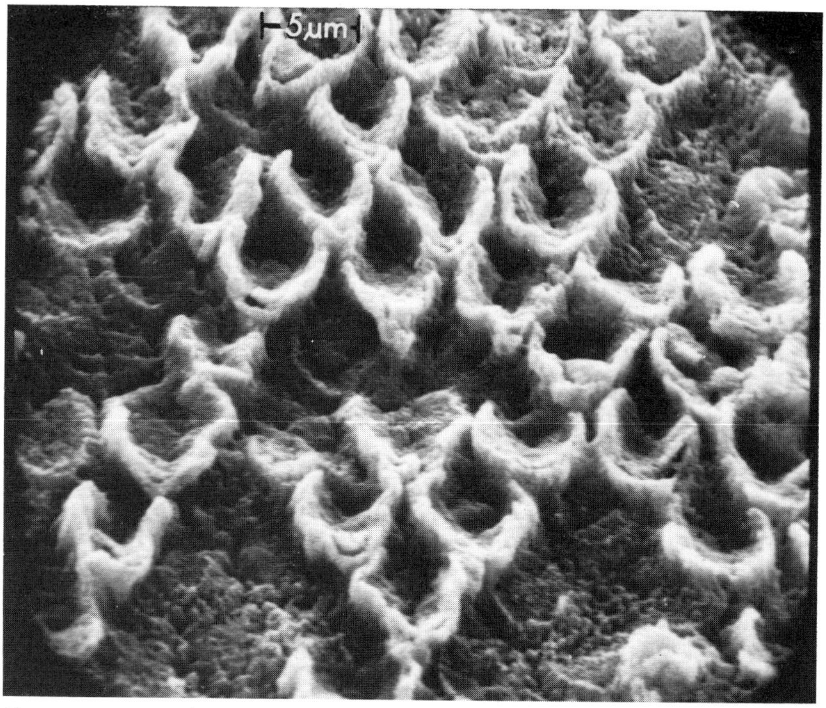

Figure 18–2 Scanning electron photomicrograph of an enamel surface after etching for 1 min. with 30 per cent H_3PO_4. Typical Type 1 etching pattern, where prism core material has been preferentially removed leaving the prism peripheries relatively intact, can be seen.

The etched surface is of critical importance to the strength of the bond, for it is into this roughened surface (see Fig. 18–2) that the resin flows, forming the "tags" that are the basis for retention (Fig. 18–3). The surface not only must be etched for the correct time with the ideal strength of the best acid, it also must be dry and free of contaminants when the resin is applied. It has been suggested by Ibsen and Neville (1974) that after etching the patient should rinse, although in the same book the authors stress "isolation to prevent contamination." How these factors (that is, rinsing and noncontamination) are compatible is hard to understand. Most authors presently agree that rinsing by the patient after etching should not be allowed and that the sealant should be applied as soon as possible after etching, washing and drying with air that is not contaminated by oil or water. It was Rock's (1974) impression that "bond strength was more related to the nature of the adhered surface than to the resin used."

Deciduous enamel has been described as prismless by Gwinnett (1973) and by Ibsen and Neville (1974). Silverstone (1975) found that decidous enamel was not, in fact, prismless, but that it did require an increase in etching time to 2 minutes to produce a comparable etch to adult enamel, using H_3PO_4 in a concentration range of 20 to 50 per cent. Correctly etched enamel, whether adult or deciduous, has a characteristic chalky or frosty appearance. The luster is removed, and if the enamel does not appear frosty after the correct etching time the etch should be repeated, for intrinsic factors such as the age of the tooth, or the fluoride content of the enamel could have prevented a satisfactory etch. The incidence of prismless enamel and its effect on etching in both deciduous and permanent teeth is still an area of disagreement among authors.

RESIN MATERIAL

There are two basic types of resin material on the market today: those that con-

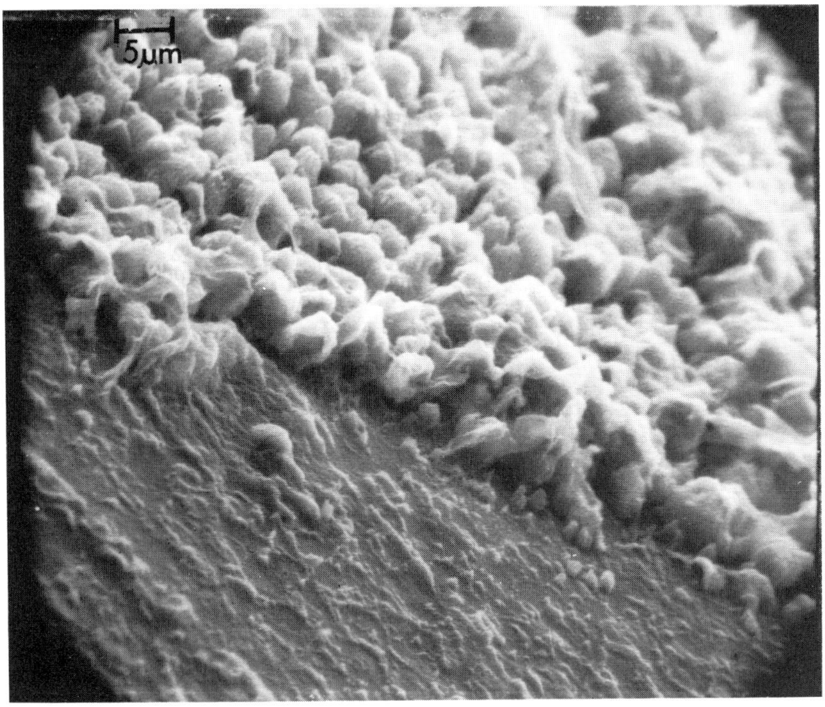

Figure 18–3 Scanning electron photomicrograph of a resin surface showing "tags." The specimen was prepared by coating a partially etched enamel surface with an unfilled resin and then decalcifying the enamel with 10 per cent HCL. The margin where etched met unetched enamel can be clearly seen.

tain an ultraviolet catalyst and are polymerized by exposure to ultraviolet light, and those that when mixed polymerize chemically. The main advantage of the latter is the cost savings in not having to invest in an ultraviolet light; the main advantage with an ultraviolet light is that the operator can completely control the setting time. This, as any experienced user of both systems will testify to, is a major advantage and a very useful characteristic of the ultraviolet systems. The forerunner of the ultraviolet systems has been the Nuva System (L. D. Caulk Company, Milford, Delaware). In this system, some problems of ultraviolet light delivery have recently emerged (1975). An alternative ultraviolet sealant is the Alpha System (Amalgamated Dental, London). This system is not presently (1976) available in the United States. The Alpha System uses a quartz fiberoptic for delivery of the ultraviolet light. The handpiece is no larger than a pen, and the ultraviolet bulb, which gets quite hot, is not close to the patient's face (see Fig. 18–4). Thus, the problems of overheating and scatter radiation are overcome in the Alpha system.

The chemically curing fissure sealants

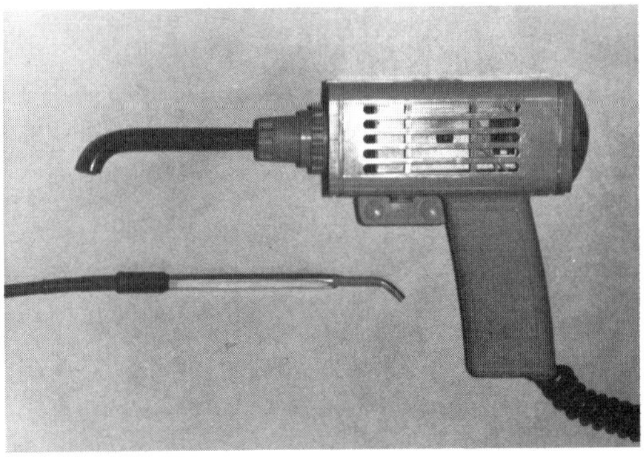

Figure 18–4 This photograph clearly shows the size difference between the NuvaLite (L. O. Caulk Co., Milford, Delaware) and the AlphaLite (Amalgamated Dental, London, England). The Nuva system houses the ultraviolet bulb within the handpiece, whereas the bulb in the AlphaLite is in the main unit and the ultraviolet light is transmitted via a quartz fiberoptic system to the pencil-sized handpiece.

have been many in number and variable in quality over the years. Because the best to emerge are basically very similar, a detailed description of one chemically curing sealant will be presented.

The Concise Enamel Bond System (3M Company, St. Paul, Minnesota) comes with both an unfilled and a filled resin, designed to be used together or independently. Basically, for fissure sealing, only the unfilled resin is used. A technique of diluting the filled resin will be described later.

The Concise Enamel Bond System uses a 37 per cent orthophosphoric acid solution (by weight), which falls within the ideal range quoted by Silverstone (1974). A 60 second etch time is recommended for adult enamel. The approximate surface loss of 8 to 10 microns after etching for 60 seconds can be compared to, for example, the 5 to 10 microns that are lost during a pumice prophylaxis. (Normal enamel is between 1000 and 2000 microns thick.)

The Enamel Bond System consists basically of a resin from the Bowen formula; that is, the dimethacrylate addition reaction product of bis-phenol A and glycidyl methacrylate. To decrease the viscosity of this resin, an active diluent, triethylene glycol dimethacrylate, is added. In an Enamel Bond kit, this resin comes in two parts, to one part a benzoyl peroxide catalyst is added, to the other an aromatic amine accelerator is added. When the two parts are mixed in equal volumes for 10 seconds there is approximately 50 seconds of working time. The resin will have a greasy appearance on polymerization, as the surface layer is inhibited from curing by oxygen in the atmosphere.

The Enamel Bond System resin will form a chemical bond with its composite filling material counterpart, Concise, because of the similarity of resin and curing agents. Most presently available filled resin systems can be used in conjunction with any unfilled resin.

QUESTIONS FREQUENTLY RAISED CONCERNING ACID ETCH

1. What happens to etched areas that are not covered by sealant?

It appears that remineralization of these areas takes place quite rapidly, the enamel gaining a normal appearance within 24 to 48 hours. This remineralization is caused by deposition of the organic and mineral components of saliva into the etched surface layer of enamel. No study has shown increased caries susceptibility as a result of a single etching exposure, and there is nothing to suggest that the enamel is more liable to attack for more than a few days than adjacent unetched enamel.

2. Why does a stronger solution of phosphoric acid create a less desirable etching pattern than a weaker solution?

This question is still unanswered. Silverstone (1975) has suggested that it "may be related to the degree of ionization of the acid. The weaker the acid the greater the ionization, and therefore the greater effect of diffusion into the tissue. In addition, one must consider the formation of other phases, in this way soluble or insoluble precipitates will affect further the dissolution rate."

3. If the sealant is lost, will the tooth be more susceptible to caries?

If the technique has been correctly performed the "tags" of resin will remain within the enamel latticework after the sealant is removed. (If the sealant is lost there probably were few "tags," and the enamel will return to its original state.) The "tags" will have a certain anticariogenic effect, thus decreasing caries susceptibility.

4. How long will sealants last?

Again, if the technique has been correctly performed, there is at present no answer to this question. Clinical studies have shown excellent results over periods of three years and longer. Failures may result from faulty technique, as they usually occur within the first six months, and after that the retention rates are relatively stable. Longer term clinical studies are still underway but there is really no reason to doubt that sealants that have lasted three years will last much longer.

TECHNIQUE FOR FISSURE SEALING

1. The tooth must be initially clean. A pumice and water mix is good for clean-

ing debris or plaque from the tooth. Oil-based mixtures or those containing fluoride should be avoided, as these will hinder etching of the enamel.

2. The tooth must be isolated. Rubber dam isolation is ideal; however, cotton rolls are more frequently used. This avoids the use of anesthesia where rubber dam retainer discomfort is not tolerable. In cases where a quadrant is isolated under rubber dam for restorations the opportunity should be taken to include any teeth requiring sealant under the dam. In the case of partially erupted permanent molars, where possibly a flap of tissue covers the distal marginal ridge, a combination of anesthesia, Ivory #14A retainer and rubber dam (slipped under the distal flap of tissue) will usually provide excellent working conditions for sealant application in an otherwise impossible area.
3. When salivary contamination has been eliminated, the phosphoric acid can be applied to the areas to be etched. The acid is best applied with a small sable brush, with which one can better control the amount and flow of acid. (Sometimes areas that are not to be sealed will be unavoidably etched or acid will be spilled onto tissue. In these cases the acid can be washed off quickly with water, resulting in no after effects.) Once the acid has been initially applied, fresh acid should be continually brought into contact with the enamel surface. The etching should be continued for one minute for adult teeth, and two minutes for deciduous teeth or adult teeth showing little etching effect after one minute (such as teeth of the elderly or of those living in a heavily fluoridated area).
4. After etching, the tooth is washed with a copious amount of water. In a water-air combination spray, the amount of water can be gradually reduced as the air is increased, thus going from pure water to spray to pure air. The tooth is then thoroughly dried with air. Care must be taken that the air hose does not have a water leak or any oil contamination, as it is imperative to the success of the sealant retention that the etched area is completely dry prior to sealant application and that no contamination of oil (from air hose) or saliva is permitted. High speed evacuation greatly facilitates the removal of water and is almost a necessity in the routine application of sealants. By placing the beveled aspirator tip adjacent to the etched tooth, one can in almost every case direct the phosphoric acid and water straight into the suction area. This can frequently eliminate the need to change cotton rolls. Should, however, the cotton rolls be soaked at this time, a change is indicated. Lingually to the lower molars, it is often possible to simply place a fresh cotton roll on top of the old one, thus reducing the possibility of salivary contamination.
5. When the tooth is thoroughly dry, sealant is applied to the occlusal grooves either with a small sable brush, in the case of ultraviolet polymerizing sealants, or with small sponges. For curing times refer to the individual manufacturer's instructions. If sealant interferes with occlusion it can be trimmed down or in minor cases it is sufficient simply to inform the patient that in a few days occlusal forces will wear the sealant down.

Indications for Use of Sealants

1. Deep pits and fissures on molars (or bicuspids) that are likely to become carious.
2. Minimal or questionable fissure caries. Technique described on page 332.
3. Patient is unable to maintain ideal oral hygiene.

Contraindications to Use of Sealants

1. Rampant or moderate decay where interpoximal caries is probable in the future.
2. Rounded fissures where decay is unlikely.

The question of whether decay exists in posteruptive fissures is influenced by many variables, including the skill and diagnostic criteria of the examiner and even the sharpness of his instruments. If decay is minimal and is sealed successfully the bacterial count will decrease and the caries activity cease. However, it is not presently recommended to seal caries.

One technique that has been used successfully by this author, in an as-yet-unpublished study, is to combine fissure sealing with the restoration of the decayed occlusal lesion. A very small bur is used to remove only the decayed tissue, thus leaving most fissures intact and saving considerable tooth structure. If dentin is exposed, a calcium hydroxide base is applied. The enamel margins of the restoration are slightly beveled, and all remaining pits and fissures are then etched and sealed along with the cavity preparation.

Although pure unfilled resin was initially used in attempts with this method, at the present a diluted filled resin, Concise Enamel Bond System (3M Company, St. Paul, Minnesota) is also being used for these sealant restorations. This combines, I believe, the advantages of both systems, for sufficient unfilled resin is available for the prevention of microleakage and for the production of the viscosity necessary for penetration and tag formation. At the same time, the added filled resin increases abrasion resistance and decreases creep. The size of the preparation determines whether pure unfilled resin or a combination of unfilled and diluted filled resin is used.

The Concise filled resin can be easily diluted or thinned with the Enamel Bond unfilled resin in several different ways. The most successful appears to be to dilute the universal paste with a drop of universal resin, and the catalyst paste with a drop of catalyst resin. Depending on the amount of filled resin used, when mixed together this produces a filling material and sealant that flows nicely when placed on the occlusal etched surface. Ulvestad (1975) has the only published study to date concerning the use of diluted Concise as a fissure sealant. Ulvestad's results show 100 per cent retention after 15 months. One of the big advantages he cites in the use of diluted Concise is the ease with which the sealant can be seen on recall appointments. An unfilled resin can sometimes remain in the deepest portions of the fissure without being visible, and this may contribute to some of the poorer retention results other authors have published. Ibsen (1973) also reported nearly 100 per cent retention (one failure in 439 cases) after one year of using a filled diacrylate (Enamelite). It would seem that the use of a filled resin for fissure sealing deserves further clinical investigation, as does the incorporation of a color into the unfilled resin. The addition of color would greatly facilitate recall visualization of the sealant. The fissure sealant is a necessity for any successful preventive program. Improvements will undoubtedly continue in technique and materials. The only area of question in the technique, is to whom does one apply the sealant? A sealant cannot be judged successful if decay on another surface necessitates the sealant's removal in six months even if it could have been retained for a lifetime under other circumstances.

RESTORATIVE PROCEDURES

In the development of the acid etch technique as a preventive procedure, it was not fully understood just how clinically strong the etched bond would be until successful attempts were made at anterior fracture repair. The results showed not only strength but also maximum preservation of tooth structure and a highly aesthetic restoration. This initial success has led to several other uses of the technique, which will be discussed here.

Restoration of Fractured Incisors. With the spreading use of the acid etch technique in restoration of fractured incisors the days are gone when a budding young athlete was destined to spend his adolescent years with a stainless steel crown or a three-quarter gold crown with acrylic facing on a central incisor. The very poor aesthetics frequently associated with these restorations made them quite harmful psychologically to the adolescent. The chronic gingivitis created by mediocre or poor adaptation of the stainless steel crown is also a drawback, for frequently, when the time came for a porcelain jacket crown, gingival recession had taken place. Although the acid etch incisal angle has up until now been regarded as a temporary restoration, the time has come to look upon it as a permanent restoration requiring occasional refinishing.

TECHNIQUE. Only very minimal preparation is needed. When less than one third to one half the crown has fractured it is sufficient to merely bevel or chamfer the enamel with a fluted finishing bur or bullet-nosed diamond in the high-speed handpiece. Approximately $1\frac{1}{2}$ millimeters are beveled at about 45 degrees in order to provide the correct orientation of the enamel prisms for etching. Enamel fractures occur most frequently along the longitudinal axis of the enamel prisms, and this does not create an ideal area for etching. The prisms need to be "end-on" for an ideal pattern. After beveling, the dentin is covered with a calcium hydroxide base. The enamel is etched, and an intermediate sealant layer is applied. The filled resin is mixed at the same time and added with the aid of a clear plastic crown, or some other matrix form, before the sealant has polymerized. This ensures sufficient unfilled resin to form the "tags" necessary for mechanical retention. The filled and unfilled resins are, when polymerized together, not distinguishable as separate layers.

There is some disagreement as to the necessity of an intermediate sealant layer. Authors such as Raadal (1975) and Dryer Jorgenson (1975) have found "tag" lengths from the filled resin to be equal to those from an unfilled resin on etched enamel. This is explained by the fact that there is sufficient unfilled resin present in the filled resin for tag formation. Dogon's studies (1975), however, show that microleakage, which is present when only the filled resin is being used, is eliminated when an intermediate layer is used. This intermediate layer can be polymerized before the filled resin is added (as is necessary in the ultraviolet systems) or used as described above.

It is significant that no study purporting equal tag lengths from filled and unfilled resins shows the very fine long tags (up to 100 microns) that can be seen from careful preparation of unfilled resin specimens. These fine tags are almost invariably broken in specimen preparation, leaving the commonly seen "base tags" of 10 to 20 microns. Such base tags can also be seen from filled resin but it is doubtful if the fine tags are present in the same length or number as with an unfilled resin. This could explain the microleakage seen by Dogon (1975) on specimens not using an unfilled resin layer directly on etched enamel. Most authors presently agree that the intermediate layer is desirable.

When the filled layer has polymerized it can be trimmed using discs, strips, fluted finishing burs in a high-speed handpiece, or any finishing technique preferred by the individual operator. With the range of color choices available and with skillful placement of anatomy, these acid etch anterior trauma restorations can frequently be made indistinguishable from the original tooth.

Double Etch. On all acid etch restorations, the author suggests re-etching approximately 2 to 3 millimeters of enamel adjacent to the enamel resin interface after all finishing has been completed. A layer of unfilled resin is then flowed over the whole restoration and the adjacent etched enamel. This insures (initially at least) the very smooth finish, and doubly insures against marginal leakage. The unfilled resin will chemically bond with the filled resin, and even though it will wear down through abrasion it can be easily reapplied. Simonsen and Stallard (1976) found unfilled resin applied as a "glaze" layer present over most of the labial surfaces of anterior fractures one year after application. Where the resin was not present, initial non-polymerization rather than subsequent abrasion was hypothesised as being the cause.

If more than one third to one half of the crown has been fractured, one is frequently forced into endodontic therapy as well as crown restoration. If this amount of crown is fractured, more of the remaining labial and lingual surfaces will have to be utilized for retention. Approximately 1 millimeter of surface enamel can be removed and the bevel placed up to or into the gingival sulcus if necessary.

Some authors recommend complete coverage of labial and lingual surfaces for even relatively minor fractures. However, this author has found that finishing the restoration to a small bevel provides more than adequate retention. This method should be utilized whenever possible in order to maximize the saving of tooth structure.

One great advantage of the acid etch system is that it can be added to at any time. For example, colors that are not quite perfect can be changed by removing a thin surface layer of resin and applying a new layer of the desired color. Similarly, a crown can be made directly on top of an acid etch bandage.

When fractures occur there is frequently not time in a busy office schedule to permit making the complete crown, so a temporary "bandage" can be applied to protect the pulp from further insult. The procedure is the same as that for a crown; that is, bevel, base, etch, and apply unfilled and filled resin. However, for expediency, only a small amount of filled resin is used to protect the fractured area. The patient is then sent home and the finished crown made on top of the bandage at a later date.

It should be noted that a tooth that is mobile or displaced as well as fractured can easily be stabilized by etching areas on adjacent teeth and flowing the material into these areas. When the time necessary to ensure stability has passed, a fluted finishing bur can be used to cut away the excess on the adjacent teeth, and the crown can be finished.

Restoration of Anterior Tooth Caries. The same principles apply here as have been noted previously. The main advantage to acid etching all anterior tooth caries is the great increase in marginal integrity. The acid etch bond has given us the means to eliminate "leaky" composites.

No retention is necessary apart from that obtained by etching enamel margins. This minimizes tooth preparation to the removal of caries and the beveling of enamel. A base is carefully applied, and the restoration is completed as previously described. A "double etch" is also almost always utilized.

Restoration of Defects. The following defects can be easily remedied using techniques previously described.

1. *Tetracycline stains*
   The typical discoloration from ingestion of tetracycline during the calcification stage of tooth development can be hidden by removing approximately 1 millimeter of labial surface enamel and using an opaque filled resin initially to mask the underlying dark color. The color of choice is then utilized on the surface layer of filled resin for the finished restoration.
2. *Peg laterals*
   This defect can be eliminated by etching the whole peg and using it as a stub upon which a crown is etched.
3. *Fluorosis*
   Depending upon severity, this defect can be treated as a tetracycline stain or as a hypocalcification defect.
4. *Hypocalcification marks*
   The defective areas are scooped out as much as is necessary to remove the discolored enamel. Calcium hydroxide is utilized if dentin is exposed, and an opaque layer of filled resin is applied when required.

Splinting of Teeth. Splinting is done simply by etching interproximally for as many teeth as one needs stabilized. Unfilled resin and then filled resin are applied for stability. For aesthetic reasons, the filled resin is utilized mostly on the lingual surface but also sparingly in labial embrasures. This creates a firm bond if conditions for etching are adhered to, although it must be noted that frequently in trauma cases a dry field is very difficult to maintain. Small wedges can be used interproximally to prevent the unfilled resin from flowing onto the tissue and into the sulcus. When using the wedges care must be taken not to displace a mobile tooth from its normal position.

Construction of Temporary Bridges. A whole chapter could be written on this aspect of the acid etch system, but it is sufficient at this time to say that acid etch bridges are not only possible but in many cases desirable. Their time of retention has yet to be fully determined, but this author already has 18-month-old retention results with many cases, and other authors have reported similar success. A plastic denture tooth (with retention grooves cut in) or a tooth made entirely of composite material is etched into the place of the missing tooth.

Hailed by some, greeted with skepticism by others, the acid etch principle is nevertheless the single most important development for the future practice of dentistry to come from the last 50 years of research. It is doubtful if Michael Buonocore, when he published his initial thoughts on the etching of tooth enamel (1955), was fully aware of the potential scope of his discovery, which can already be applied to all facets of clinical dentistry.

REFERENCES

1. Ast, D. B., Smith, D. J., Wachs, B., and Cantwell, K. T.: Newburgh-Kingston Caries-Fluorine Study XIV. Combined clinical and roentgenographic dental findings after ten years of fluoride experience. J.A.D.A. *52*:314–325, 1956.
2. Buonocore, M. G.: A simple method of increasing the adhesion of acrylic filling materials to enamel surfaces. J. Dent. Res. *34*:849–853, 1955.
3. Dogon, I. L.: Studies demonstrating the need for an intermediary resin of low viscosity for the acid etch technique. Proceedings of International Symposium on the Acid Etch Technique. St. Paul, Minnesota, North Central Publishing Co., 1975, pp. 100–118.
4. Dryer Jorgensen, K.: The adaptation of composite and non-composite resins to acid etched enamel surfaces. Proceedings of International Symposium on the Acid Etch Technique. St. Paul, Minnesota, North Central Publishing Co., 1975, pp. 93–99.
5. Gwinnett, A. J., and Buonocore, M. G.: Adhesives and caries prevention: A preliminary report. Br. Dent. J. *119*:77–80, 1965.
6. Gwinnett, A. J., and Buonocore, M. G.: A scanning electron microscope study of pit and fissure surfaces conditioned for adhesive sealing. Arch. Oral Biol. *17*:415–423, 1972.
7. Gwinnett, A. J.: The bonding of sealants to enamel. J. Am. Soc. Prev. Dent. *1*:21–29, 1973.
8. Ibsen, R. L., and Neville, K.: Adhesive Restorative Dentistry. Philadelphia, W. B. Saunders Company, 1974.
9. Ibsen, R. L.: Use of a filled diacrylate as a fissure sealant: One year clinical study. J. Am. Soc. Prev. Dent. *4*:62–65, 1973.
10. Raadal, M.: Mikroretensjon av Plastfyllingsmatrialer paa Syreetset Emalje. Den Norske Tannlaegeforenings Tidende. *10*:404–413, 1975.
11. Rock, W. P.: The effect of etching on human enamel upon bond strengths with fissure sealant resins. Arch. Oral Biol. *19*:873–877, 1974.
12. Scheer, B., and Silverstone, L. M.: Replacement of missing anterior teeth by etch retained bridges. J. Int. Assoc. Dent. Child. *6*:17–19, 1975.
13. Silverstone, L. M.: Fissure sealants: Laboratory studies. Caries Res. *8*:2–26, 1974.
14. Silverstone, L. M., Saxton, C. A., Dogon, I. L., and Fejerskov, O.: Variation in the pattern of acid etching of human dental enamel examined by scanning electronmicroscopy. Caries Res. 9:373–387, 1975.
15. Silverstone, L. M., and Dogon, I. L. (Eds.): Proceedings of an International Symposium on the Acid Etch Technique. St. Paul, Minnesota, North Central Publishing Company, 1975.
16. Silverstone, L. M.: Personal communication.
17. Simonsen, R. J.: Unpublished data.
18. Simonsen, R. J., and Stallard, R. E.: Surface characteristics of composite restorations. I.A.D.R. abstract #314, Feb. 1976.
19. Ulvestad, H.: Clinical trials with fissure sealant materials in Scandinavia. Proceedings of an International Symposium on Acid Etch Technique. St. Paul, Minnesota, North Central Publishing Company, 1975, pp. 165–175.
20. Ulvestad, H.: Personal communication.

ADDITIONAL READING LIST

1. Albert, N., and Grenoble, D. E. An in vivo study of enamel remineralization after acid etching. J. South Calif. Dent. Assoc. *39*:747–751, 1971.
2. Backer Dirks, O.: The assessment of fluoridation as a preventive measure in relation to dental caries. Br. Dent. J. *114*:211–216, 1963.
3. Bowen, R. L.: Adhesive bonding of various materials to hard tooth tissues. One method of determining bond strength. J. Dent. Res. *44*:690–695, 1965.
4. Buonocore, M. G., Wileman, W., and Brudevold, F.: A report on a resin composition capable of bonding to human dentin surfaces. J. Dent. Res. *35*:846–851, 1956.
5. Buonocore, M. G.: Principles of adhesive retention and adhesive restorative materials. J. Am. Dent. Assoc. *67*:382–391, 1963.
6. Buonocore, M. G., Matsui, A., and Gwinnett, A. J.: Penetration of resin dental materials into enamel surfaces with reference to bonding. Arch. Oral Biol. *13*:61–70, 1968.
7. Buonocore, M. G.: Adhesive sealing of pits and fissures for caries prevention, with use of ultraviolet light. J. Am. Dent. Assoc. *80*:324–328, 1970.
8. Buonocore, M. G.: Caries prevention in pits and fissures sealed with an adhesive resin poly-

merized by ultraviolet light: A two-year study of a single adhesive application. J. Am. Dent. Assoc. *82*:1090–1093, 1971.
9. Buonocore, M. G.: Adhesives for pit and fissure caries control. Dent. Clin. North Amer. *16*:693–708, 1972.
10. Cueto, E. I., and Buonocore, M. G.: Sealing of pits and fissures with an adhesive resin: Its use in caries prevention. J. Am. Dent. Assoc. *75*:121–128, 1967.
11. Gwinnett, A. J.: The ultrastructure of the "prismless" enamel of deciduous teeth. Arch. Oral Biol. *11*:1109–1115, 1966.
12. Gwinnett, A. J.: The ultrastructure of the "prismless" enamel of permanent human teeth. Arch. Oral Biol. *12*:381–387, 1967.
13. Gwinnett, A. J., and Matsui, A.: A study of enamel adhesives: The physical relationship between enamel and adhesives. Arch. Oral Biol. *12*:1615–1620, 1967.
14. Gwinnett, A. J.: Histologic changes in human enamel following treatment with acidic adhesive conditioning agents. Arch. Oral Biol. *16*:731–738, 1971.
15. Gwinnett, A. J.: Caries prevention through sealing of pits and fissures. J. Canad. Dent. Assoc. *37*:458–461, 1971.
16. Gwinnett, A. J.: Morphology of the interface between adhesive resins and treated human enamel fissures as seen by scanning electron microscopy. Arch. Oral Biol. *16*:237–238, 1971.
17. Gwinnett, A. J., Buonocore, M. G., and Sheykholeslam, Z.: Effect of fluoride on etched human and bovine tooth enamel surfaces as demonstrated by scanning electron microscopy. Arch. Oral Biol. *17*:271–278, 1972.
18. Gwinnett, A. J.: Human prismless enamel and its influence on sealant penetration. Arch. Oral Biol. *18*:441–444, 1973.
19. Gwinnett, A. J., and Ripa, L. W.: Penetration of pit and fissure sealants into conditioned human enamel in vivo. Arch. Oral Biol. *18*:435–439, 1973.
20. Gwinnett, A. J.: Structural changes in enamel and dentin of fractured anterior teeth after acid conditioning in vitro. J. Am. Dent. Assoc. *86*:117–122, 1973.
21. Handelman, S. L., Buonocore, M. G., and Schoute, P. C.: A preliminary report on the effect of fissure sealant on bacteria in dental caries. J. Prosthet. Dent. *27*:390–392, 1972.
22. Horowitz, H. S., Heifetz, S. B., and McCune, R. J.: The effectiveness of an adhesive sealant in preventing occlusal caries: Fingings after two years in Kalispell, Montana. J. Am. Dent. Assoc. *89*:885–890, 1974.
23. Laswell, H. R., Welk, D. A., and Regenos, J. W.: Attachment of resin restorations to acid pretreated enamel. J. Am. Dent. Assoc., *82*:559–563, 1971.
24. McCune, R. J., Horowitz, H. S., Heifetz, S. B., and Cvar, J.: Pit and fissure sealants: One year results from a study in Kalispell, Montana. J. Am. Dent. Assoc. *87*:1177–1180, 1973.
25. Nelson, S. R., Till, M. J., and Hinding, J. H.: Comparison of materials and methods used in acid etch restorative procedures. J. Am. Dent. Assoc. *89*:1123–1127, 1974.
26. Retief, D. H.: Effect of conditioning the enamel surface with phosphoric acid. J. Dent. Res. *52*:333–341, 1973.
27. Ripa, L. W., and Cole, W. W.: Occlusal sealing and caries prevention: Results 12 months after a single application of adhesive resin. J. Dent. Res. *49*:171–173, 1970.
28. Roberts, M. W., and Moffa, J. P.: Restoration of fractured incisal angles with an ultraviolet activated sealant and a composite resin—A case report. J. Dent. Child. *5*:30–31, 1972.
29. Rock, W. P.: Fissure sealants: Results obtained with two different sealants after one year. Br. Dent. J. *133*:146–151, 1972.
30. Rock, W. P.: Fissure sealants: Results obtained with different bis-GMA type sealants after one year. Br. Dent. J. *134*:193–196, 1973.
31. Rock, W. P.: Fissure sealants: Further results of clinical trials. Br. Dent. J. *136*:317–321, 1974.
32. Sheykholeslam, Z., and Buonocore, M. G.: Bonding of resins to phosphoric acid-etched enamel surfaces of permanent and deciduous teeth. J. Dent. Res. *51*:1572–1576, 1972.
33. Silverstone, L. M.: Etching teeth with acids. Br. Dent. J. *135*:95, 1973.
34. Taylor, C. L., and Gwinnett, A. J.: A study of the penetration of sealants into pits and fissures. J. Am. Dent. Assoc. *87*:1181–1188, 1973.
35. Wei, S. H. Y.: Remineralization of enamel and dentin—A review. J. Dent. Child. *34*:444–451, 1967.

chapter 19

THE COMPOSITE RESIN: A PREVENTIVE OPERATIVE PROCEDURE

by
C. H. PAMEIJER, D.M.D., M.Sc.D., D.Sc.

Operative procedures have been carried out since the turn of the century basically in accordance with the principles advocated by G. V. Black. Black's investigations were thorough and impressive, and carried out in a time when dental research was in its early stages. His knowledge of clinical dentistry and research has influenced every aspect of dentistry. Improvement of research facilities and an increased knowledge in the areas of physics, microstructure, and biological science have stimulated interest and challenged many established techniques which were practiced for years. During recent decades, the refining of existing research equipment and the invention of new equipment have enabled investigators to obtain more accurate and detailed data. High magnifications with better resolution may now be obtained. All these have contributed greatly to a better understanding of the many problems encountered in dental research.

Extensive research, by numerous people, has resulted in the production of dental restorative materials with improved mechanical and esthetic properties. This is important, since the major objectives in restoring teeth are (1) the restoration of function, and (2) the creation of or improvement in esthetics. Ironically, most materials have been developed to satisfy the need to restore carious lesions. Prevention of these lesions would more effectively serve the patient and allow time and effort to be devoted toward other areas in dentistry that have not received the proper attention. Prevention does not receive the attention it deserves, and the profession is concerned with the existing situation. There are, however, many positive aspects involving unusual and often demanding situations; for instance, the repair of a fractured incisor. Esthetically and functionally, this type of restoration (depending on the severity of the case) has usually been a compromise. With the new materials and techniques, the final results can sometimes be so sophisticated that one wonders how these problems could have been solved in the past.

Another example is the treatment of enamel hypoplasia. Today, with the development of adhesive restorative materials, these lesions can be treated so that the esthetic value is remarkable. More attention to the actual operative procedures will be given later in this chapter.

For many years, anterior teeth were restored with silicate cements, which were developed in Europe around the turn of the century. They were noted for their esthetic value but criticized for the irritative effects caused by their release of phosphoric acid. Improvements in the composition of the material and the use of cavity liners to protect the pulp have lessened the chances of jeopardizing the intercoronal structure. The esthetic results when the materials are properly handled are unequalled by any other restorative material. The advantage of incorporating fluoride in silicates,[14] to reduce secondary decay is attributed to the solubility of the filling material, thus resulting in release of the fluoride. Since this is a long-term process, a continuous topical application protects the surrounding enamel by increasing its resistance to acid solubility.

In the early 1940's a group of filling materials were introduced which were completely different from the silicate cements. For all practical purposes, these materials can be classified as unfilled resins to distinguish them from composite resins, which were developed later. The particle shape of these resins is usually spherical and their diameter varies individually (Fig. 19–1). They are chemically accelerated and can be polished to a smooth surface. Immediately after placement and for a short period thereafter the esthetic value is high; however, marginal discoloration due to percolation, and darkening over a period of time yield an inferior restoration. This is due to the porous nature of the material coupled with other factors such as a high coefficient of thermal expansion, which causes the resin to shrink and expand seven or more times as much as tooth structure for every degree of temperature change.[17]

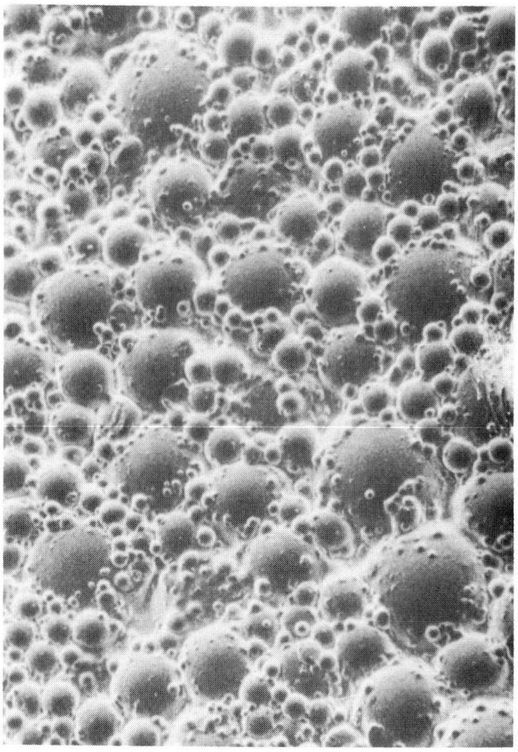

Figure 19–1 A scanning electron micrograph of an unfilled resin. Note the variety in size of the spherical polymer particles (× 200).

The introduction of composite resins brought us to a new era in restorative dentistry. Its application has gained tremendous popularity over existing filling materials. Initially, composites were utilized only in Class III and V restorations. The physical properties were so favorable, however, that other possibilities were readily recognized.

The composites are made of a resin matrix, which is a cross-linked organic mixture of polymer and monomer, and inorganic filler particles. The filler has been added up to 75 per cent by weight and varies depending upon the restorative material. Filler particles include glass beads, glass rods, quartz, lithium aluminum silicate, and boro silicate. In order to promote the bond of the resin to the filler, the particles are coated with a coupling agent, for which usually silane is utilized.

The bases of the copolymer resin matrix is a reaction product of bisphenol-A and glycidyl methacrylate. The polymerization process is accomplished by a peroxide amine system utilizing a catalyst of benzoyl peroxide and an accelerator of *n n*-dimethyl-*P*-toluidine.[13, 18] Thus, these materials are, with reference to mechanical properties, superior to the conventional resins. Factors which are improved include (1) greater compressive and tensile strength, (2) higher modulus of elasticity, (3) superior hardness and resistance to abrasion, (4) lower polymerization shrinkage, and (5) a reduced coefficient of thermal expansion.[17]

The first composite resin commercially introduced was Addent 35. Its filler consisted of glass balls and glass rods. After the introduction of Addent 35, other brands appeared on the market. The main difference consisted of the type of filler particles. Wetting properties were improved. The convenience was enhanced in that the composites do not have to be stirred prior to use. In the past, particles precipitated over a period of time, causing the filler concentration of the bottom layers to increase. It can easily be understood that when small quantities were taken from the top without stirring the contents of the jar, the final mixture was low in particle concentration and, therefore, did not produce the optimal physical properties, while, at the same time, the bottom layers were saturated with particles.

The marginal adaptability of commercially available composite resins has been investigated by means of microleakage techniques and scanning electron microscopy. In addition, specimens have been subjected to thermal cycling.[12] Although the composite resins are definitely superior to the conventional filling materials, one should bear in mind that several so-called "improved" properties, such as increased hardness and abrasion resistance, have never been proven to be of clinical significance. Like many new materials, there are many inherent problems associated with composite resins. The presence of the filler, for instance, determines the surface characteristics and always produces a rough surface, regardless of the type of filler that is used. A study conducted by Johnson *et al.*[9] to investigate the effect of different finishing burs on the surface of composite resins revealed that, in the opinion of the writers, the 12-fluted bur produced the smoothest surface. Another study evaluating 15 different finishing procedures[5] concluded that the smoothest surface was obtained when the material polymerized in contact with a Mylar matrix strip. Regardless of the finishing procedures tested, that surface smoothness could not be equalled. According to the authors, a white stone produces the best finished surface characteristics. A special diamond disc was developed by Chandler, *et al.*[4] which, according to their findings with a scanning electron microscope, produced a smoother surface than commercially available composite finishing burs.

A first concern when using a new restorative material should be its irritative potential to the underlying pulp. As discussed previously, the release of phosphoric acid from silicate cements may cause symptoms that range from mild inflammation to pulp death. Several investigators have histologically studied the effects of composite resins on pulp tissue.[2, 8] Among other findings, it was observed that the amount of thickness of the remaining dentin was important. In these cases, the pulp inflammation caused by most of the resins appeared to be reversible. The inflammatory reaction was attributed to (1) chemical irritation from the material, and (2) poor adaptation of the restorative material. The space between the material and pulpal wall allows percolation of microorganisms from the oral cavity to the pulp chamber. A significant improvement was accomplished when cavity liners were applied to the walls of the cavity preparation. It is, therefore, generally recommended that these cavity sealers be used beneath composite resins.

Another matter of concern is the reaction of the filling material to the gingival tissues. Several studies reported a favorable reaction.[3, 19] The presence of marginal gingivitis was observed by Larato[11] and was attributed to the fact that the resin was under the gingival surface. It was felt, however, that the main cause of the inflammation was the ready collection of plaque on the rough surface of the composite resins rather than the roughness of the material and retention per se. It is, therefore, advisable to place the gingival margin of a composite restoration 1 millimeter away from the gingival margin. In practice, however, this may not always be possible. Careful finishing of the restoration, blending the contour with the natural anatomy of the tooth, enables the patient to clean the restoration adequately, which will prevent the accumulation of plaque. The application of a thin layer of pit and fissure sealant to prevent microleakage[5] may be beneficial. The principle of sealing composites is based on the following technique. After placement and contouring of the restoration, the surface of the restoration and approximately 1 to 2 millimeters of the surrounding enamel are prepared with the conditioner. Sixty seconds after the acid has been applied, the preparation is thoroughly washed and air dried. With a fine camel's-hair brush, a thin layer of sealant is painted over the restoration and the conditioned enamel; by means of ultraviolet light this material hardens, and a protective shell of plastic covers the tooth. For as long as this protective layer is present, microorganisms from the oral environment will not have access to the interface filling material and enamel, thus preventing microleakage. An *in vitro* study by the aforementioned authors, in which bovine teeth were boiled for 24 hours after application of the sealant, revealed that no microleakage had occurred. One must bear in mind, however, that the circumstances to which these specimens were exposed, and *in vitro* experiments in general, differ totally from the *in vivo* situation. Factors such as saliva, bacteria, pH, plaque, and masticatory forces may all together or individually determine the longevity of the applied principle. An *in vivo* and *in vitro* study of this sealing principle was done by Kun and Pameijer.[10] After 12 months, a clinical evaluation of 57 teeth indicated that 78.4 per cent of the experimental teeth were still completely covered with the protective layer. In 21.6 per cent the sealant was either completely or partially absent. Additional *in vitro* experiments revealed that no leakage of basic fuchsin dye was observed in cross sections of the experimentally treated teeth. In other words, the material provided a perfect seal against microleakage. Scanning electron micrographs demonstrated the intimate relationships between adhesive and sealant, as well as that of sealant and restorative material.

The clinical manipulation of composites is sometimes complicated by their tendency to adhere to the instruments. This may result in voids in the material or poor adaptation of the material to the cavity walls. Without any question, the use of a matrix band is recommended during insertion of the composites. A very valuable adjunct in inserting composite resins is a specially designed syringe. The instrument has proved to be ideally suited for poorly accessible areas. The fabrication of a composite core when pins are used for retention is a clear example for the use of the syringe. The tip of the nozzle can be inserted into the matrix to the floor of the cavity. Injection of the material is quick and usually guarantees a perfect adaptation. Overfilling with subsequent finger pressure thus yields a well condensed composite restoration. After removal of the matrix, the cylindrical tooth is immediately ready to be cut to a crown preparation. The composite is mixed as directed, and packed in a disposable plastic nozzle. A self-lubricating rubber plug is inserted in the nozzle, and this assembly is placed into the syringe. The plunger of the syringe will push the plug, and the material can then be ejected into the cavity (Fig. 19–2). The working time is limited, but adequate. No maintenance is required, as the plastic nozzle with the rubber plug is disposable.

The instructions for handling composite resins vary considerably among manufacturers. A majority of composites consists of two pastes which are mixed in equal portions. Another brand has to be mixed on a

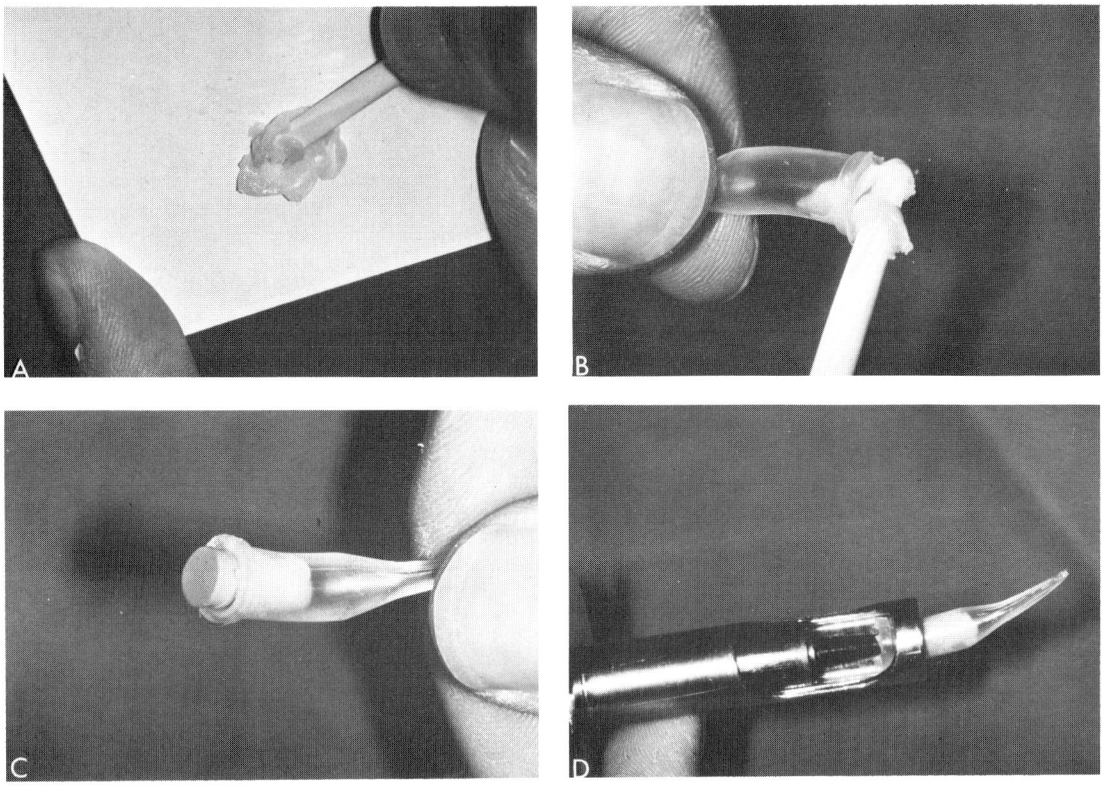

Figure 19–2 *A*, The composite restorative material is mixed as recommended in the manufacturer's instructions and subsequently packed into a plastic nozzle (*B*). *C*, A rubber self-lubricating plunger is inserted in the nozzle, and this assembly is mounted in the syringe (*D*). Practical experience has demonstrated that the opening of the nozzle should be trimmed at the end to widen its orifice, allowing for the low viscosity of some composite materials which may cause too much tension in the nozzle. The result is that the nozzle may "pop" and the material escapes through other openings.

special, catalyst-impregnated mixing pad in order to set. Also available is the paste–liquid combination. In general, it is recommended that composite resins be allowed to polymerize against a matrix band of Mylar. Findings in this laboratory confirm the results of Dennison and Craig[5] that the matrix band in close contact with the composite resin produces the smoothest surface. Our studies were carried out utilizing a scanning electron microscope, which, because of its great depth of field and excellent contrast, together with the three-dimensional image, provides detailed information about surface texture. In contrast to the excellent results obtained under laboratory conditions, the clinical picture demonstrated other features. In order to study the behavior of composite resins *in vivo* a replica technique was developed for use with scanning electron microscopy.[15]

Under the stated ideal laboratory conditions, composite resins exhibited a smooth surface where intimate contact had been present with the matrix band. Occasionally, however, surface defects in the form of voids could be observed (Fig. 19–3). The surface defects were attributed to the trapping of air during the mixing of materials. Clinically, however, the results differed considerably. Working time, type and size of restoration, use of rubber dam, and patient cooperation were all factors that greatly influenced the ultimate success and quality of the restoration.

A clinical experiment to study marginal adaptation and surface characteristics of composite resins was conducted by Pamei-

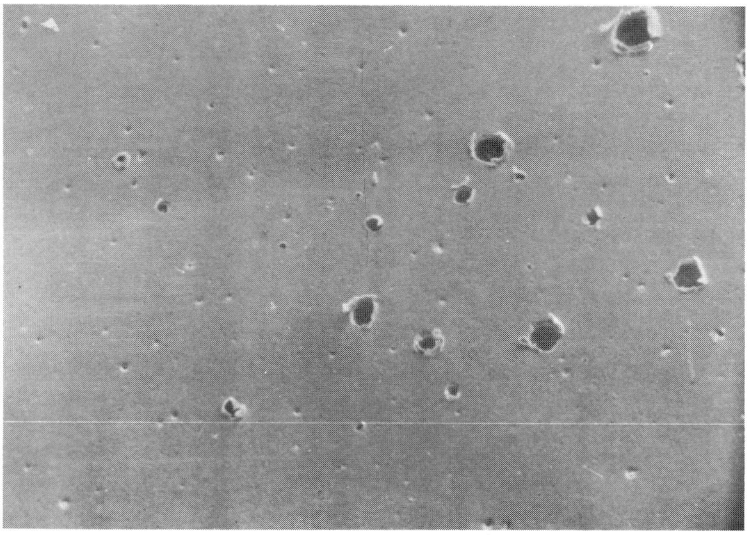

Figure 19–3 Surface texture of a composite resin, cured against a matrix band under laboratory conditions. Note the smooth surface, and several small and large voids (× 50).

jer and Stallard in 1973.[16] Several commercially available composite resins were tested. The preparations were standard, and carried out under rubber dam. The restorative materials were inserted with a plastic instrument and allowed to cure against a Mylar matrix band. Upon removal of the matrix band it was noticed that flash was present and extended over the enamel surface. This could easily be removed with a sharp instrument. No attempt was made to correct the contour or the margins of the restoration. Prior to removing the rubber dam, the restorations were duplicated, utilizing a replica technique reported previously. By means of this technique an exact copy of the restoration was obtained, which was prepared for scanning electron microscope investigation. The results appeared to be rather uniform, and regardless of the composite restorative material used the following could be observed. Upon clinical examination all restorations appeared to be clinically acceptable and were considered successful; the smooth, shiny appearance which was characteristic for the *in vitro* prepared samples was not always observed, however. On a microscopic level, pits and voids and surface irregularities were usually present and were attributed to the fact that

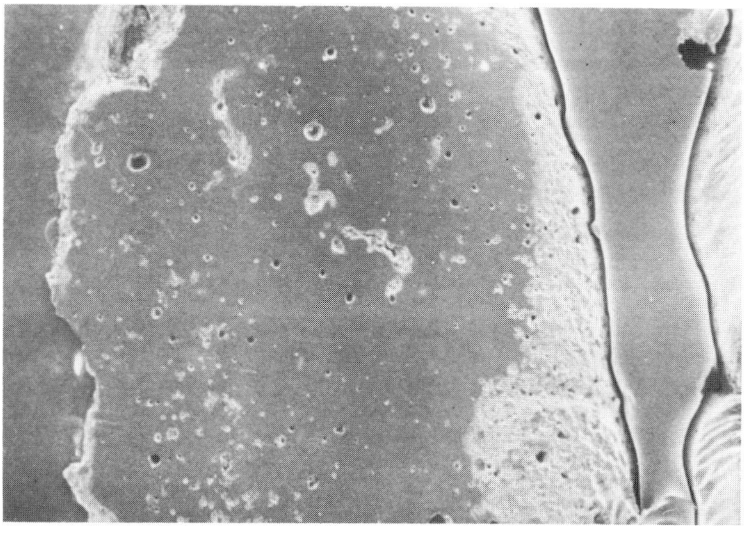

Figure 19–4 A low power micrograph (× 25) of a replica of an *in vivo* duplicated restoration (Cl. III). Note the overhang, the void at the margin and the multiple surface defects.

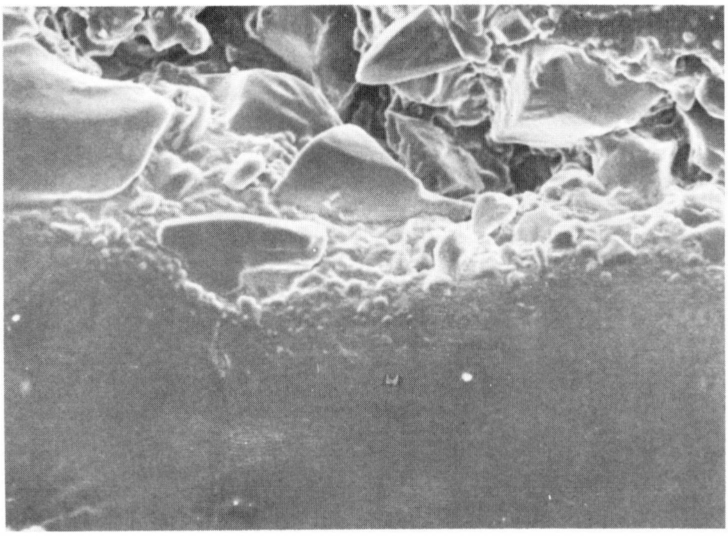

Figure 19–5 This is a high-power magnification (× 1000) of one of the surface defects shown in Figure 19–4. The filler particles are immediately below the smooth surface.

the matrix band cannot be completely immobilized during the polymerization process (Fig. 19–4). On areas where no contact with the matrix band was accomplished, or where movement had occurred, filler particles could clearly be seen penetrating the resin matrix (Fig. 19–5).

Most disconcerting, however, was the presence of either partial or total overhanging margins, with a surface that was elevated in relation to the enamel surface. No attempt was made to correct these margins, since it was of interest to observe this situation again after periods of weeks and months. Therefore, the replicating procedure was repeated at intervals ranging from weeks to months, with no special home care instructions given to the patient. These replicas provided a series of samples which permitted analysis of the surface changes on a sequential basis. Figure 19–6 shows a series of scanning electronmicrographs obtained from replicas of a freshly placed restoration to the post-insertion appearance after a period of seven weeks. As can be seen in Figure 19–6*A*, the fact that a matrix band was utilized provided no guarantee that a smooth surface would be produced. Overhanging margins and voids mar the surface of the restoration. A replica made one week after insertion demonstrated a completely different surface appearance. In the areas where a smooth surface was present immediately after operation, filler particles could now be observed penetrating the resin matrix. In other words, after one week all superficial resin matrix had disappeared, presumably by abrasion. The results after seven weeks were essentially no different from those after one week.

It is of interest to note that after the initial disappearance of the resin matrix, the materials demonstrate a much higher resistance to abrasion. For example, in Figure 19–6*B* a specific filler particle was observed which could be replicated in the same detail after a period of seven weeks. Another example is presented in Figure 19–7. This time a different composite resin was utilized and clinically the restoration demonstrated an acceptable result. Figure 19–7*A* depicts the enamel-composite interface. It is of particular interest to note that this time, although a matrix band was utilized, no smooth surface was created whatsoever. At a higher magnification (× 150) a surface saturated with quartz filler was shown. Note the detail of enamel rods in the damaged margin of the cavity wall. Figure 19–7*C* shows the surface after a period of seven weeks. Plaque has now accumulated at the margins (see arrow) and has filled the enamel defect of the cavity wall (Fig. 19–7*D*). Only a small amount of the superficially present quartz filler was re-

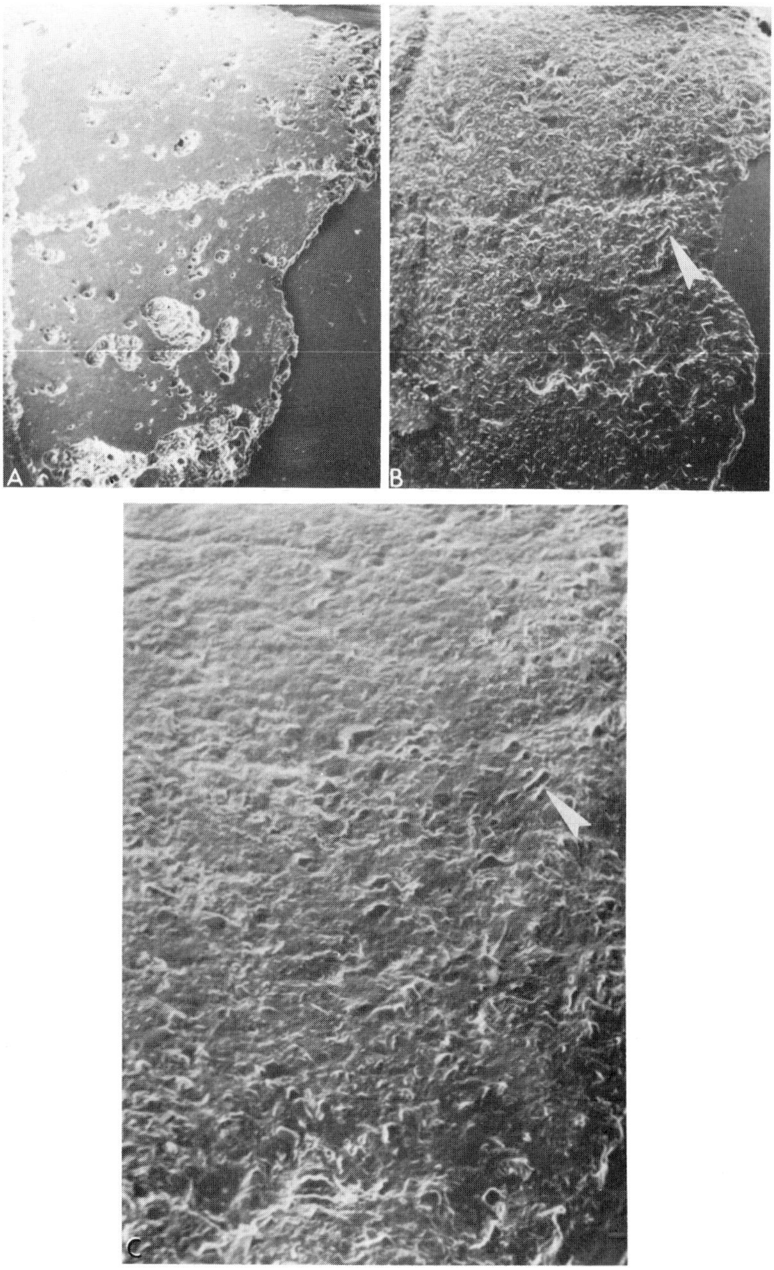

Figure 19–6 *A*, This replica of a Class V restoration demonstrates the surface characteristics of an *in vivo* placed restoration. Numerous surface defects can be seen along with smoother areas, together with overhanging margins. Note the crossed grooves which serve as reference lines between the different replicas (× 50). *B*, Appearance of the same restoration of *A* after one week. Over the entire surface, exposure of filler particles has occurred, owing to abrasion of the superficial resin matrix (× 50). *C*, After seven weeks the appearance is similar to that demonstrated after one week. The arrow shows a particular filler, among others, which also could be observed after one week. This proves that initial abrasion of the resin matrix is a rapid process, but that once the filler is exposed composite resins exhibit a high resistance to abrasion.

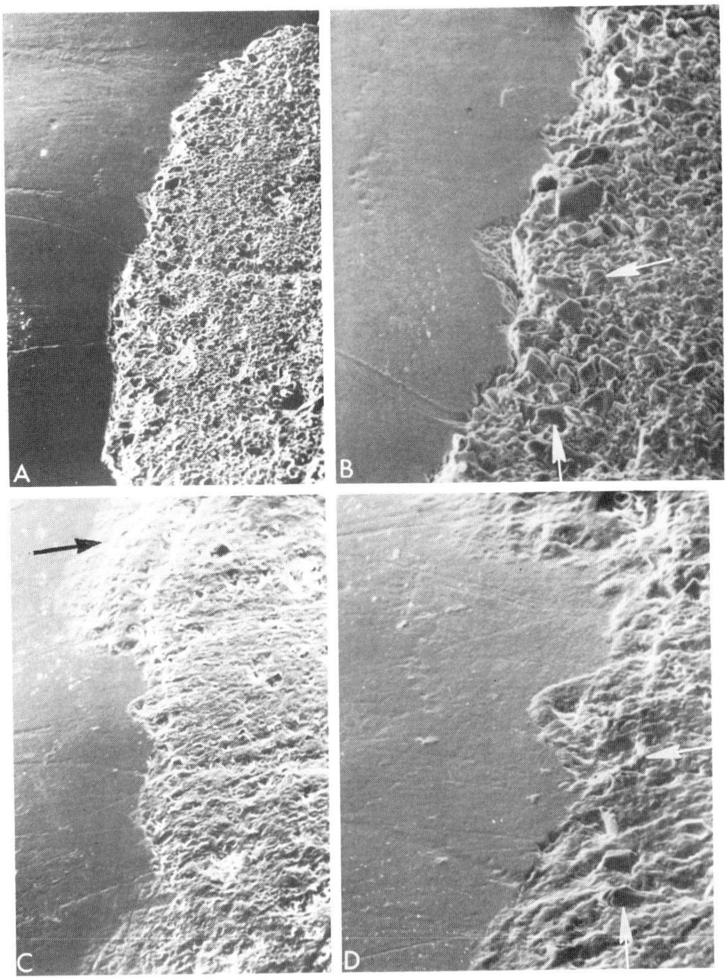

Figure 19–7 *A*, A replica of a composite resin immediately after placement. Although a matrix band was utilized, no smooth resin surface was obtained. *B*, A high-power view demonstrating the abundance of quartz particles at the surface. *C*, The appearance of the restoration after a period of seven weeks. Note the accumulation of plaque (see arrow), bordering the interface enamel composite resin. *D*, A high-power view of the same area of *B* after a period of seven weeks. With a few exceptions (see arrows) most superficial filler particles are washed away.

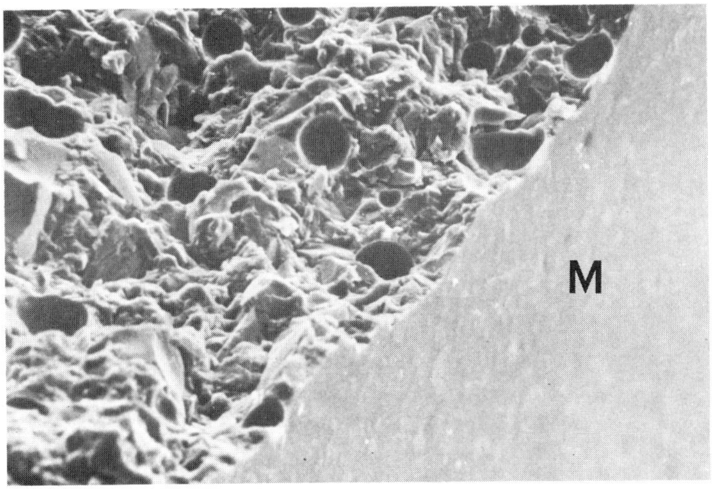

Figure 19–8 Fractured sample of Adaptic. The smooth surface of the resin matrix (M) can be seen, with immediately below it numerous quartz particles and several voids, caused by trapping of air.

tained; the majority has been washed away by saliva.

A fractured sample of a composite material (Fig. 19–8) demonstrates the smooth, superficial resin material underneath which the filler can be seen. Deeper layers are composed of resin matrix surrounding the filler, and occasional voids caused by trapping of air. The pure resin of the surface layer disappears in a matter of weeks, exposing the filler, which is extremely hard and resistant to abrasion. Continuous loss of filler particles proceeds, however, owing to abrasion of the surrounding matrix or to other, as yet unknown factors.

These clinical findings confirmed the *in vitro* experiments of Eames (1971), and Eames et al (1971). Similar studies had been conducted by the author in which samples were prepared *in vitro* and polymerized against a matrix band. The specimens were brushed for five, 10 and 30 minutes with an electric toothbrush. Examination with a scanning electron microscope revealed that basically no differences in surface characteristics were observable. The results of five minutes of brushing caused abrasion of the surface resin layers and protruding of filler particles (Fig. 19–9). In other words, brushing for five minutes is sufficient to abrade the superficial layer of resin, thus exposing the underlying filler. Even if clinically a smooth, shiny surface could be obtained, it would be of very short duration once the restoration was exposed to the oral environment.

It can be concluded from the foregoing that the overhanging margins are undesirable, as they create food traps (Fig. 19–4). What, then, are the alternatives to finish these surfaces? A variety of finishing burs and stones were designed, among which

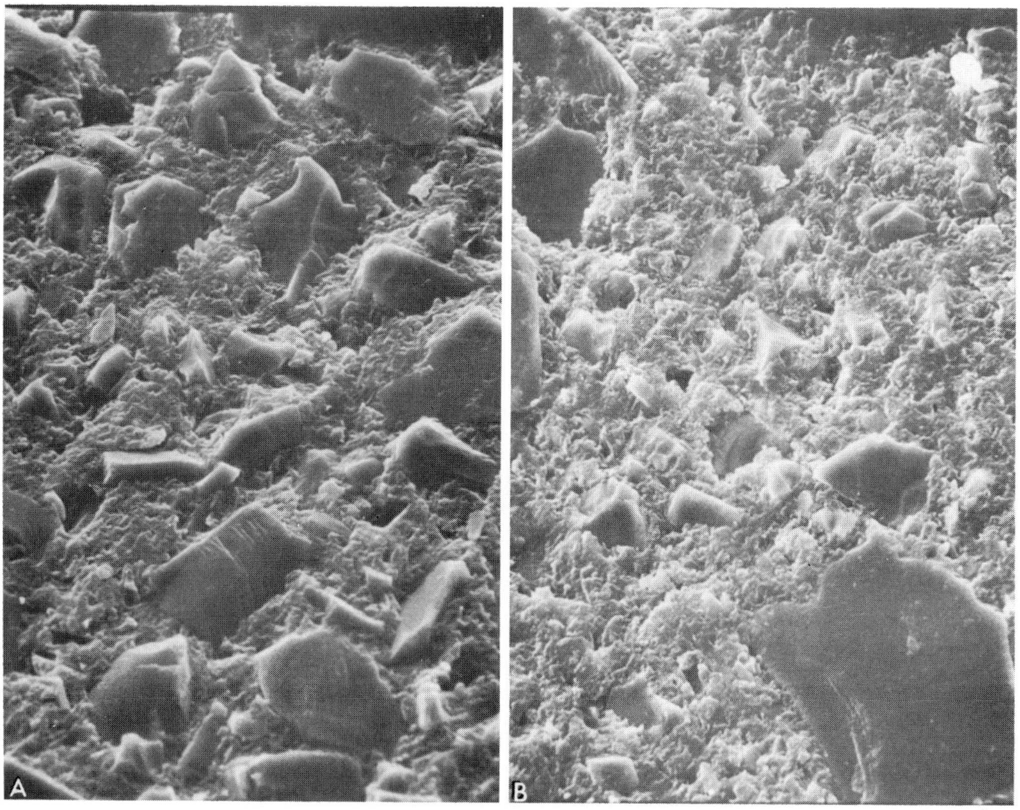

Figure 19–9 *A*, Example of a specimen of Concise, cured against a matrix band and brushed for five minutes with an electric toothbrush (× 1000). *B*, The same resin but now brushed for 30 minutes with an electric toothbrush. Essentially, no difference can be noted as the only change occurs after the resin matrix is worn out (× 1000).

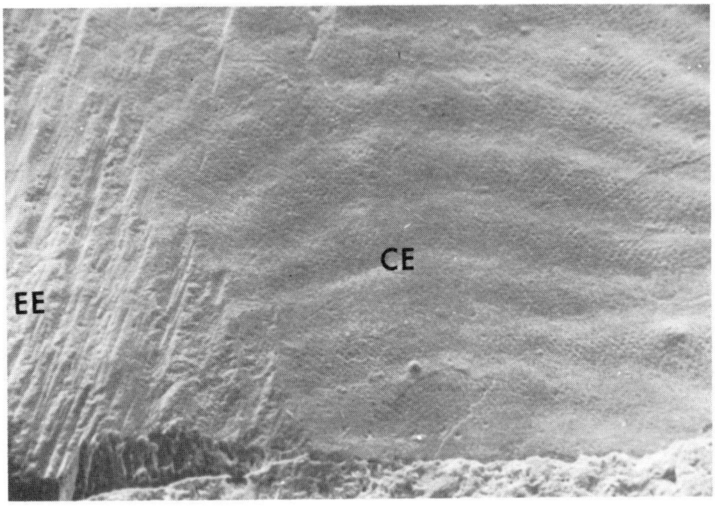

Figure 19–10 The result of the use of a superfine finishing bur on the surrounding enamel. Note the grooves and scratches on the experimental side (EE) compared to the smooth appearance of the control side. (CE) (× 127).

were special paper discs, white stones, and superfine high-speed diamond finishing burs. The most efficient bur in finishing and contouring resins was found to be the diamond bur. However, the devastating effect on the surrounding enamel, causing grooves and scratches, should be considered highly undesirable. A similar effect, although perhaps to a lesser extent, was observed with all finishing burs. Figure 19–10 is a scanning electron micrograph of a composite resin finished with a superfine diamond bur. Note the roughening of the enamel surface (EE) compared to the other half of the tooth which was not touched (CE).

Ironically, no improvement of surface smoothness of the composite resins was accomplished. It is, therefore, of importance to always finish the contoured restoration with pumice or polishing paste. This will polish the grooves and scratches in the enamel caused by finishing burs or discs, but is not intended to polish the composite. It is essential that these grooves be eliminated, since their retention of plaque will promote microleakage, which may subsequently cause a discoloration of the margins and finally result in failure of the restoration.

New methods have recently been introduced which by-pass the problems encountered with the rough surface of composite resins. One method utilizes the principles of pit and fissure sealants. After the restoration is contoured and finished to the operator's satisfaction, 1½ to 2 millimeters of surrounding enamel is conditioned with phosphoric acid. The conditioner will etch the enamel and clean the composite resin. The 50 per cent phosphoric acid is commercially termed "conditioner," since this term sounds less alarming than 50 per cent acid. After one minute the acid is thoroughly washed away and the preparation air dried. Using a fine camel's-hair brush, a thin layer of sealant is painted on the restorative material and the 1½ to 2 millimeters of surrounding enamel. By means of ultraviolet light the material is polymerized, and the excess monomer is wiped off with a wet cotton roll. An esthetically superior restoration is obtained, and chances that microleakage will occur are diminished if not eliminated for as long as the sealant is present. Figure 19–11 represents a clinical case of two Class V restorations. It can be observed that the dull appearance of the surfaces has disappeared upon application of the sealant. The composite restoration on the canine shows the "highlight" which is so characteristic of wet enamel and determines esthetics of natural teeth.

It should be clear from the foregoing that the numerous advantages which accrue with the addition of filler particles become drawbacks when it comes to finish-

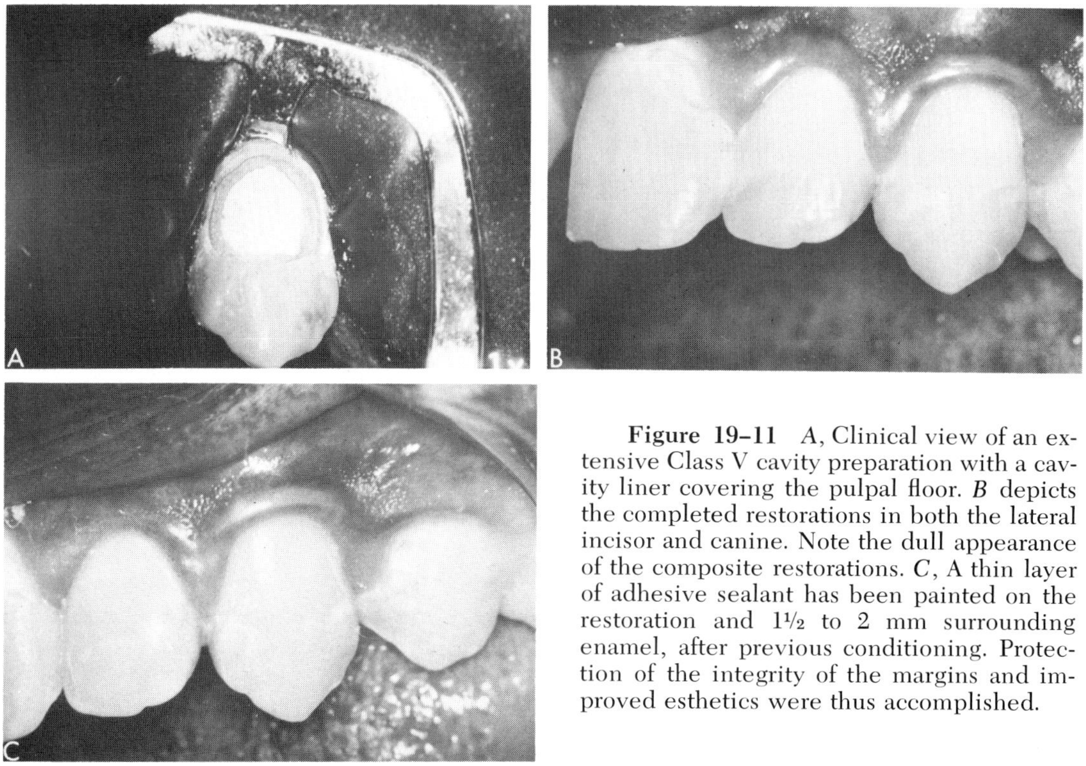

Figure 19–11 *A*, Clinical view of an extensive Class V cavity preparation with a cavity liner covering the pulpal floor. *B* depicts the completed restorations in both the lateral incisor and canine. Note the dull appearance of the composite restorations. *C*, A thin layer of adhesive sealant has been painted on the restoration and 1½ to 2 mm surrounding enamel, after previous conditioning. Protection of the integrity of the margins and improved esthetics were thus accomplished.

ing the restorations to a smooth surface. That diamond particles could polish fillers such as glass balls or quartz appeared to be clinically impossible. Diamond can polish glass, but not the combination filler and resin, the last constituent of a significant lower hardness.

Recently, new polishing stones and pastes have been developed which are capable of polishing filler particles. It requires only minutes to smooth the particles at the surface. This can be illustrated by scanning electron micrographs made from the following samples. A representative sample was replicated by means of the hard replica technique[15] and subsequently polished for 30 seconds. At this time another replica was made, followed by a second period of 60-second polishing. A third replica was then made, representing the total surface changes after 90 seconds. The original and two replicas were compared and can be seen in Figure 19–12*A*, *B*, and *C*. The scanning electron micrographs show that only a short time is required to polish the filler particles. That particles are actually polished is demonstrated by the flat appearance. With this type of surface, essentially composed of filler, a considerable resistance against abrasion can be anticipated. Whether in the long run this surface will prove to be satisfactory depends on the rate of abrasion of the interparticle resin matrix. Wear will eventually cause the release of polished particles, thus exposing new ones which have their original sharp and pointed appearance. Over how long a period of time this will happen remains to be seen and needs further investigation. In conclusion, it can be said that (1) from a clinical point of view, the use of a matrix strip with composite resins to produce a smooth surface is not realistic. The matrix band keeps the restorative material within the basic contours of the preparation, yet rarely produces a clinically microscopically smooth surface. (2) Routinely, overhanging margins and an elevated resin surface to the enamel level exist in what appears to be a clinically acceptable restoration. Theoretically, even if an ideal, smooth surface could be obtained with perfect marginal

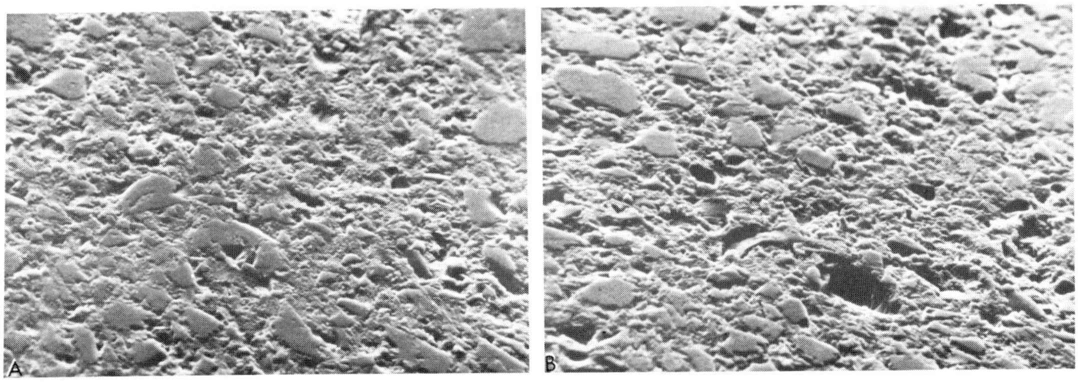

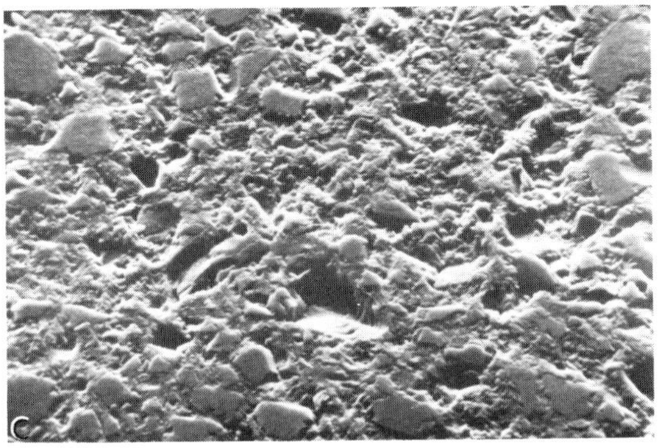

Figure 19–12 A sequence of replicas representing the effect of a composite finishing stone. *A* demonstrates the effect of polishing during 30 seconds. The filler particles appear to be definitely flattened and polished. The effect of another 30 seconds (*B*) caused the release of several fillers, and the same occurred with an additional 30 seconds (*C*) (× 220), without significantly improving the surface smoothness.

adaptation, utilizing a matrix strip, exposure to the oral environment would still cause the surface resin layer to wear in a short period of time, thus exposing the deeper filler particles and resulting in a rough surface. (3) Diamond finishing burs or discs do not polish composite resins, but rather are effective in contouring restorations; at the same time they cause damage to the surrounding enamel. (4) The rough enamel surface thus created retains plaque better, and promotes marginal leakage and discoloration. (5) Subsequent polishing with pumice or polishing pastes creates a smoother enamel surface, which can be maintained more easily and is less prone to plaque retention. (6) The application of a thin layer of pit and fissure sealant not only improves the esthetics but also prevents microleakage as the porte d'entree is sealed off. Thus the composite resin restoration must be considered a tremendous addition to the armamentarium of the dentist in preserving and restoring natural teeth.

REFERENCES

1. Buonocore, M. G., and Sheykoleslam, Z.: Effect of enamel adhesives on marginal leakage. I.A.D.A. Abstracts No. 711, March 1972.
2. Brannstrom, M., and Nyborg, H.: Pulpal reactions to composite resin restorations. J. Prosthet. Dent. 27:181–189, 1972.
3. Chan, K. C., Soni, N. N., and Khowassah, M. A. F.: Fissure reactions to two composite resins. J. Prosthet. Dent. 27:176–180, 1972.
4. Chandler, H. H., Bowen, R. L., and Paffenbarger, G. C.: Method for finishing composite restorative materials. J. Am. Dent. Assoc. 83:344–349, 1971.
5. Dennison, J. B., and Craig, R. G.: Physical properties and finished surface texture of composite restorative resins. J. Am. Dent. Assoc. 85:101–108, 1972.
6. Eames, W. B.: Finishing and polishing restoratives. J. Tenn. Dent. Assoc. *51*:(No. 1) Jan. 1971.
7. Eames, W. B. et al.: The effect of brushing on the surfaces of filled resins. J. Alabama Dent. Assoc. 55:22–25, 1971.
8. Goto, G., and Jordan, R. E.: Pulpal response to composite resin materials. J. Prosthet. Dent. *28*:601–608, 1972.
9. Johnson, L. N., Jordan, R. E., and Lynn, J. A.: Effects of various finishing devices on resin surfaces. J. Am. Dent. Assoc. 83:321–332, 1971.
10. Kun, W. B. and Pameijer, C. M.: An adhesive for

sealing composite resins. J. Dent. Childr. pp. 25–31, March. April, 1975.
11. Larato, D. C.: Influence of a composite resin restoration on the gingiva. J. Prosthet. Dent. *28*:402–404, 1972.
12. Lee, H. L., and Swartz, M. L.: Scanning electron microscope study of composite restorative materials. J. Dent. Res. *49*:149–158, 1970.
13. Mosteller, J. H.: Composite resin restorations. J. Ala. Dent. Assoc. *56*:27–31, 1972.
14. Norman, R. D., Phillips, R. W., and Swartz, M. L.: Fluoride uptake by enamel from certain dental materials. J. Dent. Res. *39*:11–16, 1960.
15. Pameijer, C. H., and Stallard, R. E.: Application of replica techniques for use with scanning electron microscopes in dental research. J. Dent. Res. *51*:672, 1972.
16. Pameijer, C. H., and Stallard, R. E.: The fallacy of polishing composite restorations. Dent. Surv. 33–37 April, 1973.
17. Phillips, R. W.: Science of Dental Materials. 7th ed., Philadelphia, W. B. Saunders Co., 1973, p. 228.
18. Phillips, R. W., Swartz, M. L., and Norman, R. D.: Materials for the Practicing Dentist. St. Louis, C. V. Mosby Co., 1969, Chap. 11.
19. Trivedi, S. C., and Talim, S. T.: The response of human gingiva to restorative materials. J. Prosthet. Dent. *29*:73–80, 1973.

SUGGESTED ADDITIONAL READING

Ast, D., Bushel, A., and Chase, H.: A clinical study of caries prevention with zinc chloride and potassium ferrocyanide. J. Am. Dent. Assoc. *41*:437–442, 1950.

Bodecker, C.: Enamel fissure eradication. N.Y. State Dent. J. *30*:149–154, 1964.

Buonocore, M. G.: Caries prevention in pits and fissures sealed with an adhesive resin polymerized by ultra-violet light: A two year study of a single adhesive application. J. Am. Dent. Assoc. *82*: 1090–1093, 1971.

Hyatt, T. P.: Prophylactic odontotomy. Dent. Cosmos *65*:234–241, 1923.

Klein, H., and Knutson, J.: Effect of ammoniacal silver nitrate on caries in first permanent molars. J. Am. Dent. Assoc. *29*:1420–1426, 1942.

Miller, J., and Pameijer, C. H.: A clinical investigation in preventive dentistry. Dent. Pract. *1*(3):66–75, 1950.

Walter, O., and Moreira, B.: Effectiveness of acetic acid and chromic anhydride in prevention of dental caries. J. Dent. Child. 38:70–72, 1971.

chapter 20

PREVENTION OF MALOCCLUSION AND MINOR ORTHODONTICS

by

T. K. BARBER, D.D.S., M.S.

INTRODUCTION

Twenty years ago the general dentist asked, "How do you make a space maintainer? How do you bend a labial wire for a Hawley retainer?" or "How do you use rapid cure acrylic?" We were technique-oriented and what appeared important to the practitioner was his learning to use materials, instruments and appliance construction.

Manual skill technique is still important, but today's graduate and today's general dentist more frequently ask questions related to what, why and when. What is the status of this child's occlusion? What can be expected to occur if I do not treat it? Why are these crowded? Why has the deciduous cuspid space closed? When can I expect to see a growth change? When is it necessary to open the bite? These and many similar questions point out the desire on the part of the busy practitioner to gain greater insight and a depth in understanding the dynamics of growth and dental development of the child. In addition, he seeks practicality—How do I apply this knowledge to everyday use in my practice?

Equally important are the frustrations of the practitioner who feels insecure in the great desire to include minor orthodontic service in his dental practice yet lacks confidence in his ability to discriminate between those types of problems he can treat and those with which he needs help or which he should refer to a specialist. It all depends upon his individual diagnostic skill.

Prevention of malocclusion and the success of minor (or major) orthodontic intervention of a developing malocclusion depend almost entirely upon diagnostic skill and the ability of the general dentist to recognize his capability to reverse the process of dentition maldevelopment. Thus, the objectives of this chapter are to:

1. Define the needs for general practice participation in preventive and minor orthodontics.

2. Provide an overview of the types of common problems encountered in mixed-dentition development.

3. Present and discuss diagnostic aids, their uses and application by the general dentist.

4. Provide a guide for his discrimination as to the types of dental maldevelopment that he can expect to manage alone, those he might manage with orthodontic specialist consultation and those which can be treated only by the specialist.

5. Suggest treatment needs for a sample of the most common problems.

THE SCOPE OF PREVENTABLE MALOCCLUSION

Undoubtedly, the major reason parents desire orthodontic care for their children is aesthetic—a pretty smile on a pleasant face. However, this is not the only reason. Parental concern for caries prevention and periodontal disease prevention extends beyond the aesthetics of a good occlusion to the recognition that an acceptable occlusion relates to these other disease entities. Not all minor malocclusions should, or even could, be treated. The general dentist can be expected to discriminate between acceptable and unacceptable occlusion and advise the parent on the child's needs for treatment.

WHAT IS MALOCCLUSION?

Normal occlusion generally implies the acceptable relationship of the teeth in one jaw to each other and to those of the opposing jaw. Stated in another way, malocclusion is broadly of two types:

1. The relationship of the upper and lower jaws to each other is quite acceptable, but *within* the jaws the teeth are in malrelation. This is a *dental malocclusion.*

2. The teeth may or may not be in an acceptable relation within each jaw, but the jaws are in malrelation. The malocclusion is thus the fault of the skeletal malrelation. This is a *skeletal malocclusion.*

The generally accepted key to occlusion and means of classification lies in the relationship of the first permanent molars in occlusion. As the lower molar relates to the upper, Dr. Angle[1] described occlusion as (1) normal, (2) Class I malocclusion, (3) distal or Class II malocclusion, and (4) mesial, or Class III malocclusion.

There is an important discrimination to be noted in the above classifications which often goes unnoticed and is graphically illustrated in Figure 20–1. "Normal" means that both the jaw relations to each other and the occlusion of the teeth within these jaws are normal (or desirable). A "Class I malocclusion" means that the jaws relate to each other desirably, but the teeth within these jaws are in malrelation. Thus, a Class I malocclusion is a *dental malocclusion.* It must be recognized that molar relations to each other can be altered locally through migration of one or both of the permanent molars. Thus, the molars could relate to each other in a Class II position but still be a Class I malocclusion.

Both Class II and Class III malocclusions are the result of jaw malrelation. They are the *skeletal malocclusions.* As in the former example, the molars in a Class II or III skeletal relation can migrate to a Class I molar relation, but the malocclusion still has as its basis a skeletal malrelation and classification (Figs. 20–1B and 20–1C). It will be one of our important objectives to learn to discriminate between these differences, for there is a strong relation to treatment by the general dentist.

ETIOLOGIC CONSIDERATIONS

To relate the malocclusion to its etiologic factors is a step toward reaching our objective of discrimination, or the development of diagnostic skill. Our knowledge and understanding of the etiology of malocclusion have a strong bearing on treatment. The point has been made that malocclusion is either the result of tooth migrations within the jaw base (dental malocclusion) or a malrelation of the jaw bases themselves

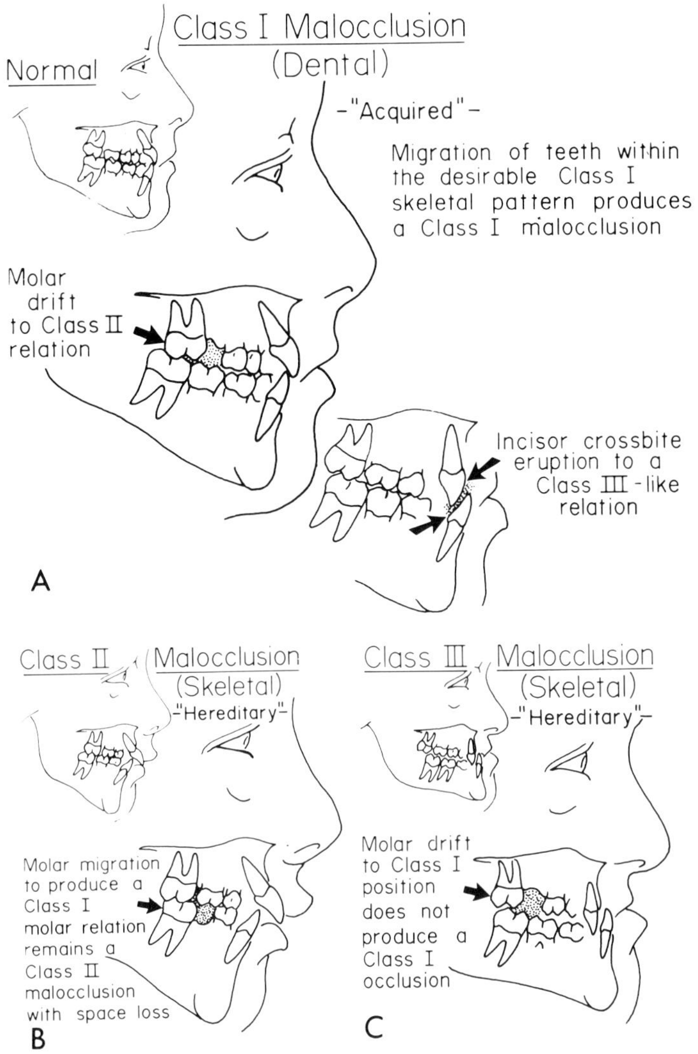

Figure 20–1 Discrimination between "dental" malocclusion of teeth alone on a normal skeletal relationship *(A)* and those of retrognathism, Class II *(B)* and prognathism of Class III *(C)* commonly termed "skeletal" malocclusion. Note that individual teeth may drift to alter the molar or incisor relation without changing the basis for the type of malocclusion.

(skeletal malocclusion). The latter is strongly related to jaw growth and anatomy.

Class II Malocclusion. Referring again to Figure 20–1B, the child with a true Class II malocclusion pattern gives the impression that the mandibular anatomy is one of a lengthened ramus and shortened body. At least, when compared to the maxillae and the profile, a mandible of this shape would produce a facial profile showing a retruded (retrognathic) chin. The result is the distocclusion of the molar relation and a wide variety of incisor relations, the most common being an apparent maxillary protrusion.

Class III Malocclusion. In contrast, the reverse anatomic variation is seen in the true Class III occlusion, i.e., the characteristic mandibular anatomy is one of shortened ramal height and a lengthened body. The result is a mesiocclusion of the molars with a protrusive chin profile (prognathic). The common incisor relation in a Class III case is one of crossbite. Quite frequently the entire maxillary dental arch is contained (crossbite) within the mandibular arch and almost gives the impression of an underdeveloped maxilla (Fig. 20–1C). Both true Class II and Class III are related to skeletal jaw growth patterns and are regarded as having a *hereditary* etiology. Consider for a moment our inability to treat or correct a jaw growth malrelation caused by heredity.

Such is outside the scope of general dental practice.

I want to emphasize once again that the teeth *within* the Class II and Class III jaw relations can migrate to produce a Class I molar relation, but the occlusion remains a Class II or III malocclusion. It is not a Class I malocclusion and the practitioner must learn this discrimination (Figs. 20–1B and 20–1C).

Class I Malocclusion. The Class I malocclusion has been labeled the *dental malocclusion.* The skeletal relation of upper to lower jaw is normal (desirable), but as a result of dental developmental disturbances, the teeth migrate to malrelationships. The child *acquires* his malocclusion as distinguished from an inherited malocclusion (Fig. 20–1A).

Dental development, from birth to adulthood, depends upon a finely integrated and balanced oral environment. The normal growth process must continue unencumbered by traumatic accidents or other internal or external environmental influences. The environment includes a muscular influence as teeth erupt. When the oral musculature is imbalanced by abnormal muscular forces, the teeth migrate to undesirable positions in response to the pressures or lack of pressure. Actively erupting teeth exert a force upon the already erupted teeth sufficiently strong as to be capable of altering their dental arch position, should the environment permit. Unopposed, the erupting tooth will migrate to a malposition in the arch. Once in place, and in occlusion, each tooth is subject to forces of occlusion sufficient to drive teeth into positions of malrelation, should they be unopposed or out of contact or rotated.

The practitioner must be able to recognize those molar teeth that have migrated to a Class II or Class III *molar relation* in a Class I case. It is still a Class I case and because the teeth have migrated, it becomes a "Class I malocclusion," not a Class II or III malocclusion.

In summary, Class I (dental malocclusion) is a desirable jaw relation on top of which the teeth have *acquired* a malocclusion as the result of disturbances in the timing, pattern or sequence in (1) normal growth, (2) muscular balance, (3) eruption forces, and (4) occlusion forces.

THE FREQUENCY OF MALOCCLUSION

Our attention is drawn to statistical surveys of the types of malocclusion and their frequency in the child population, since they have bearing on a program of preventive or minor orthodontic care. If we accept the concept that the "skeletal" malocclusions require fully corrective orthodontic procedures rendered by the specialist, then the dental malocclusion remains as a limiting classification for preventive or minor orthodontic guidance. The non-specialist, or general practitioner, may be expected to render a significant dental service to that segment of the child population whose developing malocclusion is the result of developmental disturbances in timing, sequence or pattern. Thus, the Class I malocclusion *may* be prevented or may respond favorably to minor orthodontic guidance for correction.

The dental literature contains numerous reports of isolated surveys tabulating the variability of normal and abnormal occlusion in the child population.[2-14] The data from the older literature are difficult to compare because of the wide diversity of criteria used, the wide range of ages examined and the irregular intermixing of data from both deciduous and permanent dentitions. The more recent data tend to identify the incidence of malocclusion based upon Angle's[1] classification.

In general, the prevalence of Class I, or dental malocclusion types, will vary between 50 and 60 per cent of the child population at almost any age. At the same time, Class II malocclusion will range from 30 to 45 per cent, while Class III malocclusions are seen from 0 to 10 per cent in the child population. Both Classes II and III are termed skeletal malocclusions, arising as the result of skeletal growth patterns and strongly based on heredity.

WHAT IS PREVENTABLE?

It seems reasonable to expect that little, if anything, might be contemplated by the general dentist to prevent or intercept, by minor orthodontic therapy, a malocclusion developing as part of a basic and hereditary skeletal pattern. Graber[15] states that "unless we can change cranial and facial superstructures and reorient the bony trabeculae, stress trajectories, and supporting pillars and buttresses, along with their muscle attachments, we cannot significantly change arch form, much as we would like to, in an attempt to accommodate the teeth."

A preventive or minor orthodontic program of dental service rendered by the general dentist should be limited to the Class I (or otherwise normal occlusion) desirable skeletal growth pattern, in which minor and local dental developmental etiologic factors may lead to a more gross malocclusion if uncorrected. The Class I malocclusion is the most frequent (50 to 60 per cent) and represents the largest portion of the child population with malocclusion. This is the group in which the general dentist can expect to exercise a successful preventive or minor orthodontic program.

DIAGNOSTIC AIDS

THE IMPORTANCE OF DIAGNOSIS

Treatment of the preventable or minor orthodontic problem by the general dentist depends upon his ability to distinguish between the Class I, II and III malocclusions. He must be able to reasonably diagnose a skeletal pattern (non-preventable) from a dental pattern (acquired-preventable) of malocclusion. In addition, his diagnosis will depend upon the ability to identify the acquired pattern and to determine what, when and how he can intervene to reverse the aberrations of normal dental development.

An experienced diagnostician can usually distinguish between skeletal and dental malocclusions in some percentage of cases by his clinical examination alone. In some additional percentage, he will call upon diagnostic aids for further information to help him make his decisions. In another percentage of cases, he will still not be certain of his diagnosis even with the use of diagnostic aids, but he will speculate. He will repeat the diagnostic tests at yearly intervals to help him determine more accurately the value of his speculations. And in some percentage of cases, he will never be sure of his diagnosis.

The inexperienced diagnostician will need to use diagnostic aids as learning tools. With their repeated use he gains experience. With experience his diagnostic abilities improve, and as an experienced diagnostician he will still be faced with the superior "batting average" of the more experienced man, but his own will have markedly improved and he will have learned more clearly what his own limitations are. To be an effective general dentist employing preventive and minor orthodontic services in the child patient requires study and practice—there are no short cuts.

CLINICAL EXAMINATION OF THE PATIENT

The clinical examination of the child patient is probably the most essential element of diagnosis. Dental study casts, or models, intraoral or cephalometric radiographs and photographs are aids to the diagnosis made clinically. Generally, these aids are used to confirm or deny the impressions gained by the clinical examination. They add information not observed clinically by allowing a better or more complete view of the clinical material as it relates to occlusion. In any event, a systematic clinical examination of the state of occlusion should be performed so that important signs will not be overlooked. A suggested order of examination is discussed below.

EXAMINATION OF THE FACE

The facial characteristics of the child reveal information relative to his dental occlusion, and quite frequently the examiner is able to gain a solid impression of the skeletal growth pattern by this examination alone. The dentist should examine the facial morphology carefully and by employing a few simple procedures, he can identify quite accurately the facial type, its symmetry and the facial proportions of vertical dimension.

Facial Type (Frontal and Profile)

One of our major objectives is to distinguish between Class I, II and III skeletal patterns. Begin by examining the full face from in front. It generally holds true that a narrow face will contain narrow dental arches; a broad face, broad arches. Frequently, one is able to view a broad face which contains narrow dental arches and would lead the examiner to be suspicious of dental crowding possibly due to muscle patterns or habits.

Frontal View. Of particular interest is the symmetry of the right and left sides of the face. Are they equal in size and do they display similar contours? If not, explore the possibilities. Perhaps there has been unequal growth, a traumatic accident or other factors, all of which may be reflected in the shape or size of the dental arches. Examine the midline of the face and its relation to the incisor dental midline.

Figure 20–2 illustrates how the examiner may take any straight-sided card or paper and, standing directly in front of the patient, hold the edge of the card in front of the face so that it coincides with the center of the bridge of the nose and filtrum of the upper lip. Now ask the patient to close on the back teeth. Part the lips and note whether the edge of the card coincides with the interproximal line between the upper incisors. Let us suppose it does not. Ask the patient to relax, that is, to part the teeth slightly, and note the relation of the card to the lower incisor midline. If it coincides with the card, the upper dental arch is not symmetrical and deviates to one side, but the lower arch is symmetrical with the face. If the upper has been found correct and the lower midline coincides with it, both are

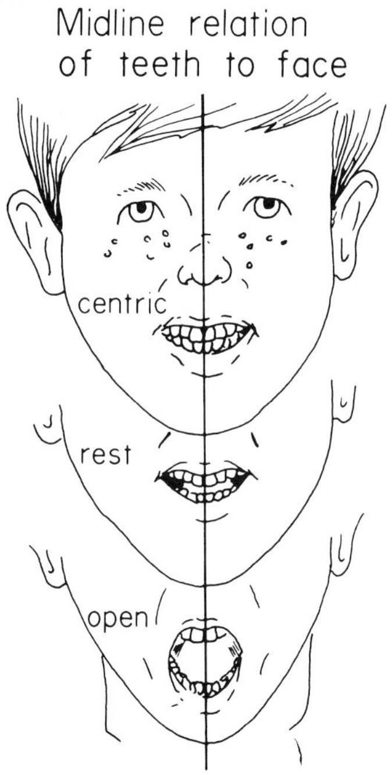

Figure 20–2 Identification of the facial midline and examination of right and left facial symmetry. Note the relation of upper and lower dental midline in occlusion, rest and wide open positions.

correct. If the upper is correct but the lower does not coincide with it, the lower dental arch is not symmetrical. Be sure to note all relations exactly because all manner of variations are possible; that is, both may deviate to the same side or upper and lower may deviate to opposite sides. The information has considerable value when related to the dental examination and the need for minor corrective orthodontics.

Other factors of facial symmetry that should be examined for in the frontal view include the parellelism of the eyes, ears and dental occlusal plane. Figure 20–3A illustrates the transporionic, transorbital and occlusal plane axes. Examine to determine if the ears and eyes are in a level with one another. Use the midplane of the face for reference and determine if the horizontal plane of the iris of the eye is at right angles to the mid-facial plane. Ask the child to place one of his fingers in each ear and examine to determine if the external auditory canals are similarly horizontal and perpendicular to the midplane of the face (transporionic axis).

One can expect symmetry of the face to display symmetry in the dental arches. Conversely, asymmetry of the face may display asymmetry in the dental arches. Next, examine the horizontal relation of the occlusal plane. Ask the child to bite on a straight edge such as a heavy card or small ruler in such a way as to allow for observation of the horizontal parallelism of the occlusal plane in relation to the eyes and ears and vertical to the mid-facial plane. Do they all coincide and are they in symmetrical relation to each other? Let us, as an example, find that they do not. The possible reasons cannot be explored fully, but these side-by-side asymmetries relate to maxillary and mandibular growth and development and very frequently display relations to dental findings.

The Lateral Profile. With the patient sitting upright in the chair, examine the lateral profile by visualizing two planes: the Frankfort horizontal plane and the facial plane. Figure 20–3, the lateral profile, illustrates each. The Frankfort horizontal plane extends horizontally from the upper border of the external ear canal forward to the palpated lower border of the bony orbit. The facial plane is visualized vertically as a plane from the bridge of the nose to the chin.

Vertical Dimension. Does the patient show a balanced (Class I) pattern as in Figure 20–3B, where the facial and Frankfort planes form nearly a right angle? Or does the profile appear retrognathic as in Figure 20–3C, where the maxillae look protrusive and the mandible retrusive with a receding chin (Class II). The reverse may be seen as in Figure 20–3D with the maxillae straight or retrusive and the mandible protrusive (Class III). It is often helpful to hold a right-angle card, such as the patient's record folder, next to the face to aid in this visualization.

Note that in Figures 20–3B, 20–3C and 20–3D the profile examination includes an assessment of the facial convexity. Note the relation or the angulation formed from the bridge of the nose to the upper lips and from

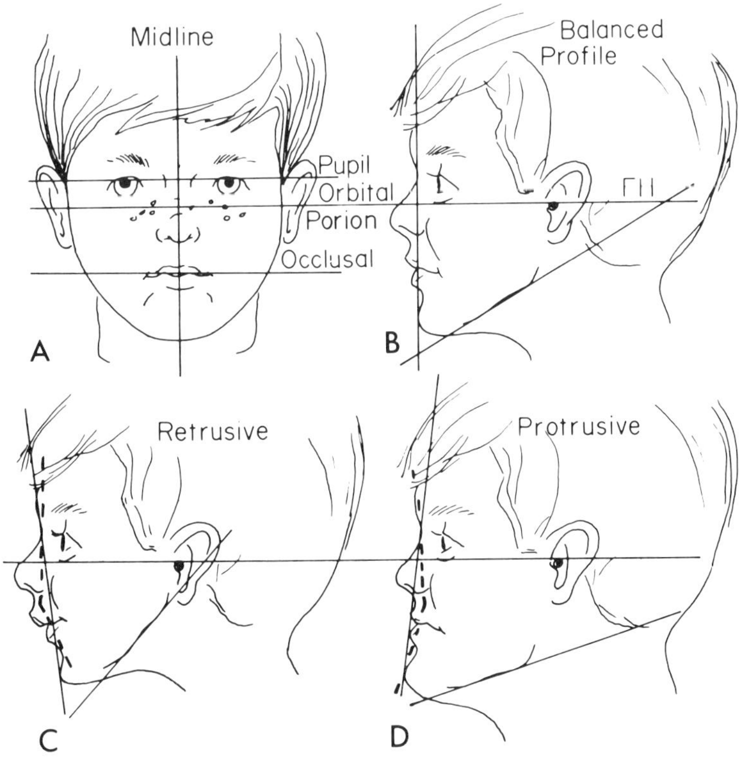

Figure 20–3 Parallelism of the transverse pupillar, orbital, porionic and occlusal plane axes with each other and their perpendicular relation to facial midline *A*. Lateral profile views in *B* show orthognathic or balanced features of Class I while *C* illustrates the steep mandible, convex and retrognathic face of the Class II and *D* the concave and prognathic face of the Class III skeletal patterns.

the lip to the chin. A straight line or plane is part of the balanced Class I skeletal pattern (Fig. 20–3B), while the Class II pattern (Fig. 20–3C) displays convexity and the Class III pattern (Fig. 20–3D) is concave or shows an excessively long face.

The lateral profile examination should also include an assessment of the angulation of the lower border of the mandible. Using a straight edge, such as a card, placed along the lower border of the mandible, examine this mandibular plane in relation to the Frankfort horizontal (ear-eye) plane. A steep (excessively angled) mandibular plane, as seen in Figure 20–3C, usually relates to the downward and less forward-growing mandible of the Class II patient.

Clinical data of this type can usually be correlated quite well with cephalometric data obtained from careful measurement of oriented lateral radiographs to be discussed later. The clinician is frequently able to identify the skeletal pattern of Class I, II or III on the basis of the clinical examination alone. As stated in earlier discussions, the management of minor dental occlusion maldevelopment by the general dentist is limited to the dental malocclusions seen in Class I, and all of the Class II and III skeletal types will require clinical management of the specialist. Thus, the separation or identification becomes very important.

Functional Examination

The purpose of this phase of the examination is to determine the symmetrical function of right and left temporomandibular joints and their functional relation to the dental occlusion. Stand in front of the patient and lightly palpate each TMJ. While doing this, have the patient open his mouth wide and slowly close to centric occlusion as seen in Figure 20–2. You should palpate a bilaterally symmetrical initial hinge action on opening to rest position followed by a forward glide of the mandibular condyle. Carefully observe the behavior of the upper and lower dental midlines during function. They should continue to coincide from occlusion to a wide-open position and return in a symmetrical pattern.

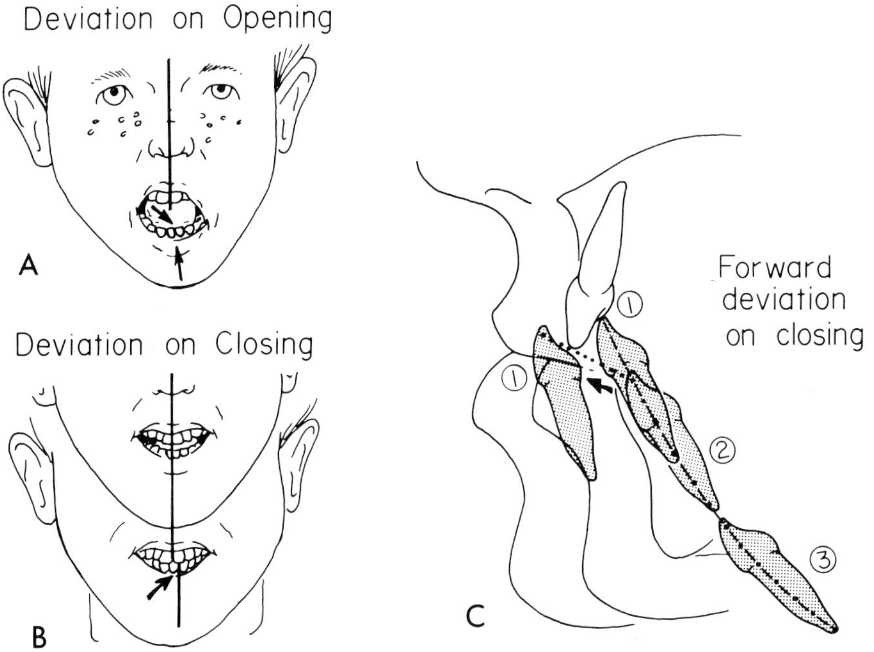

Figure 20–4 Alterations in occlusion pattern during function as in *A* where the mandible skews to the left upon opening and *B* where the skewing occurs upon closure. In *C* the pattern is one where the child closes in a forward pattern. In each, the dental pattern may affect function.

Occasionally, a child will demonstrate asymmetry of mandibular function either upon opening or upon closing. In Figure 20–4A the child deviates his mandible to the left upon opening. This may occur as the result of asymmetrical mandibular growth with related dental findings. In Figure 20–4B the child shows a deviation of mandibular closure from rest position to centric occlusion. This is a fairly common occurrence and most frequently relates to dental findings wherein the dental occlusion shows a deviate midline and a unilateral crossbite. It can be speculated that at some time the young child experienced a dental cuspal interference and developed a "convenience" bite to one side. Clinically, the picture is one of a crossbite, whereas in reality the fault is not dental, it is functional.

Dental treatment usually consists of maxillary expansion to accommodate the mandible in occlusion.

Functional crossbites are seen also as illustrated in Figure 20–4C. In this case the child appears to show a Class III pattern in centric occlusion. Dentally, he may exhibit a crossbite of the total maxillary-mandibular occlusion. As in the previous example, his pattern of mandibular closure might be quite smooth from a wide-open position to rest position; but from there to full occlusion, he can be seen to thrust the mandible forward to produce an anterior crossbite, and the TMJ is palpated to exhibit a forward thrust of the mandible. Here, too, the child may be demonstrating a "convenience" bite and, while resembling a Class III patient initially, may not be at all.

Dental treatment usually consists of maxillary expansion to accommodate the mandible in occlusion.

Facial (Soft Tissue) Physiology

The clinical examination of the face includes an assessment of muscle tone, particularly of the lips and tongue, and of the patient's facial habits, breathing, swallowing and speech. Since each constitutes a part of the muscular environment of the teeth and dental arches, several points should be noted during the initial examination to distinguish an acceptable pattern from one which may affect the dental occlusion.

Lips

The level of the lip line, their size, tonus and any evidence of abnormal function should be noted.

Figure 20–5 illustrates the usual anatomic variable observed in lip level. It may vary from the edge of the upper incisor teeth (Fig. 20–5A) to a level well up on the labial surface of the alveolar process above the incisors (Fig. 20–5C). The average lip level is about one-third up from the maxillary incisal edge (Fig. 20–5A). A shortened upper lip, as seen in Figure 20–5D, will

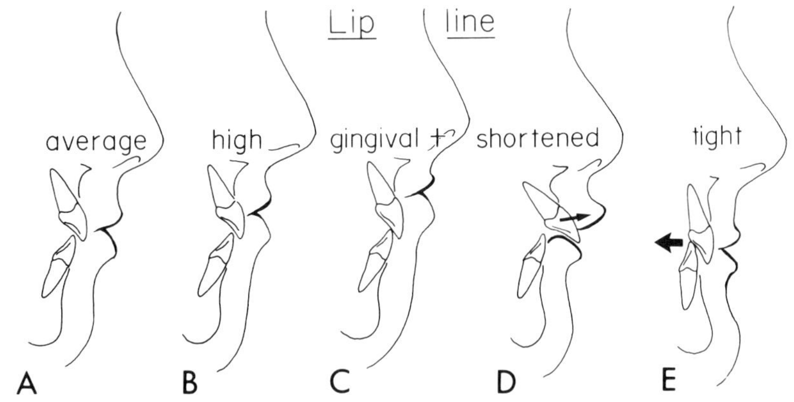

Figure 20–5 The level of the lipline, their size and functional tone provide muscular force to retain tooth position. In *D* the incisors are protrusive due to muscular imbalance typical of thumb and tongue habits. *E* illustrates the upright incisor position attending excessive labial pressures.

often require the patient to close the lips with difficulty. Frequently, such patients have an "open-mouth" habit and are mouth breathers. The occlusion may demonstrate protrusive incisors with spacing due to the migration of the teeth unopposed by a normal lip musculature.

Lip *tonus* relates to tension and is usually described as flaccid (loose), rigid, or average. Through experience, the dentist may develop an impression of tonus by gently pinching the lip with thumb and forefinger and gently pulling the lip forward. There is a definite feeling of a loose and rather fatty lip with little tone. The incisors will often protrude, evincing deficient muscle tone (Fig. 20–5D). Others will be crowded and forced lingually with hyperactive lips (Fig. 20–5E).

In a relaxed state (in the rest position), a child may have his lips apart (open-mouth habit), thus producing a lack of *lip seal.* In such cases the lips are usually flaccid and produce no external pressure forces on the upper anterior teeth. The upper anterior teeth may then tend to protrude as a result of the lack of lip pressure. Occasionally, a child may develop habits of chronic breathing through the mouth. The gingivae may then become dried and inflamed due to constant exposure to air.

The mentalis habit is that of chronic puckering of the chin muscle. It is quite strong and produces a severely crushed and crowded lower dental arch. Usually the habit is formed by forcing the lower lip to reach for a shortened upper lip because of a lack of lip seal. Such an abnormal and constant pressure may collapse the lower anterior teeth lingually and prevent full eruption of the upper anteriors. The dental effects are profound and treatment consists of applying a "lip bumper" to reduce the labial pressures on the teeth. (See Figure 20–21.)

Tongue

Little is known of the physiologic-neuromuscular synergism between the lips and tongue, although a great deal of clinical importance is attached to their muscular balance and related tooth position. Examination of the face should include an examination of the tongue. However, dental findings will often remind the dentist to examine the lips and tongue for their influence on tooth position.

The absolute *size* of the tongue is not as important as its size relative to the oral cavity. While true macroglossia is rare, relative macroglossia is not infrequently encountered in children, especially those with Down's Syndrome. An overly large tongue will almost invariably be accompanied by spacing of the teeth. This may be seen in both arches or only in the lower. If in the lower alone, it may indicate that the tongue habitually lies low in the floor of the mouth, whereas if both upper and lower teeth, and particularly the anterior, are spaced, it indicates a tongue that completely fills the mouth.

The so-called physiological spacing that occurs in many children coincident with, or just prior to, the eruption of the permanent successors can usually be distinguished quite easily from the spacing caused by an oversized tongue. In the former, the arch will be typical in form and only the anterior teeth will exhibit the spacing, whereas in the latter the arch will be rounded out in the buccal areas and the buccal teeth will also show spacing.

The tongue may also be seen to function in other positions and habits which reveal themselves through the position of the teeth. One of the most frequently encountered is that in which the tip of the tongue is habitually held between the roof of the mouth and the edges of the lower incisor teeth. The incisor teeth will be prevented from fully erupting and a significant space will be noted with the teeth in occlusion (Figs. 20–6A and 20–6B). This tongue position results in a perfectly even mandibular incisal line but one which is below the occlusal plane of the other lower teeth. The upper arch may show no deviation from the normal or the upper incisors may also be prevented from erupting.

Occasionally, a child will be seen in whom both upper and lower incisors have been pushed forward by either an excessively large tongue or by a habit of thrusting the tongue against these teeth while swal-

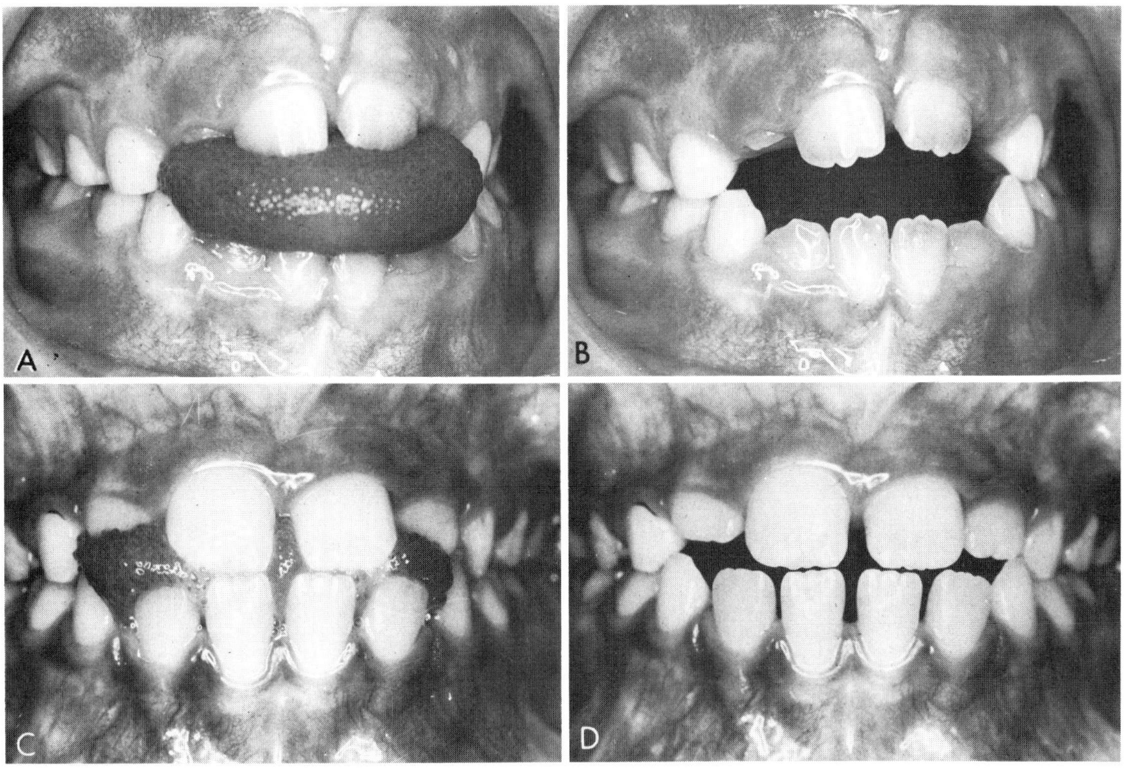

Figure 20–6 Dental effects of abnormal tongue habits. *A* and *B* illustrate tongue "resting" while *C* and *D* show incisor protrusion from tongue "thrusting" associated with the visceral swallowing pattern of the young child.

lowing (Figs. 20–6C and 20–6D). These can usually be differentiated by noting the form of the dental arch. The large tongue is usually found in an arch that is wide as well as spaced, the thrusting habit is frequently associated with an abnormally narrowed arch. Treatment of these minor malocclusions usually encompasses muscular retraining, often performed by a speech therapist, or the use of dental appliances to inhibit or retrain the muscular habit pattern (see Figure 20–20).

Speech

The only speech deviation that has ever been shown to be caused by disarrangement of the anterior teeth is the lisp. Lisping results frequently from the inability of the patient to seal the front of the mouth with the tongue or lips when pronouncing *S*, *Sh*, or related sounds. Spaces between the teeth of the two arches permit air leakage and cause the lisp. Parents frequently ask the dentist for his opinion regarding the speech of their children, particularly those under the age of six. Spacing of teeth with minor effect on speech patterns is common but not abnormal. It nonetheless is part of a thorough clinical examination to relate aural observations with dental patterns to identify the presence or absence of a relationship. Usually no dental treatment is necessary.

INTRAORAL EXAMINATION OF OCCLUSION AND DENTAL DEVELOPMENT

To clinically examine the child and determine the relationships of his teeth to each other within each arch and to the arches together, it is necessary to systematize the examination so as to minimize overlooking any one factor of importance. Many details are observed more thoroughly through study of a set of dental casts, or models. This technique will be discussed separately.

First, count the teeth in each arch. This seems like an unnecessary step, especially to a trained examiner, yet is is remarkable how frequently supernumerary teeth will occupy space in an arch, and their presence will most often adversely affect the positions of adjacent teeth and the occlusion and go unnoticed. Most often the supernumerary tooth should be removed. Teeth that are absent, either for congenital reasons or lost through normal exfoliation or through extraction, will also adversely affect the spacing of the dental arch. Usually, space loss and ultimate crowding result. Frequently, the need to open, or regain, lost space is identified through the simple process of counting the teeth.

Secondly, examine each arch, upper and lower, to identify the deciduous and permanent components. Try to establish the dental age of the child as compared to his chronologic age. Frequently, the dental age will be advanced, i.e., he is erupting permanent teeth earlier than normally expected. Occasionally, some crowding will be present. What is the relation of tooth size to his growth status? Large teeth in small jaws lead to crowding, while smaller, even peg-shaped, teeth will result in generalized interdental spacing. Do the arches look symmetrical in shape from right to left side? Do they appear collapsed, too narrow, too wide? Do they appear to correspond to the wide or narrow face?

An important part of this preliminary observation of the arches is to examine the mid-palatine suture or median raphé of the palate. It should coincide with the middle of the face. The later examination of the dental study casts will use this raphé as a plane of reference. Any skewing of the raphé to one side should be noted for future reference.

THE ARCHES AND TEETH IN OCCLUSION

It can be expected that the child with a Class I skeletal pattern will show Class I dental relationships, *unless* they have migrated to malposition (Fig. 20–1). This would then be the *dental malocclusion*, susceptible to preventive or minor corrective treatment.

It follows that the Class II and Class III skeletal patterns will exhibit a corresponding occlusion, *unless* the teeth have migrated. Thus, a careful examination of occlusion is made and must be related to the skeletal pattern before any treatment is determined or instituted.

Molar Relation

The child should be instructed to close his back teeth together and hold them tight. Occasionally, the young child will close on the incisors and no attempt by the dentist to move his mandible back is successful. The operator finds it difficult to gain the child's understanding and cooperation.

Place a small piece of paper on the lower molar on each side, asking the child to bite on the paper. He will usually accomplish centric occlusion with the aid of the tactile sensations provided by the presence of the paper. Retract the corners of the mouth and examine the molar relation directly from a side view. At the same time, examine the relation of the deciduous second molars and deciduous cuspid teeth.

Figure 20–1 illustrates three of the four anteroposterior molar relationships. In the small diagram labelled "normal," the tip of the mesiobuccal cusp of the upper molar and the buccal groove of the lower molar coincide. The examination of the second primary molars is the same as for the permanent molars. A Class I relation finds the mesiobuccal cusp of the upper molar falling into the buccal groove of the lower molar. In a Class II relation the distobuccal cusp of the upper first permanent molar (or second primary molar) drops into the buccal groove of the corresponding lower molar. In Class III, the mesiobuccal cusp of the upper may occlude anywhere from the distobuccal groove of its normal antagonist back to complete lack of contact with it. The fourth possibility is termed "cusp to cusp" or "edge to edge" (not illustrated). The cusp-to-cusp relation is halfway between Class I and Class II, i.e., the tips of the mesial buccal cusp of the upper molar coincide with the

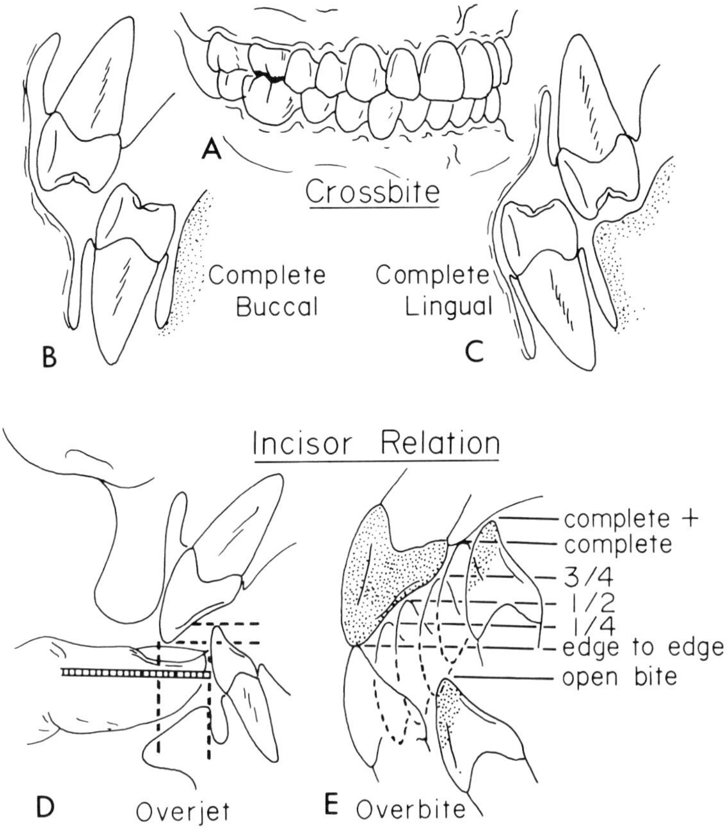

Figure 20–7 A crossbite is evidenced when opposing teeth meet so that the buccal cusp of the upper tooth occludes with the central fossae of the lower as in *A*. In *B* and *C* the crossbite is either completely buccal or completely lingual when the teeth fail to occlude centrally. *D* illustrates incisor overjet measurement using a millimeter scale while *E* provides a means of defining the amount of overbite or closed bite.

mesial buccal cusp of the lower molar. Remember, the molar relationship can be "true" or "false" due to migration. As an example, the molar relation could be Class I in a Class II skeletal pattern due to space loss in the mandibular arch and forward migration of the lower molar into a Class I position.

Figure 20–7 illustrates the *buccolingual* relation of teeth. Ordinarily, the upper teeth overhang the lower throughout the entire extent of the arch from molar to molar. The upper incisors pass in front of the lowers and the buccal cusps of the upper posterior teeth overhand the buccal cusps of the lowers. The lingual cusps of the upper posterior teeth thus drop into the fossae between the buccal and lingual rows of lower cusps.

Crossbite is the term given to any departure from normal buccolingual or labiolingual relation of the upper to the lower teeth. Occasionally, one or more of the upper incisors will be found to close lingual to the lowers (See Fig. 20–17A). Such teeth are said to be in (incisor) crossbite. Similarly in the buccal segment, one or more teeth of the upper arch may be so positioned that the buccal cusp of the upper is caught between the buccal and lingual cusps of the lower teeth (molar or bicuspid crossbite, Fig. 20–7A). The crossbite may be so marked that the upper molars are completely buccal to the lower, as in Figure 20–7B (or lowers in complete lingual relation to the uppers, as in Figure 20–7C).

Most frequently, the crossbite is the manifestation of an ectopic or deviate eruption pattern and easily correctable by the general dentist. On some occasions the crossbite is produced by a deviation of the mandible during function (see previous section). Suggestions for treatment will follow in a later section.

Incisor Relation

Incisor relationships are measured in *overbite* and *overjet,* as illustrated in Figures 20–7D and 20–7E. Anterior overbite relates to the distance by which the upper incisors overhang the lower, vertically or in a superoinferior direction. It may range from a condition of no contact (open bite) to one in which the upper teeth completely obscure the lower when the jaws are together (Fig. 20–7E). To arrive at a judgment of the overbite of the anterior teeth while in occlusion, mark the position of the incisal edge of the upper right central incisor on the lower central with a pencil. Note the degree of overbite in estimated fractions of the amount of the lower incisor crown which was covered, as follows: open bite; edge to edge: 1/4; 1/2; 3/4; complete; complete +. If the incisal edge of the upper closes to a position *below* the gingival margin of the lower, this is considered complete ++. The open bite exists during the early stages of incisor eruption persists as a consequence of several oral habits and muscle imbalances. The closed bite is seen after eruption is complete and is normal during the early stages of growth and dental development. The closed bite of the young child is reduced through mandibular growth. It persists as a treatable phenomenon, usually because of supraeruption of the incisors and as a consequence to arch collapse. Treatment suggestions follow in a later section.

Overjet relates to the distance by which the upper teeth fail to contact the lowers in a horizontal or posteroanterior direction (Fig. 20–7D). To measure the overjet insert a millimeter scale horizontally in the same way the pencil was used to measure overbite. Measure the distance in millimeters after making sure that the zero mark is at the end of the scale.

Both overbite and overjet can be made more accurately from study models, but satisfactory approximations can be made directly on the patient. Overjet will frequently be excessive when the child exhibits an oral habit, such as finger sucking. Many times the protrusive incisors relate to the closed bite, while in other instances the excessive overjet will be a part of the Class II skeletal and molar relation.

In summary, the objectives of the clinical examination are to:

1. Attempt to identify the skeletal pattern from the observation of the frontal and lateral profile of the face.
2. Identify the occlusion and its relation to the clinical assessment of the facial variants.
3. Develop a preliminary appraisal of the need for minor orthodontic correction and the feasibility of its treatment by the general dentist.

CEPHALOMETRIC RADIOGRAPHY

Growth and development of children are difficult to predict. Physical growth of young children is usually a continuous process, but between children there exists manifold variation in patterns and rates of growth.

The dentist must appreciate the changes that occur during jaw growth and the changes that occur during dental development. The ultimate occlusion of the grown child is the result of these two factors and, since each has an affect on the other, their influence is difficult to separate. Jaw growth affects the occlusal relation of the total upper and lower dental arches to each other, thereby producing the "skeletal malrelations" of occlusion. Dental development *within each arch* often has much the same effect. However, these "dental malrelations" may be prevented or guided with some measure of success if we can distinguish between skeletal effect and dental developmental pattern. The careful clinical examination of the growing child provides limited insight to growth. Cephalometric roentgenography provides an additional tool whereby the student, general practitioner and orthodontist may continuously appraise the growing jaws in several ways.

Cross-sectional cephalometry is the comparison of the data obtained from a child's head film with like data obtained from a population of children at the same age. Stated another way, how does this child's skeletal pattern differ from those of other children, particularly those who exhibit a normal, desirable jaw growth and relationship? *Longitudinal* or *serial* cephalometry allows the comparison of a given child's skeletal pattern from one year to the next. Stated another way, how is he growing when you compare his data from year to year? Cephalometry provides a means for evaluating the pattern of jaw growth, the roles and direction of jaw growth and some related facets of dental development. Superimposed tracings of head films permit an analysis of the changes occurring in jaw relation and give evidence of accompanying dentitional change.

CEPHALOMETRIC TECHNIQUE

There are a variety of cephalometric "analyses" utilized to appraise skeletal and dental growth patterns from a lateral head film. Each employs measurement of planes and angles determined from anatomic landmarks of the skull and facial structures. The reader will find a fairly comprehensive presentation of cephalometric technique in Graber's text of orthodontics[16] and is referred to individual reports and studies[17-41] for more detailed information.

In general, desirable skeletal patterns will fall within a range of acceptable "norm values." These are regarded as Class I skeletal patterns. Class II and Class III skeletal malocclusions demonstrate various deviations in growth pattern from the normal, desirable range. Thus, the skeletal analysis provides a means to appraise the facial type and the anteroposterior relationships of the denture base. Examination of the opposing incisor teeth in relation to each other and to their individual bony bases provides information on tooth position and its relation to dental arch space availability.

Skeletal Patterns

In general, "norm standard values" for cephalometric data are available for a young adult age range[18, 26, 28, 40] with markedly limited data for the younger childhood ages.[17, 19, 21, 22, 25, 30, 31, 33] Figure 20–8 depicts a generalized gross differentiation between the skeletal profiles of Class I, II, and III types. In Figure 20–8A the normal pattern of skeletal jaw growth illustrates that the slightly convex face of the young child grows to become a straight profile. The mandible grows downward and forward faster than the maxillae, bringing the profile of the young child to the balanced profile of the adult. This is seen as the angle SNA (maxillae) and SNB (mandible) increase with time; the mandibular SNB often increases more than the maxillary SNA. The chin follows a downward and forward pattern depicted by the "Y" axis within acceptable range (59°). In the Class I pattern, the face "swings out from under" the cranium. The steep mandibular plane and occlusal plane flatten or become less acute. The face develops at a right angle to the Frankfort plane and facial convexity is reduced.

In Figure 20–8B, the growth pattern is that of a Class II. The original profile shows factors wherein the mandible is retrognathic and the maxilla is protrusive. The growth vector of the mandible continues more downward than forward. The "Y" axis angle (64°) is less acute than the Class I case in Figure 20–8A. The facial profile becomes more convex and the angulation of the mandibular and occlusive planes become more steeply angled.

Figure 20–8C represents a converse picture for the typical Class III growth pattern. The straighter or concave face of the young child becomes more concave with growth. In this case, the mandible grows more forward than downward. The chin point and "Y" axis are generally more acute than the Class I profile; the mandibular and occlusive planes are flattened.

Limited cephalometric values for the young child[17, 21, 25, 30] make early skeletal comparisons difficult. However, the age range from three to seven years will generally appear to have some Class II skeletal characteristics when compared to cephalometric data of the young adult. The child grows to become the young adult. Thus, only the marked Class II and III patterns are identified with some ease at the younger ages. The Class I skeletal pattern of the young child has some Class II-like ele-

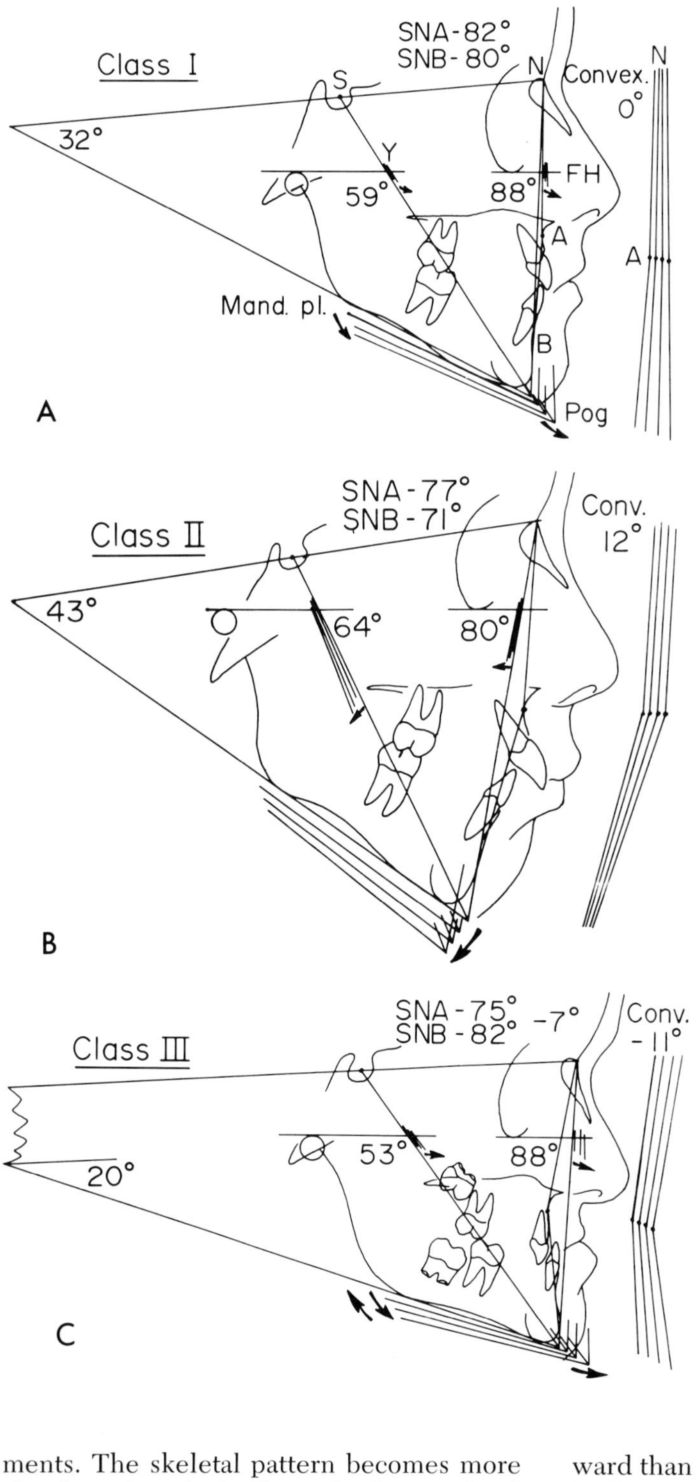

Figure 20–8 The fundamental differences between Class I *(A)*, Class II *(B)* and Class III *(C)* skeletal patterns as viewed via cephalometric tracings. In *(A)* the Class I pattern shows a straight profile which grows to reduce the slight convexity. In *B* the Class II pattern increases convexity during growth while in *C* the Class III pattern is one of increasing concavity and prognathism.

ments. The skeletal pattern becomes more clearly identified through longitudinal study, i.e., as films of the child are compared at yearly intervals. The skeletal change from one year to the next (serial study) begins to show that he is "becoming a Class I" or that he is growing like a Class II (more downward than forward) or like a Class III (markedly more forward than downward, beyond the range of Class I).

Purpose of Skeletal Assessment. The skeletal analysis of the young child is made to identify his jaw relationships and predicted growth pattern. If he shows a Class II

Dental
Pattern

Norms

$\underline{1}$ to NA°		22°
$\underline{1}$ to NA mm.		4 mm.
$\overline{1}$ to NB°		25°
$\overline{1}$ to NB mm.		4 mm.
$\underline{1}$ to $\overline{1}$		130°
$\overline{1}$ to MPA		90°

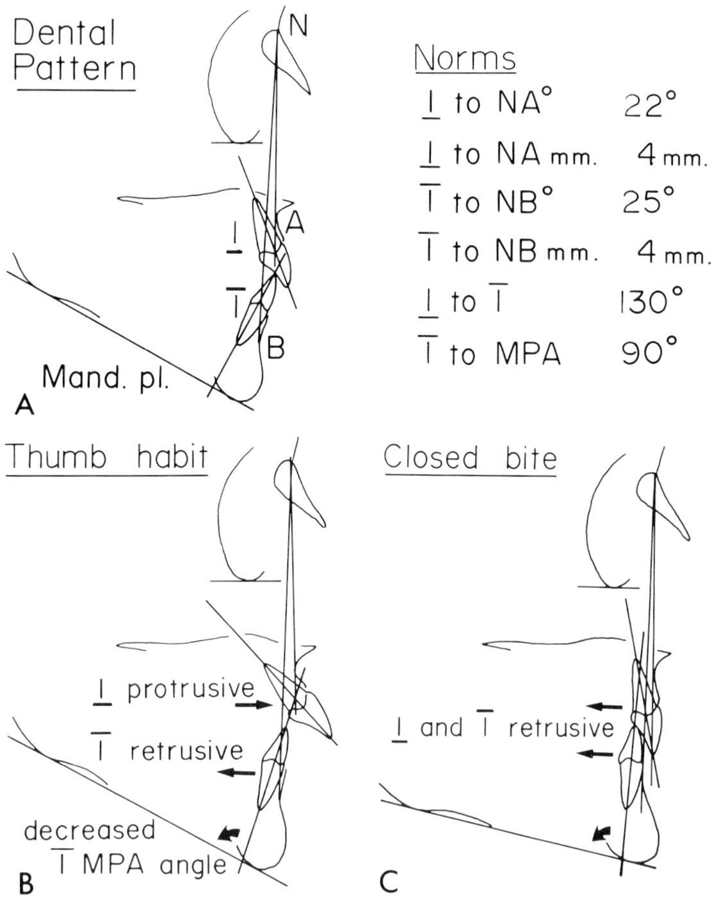

Figure 20–9 *A* depicts the generally acceptable dental pattern of incisal relation along with the norm values of angular and linear measurement. *B* illustrates a typical angular change coincident with the thumb habit while *C* depicts the incisor angulation frequently associated with a closed bite or an excessively active lip musculature.

Mand. pl.

A

Thumb habit

$\underline{1}$ protrusive

$\overline{1}$ retrusive

decreased
$\overline{1}$ MPA angle

B

Closed bite

$\underline{1}$ and $\overline{1}$ retrusive

C

or III skeletal growth pattern, it follows that his developing dental malocclusion will require fully corrective orthodontic therapy by the specialist. The non-orthodontist may wish to engage in managing space loss, oral habits and other problems of dental development in these youngsters but of limited value in the total orthodontic need. It may be more wise to recognize this greater need and thus defer any consideration of minor tooth guidance.

Dental Pattern

The cephalometric analysis of dental pattern refers mainly to the incisors. Figure 20–9 illustrates a common method of appraising incisor relations and represents the combination of the work of Steiner[40, 41] and Downs.[26, 27] The standard norm values represent average values of desirable relations at maturity for the young adult and bear little relation to the unknown values for the deciduous teeth of the child. In Figure 20–9A the incisors are in balance with good overjet and overbite; the lower incisor stands relatively upright on the mandibular base, as represented by the mandibular plane angle.

Graber[16] points out that it is unwise to attach too much significance to any one criteria, such as the axial inclination of the lower incisor, since a wide range of acceptable inclinations have been reported. However, in the individual case the incisor angulations present give useful information when some form of desirable treatment is contemplated. For example, in Figure 20–9B the upper incisors are found to be quite protrusive and the lower incisors are inclined lingually in the thumbsucking child. In Figure 20–9C the incisors are upright and inclined lingually in an overbite (closed bite) example. With the knowledge of where these teeth would more desirably be positioned in a normal relation, the dentist is often able to determine how far he may adjust these labiolingual relations and still remain within normal limitations. Frequently, the analysis of incisor position provides considerable data in determining the adequacy or inadequacy of available arch space and its regulation.

In summary, the use of cephalometric data to determine skeletal pattern and appraise dental relations to support the data obtained from the clinical examination will aid the practitioner in deciding whether he should involve himself in the treatment of the existing developing malocclusion. As a generalization in the broadest possible terms, the skeletal malocclusions of the Class II and III variety require management by the specialist. In addition, many Class I malocclusions are complicated and severe, requiring multiple tooth movements in multiple directions for correction. Many of these are more difficult to manage in correction than the typical Class II. The general practitioner should limit his clinical involvement in correcting or guiding minor malocclusions to those cases for which he has developed adequate diagnostic data after practice and skill in their application and generally with the consultation of the specialist.

ANALYSIS OF DENTAL STUDY CASTS

One of the most important diagnostic aids is a set of accurate dental study casts or models. They provide a view of the occlusion not readily obtained from clinical examination alone and enhance the data obtained through cranial radiographs. Unfortunately, the average dental practitioner has neglected to appreciate the importance of diligently obtained dental study casts as a form of dental record and as a source of useful and detailed information. Any consideration for minor tooth guidance during dental development requires repetitive record-taking on study models. Dental casts, when taken at periodic intervals, provide a basis for comparison from period to period and allow the appraisal of such problems as space loss, diastemata, tooth size differences, malpositions, arch shape and symmetry, the relation of one arch to the other and many others.

SYMMETRICAL ANALYSIS

The technique is to examine the dentoalveolar complex, comparing dental arches and antimere teeth positions for symmetry. It is a technique of "seeing." Once an asymmetry is seen, the examiner can apply his knowledge of the possible causes for the asymmetry and add to his diagnostic data. When he can see what is wrong, his plans for treatment become more valid.

In addition to a properly trimmed set of dental casts, the materials used are a pair of double-pointed dividers with the points adjustable for length and a Boley gauge. Dividers of this type are available at most drawing supply and art stores.

Overview. To begin the study cast analysis, examine the overall appearance of the models in occlusion, as illustrated in Figure 20–10A-C. Take note of any crossbite, an open bite or the presence of malposed teeth and the general appearance of occlusal symmetry. From frontal view, as in Figure 20–10B, draw a vertical line between the maxillary and mandibular central incisors. This is the *dental midline.* Compare how the upper and lower dental midlines relate to one another. When they do not coincide, it suggests that either one or the other deviates to one side or there may be a combination of both.

Rotate the casts to view the right side, as seen in Figure 20–10A. Draw a vertical line through the mesial buccal cusp of the upper first molar and another line through the central groove of the lower molar. Note the molar relationship as Class I, II, III or cusp to cusp. While viewing each side, examine the relationship of the upper and lower canine teeth. In a balanced occlusion, the maxillary canine occludes with the interproximal space distal to the mandibular

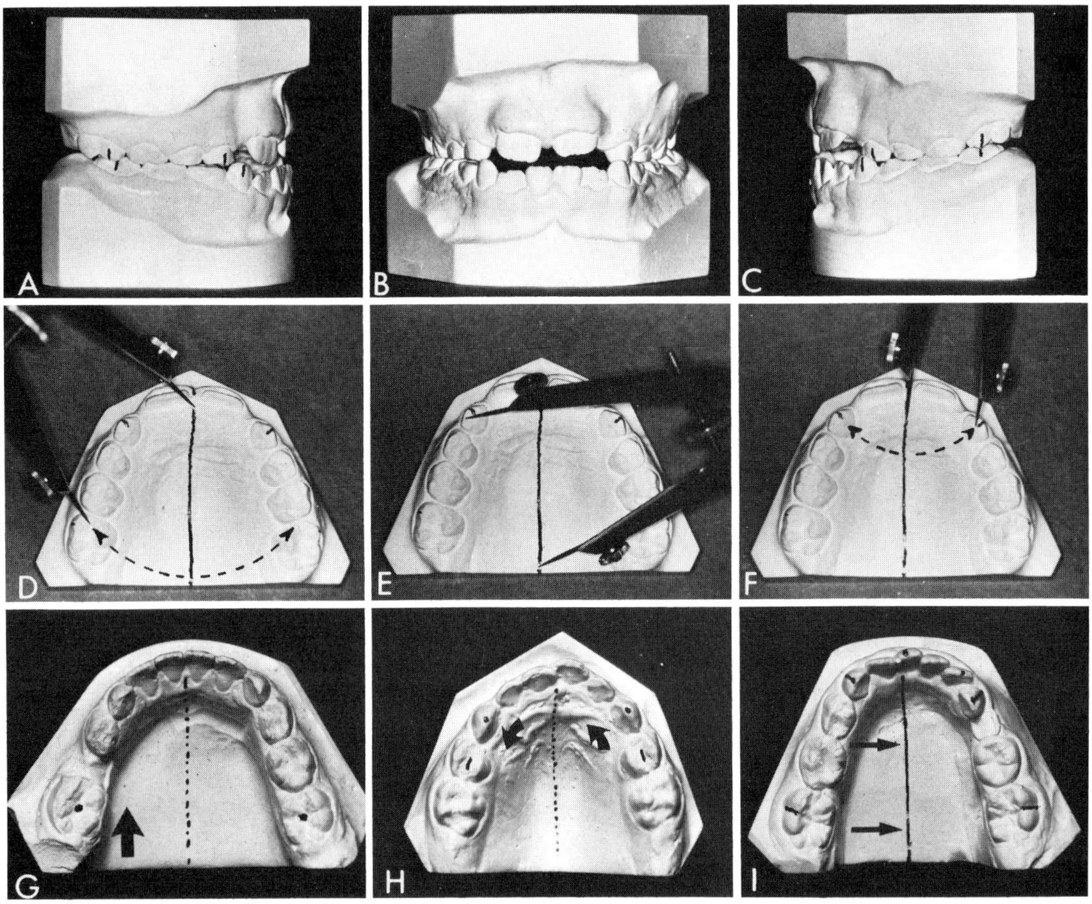

Figure 20–10 Study cast (model) analysis. *A–C* depict the preliminary examination of the casts from frontal *B* and lateral *A, C* aspects noting molar and canine relationships in occlusion. *D–F* illustrate the method of comparing right and left tooth positions for symmetry using a double pointed divider. Molar position *(D)* is tested for anteroposterior symmetry while the canine teeth *(E)* are similarly examined. In *F* the lateral position of opposite teeth may be estimated. An example of anterior molar asymmetry is seen in *G* while in *H* an asymmetry in canine position can be noted. In *I* the left buccal segment is seen to be closer to the midline than the right side.

canine. This is a Class I canine relation. Compare canine and molar relations on the same side. Are they the same? If they differ, is there a readily explainable reason such as the loss of a tooth between the canine and molar in either arch with evidence of tooth migration to close the space?

Rotate the casts to view the opposite side, as seen in Figure 20–10C, and repeat the examination of the molar and canine relationships. The profile examination of incisor overbite and overjet can also be performed to support the information gained during the clinical examination of the patient.

The cast overview provides a general impression of the occlusion. We generally ask ourselves, were the two buccal sides symmetrical? If not, was there an impression of space loss, a right and left discrepancy suggestive of a skeletal or dental shift in the arches? How did right and left buccal relations relate to any shift in dental midline? A deviation in one is reflected often in the other two.

Examination of Separate Casts. The study models are examined separately from a view of the occlusal surfaces beginning with the maxillary cast. First, do the arches appear symmetrical from side to side or is there evidence of a skewed shape in the outline of the circumference? The midpalatine suture, or raphé, serves as the skeletal midplane for reference. The suture is the base for comparing right and left arch symmetry and individual tooth position both buccally and anteroposteriorly. When transferred to the mandibular arch, the midpalatine suture serves the same purpose for the mandibular teeth and provides a clue to the way the mandible relates to the maxilla in occlusion. The line serves as a skeletal reference. For example, a right-angle square could be placed along the suture with the intersecting right-angle plane placed to correspond to the mesial surface of antimere molar teeth. If the molars are equidistant anteroposteriorly, their mesial surfaces could be expected to lie in the same plane at right angles to the midpalatal suture.

The principles of simple geometry can be applied to examine tooth and arch symmetry using an adjustable double-pointed divider for measurement. Figure 20–10D illustrates how one leg of the divider is placed on the midline at an anterior point and the divider is adjusted to correspond to an easily identifiable anatomic landmark on one first permanent molar. While maintaining the anterior divider position, the divider is rotated to compare the position of the molar on the other side (antimere) using the same anatomic landmark. Thus, the anteroposterior molar positions can be compared. Figure 20–10E illustrates the comparison of canine teeth for anteroposterior position using a point distally on the midline for reference. In the same fashion, a buccolingual symmetrical determination of antimere teeth can be made, as seen in Figure 20–10F.

Examples of the kinds of information revealed from the symmetrical appraisal are illustrated in the remainder of Figure 20–10. In 20–10G one of the molar teeth has migrated mesially and is identified through the asymmetry. In 20–10H the canine asymmetry identified indicates a space loss due to distal migration of one canine and similarly shows collapse of the anterior segment with a midline deviation. Figure 20–10I shows the type of buccolingual asymmetry that might accompany a crossbite on one side.

When the casts are placed in occlusion, it is relatively easy to transfer the median raphé line to the lower cast. The anterior point will be most accurate. The symmetrical appraisal can then be repeated for the mandibular cast, revealing similar information for that dental arch.

Another useful aid is to draw a line on the occlusal surfaces and incisal edges of each tooth extending from one contact point to the other. As the "contact line" for each arch is viewed, any minor rotations of individual teeth become readily apparent.

Review. The final step in symmetrical cast analysis is to compile the information into usable form. The technique is to "see" the differences after which we need to assess the findings with the following questions in mind:

1. *What* asymmetries were observed that can be considered normal for the stage of dental development?
2. Having observed what is out of the ordinary, we must next establish *why* the condition is there.
3. Bring the data together by asking *how* the irregularities occurred. Such influences as muscular imbalances, loss of space, crowding, crossbites, and others have a profound effect on the developing occlusion.

By attempting to answer what, why, and how the developing irregularities have occurred, the examiner may improve his diagnosis and approaches to dental therapy.

MIXED-DENTITIONAL ANALYSIS

In any examination of the child's developing occlusion, it is necessary to analyze the relation of tooth size and dental arch size. This is especially important during the transition from the deciduous arch to the permanent arch from 6 to 12 years. These measurements are most accurately made on the plaster dental study casts. The desire is to determine if each dental arch contains enough space (arch length) to accommodate the yet-unerupted remaining permanent teeth. Usually, the need to do an arch length analysis arises following eruption of the first permanent molars and at the time when the permanent incisors have erupted in their most common crowded position. The dentist would like to determine at that point if there is sufficient room (arch length) to allow for straightening of the incisors with enough remaining space for the unerupted canine and premolar teeth.

There are several popular methods for determining the space needs of the arch, namely the Nance,[42] Hixon-Oldfather,[43] and Moyers-Michigan[44] analyses. The latter, Moyers Mixed Dentition Analysis, is the most commonly used technique, offering a high degree of accuracy and reliability. Based upon the concept that the sizes of one group of teeth bear relation to the sizes of another group of teeth in the same mouth, Moyers has supplied a table of prediction measurements based upon the mesiodistal widths of the lower permanent incisors.

Technique

1. Measure the mesiodistal widths of the lower central and lateral incisors, as in Figure 20–11A. The sum of these four measurements represents the arch length (space) needed to properly align the four permanent incisors.

2. One-half of this total sum is the space needed in each incisor quadrant on either side of the midline. Note that in some cases the "dental midline" does not coincide with the "skeletal midline." Thus, one-half of the sum is the space needed on either side of the *corrected* midline to

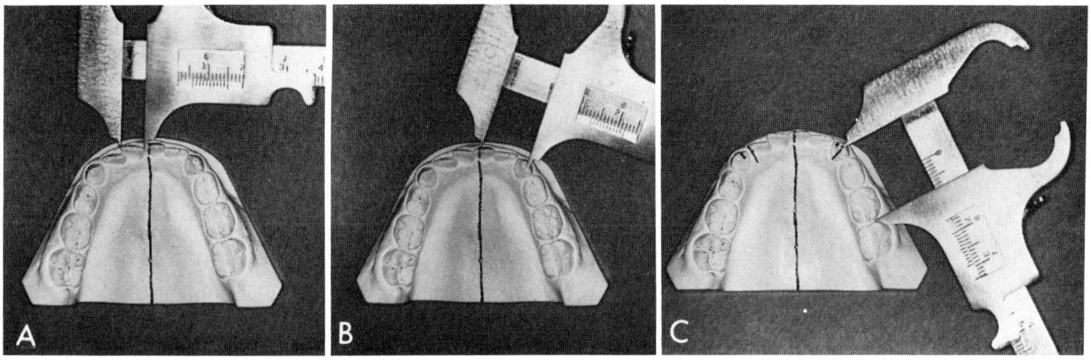

Σ21|12	19.5	20.0	20.5	21.0	21.5	22.0	22.5	23.0	23.5	24.0
Max. 75%	20.6	20.9	21.2	21.5	21.8	22.0	22.3	22.6	22.9	23.1
Mand. 75%	20.1	20.4	20.7	21.0	21.3	21.6	21.9	22.2	22.5	22.8

Figure 20–11 Mixed Dentition Analysis (Michigan-Moyers) is utilized to estimate the space available in the deciduous arch to accommodate the unerupted permanent canine and premolar teeth. In *A* the four lower permanent incisors are measured. In *B* the illustration indicates the space needed to accommodate one-half the sum of the incisors. Note that a portion of the canine space is needed and called "incisor liability." *C* is the space available from the point of incisor liability to the permanent molar for the canine and premolars. The chart below provides an estimate of the unerupted canine and premolar size. Find the sum of the four measured lower incisors in the top row labeled Σ21|12; next, locate the maxillary or mandibular "predicted" size for the unerupted teeth in the column beneath the sum of the incisors measured. Comparison of "space needed" (predicted tooth size) with "space available" (measured on the cast) materially aids space management.

properly position the central and lateral incisors.

3. When the incisors are normally crowded, some of the space necessary to align the incisors is occupied by the deciduous canine tooth. Thus, the Boley gauge is adjusted for one-half the total sum of the incisors and with one point of the gauge placed at the *corrected* midline the other is held along the arch circumference to make a mark on the deciduous canine (Figure 20–11B). This represents the space needed for the incisors, and the amount of canine space used is termed the *incisor liability*.

4. The space remaining between the mark on the deciduous canine and the mesial surface of the permanent molar is the *space available* for the unerupted permanent canine and premolar teeth (Fig. 20–11C).

5. Having determined the space available in each arch, the next step is to determine the space needed, or to predict the sum of the sizes of the unerupted teeth. Moyers has provided a probability chart for each maxillary and mandibular set of teeth.[44] The purpose is to locate the predicted sizes of the unerupted teeth on the chart, based upon the total sum of the mandibular incisor widths of the case being measured. The sum of the mandibular incisor teeth is used to locate predicted canine and premolar widths for both maxillary and mandibular arches. Since the 75 per cent level of probability has been shown to be the most accurate, only that level is presented in Figure 20–11D. This level has the highest confidence and is generally the only set of numbers used. Referring to Figure 20–11D, locate the sum of the four mandibular incisor widths in the top line closest to the measurement in your case. The corresponding numbers beneath this sum of incisor widths are the predicted total mesiodistal widths of the canine and premolar teeth for your case. A separate value is given for the maxillary and mandibular arches.

6. By comparing the space needed (predicted tooth size) with the measured space available (Fig. 20–11C), you can readily determine the needs for total space in each quadrant.

At this point, it should become obvious that space deficiencies may relate to the forward migration of molar teeth (often observed on study cast symmetry analysis) or the collapse of the anterior segment (often seen on lateral head-film incisor analysis). On other occasions lateral collapse of the arches (frequently with crossbites) will produce loss of needed space and, finally, the teeth may be too large for the arch. It would appear that minor adjustments of malposed teeth can frequently regain the needed space. On the other hand, when the adjacent teeth will not allow adjustment for space regaining, it may be necessary to consider extraction of bicuspid teeth. Determine *first* if tooth adjustment is possible before resorting to extraction to gain necessary space. This is the conservative approach.

SUMMARY TO DIAGNOSTIC TECHNIQUES

A fairly thorough examination of the patient provides a visualization of the denture in its surrounding bony and soft tissue framework. In addition to providing a gross overview of the occlusion, it allows for an examination of function and muscular environment and the relation of each to tooth position. Cephalometric analysis may be utilized to confirm the clinical appraisal. At the same time, the cephalometric appraisal provides a more finite method of assessing skeletal and dental patterns. It gives a basis for discriminating between skeletal growth patterns.

The critical appraisal of dental study casts for symmetry provides information about the arches as a whole and the positions of the tooth units within each arch. The mixed dentition analysis allows for the accurate description of space needs within each dental arch. Together, these diagnostic aids give the practicing dentist a base upon which he can learn to distinguish between those problems of a minor malocclusion nature, which his efforts in treatment may help to correct, and those which most certainly require treatment by the specialist.

TREATMENT NEEDS

The general dental practitioner cares for the dental needs of the vast majority of growing children. He is the first dentist to examine most children and relies upon referral to the pedodontist for some special problems and to the orthodontist for the vast numbers of children requiring occlusion management. It has been said that orthodontic manpower is insufficient to accommodate the growing public demand for specialized care. It seems natural that the general dentist and pedodontist may serve as the "dental auxiliaries" of the orthodontist and may elect to expand the range of their practices through the care of many minor occlusal developmental problems.

The competence of general dentists and pedodontists in providing orthodontic care has been questioned by some in the profession.

Only through cooperation, guidance and education between the disciplines in dentistry will doubts and suspicions pass. Only through cooperative professional effort will our child population be better served. Toward this end, the following table is presented as a guide to the types of treatment needs with suggestions for their care through an interdisciplinary approach:

A. *General Dentist Care and Guidance*
   1. Guiding normal dental development
      a. Passive Treatment—Arch-length maintenance
         1. Restorative dentistry
         2. Space maintenance
      b. Active Treatment—to preserve and restore arch length
         1. Regaining small losses in arch length
         2. Minor ectopias
         3. Crossbites
         4. Oral habits
         5. Uncomplicated spacing
         6. Rotations with available space

B. *General Dentist with Orthodontic Specialist Guidance*
   1. The "interim patient"—long-range need
      a. Questionable growth diagnosis
      b. Closed bite
      c. Questionable arch-length needs
         1. Excessive loss
         2. Expansion—anteroposterior and/or buccolingual
         3. Serial extraction
      d. Difficult ectopia
      e. Congenital problems
         1. Absent teeth with ultimate orthodontic-prosthetic need.
         2. Others requiring restorative, minor guidance, and ultimate prosthetic needs

C. *Orthodontic Specialist*
   1. Physical and esthetic handicapping malocclusion
      a. The skeletal discrepancies
         1. Class II
         2. Class III
      b. The dental discrepancies
         1. Class I with multiple problems
         2. Treatment needs following bicuspid extraction
      c. Surgical-Orthodontic coordination
      d. Orthopedic-Orthodontic coordination

PREVENTIVE ORTHODONTICS IN GENERAL PRACTICE

ARCH-LENGTH MAINTENANCE

Arch length is a measure of the total mesiodistal diameters of the teeth. This is the total space necessary to properly align the teeth in the dental arch. The total space in a young child's deciduous arch gives way to the erupting permanent teeth to form the permanent arch. Thus, the transitional period and the space available is a combination of tooth size and jaw growth. The segment of the arch concerned during this period is from the mesial surface of the erupting first permanent molars through the arch contacts to the mesial surface of the first permanent molar on the opposite side. This dimension must provide sufficient space in which to position the unerupted permanent segment of incisors, canine and premolars. It is the segment that gives us the greatest concern.

MESIODISTAL WIDTHS OF TEETH

In 1947 Nance[42] provided the concept of *leeway space.* He described the difference of 1.7 mm found in size wherein the deciduous mandibular canine and molar teeth were that much larger than their successors. The maxillary deciduous group are 0.9 mm larger than their successors. In application through the years, it meant that the permanent molars could be allowed to migrate forward 1.7 mm and there would still be sufficient room for the permanent successors. Nance did not take into account the difference in deciduous or permanent incisor sizes.

In 1959 Moorrees[45] measured the widths of deciduous and succedaneous permanent teeth in a representative group of children, which included the incisors and showed that the average *mandibular* deciduous and permanent arches are nearly the same size (< 1.0 mm total). The deciduous tooth group was slightly larger than the permanent group. In this study[45] the comparison of deciduous and succedaneous *maxillary* teeth showed the permanent tooth group to average 3–5 mm larger than the deciduous group. Thus, the credibility of the leeway-space concept must be questioned. Various factors of arch growth and change in shape contribute to ultimate space available for the permanent teeth, but as leeway space was built on the concept of tooth size, so it must be questioned on that same basis. It appears that the 1.7 mm of leeway space described by Nance is taken up by the larger permanent anterior teeth, as seen in Figure 20–12A. Also noted in 20–12A is that the larger permanent incisors require the eruption of the permanent canine tooth in a position more distally on the dental arch than was the position of the deciduous canine. This will allow for reduced incisor crowding. At the same time the old leeway space is used by the more distal position of the canine. Figure 20–12B illustrates that the distance from the mesial surface of the permanent molar to the tip of the deciduous canine on the left model is greater than the same distance to the permanent canine on the right model taken off the same child at a later age. Thus, the perma-

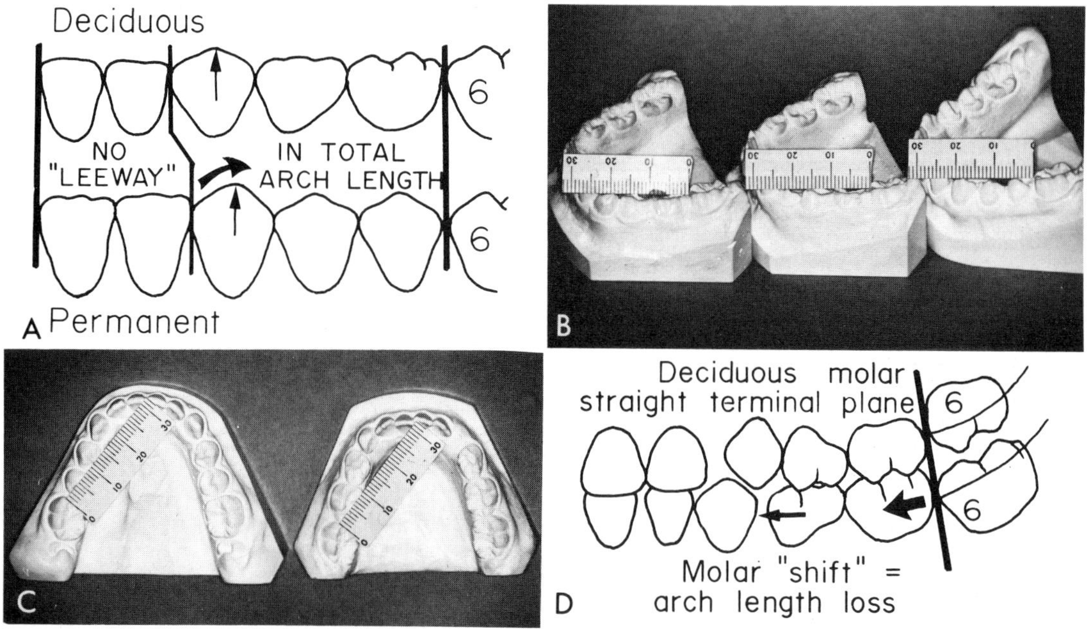

Figure 20–12 Comparison of the deciduous mandibular quadrant with the permanent replacements. In total measurement they are similar *(A)*. The larger deciduous molars are counteracted by the larger permanent incisors for total arch length similarity. Note that the permanent canine will be further distal on the arch than was the deciduous canine *(A)* and as illustrated in *B* where the cast on the left is of a seven-year-old girl and the cast on the right is at 11 years of age. In *C* these same casts show little length difference. In *D* the deciduous terminal plane when forming a straight line does not automatically indicate that the lower molar should move forward. Such may produce a loss in needed arch length.

nent canine is positioned more distally, using the leeway space to allow incisor alignment. Figure 20–12C compares these same two casts, indicating a negligible difference in overall molar to incisor distance. The molar has not moved forward. Instead, the canine is positioned more distally. Thus, any migration of the first permanent molars forward *in the dental arch* would reduce available necessary space.

In 1950 Baume[46] described the occlusal relation of the deciduous second molars, whereby their distal surfaces form a straight line (straight terminal plane), as in Figure 20–12D. This relation is seen particularly in the younger age ranges. He noted that the permanent molars erupted into an end-to-end or cusp-to-cusp occlusion which was corrected by the mandibular molar migrating forward *in the dental arch* to close any existing space or utilizing the leeway space as the second deciduous molar exfoliates.

Since this migration could contribute to loss in space, perhaps it would be premature to expect that the permanent molar relation will adjust itself as the result of the downward-forward growth of the mandible which is accelerated over that of the maxilla. That this molar relation change occurs as the result of mandibular growth has not yet been shown through longitudinal cephalometric study. However, the dental changes described by Baume,[46] based upon examination of dental casts alone, did not take into account that the observed molar shift did not occur as the result of jaw growth.

ARCH-LENGTH LOSS

As was noted earlier, the eruptive and occlusal forces of the permanent molars tend to drive them forward in arch position. Should this occur as the result of caries in the deciduous arch, then arch length is lost, as in Figure 20–13A. Similarly, if a deciduous tooth is lost through extraction, the first permanent molars may migrate mesially a considerable amount, as in Figure 20–13B. This mesial movement of the molars is acceptable to many dentists in the belief that there is leeway space.

Total arch length is lost in other ways. Occasionally, the incisor segment will be forced lingually, due to a lip habit, a closed bite or through the early loss of a deciduous canine tooth, as in Figure 20–13C. Frequently, this excessive lingual tipping of the incisor segment can be demonstrated by analyzing the position from a lateral head film. Many times it can be clearly visualized on clinical examination alone. In some cases, total arch length is decreased by the collapse, or lingual tipping, of the buccal segments, as in Figure 20–13D. This is more difficult to diagnose since clinical judgment is applied in place of a valid diagnostic measurement technique.

Lastly, arch length can be inadequate because the erupting permanent teeth are genuinely too large by comparison to the deciduous predecessors. This is generally referred to as a "tooth size-jaw base discrepancy." Lacking a diagnostic method for measuring jaw base size, it becomes difficult to justify with assurance.

ARCH-LENGTH MANAGEMENT

There are two main approaches to guiding the individual arch-length needs of the child patient—conservative and sacrificial. The conservative approach has as its goals the preservation of all permanent teeth in the dental arch (if possible), while the sacrificial approach "sacrifices," through extraction, tooth units (usually first premolars) to alleviate the needs for arch length. Each approach has a need, and there is overlapping between each such that management of the individual child's needs for arch length should be carefully examined. It should be our goal to preserve the permanent segment *in toto* (conservative) wherever possible and employ extraction as a means of treatment (sacrifice) only when necessary. Even so, as Graber[16] points out in his chapter on extraction, the decision to extract teeth in a Class I malocclusion is an orthodontic decision and requires the expert clinical experience of the orthodontist,

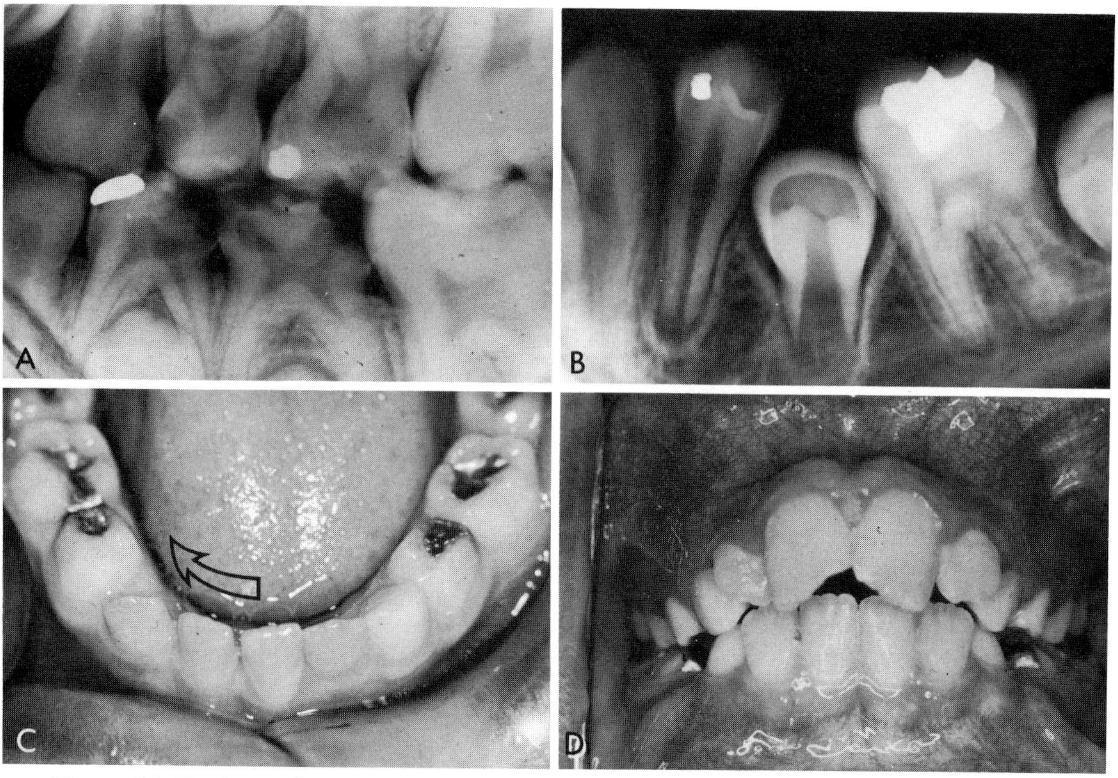

Figure 20–13 Loss of space or decrease in needed arch length through caries *(A)*, molar migration *(B)*, incisor segment collapse or migration *(C)*, and buccal segment collapse *(D)*. Each decreases space availability in the arch for the remaining unerupted permanent teeth.

who must ultimately complete the therapy. In addition, Moyers[44] has suggested that when space loss is slight (e.g., 1–3 mm), it may be recovered if treatment can be accomplished before the second permanent molar erupts. Moyers continues to express that when the amount of space to be regained is excessive (e.g., 5–7 mm), it may be necessary to consider removal of a tooth, and "when in doubt, a sound plan for the average nonspecialist is never to extract but instead to try all of the suggested procedures for regaining the length of the arch."

SPACE MAINTENANCE

Space maintainers begin with restorative dentistry. The loss in arch length, pictured in Figure 20–13A, is prevented by operative dentistry applied before space loss occurs. After loss of space has occurred, the problem becomes one of space regaining. Space maintainers are but one facet of arch-length preservation. Our goal should be to preserve the total arch of which one space is but a part of the whole.

When do you place a space maintainer? Before there has been any arch length loss. Any factor that leaves the arch vulnerable to diminution (e.g., caries, loss of a tooth, possible incisor collapse from lip habits and the loss of a deciduous canine tooth) should be counteracted with a holding appliance. Figure 20–14 illustrates the most commonly employed holding appliances. The band-loop space maintainer in Figure 20–14A has fallen into disfavor today, for it usually has to be removed too early and replaced by a lingual arch. This is usually due to exfoliation of the deciduous abutment tooth or because the bicuspid erupts through the loop, lulling the practitioner into the belief that the job is done. The permanent molar can then begin its mesial migration with insiduous space loss after the band-loop is removed.

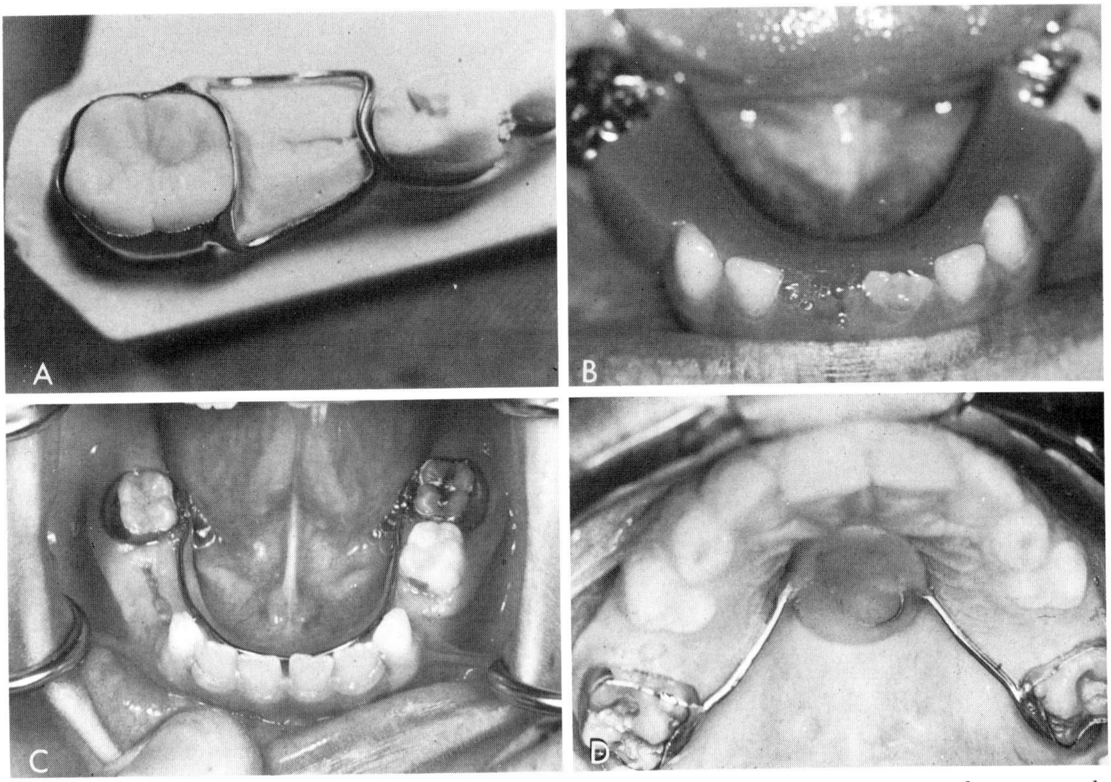

Figure 20–14 Space (arch length) maintenance to prevent molar migration and incisor collapse. *A* shows the band-loop space maintainer for single deciduous tooth loss while *B* is the acrylic space maintainer commonly used for bilateral loss. Fixed appliances commonly employed are the lingual arch *(C)* which passively holds the entire arch in place and the Nance holding arch *(D)* employing a "button" of acrylic adapted to the palatal vault to resist forward molar movement.

In Figure 20–14B is illustrated the removable acrylic space maintainer, useful when there has been multiple deciduous tooth loss. The acrylic appliances readily adapt to most space management problems, are easily modified to accommodate erupting permanent teeth, provide opposing occlusal function but retain the disadvantages of breakage, loss by the child, and occasionally increase caries activity, especially when the child is careless with his oral hygiene. Nevertheless, the general practitioner will find it one of his most useful appliances for arch-length maintenance, especially when he experiences discomfort in working with banded appliances.

Figures 20–14C and 20–14D illustrate fixed-wire lingual arch appliances which provide a maximum of arch-length control. Since they are fixed appliances, they do not rely on the child's cooperation as do the removable appliances. The passive lingual arch for the mandibular segment (Fig. 20–14C) serves the multiple purposes of retaining molar position, preventing anterior segment collapse, holding deciduous canine spaces and preserving total arch length during serial extraction procedures. The lingual arch is sometimes referred to as the "antibiotic of preventive orthodontic procedures" in that it is likely the most universal appliance for all problems of mandibular arch maintenance. The maxillary molar holding arch in Figure 20–14D utilizes a "button" of acrylic processed to fit the palatal vault. The palatal vault provides superb anchorage, or resistance, to prevent the mesial migration of the maxillary molar teeth. At the same time, the remainder of the arch may undergo adjustments in tooth position, uninhibited by possible interference of an appliance.

INDICATIONS FOR ARCH MAINTENANCE AND REGAINING

Utilizing the diagnostic aids previously described, the general practitioner will need to perform an arch-length assessment of every child in his practice. The needs for arch length are determined by the mixed dentition analysis. The study casts are further analyzed to identify asymmetry and the possibility of tooth migration. If anterior tooth collapse is suspected, he may elect to utilize cephalometric data. Mesial molar migrations are most commonly visualized by model analysis with the aid of clinical examination and intraoral radiographs. Any potential environmental factor of the deciduous arch that may lead to space loss should be counteracted by the placement of holding appliances.

Once it has been determined that arch length has been lost, the problem requires answers for how much has been lost, where has the loss occurred and why did it occur? Application of the diagnostic examinations described earlier will frequently identify how much loss and where it has occurred. Why the space loss has happened will require the application of basic knowledge coupled with a reexamination of the patient and his dental history.

Mesial migration of the molar teeth usually follows caries attack in the deciduous teeth, as seen in Figure 20–13A, or the loss of a deciduous molar, as in Figure 20–13B. In each instance the task is to move the molar distally to regain the space. It is important to initiate this treatment *before* the second permanent molar has erupted far enough to contact the distal surface of the first molar. The contact of the second molar compounds the problem, space regaining becomes quite difficult and may not be accomplished at all by the general practitioner. Frequently, it will be necessary to extract a biscuspid tooth if the space loss is great and the second permanent molar is fully erupted. Therefore, regain molar space as early as possible.

A common occurrence in permanent molar eruption is the ectopia associated with impaction beneath the second deciduous molar, as seen in Figure 20–15A. Occasionally, the deciduous tooth requires extraction because of pulpal involvement, in which case care should be taken to insure that the upper permanent molar is tipped distally to its desirable position. An acrylic palate with an embedded light wire (0.020″ steel) is useful for this purpose (Fig. 20–15E). When pulpal involvement does not require extraction of the deciduous molar, the placement of a brass separating wire (Fig. 20–15B) will exert a force against the permanent molar sufficient to tip it distally, unlock the impaction and free it to continue its normal eruption path. Longitudinal radiographic studies have shown that the antagonistic resistance provided by the deciduous arch is quite sufficient to prevent forward movement of the deciduous teeth. Similar technique may be employed with impacted lower permanent molars, as in Figure 20–15C. However, the occurrence with lower molars is far less than that found in maxillary molar eruption patterns.

When deciduous molars have been lost through extraction, after which the permanent molar tips mesialward because of its eruptive path or the forces of occlusion (Fig. 20–13B), the regaining of modest amounts of space may be accomplished with a split-saddle acrylic space maintainer, as illustrated in Figure 20–15D. The appliance utilizes two loops of wire (0.020″ steel), one buccal and one lingual to the edentulous area requiring expansion and contained to avoid tissue impingement. Spring action is accomplished by opening the loops attaching the two halves of the saddle. The saddle is then compressed for placement. When in place, the spring loops push distally against the molar tooth and are counterposed, or the resistance and anchorage is provided by the adaptation of the appliance lingual to the entire anterior segment.

The lingual arch described previously may be modified to perform the same task as the split-saddle acrylic appliance, should a fixed type of appliance be desired. The lingual arch may be adapted with a coiled push spring activated against the molar tooth. In addition, the arch wire may be bent to utilize the loop principle for activa-

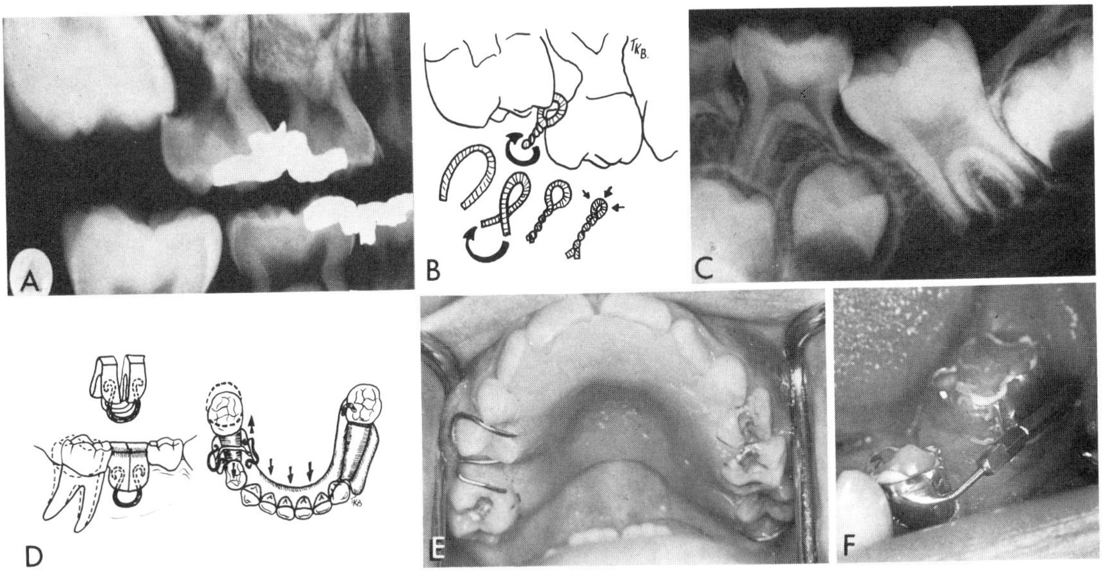

Figure 20–15 Space regaining by distal molar movement in small amounts. The molar impaction in *A* and *C* may be unlocked by employing a ligature wire passed and tightened around the contact. *D* and *E* show methods of applying spring pressure against the molar tooth while using the rest of the arch or palate for reciprocal resistance. The "jack-screw" in *F* is to be avoided for the weaker anterior tooth can be expected to move forward instead of the desired molar movement.

tion. In each case, the entire anterior segment is utilized for resistance or anchorage to insure distal molar movement.

The type of appliance illustrated in Figure 20–15F, employing a jack-screw or coiled push spring, is to be discouraged for, unlike the split saddle appliance just described or a lingual arch that utilizes the entire anterior segment for achorage and resistance, not enough reciprocal anchorage or resistance is present. In the illustration of Figure 20–15F, it can be visualized that the "weaker" of structures will move. In this case, the deciduous teeth anterior to the space can be expected to be driven forward. Often the deciduous canine is driven forward to destroy the contact with the lateral incisor. Instead of the desired distal movement of the molar tooth, the teeth anterior to the space are driven forward.

INCISOR CROWDING AND SERIAL EXTRACTION

Crowding of the incisor segments is a normal part of early dental development and must be carefully assessed in each child as to its effect on the total arch-length availability. Basically, incisor crowding must be regarded as:

1. Temporary, the arch length is adequate and will be self-correcting;
2. Artificial, the arch length has been decreased through incisor tipping or collapse, is correctable through adjustment of tooth position and may lead to ultimate bicuspid extraction if left untreated; and
3. Permanent, the incisors are in their proper labiolingual position, the crowding can be corrected, and the total arch length is still inadequate.

We can expect to see some degree of crowding in almost every child's dentition during the emergence of the permanent incisor segment. The presence of this crowding should not automatically be diagnosed for bicuspid extraction without determining why the crowding exists. Graber[16] states "when an orthodontist sees a child of five or six years of age with all the deciduous teeth present in a slightly crowded state or with no spaces between them, he can predict with a fair degree of certainty that there will not be enough space in the jaws to accommodate all the permanent teeth in their proper alignment." An additional thought on the part of many practitioners is that *any* crowding of the permanent incisors is an indication for bicuspid removal. Throughout these concepts is the belief in the presence of the 1.7 mm of leeway space. That is, if you believe that the permanent molars are supposed to migrate forward 1.7 mm, and allow it to happen, you automatically reduce available total arch length. Then the normal crowding of the incisor segment has less room for final adjustment and self-correction. When considering the total arch length, a diagnosis of bicuspid extraction on the basis of *any* incisor crowding must be fallacious. It is imperative that we diagnose *why* the crowding is present.

Temporary (normal) crowding is almost universal. The permanent incisors cannot fit in the same arch space as the smaller deciduous incisors did. In Figure 20–12A we saw that the posterior leeway space is taken up by the larger permanent incisors. Figure 20–11 B shows the need to determine "incisor liability," and 20–11C indicates the remaining space available for the permanent canine and premolars in Figure 20–12A. Should the molars be allowed to come forward, decreasing available arch length, the incisor segment will not have enough room for self-correction of its temporarily crowded state. Assuming that incisor crowding is present in a hypothetical case, and the mixed dentition analysis shows that arch length is adequate, it then follows that the crowded incisor segment will gain room for proper alignment in the future as the deciduous canine exfoliates and is replaced by the permanent canine which erupts in a more distal position. This alignment is seen in Figure 20–13A and is illustrated in Figure 20–13B. Thus, the leeway space is utilized by the more distal position of the permanent canine, allowing the incisors to be relieved of their crowding. Again, if the molars are allowed to come forward, the distal shift of the canine is prevented and the incisor crowding remains. Mesial molar movement *in the dental arch* reduces arch length and encourages incisor crowding. Examine each case carefully. Use a lingual arch.

Artificial incisor crowding can be seen when arch length has decreased due to incisor collapse. An example is seen in Figure 20–13C. In this example, the erupting lateral incisor has caused resorption of the deciduous canine root; the canine exfoliates early and the incisor segment collapses toward that side with a loss in total arch length as the result. Figure 20–16A is a similar example of collapse and caused by the closed bite, as illustrated in Figure 20–16B. Instead of diagnosing only from the occlusal view of the teeth and deciding that bicuspid teeth need to be removed, it would seem more proper to visualize the arch from all aspects. Frequently, the collapsed segment can be demonstrated by examination of the lateral cephalograph. As in Figure 20–9C, the effect of the closed bite on incisor crowding or collapse of the arch length availability can readily be visualized. This being the case, the bite should be opened by means of an acrylic bite plane, as in Figure 20–16C, recreating the lost interincisal space and thus regaining the lost arch length through forward movement of the incisors seen in Figure 20–16D. The tongue may push the incisors forward naturally; however, it may be necessary to place a lingual arch appliance, to which a lingually placed finger spring has been added, to aid the forward movement of the incisors.

Similar incisor collapse can be produced by muscular pressures from the labial side, such as is seen in lip-wetting and sucking habits and the thumb and mentalis habits. In each instance, the cause of the incisor collapse and crowding should be corrected. It is improper to resolve all crowding through biscuspid extraction on the basis that "just because crowding is present, extraction is necessary."

On the other hand, incisor crowding may actually be visualized in a true arch-length discrepancy. In this instance, the incisor crowding is *permanent,* unless extraction is performed. Here the incisors can be demonstrated to be in their proper labiolingual positions; the molar teeth have not drifted forward and the total arch-length is

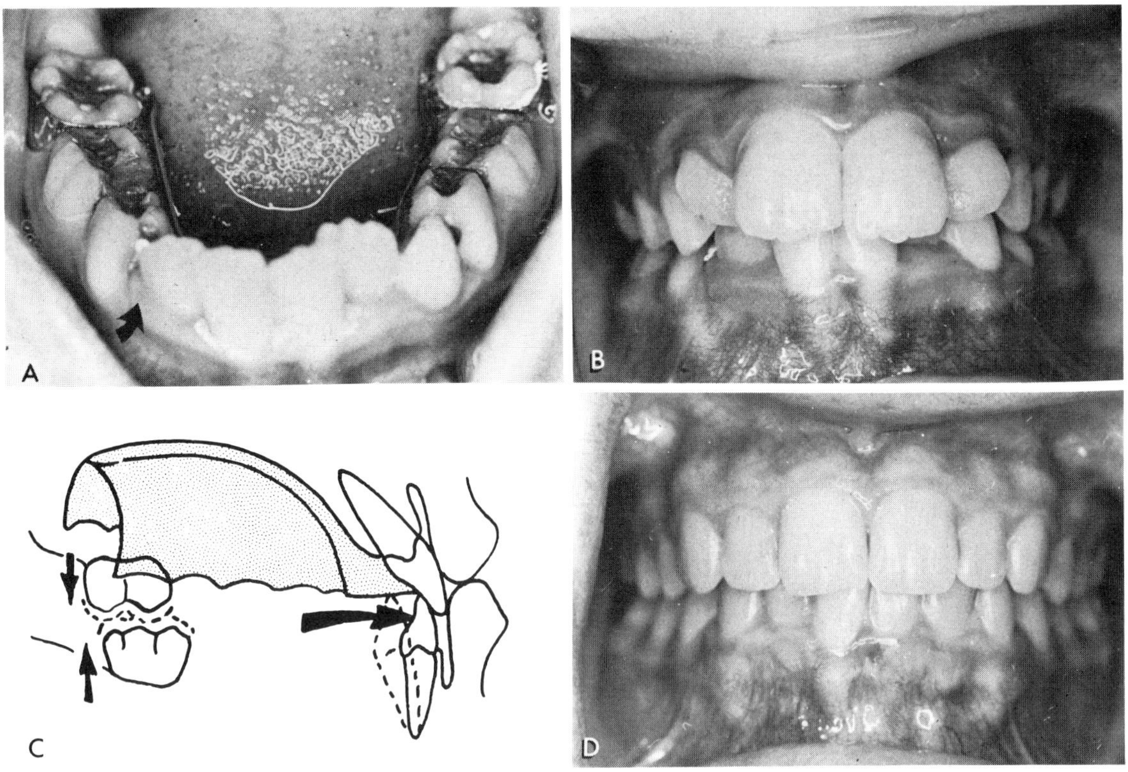

Figure 20–16 Closed bite effects on arch length. In *A* the arrow indicates space loss through early loss of the deciduous canine. *B* illustrates the resultant closed bite. *C* represents the method of opening the bite with an acrylic palate allowing the molars to erupt and the creation of interincisal space to allow forward incisor movement in the mandible, thereby recreating the canine space. *D* shows modest bite opening from *B* and the successful eruption of all permanent mandibular teeth.

shown to be inadequate. There is truly a tooth-size arch length discrepancy and bicuspid extraction will be required. All cases will eventually require full orthodontic management and should thus be performed by the specialist. When in doubt, consult and seek justification for extraction in the individual case.

Serial extraction was originally designed[47-50] to provide room in the arch for the erupting lateral incisors by extracting the deciduous canines early so that the incisors do not become crowded. Following this, sequential extraction of the deciduous molars allow for the uncrowded eruption of the remaining permanent teeth. Graber[16] provides a thorough and excellent review of the procedure. Without support, the arch will frequently collapse and when the molar teeth are not prevented from moving forward, loss of arch length will result. In the final stages of dental development, it is necessary to sacrifice one of the bicuspid teeth. In some instances this is desirable, especially when it has been determined that the arch was totally inadequate to begin with. However, if the mixed dentition analysis demonstrates that the total arch length is adequate and extraction of the deciduous canine teeth is contemplated to alleviate incisor crowding, the arch should be prevented from collapsing following the extraction. Thus, the placement of a lingual arch appliance might *precede* the extraction to good advantage.

Many practitioners desire to "shave" or reduce the mesiodistal widths of the deciduous canine teeth to allow the alignment of the permanent incisor teeth. This is acceptable provided caution is taken to insure that the arch will not collapse as a result. The placement of a lingual arch appliance *first* will insure that the total arch-length availability will not decrease as the result of the reduction of the size of the deciduous canine.

In summary, the presence of incisor crowding should not automatically lead to the diagnosis of a space discrepancy requiring extraction of a tooth unit. Is the available arch length adequate for all of the teeth in the arch? Is it inadequate because of incisor malposition? Can that be corrected? Have the molars tipped forward, thus contributing to the incisor crowding? Or, with the satisfaction that the arch is genuinely inadequate and there is no possibility of adjusting tooth position, will extraction of a tooth unit be the only option? The careful clinical examination of the patient, followed by the use of the diagnostic aids, such as the study-cast analysis, mixed dentition analysis and the occasional use of a lateral cephalograph, will markedly improve the plan of treatment related to incisor crowding as a clinical problem.

CROSSBITES

Crossbites refer to any departure from a normal buccolingual or labiolingual relation of the upper to lower teeth (see Fig. 20–7). They occur quite commonly during the mixed dentition and are usually related to a deviate eruption pattern of the permanent teeth. Occasionally, however,the crossbite may only be symptomatic of the child's pattern of abnormal jaw closure or mandibular function, as described with Figures 20–2 and 20–4.

The simple crossbite involving only one or two teeth has an adverse effect on arch length, serving to decrease the space available in the arch for the remainder of the teeth. Thus, crossbites generally should be corrected as soon as they are observed. An exception to this may be the simple crossbite in the deciduous dentition, for its correction, or lack of correction, may have no relation to the permanent arch development.

The common incisor crossbite in Figure 20–17A usually occurs as the result of failure of the deciduous predecessor to exfoliate in time. The permanent successor is deflected lingually. The deciduous incisor should be extracted if it is still present. Measure the space to make certain it is large enough to receive the permanent incisor in proper position before attempting to move the malposed incisor forward. Study the case further to determine the reason, should the space be inadequate. The space must be adequate before moving the malposed incisor forward. Figure 20–17B illustrates an acrylic resin bite plane cemented to a number of lower incisors. The bite plane itself is contoured to present a vertically inclined extension, serving to drive the malposed incisor forward, using the patient muscular occlusal forces as the stimulus. Figure 20–16C illustrates the corrected incisor position after treatment and the bite plane is removed. Usually, treatment can be accomplished in a period of two weeks with patient cooperation.

The simple posterior crossbite, as illustrated in Figures 20–7A, 20–7B, and 20–7C, can readily be corrected with an elastic rubber band extended across the occlusal plane from the lingual surface of one affected tooth to the buccal surface of the other tooth in crossbite (Fig. 20–17D). The rubber band is attached to hooks soldered or welded to the banded teeth. The rubber band selected (available in sizes) should be small enough to maintain tension between the hooks at all times and is to be worn 24 hours per day. It is advisable to "overcorrect" the malposed teeth so that when the bands are removed, the teeth will "settle in" to proper position, rather than to revert to the previous crossbite condition.

The buccal segment crossbite involving several teeth should be carefully examined to determine if it is merely the malposition of upper or lower teeth or the manifest symptom of a deviate pattern of jaw closure. Referring to the clinical examination of the patient and the closure patterns previously discussed and illustrated in Figures 20–2 and 20–4, it can be seen that a deviation of the mandible can produce a buccal crossbite on one or both sides. Most frequently this results from cuspal interference in the

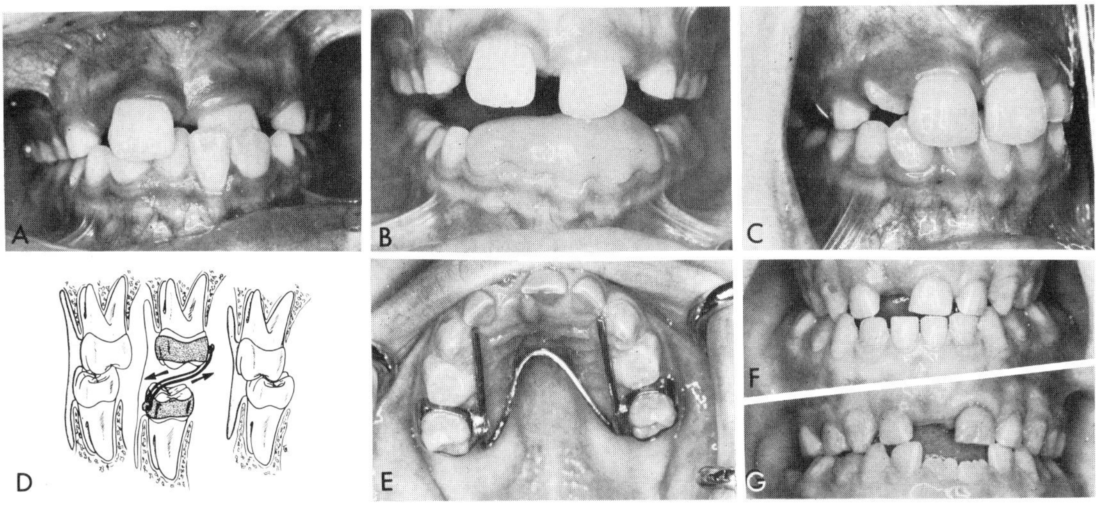

Figure 20–17 Crossbite correction using an acrylic bite plane *(B)* to correct the incisor relation in *A* to that of *C*. Single tooth buccal crossbites are corrected with an elastic band as in *D* while bilateral crossbite is more commonly corrected *(F* and *G)* using a spring "W" shaped expansion appliance as seen in *E*.

very young child and his "learning" to close his mandible to one side "for convenience." Generally, one dental arch will not fit within the other, thus requiring a modest amount of buccal expansion. The appliance seen in Figure 20–17E is one example whereby the "w-shaped" lingual arch exerts a buccally expansive force against the molar segments. The appliance is constructed on a stone model and the bends in the wire (0.040″–0.045″ steel) are "opened" slightly prior to intraoral cementation. Figures 20–17F and 20–17G illustrate before and after correction of the crossbite. As the crossbite is corrected, the child will begin to correct his path of mandibular closure and a correction of the central incisor midline deviation (Fig. 20–4B) can be noted.

Incisor crossbites should be examined in the same fashion. Occasionally, the child will close his mandible, as was shown in Figure 20–4C. In this instance, he may initially be thought to be a Class III patient. Often, his narrow maxillary arch development can be attributed to a "convenience" forward bite. Buccal expansion, as for the buccal crossbite, will often bring about a similar correction in the path of mandibular closure and a correction in the incisor relation. Examine all crossbites carefully. Are they simple tooth crossbites or related to functional paths of mandibular closure?

SPACING OF INCISORS AND ORAL HABITS

Quite frequently one can observe children with normal occlusions except for problems with anterior spacing of the incisor segment. Anterior spacing commonly relates to various oral habits or muscular imbalance patterns which can generally be diagnosed through clinical observation of the child's habits or through the history obtained from the parent. Maxillary incisor spacing may be associated with the closed-bite (overbite) problem. In some few instances spaced incisors may occur as a supernumerary tooth develops between the incisors, preventing their full eruptive closure at the midline. The same is true of the thick band of fibrous connective tissue, or labial frenum, requiring surgical removal for correction. Anomalous structures which hinder incisor development and space closure are diagnosed by periapical radiographs pointing out the need for radiographic surveys in children.

The large variety of spacing problems prevents a full description of each therapy so that a few examples with the principles of treatment will serve as a guide. In general, careful examination of the patient with the study of additional diagnostic aids is paramount.

Central incisor diastema without evidence of a frenum or hindering intrabony anomaly, such as a supernumerary tooth, may be caused by a congenitally absent lateral incisor or simply the failure of the incisors to come together. Often the permanent canine will erupt labialward with inadequate space available because of the incisor diastema. The incisors can be closed or opened with a simple removable appliance such as a retainer with embedded finger springs, as illustrated in Figure 20–18A. The type of movement is one of simple tipping of the incisor crowns. Attention should be given to the long axes of the incisors when planning treatment. If the root apices are widely separated initially, tipping will further accentuate this axis. Thus, simple tipping should be used only when the root apices are directed toward one another. Figure 20–18B illustrates banded incisors with staples (eyelets) tied together with ligature or contractile thread. This method similarly tips the crowns together without significantly changing the position of the root apices. It must be remembered that the action is reciprocal, i.e., equally effective on both teeth. Both incisors can be expected to move equally to the midline. Additional teeth should be banded and tied together to resist movement, should it be desirable to move one incisor more than the other.

An appliance should be designed to more positively control force action when bodily movement is desired, i.e., to move the root apices mesially as well as the

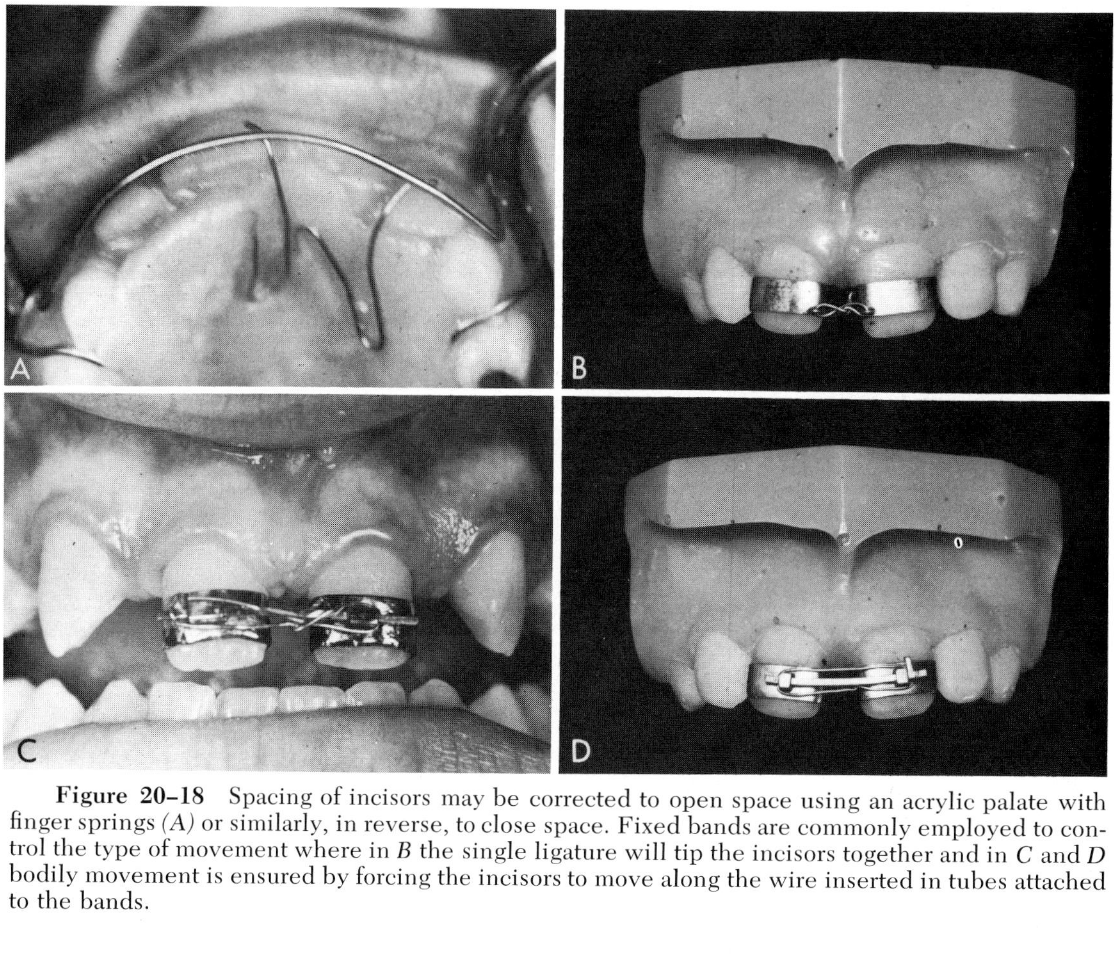

Figure 20–18 Spacing of incisors may be corrected to open space using an acrylic palate with finger springs *(A)* or similarly, in reverse, to close space. Fixed bands are commonly employed to control the type of movement where in *B* the single ligature will tip the incisors together and in *C* and *D* bodily movement is ensured by forcing the incisors to move along the wire inserted in tubes attached to the bands.

crowns, thereby retaining the vertical axes of each tooth. Figures 20–18C and 20–18D illustrate controlled movement using horizontal tubes placed on the incisor bands. A short length of wire corresponding to the inner diameter of the tube has been inserted around which is placed an elastic or contractile thread. The incisor teeth are forced along the wire in movement, thus bringing the root apices together as well as the crowns. Occasionally, it may be desirable to open a space, in which case the problems are reversed. Of course, space should be available to permit space opening. The removable acrylic retainer can be used with springs for opening, yet a fixed (banded) approach provides more control. In this instance, a coiled "push" spring is inserted between the tubes through which a length of wire of corresponding size is run. A rule of thumb is to cut the coil spring one-fourth larger than the space between the tubes. This compresses the spring to about one-fourth its total length. Minor adjustments in incisor spacing of all of the foregoing description assume that the incisor position is quite acceptable labiolingually and that the overbite and overjet are normal.

Spacing Associated with a Closed Bite (Overbite). Frequently, incisor spacing is caused by an excessively closed bite, as seen in Figure 20–19A. In most cases, the spacing is caused by protrusion and flaring of the incisors. This is the reverse effect to a closed bite causing lower incisor collapse and arch length loss as described earlier and illustrated in Figure 20–16. In the present example, upper-incisor spacing, the bite must be opened with a flat incisal bite plane (Figure 20–19D) and the incisors subsequently retracted, as in Figure 20–19C, to restore normal interincisal contact, overjet and overbite. The method of incisor retraction is to close the loops of the Hawley-type

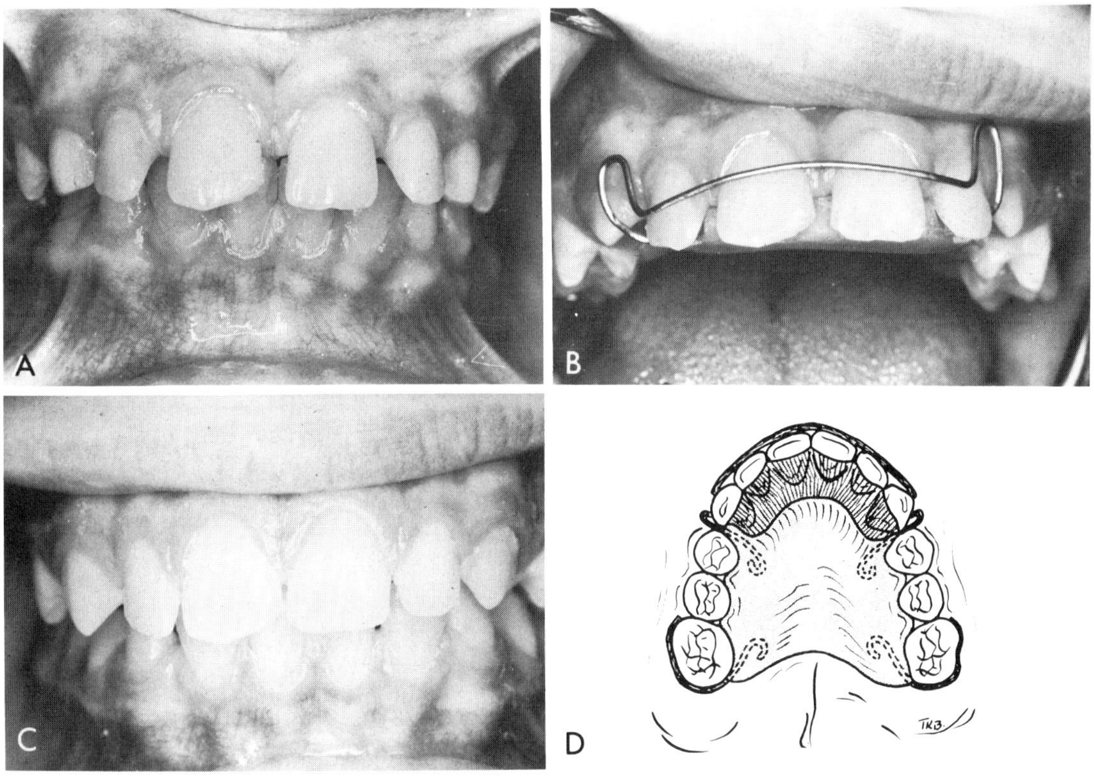

Figure 20–19 Closed bite producing (or following) spaced and protrusive incisors. The acrylic palate with flat incisal guide plane *(B* and *D)* provides for bite opening and molar eruption. Incisal space is then closed *(C)* by relieving the lingual incisal acrylic and application of lingual incisal pressure using the labial arch wire and closure of the loops.

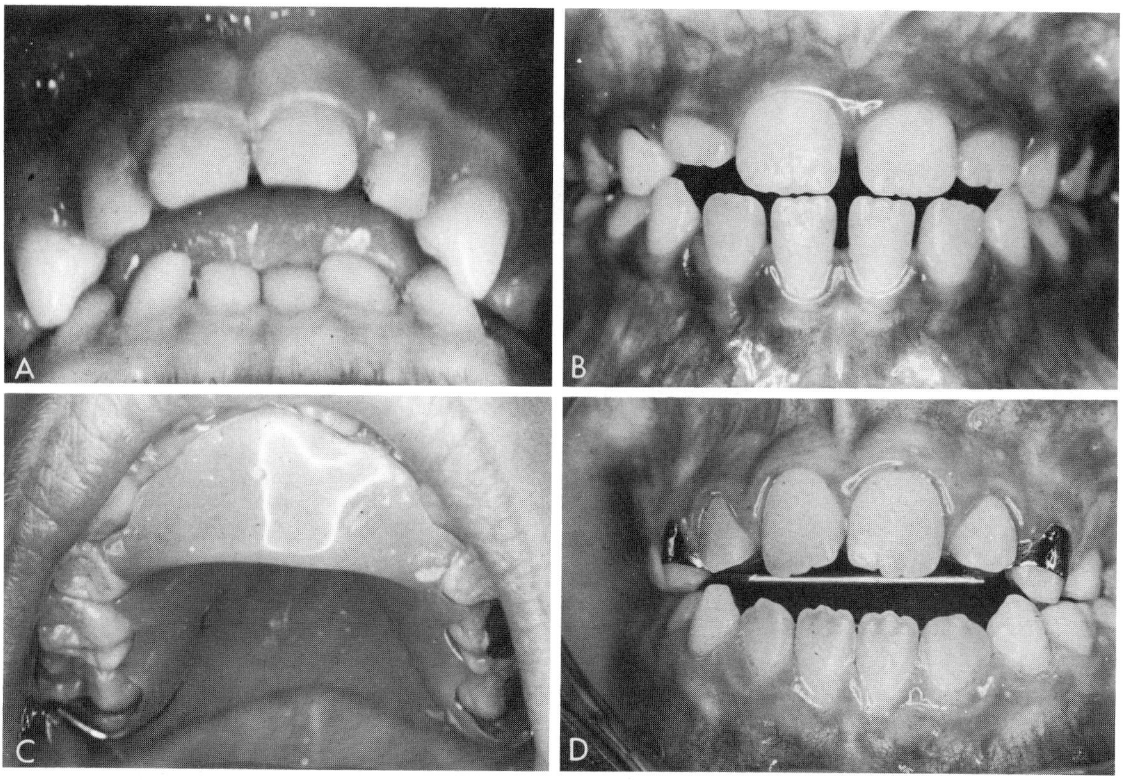

Figure 20–20 Oral habit patterns and resulting incisor malpositions. The typical thumbsucking pattern is seen in *A*, while that of a tongue-thruster is seen in *B*. Tongue habits are commonly treated using the acrylic palate and tongue barrier *(C)* or the fixed wire barrier in *D*.

labial arch wire to produce a lingually directed spring force (Figure 20–19B). Occasionally, the spaced incisors and closed-bite problem follow on the heels of a previous oral habit or muscular imbalance pattern.

Spaced Incisors and Oral Habits. Oral habit patterns in children are common. Some, such as thumb- or finger-sucking, are obvious and easily diagnosed. Others, such as tongue-thrusting, tongue-resting, lip-biting, the mentalis habit and mouth-breathing, are more difficult to diagnose but each produces a typical malocclusion.

Thumb and finger habits usually space and protrude the maxillary incisors and at the same time crush the lower incisors lingually, producing an openbite, as seen in Figure 20–20A. A discussion of thumb-habit correction is lengthy and the reader is directed to any standard text in pedodontics for suggestions of treatment. However, thumb-sucking can be disastrous to the occlusion if the child continues the habit beyond the age of six years. Psychological preparation, or motivation of the child to abort his habit, precedes successful management. Frequently, the mere placement of a tape-bandage on the thumb will successfully serve as a reminder to the motivated child and he will abort the habit pattern on his own. In most instances, the malposed teeth will return to more normal position as the lip-tongue muscle balance is restored. Frequently, an acrylic retainer with activated labial wire (Fig. 20–19B) will aid incisor retraction.

Tongue habits or abnormal swallowing patterns produce an occlusion where both maxillary and mandibular incisor segments are protrusive and spaced (Figs. 20–20B and 20–6). The patient and parents are generally unaware of the pattern which can be demonstrated by asking the child to swallow.

Immediately separate the lips, at which time the tongue is observed to be solidly thrust into the incisor spaces (Fig. 20–6C). The habit pattern may be corrected through guidance by a professional speech therapist. The dental approach is generally mechanical, i.e., a barrier against the thrusting tongue is constructed to remove the tongue pressures from the teeth. Figure 20–20C illustrates a removable acrylic palate to which has been added an extension lingual to the incisor teeth. This barrier serves to trap the thrusting tongue and directs the tip of the tongue upward and forward where the normal swallowing pattern is initiated. Some practitioners prefer a fixed type of appliance, in which case they will adapt bands to the permanent canine or molar teeth. A soldered wire barrier is constructed which extends forward from the bands to occupy the space lingual to the incisors, as in Figure 20–20D. The incisor spacing and protrusion will often be self-corrective as the normal muscular balance is restored, at which time the appliance is removed. Occasionally, the incisor retraction to close the spacing will be assisted through the activated retainer, as in Figure 20–19B.

Lip habits and an overactive mentalis muscle are capable of severely crushing the lower incisor segment and are frequently the cause of incisor collapse and loss of arch length (Figs. 20–13C and 20–16A). Lip-wetting is extremely common in young chil-

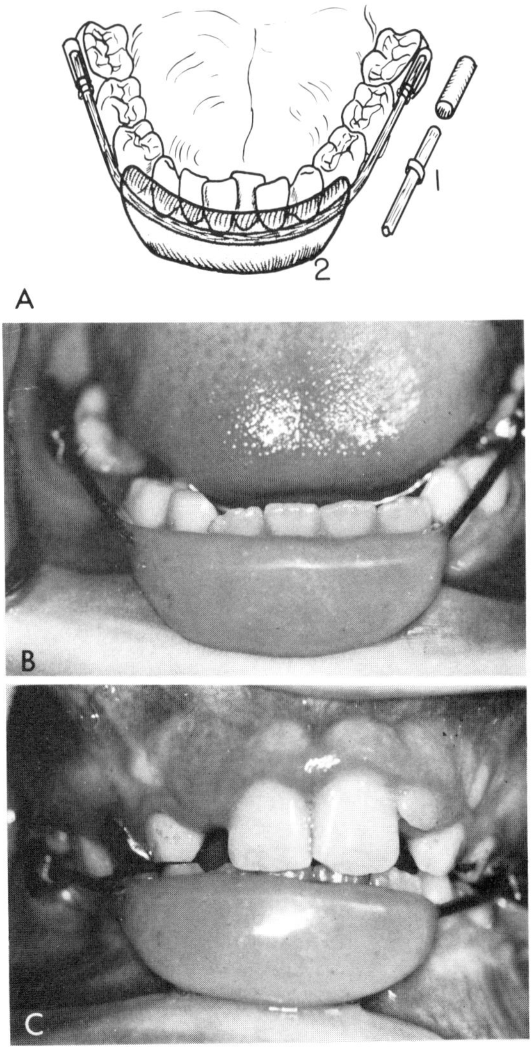

Figure 20–21 Excessive lip or mentalis muscle pressures are inhibited by a "lip bumper." Constructed as a labial arch wire *(A)* to which is processed a flat ribbon-like bumper of acrylic *(A* and *B)* and free of occlusion interference*(C)*. The lip bumper transmits the muscular force to the unyielding molar teeth, thereby reducing the force as applied previously to the incisor teeth.

dren, while the mentalis habit is uncommon. The latter is quite severe in action on the lower incisors, markedly increasing lower incisor crowding. Therapy for lip and mentalis habits consists of placing a "lip bumper" or lip guard, as illustrated in Figure 20–21. Heavy bands are adapted to the molar teeth to which are soldered 0.045-inch round buccal tubes. A section of 0.045-inch steel wire is contained to surround the dental arch, free of the teeth, and inserted into the buccal tubes. "Stops" or "rests" are soldered to the arch wire anterior to the tubes so that any force to the anterior position of the wire is transmitted to the molar teeth (Fig. 20–21A). A flat, ribbon-like, acrylic band is formed around the wire anteriorly which presents a broad, smooth, surface of the lip without contacting the teeth or interfering with the occlusion (Figs. 20–21B and 20–21C). Habit correction is accomplished by preventing the musculature of the lip or mentalis from exerting pressures on the teeth. The musculature becomes fatigued and is brought to the child's conscious level, whereupon he voluntarily ceases the activity. Again, normal muscle balance is restored and the teeth return to normal position. Occasionally, it may be necessary to place an active lingual arch wire with accessory spring attachments to aid tooth position correction labially.

SUMMARY

As stated in the earlier sections of this chapter, prevention of malocclusion or early interception through minor orthodontics depends wholly upon diagnostic skill. Truly, no orthodontics is "minor." Apparently, the notion of minor orthodontics relates to the use of simple or uncomplicated appliances. However, what may at first glance appear to be a simple problem for correction might instead be superimposed upon a more involved or complicated problem in treatment.

The orthodontist infrequently sees young children in his practice. Unless the diagnostic skills of the generalist and pedodontist are sharp enough to differentiate normal from deviant patterns of dental development in the child patient from three years of age on, interdisciplinary consultation and cooperative care will not occur.

Hopefully, the generalist will further his detailed study of diagnostic technique and the use of diagnostic aids. It can be expected that the guidance of normal dental development lies within the scope of general dental care. Careful attention to the need for restorative dentistry and problems of space management are passive measures to be employed within every dental office. Certainly, the general dentist must be skillful in the recognition of factors in dental development that act to reduce needed arch length. Such measures as regaining small losses in arch length through ectopia, crossbites, oral habits, spacing and inadequate restorative dentistry are within the scope of general dental care and correction. Our child population will be served better as the profession worries less about jurisdictional boundaries for treatment and enters a period of mutual education for more effective delivery of preventive and modestly corrective orthodontic care for vastly expanded numbers of young children.

REFERENCES

1. Angle, E. H.: Classification of malocclusion. Dent. Cosmos *41*:248–264, 350–357, 1899.
2. Thielemann, K.: Über die Laufigkeit von Stellungsanomalien der Zahne im Kleinkindersalter. Dissertation, Leipzig, 1923.
3. Korkhaus, G.: The frequency of orthodontic anomalies at various ages. Int. J. Orthod. *14*:120–135, February, 1928.
4. Stallard, H.: The general prevalence of gross symptoms of malocclusion. Dent. Cosmos *74*:29-37, January, 1932.
5. Taylor, A. T.: A study of the incidence and manifestations of malocclusion and irregularity of the teeth. Aust. Dent. J. *7*:650, October, 1935.
6. Goldstein, M. S., and Stanton, F. L.: Various types of occlusion and amounts of overbite in normal and abnormal occlusion between two and twelve years. Int. J. Orthod. and Oral Surg. *22*:549–569, June, 1936.
7. Mumblatt, M. A.: A statistical study of dental malocclusion in children. Dent. Items Interest *65*:43–63, January, 1943.
8. Sclare, R.: Orthodontics and the school child. A survey of 680 children. Br. Dent. J. *79*:278–280, November, 1945.
9. Huber, R., and Reynolds, J. W.: A dentofacial study of male students at the University of Michigan

in the physical hardening program. Am. J. Orthod. and Oral Surg. *32*:1–21, January, 1946.
10. Massler, M., and Frankel, J. M.: Prevalence of malocclusion in children aged 14–18 years. Am. J. Orthod. *37*:751–768, October, 1951.
11. Newman, G. V.: Prevalence of malocclusion in children 6 to 14 years of age and treatment in preventable cases. J. Am. Dent. Assoc. *52*:566–575, May, 1956.
12. Altemus, L. A.: Frequency of the incidence of malocclusion in American Negro children aged twelve to sixteen. Angle Orthod. *29*:189–200, October, 1959.
13. Popovich, F., and Grainger, R. M.: One community's orthodontic problem. *In* Orthodontics and Dentistry, Orthodontics in Mid-Century. Transactions of a workshop in orthodontics. (Moyers, R. E., and Jay, P., eds.) St. Louis, C. V. Mosby Co., 1959, p. 192.
14. Ast, D. B., Allaway, N., and Draker, H. L.: The prevalence of malocclusion, related to dental caries and lost first permanent molars, in a fluoridated city and fluoride-deficient city. Am. J. Orthod. *48*:106–113, February, 1962.
15. Graber, T. M.: Extrinsic Factors. Am. J. Orthod. *44*:26–45, January, 1958.
16. Graber, T. M.: Orthodontics, Principles and Practice. Philadelphia, W. B. Saunders Co., 1966.
17. Baum, A. T.: A cephalometric evaluation of the normal skeletal and dental pattern of children with excellent occlusions. Angle Orthod. *21*:96, 1951.
18. Björk, A.: The face in profile. Svensk Tandlak. Tidskr. Suppl. *40* No. 5B, 1947.
19. Broadbent, B. H.: The face of the normal child. Angle Orthod. *7*:185, 1937.
20. Broadbent, B. H.: Ontogenic development of occlusion. Angle Orthod. *11*:223, 1941.
21. Brodie, A. G.: On the growth pattern of the human head from the third month to the eighth year of life. Am. J. Anat. *68*:209, 1941.
22. Brodie, A. G.: Craniometry and cephalometry as applied to the growing child. *In* Cohen, M. M., Pediatric Dentistry. 2nd Ed. St. Louis, C. V. Mosby Co., 1961.
23. Report on the first roentgenographic cephalometric workshop. Am. J. Orthod. *44*:899, 1958.
24. Salzmann, J. A., ed.: Roentgenographic Cephalometrics. Philadelphia, J. B. Lippincott Co., 1961.
25. Coben, S. E.: Growth concept. Angle Orthod. *31*:194, 1961.
26. Downs, W. B.: Variations in facial relationships: Their significance in treatment and prognosis. Am. J. Orthod. *34*:812, 1948.
27. Downs, W. B.: The role of cephalometrics in orthodontic case analysis. Am. J. Orthod. *38*:162, 1952.
28. Downs, W. B.: Analysis of the dentofacial profile. Angle Orthod. *26*:191, 1956.
29. Dreyer, C. J., and Joffee, B. M.: A concept of cephalometric interpretation. Angle Orthod. *33*:132, 1963.
30. Higley, L. B.: Cephalometric standards for children four to eight years of age. Am. J. Orthod. *40*:51, 1954.
31. Lande, M. J.: Growth behavior of the human bony facial profile as revealed by serial cephalometric roentgenology. Angle Orthod. *22*:78, 1952.
32. Margolis, H. I.: The axial inclination of the lower incisors. Am. J. Orthod. and Oral Surg. *29*:571, 1943.
33. Moore, A. W.: Observations on facial growth and its clinical significance. Am. J. Orthod. *45*:399, 1959.
34. Reidel, R. A.: The relation of maxillary structures to cranium in malocclusion and in normal occlusion. Angle. Orthod. *22*:142, 1952.
35. Salzmann, J. A.: Limitations of roentgenographic cephalometrics. Am. J. Orthod. *50*:169, 1964.
36. Schaeffer, A.: Behavior of the axis of human incisor teeth during growth. Angle Orthod. *19*:254, 1949.
37. Scott, J. H.: Growth at facial sutures. Am. J. Orthod. *42*:381, 1956.
38. Scott, J. H.: The cranial base. Am. J. Phys. Anthropol. *16*:319, 1958.
39. Spiedel, T. D., and Stoner, M. M.: Variation of the mandibular incisor. Axis in adult "normal occlusion." Am. J. Orthod. and Oral Surg. *30*:536, 1944.
40. Steiner, C. C.: Cephalometrics for you and me. Am. J. Orthod. *39*:729, 1953.
41. Steiner, C. C.: Cephalometrics in clinical practice. Angle Orthod. *29*:8, 1959.
42. Nance, H. N.: The limitations of orthodontic treatment. I. Mixed dentitional diagnosis and treatment. Am. J. Orthod. *33*:177–223, 1947.
43. Hixon, E. H., and Oldfather, R. E.: Estimation of the sizes of unerupted cuspid and bicuspid teeth. Angle Orthod. *28*:236–240, 1958.
44. Moyers, R. E.: Handbook of Orthodontics. 2nd Ed. Chicago, Yearbook Medical Publishers, 1963.
45. Moorrees, C. F. A.: The Dentition of the Growing Child. Cambridge, Harvard University Press, 1959.
46. Baume, L. J.: Physiological tooth migration and its significance for the development of occlusion. I. The biogenetic course of the deciduous dentition. J. Dent. Res. *29*:123–132, 1950: *29*:331–337, 1950; *29*:440–447, 1950.
47. Dewel, B. F.: Serial extractions in orthodontics: Indications, objectives, and treatment procedures. Am. J. Ortho., *40*:906–926, 1954.
48. Dewel, B. F.: Serial extraction: procedures and limitations. Am. J. Ortho., *43*:685–687, 1957.
49. Mayne, W. R.: A concept, diagnosis and a discipline. Dent. Clin. N. Amer., July 1959, pp. 281–288.
50. Mayne, W. R.: Serial extraction as an adjunct to orthodontic treatment. Audiovisual sequence. American Association of Orthodontics, St. Louis, 1959.

INDEX

Note: In this index, page numbers in *italic* type refer to illustrations; page numbers followed by (t) refer to tables.